THE CIBA COLLECTION OF MEDICAL ILLUSTRATIONS

VOLUME 8 • PART II

Other published volumes of
THE CIBA COLLECTION OF MEDICAL ILLUSTRATIONS
Prepared by
Frank H. Netter, M.D.

See page 276 for additional information

THE CIBA COLLECTION
OF MEDICAL ILLUSTRATIONS

VOLUME 8

MUSCULOSKELETAL SYSTEM

PART II

Developmental Disorders, Tumors, Rheumatic Diseases, and Joint Replacement

A compilation of paintings prepared

by FRANK H. NETTER, M.D.

Richard H. Freyberg, M.D., and Robert N. Hensinger, M.D., *Consulting Editors*

Regina V. Dingle, *Managing Editor*

With a foreword by Henry J. Mankin, M.D.,
Edith M. Ashley Professor of Orthopaedic Surgery, Harvard Medical School

COMMISSIONED AND PUBLISHED BY CIBA-GEIGY CORPORATION

SUMMIT, NEW JERSEY

Copies of all CIBA COLLECTION books, ATLAS OF HUMAN ANATOMY, CLINICAL SYMPOSIA
reprints, and color slides of all illustrations contained in them are available from CIBA-GEIGY
Medical Education Division, 14 Henderson Drive, West Caldwell, NJ 07006

First Printing

ISBN 0-914168-15-0
Library of Congress Catalog No: 53-2151

Printed in U.S.A.

Book printed offset by The Case-Hoyt Corporation
Laser-scanned color separations by Daiichi Seihan USA, Inc.
Layout design by Pierre J. Lair
Text photocomposed in Mergenthaler Garamond No. 3 by Granite Graphics
Contents printed on Cameo dull text, basis 80, by S.D. Warren Company
Smyth-sewn case binding by Nicholstone Companies, Inc.
Endpapers: White Flannel text, basis 80, by Curtis Paper Division, James River Corporation
Cover material: Buckram linen cloth by Industrial Coatings Group, Inc.
Front and spine cover and front matter design by Philip Grushkin
Index by Steele/Katigbak Indexers

Foreword

In 1953, as an intern at the University of Chicago, I obtained a copy of the very first of the now world-famous CIBA COLLECTION masterpieces by Frank Netter, M.D. The subject was the *Nervous System* that, after an amazing thirteen printings, is now in its second printing of a revised edition. My colleagues and I at that time and all subsequent generations of physicians over the last 35 years marveled at the artistry and extraordinary clarity of those illustrations; and how remarkably, when coupled with the short but well-written text, they provided such a clear definition of complex three-dimensional structures and confusing relationships that we had struggled sometimes in vain to comprehend. There was little doubt in our minds that we were looking at the works of a genius—not only because he saw so much and so clearly, but because he could make us see it with equal clarity. We waited, as did the world, for subsequent volumes and were not disappointed with any of the next six. The *Reproductive System*, published in 1954, the *Digestive System* in 1957, the *Endocrine System* in 1965, the *Heart* in 1969, the *Kidney, Ureters, and Urinary Bladder* in 1973, and the *Respiratory System* in 1979 all showed the same remarkable ability to portray the anatomy and embryology, physiology, pathology, and clinical states with such extraordinary clarity and in sufficient detail as to become, for each of these disciplines, major teaching and reference texts. I wonder how many times in these past 35 years a Netter illustration has been used for a lecture or demonstration in a medical school or residency classroom, and how many copies have been made of the figures to subsequently reside in teaching collections throughout the world? Surely the number must be exceeded only by the number of physicians who hold the volumes as cherished possessions and have read them over and over in a quest for knowledge or as part of a scholarly pursuit.

Having said that, I must express a degree of disappointment on behalf of my colleagues in Orthopaedics, Rheumatology, Physiatry, and the sciences associated with connective tissue diseases, with the evident fact that with the exception of some of the plates in Volumes 1 and 4 there were few of these teaching atlases that had any relevance to our rather sizable corner of the world of medicine. It is therefore with great enthusiasm and unbridled pleasure that our specialties now greet *Volume 8: The Musculoskeletal System*. Furthermore, after consideration of the contents and study of the magnificent plates and text, I conclude that not only was the product worth waiting for but in my opinion the three parts comprising this latest work are the author's finest! Frank Netter, M.D., has not only "done it again" but he's done it better than he ever did it before!

The *Musculoskeletal System* is one of Dr. Netter's most ambitious projects. Any of the subjects covered would seem to require a separate volume, and perhaps one of the major aspects of the genius of the artist is deciding what to include. Realizing that each plate contains several main themes and multiple facts (all nicely tied together by the artistry of the author), it is not surprising that anatomy and physiology (including metabolic disorders) are included in the 214 plates that comprise Part I; and that congenital and developmental disorders can be depicted in 111 plates, neoplasms in 34, rheumatic disorders in 73, and joint replacement surgery in another 28, all in Part II. Part III on injuries (182 plates), infections (20 plates), vascular disturbances (30 plates), and rehabilitation (20 plates) completes the set. If one totals these plates, the number exceeds 700 (what a fantastic effort even for Dr. Netter!), and with the text supplied by the numerous contributors, the three parts of Volume 8 should rapidly become classic teaching texts for our specialties.

One may wonder why Volume 8 required so many plates and so much text as compared with the other disciplines, and upon consideration, I believe the answer is self-evident. The musculoskeletal system comprises most of the body's supportive and protective elements and provides movement and prehension. The tissues included vary from the undifferentiated fibrous supporting membranes to the remarkably complex organ systems of the bones and joints, and the anatomic structures are as different as the big toe and the first cervical vertebra. While trauma is almost exclusively related to the bones and joints, metabolic bone disease involves the endocrine and renal systems; genetic disorders, other multiple organ systems; arthritis, the sciences of immunology and internal metabolism; and neoplasms, the entire field of oncology. What brings these fields together in this remarkable volume and in the scientific world is the anatomic structures and, perhaps more relevantly, the entire background framework of connective tissue chemistry, mechanical engineering, and materials science, which Dr. Netter has woven so beautifully and understandably into every section.

The students, scholars, and practitioners who deal with the musculoskeletal system have been waiting along with me since 1953 for Frank Netter's Volume 8. I don't think they will be disappointed.

HENRY J. MANKIN, M.D.
Boston, July 1987

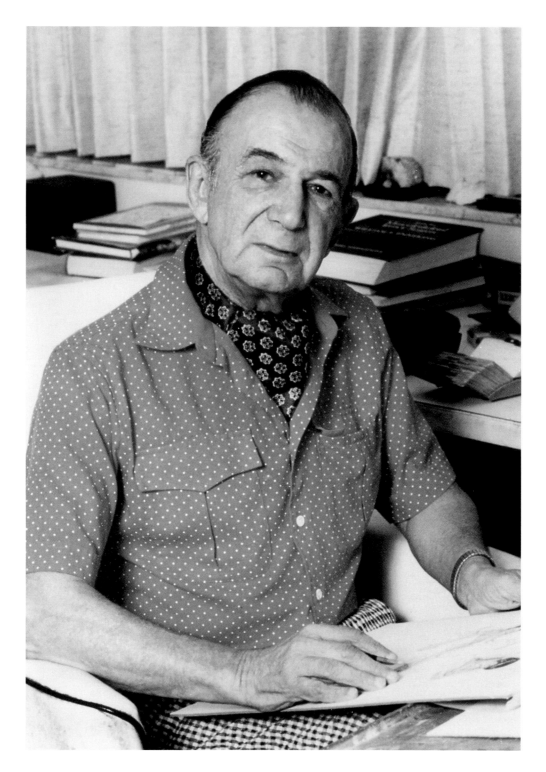

Frank H. Netter, M.D.

Introduction

In my introduction to Part I of this atlas, I wrote of how awesome albeit fascinating I had found the task of pictorializing the fundamentals of the musculoskeletal system, both its normal structure as well as its multitudinous disorders and diseases. As compactly, simply, and succinctly as I tried to present the subject matter, it still required three full books (Parts I, II, and III of Volume 8 of THE CIBA COLLECTION OF MEDICAL ILLUSTRATIONS). Part I of this trilogy covered the normal anatomy, embryology, and physiology of the musculoskeletal system as well as its diverse metabolic diseases, including the various types of rickets. This book, Part II, portrays its congenital and developmental disorders, neoplasms—both benign and malignant—of bone and soft tissue, and rheumatic and other arthritic diseases, as well as joint replacement. Part III, on which I am still at work, will cover trauma, including fractures and dislocations of all the bones and joints, soft-tissue injuries, sports injuries, burns, infections including osteomyelitis and hand infections, compartment syndromes, amputations, both traumatic and surgical, replantation of limbs and digits, prostheses, and rehabilitation, as well as a number of related subjects.

As I stated in my above-mentioned previous introduction, some disorders, however, do not fit exactly into a precise classification and are therefore covered piecemeal herein under several headings. Furthermore, a considerable number of orthopedic ailments involve also the fields of neurology and neurosurgery, so that readers may find it helpful to refer in those instances to my atlases on the anatomy and pathology of the nervous system (Volume 1, Parts I and II of THE CIBA COLLECTION OF MEDICAL ILLUSTRATIONS).

Most meaningfully, however, I herewith express my sincere appreciation of the many great physicians, surgeons, orthopedists, and scientists who so graciously shared with me their knowledge and supplied me with so much material on which to base my illustrations. Without their help I could not have created this atlas. Most of these wonderful people are credited elsewhere in this book under the heading of "Acknowledgments" but I must nevertheless specifically mention a few who were not only collaborators and consultants in this undertaking but who have become my dear and esteemed friends. These are Dr. Bob Hensinger, my consulting editor, who guided me through many puzzling aspects of the organization and subject matter of this atlas; Drs. Alfred and Genevieve Swanson, pioneers in the correction of rheumatically deformed hands with silastic implants, as well as in the classification and study of congenital limb deficits; Dr. William Enneking, who has made such great advances in the diagnosis and management of bone tumors; Dr. Ernest ("Chappy") Conrad III; the late Dr. Charley Frantz, who first set me on course for this project, and Dr. Richard Freyberg, who became the consultant on the rheumatic diseases plates; Dr. George Hammond; Dr. Hugo Keim; Dr. Mack Clayton; Dr. Philip Wilson; Dr. Stuart Kozinn; and Dr. Russell Windsor.

Finally, I also sincerely thank Mr. Philip Flagler, Ms. Regina Dingle, and others of the CIBA-GEIGY organization who helped in more ways than I can describe in producing this atlas.

Frank H. Netter, M.D.

Contributors and Consultants

George T. Aitken, M.D.*

Former Director of Area Child Amputee Clinic,
Mary Free Bed Hospital and Rehabilitation Center,
Grand Rapids, Michigan

Crawford J. Campbell, M.D.*

Former Lecturer in Orthopaedic Surgery, Harvard
Medical School; Visiting Orthopaedic Surgeon,
Massachusetts General Hospital,
Boston, Massachusetts

Mack L. Clayton, M.D.

Clinical Professor of Orthopedic Surgery,
University of Colorado School of Medicine;
Denver Orthopedic Clinic,
Denver, Colorado

Sherman S. Coleman, M.D.

Professor of Orthopaedic Surgery, University of
Utah School of Medicine; Chief of Staff,
Shriner Hospitals for Crippled Children,
Intermountain Unit,
Salt Lake City, Utah

Ernest U. Conrad III, M.D.

Assistant Professor, Department of Orthopaedic Surgery;
Director, Division of Musculoskeletal Oncology and Bone
Tumor Clinic; Medical Director, Northwest Tissue
Center, University of Washington School of Medicine and
Children's Hospital and Medical Center,
Seattle, Washington

Henry R. Cowell, M.D., Ph.D.

Lecturer,
Harvard Medical School,
Boston, Massachusetts

*Deceased

Alvin H. Crawford, M.D.

Professor of Pediatric and Orthopedic Surgery,
University of Cincinnati College of Medicine;
Director, Division of Pediatric Orthopedics,
Children's Hospital Medical Center,
Cincinnati, Ohio

William F. Enneking, M.D.

Distinguished Service Professor and Eugene L. Jewett
Professor of Orthopaedic Surgery,
College of Medicine, University of Florida,
Gainesville, Florida

Donald C. Ferlic, M.D.

Associate Clinical Professor,
University of Colorado Health Sciences Center,
Denver, Colorado

Chester W. Fink, M.D.

Professor of Pediatrics and Chief, Division of
Rheumatology, University of Texas Southwestern
Medical School at Dallas; Director, Arthritis Clinic,
Texas Scottish Rite Hospital for Crippled Children,
Dallas, Texas

Richard H. Freyberg, M.D.

Emeritus Clinical Professor of Medicine, Cornell
University Medical College; Emeritus Director, Division
of Rheumatic Diseases, The Hospital for Special Surgery;
Honorary Staff, The New York Hospital and
The Hospital for Special Surgery,
New York, New York

George Hammond, M.D.

Former Chief of Orthopaedic Department, Lahey
Clinic Medical Center, Burlington, Massachusetts;
Honorary Staff, New England Deaconess Hospital and
New England Baptist Hospital,
Boston, Massachusetts

Robert N. Hensinger, M.D.

Professor of Surgery, Section of Orthopaedics,
University of Michigan Medical School;
Chief of Pediatric Orthopaedics,
C.S. Mott Children's Hospital,
Ann Arbor, Michigan

John E. Herzenberg, M.D.

Assistant Professor of Orthopaedic Surgery,
University of Michigan Medical School,
Ann Arbor, Michigan

John N. Insall, M.D.

Professor of Orthopaedic Surgery, Cornell University
Medical College; Attending Orthopaedic Surgeon,
The Hospital for Special Surgery and The New York
Hospital; Director of Knee Service,
The Hospital for Special Surgery,
New York, New York

Hugo A. Keim, M.D.

Associate Professor of Orthopaedic Surgery, Columbia
University College of Physicians and Surgeons; Associate
Attending Orthopaedic Surgeon, New York Orthopaedic
Hospital, Columbia-Presbyterian Medical Center,
New York, New York

Thomas F. Kling, Jr., M.D.

Professor of Orthopaedic Surgery, Indiana University
School of Medicine; Chief of Pediatric Orthopaedics,
James Whitcomb Riley Hospital for Children,
Indianapolis, Indiana

Stuart C. Kozinn, M.D.

Orthopaedic Surgeon,
Scottsdale, Arizona

G. Dean MacEwen, M.D.

Chairman, Department of Pediatric Orthopaedics and
Director of Orthopaedic Education, Children's
Hospital; Professor and Chief, Section of
Pediatric Orthopaedic Surgery,
Louisiana State University Medical Center,
New Orleans, Louisiana

John A. Ogden, M.D.

Chief of Staff, Shriner Hospitals for
Crippled Children, Tampa Unit,
Tampa, Florida

Paul M. Pellicci, M.D.

Assistant Professor of Anatomy, Cornell University
Medical College; Associate Attending Surgeon,
The Hospital for Special Surgery; Associate Professor
of Surgery (Orthopaedics), The New York
Hospital—Cornell University Medical College,
New York, New York

Robert B. Salter, M.D., F.R.C.S. (C)

Professor of Orthopaedic Surgery, University of
Toronto; Senior Orthopaedic Surgeon,
The Hospital for Sick Children,
Toronto, Ontario, Canada

H. Ralph Schumacher, Jr., M.D.

Professor of Medicine, University of Pennsylvania School
of Medicine; Director, Arthritis-Immunology Center,
Veterans Administration Medical Center,
Philadelphia, Pennsylvania

Charles I. Scott, Jr., M.D.

Professor of Pediatrics and Genetics, Jefferson Medical
College of Thomas Jefferson University, Philadelphia,
Pennsylvania; Director, Medical Genetics,
Alfred I. duPont Institute,
Wilmington, Delaware

Morris H. Susman, M.D.

Orthopaedic Surgery,
Rose Medical Center and Saint Joseph's Hospital,
Denver, Colorado

Alfred B. Swanson, M.D.

Professor of Surgery, Michigan State University College
of Human Medicine, East Lansing, Michigan;
Director of Orthopaedic and Hand Surgery Training
Program, Grand Rapids Hospitals; Director of Hand
Fellowship and Orthopaedic Research,
Blodgett Memorial Medical Center,
Grand Rapids, Michigan

Genevieve de Groot Swanson, M.D.

Assistant Clinical Professor of Surgery, Michigan
State University College of Human Medicine,
East Lansing, Michigan; Coordinator of
Orthopaedic Research Department,
Blodgett Memorial Medical Center,
Grand Rapids, Michigan

George H. Thompson, M.D.

Associate Professor of Orthopaedic Surgery and
Pediatrics and Director of Pediatric Orthopaedics,
Case Western Reserve University School of Medicine,
Cleveland, Ohio

Philip D. Wilson, Jr., M.D.

Professor of Surgery (Orthopaedics), Cornell
University Medical College; Surgeon-in-Chief Emeritus,
The Hospital for Special Surgery; Attending Orthopaedic
Surgeon, The Hospital for Special Surgery and
The New York Hospital,
New York, New York

Russell E. Windsor, M.D.

Assistant Professor of Surgery (Orthopaedics), Cornell
University Medical College; Assistant Attending
Orthopaedic Surgeon, The Hospital for Special
Surgery and The New York Hospital,
New York, New York

Edward M. Wojtys, M.D.

Assistant Professor of Surgery,
University of Michigan Medical School,
Ann Arbor, Michigan

Acknowledgments

Work on Volume 8, *Musculoskeletal System* began more than a decade ago, and over the years it became evident that the original plan to publish one book was unworkable. Thus, *Musculoskeletal System* evolved from a single book of 270 illustrations into a three-part volume of more than 700.

Though Part II deals with some of the musculoskeletal system's most painful and debilitating pathology, no paintings are more touchingly presented than those of children with congenital anomalies. Dr. Netter has captured in their faces and in the way they approach their individual deficits the optimism of the human spirit they so clearly epitomize. This has helped transform an arduous task into an uplifting experience for all of us involved—an unexpected bonus to help carry us through the many years of preparation.

As in previous CIBA COLLECTION volumes, we have adopted the terminology commonly used in standard American medical texts. For consistency of presentation, our primary resource has been *Blakiston's Gould Medical Dictionary*, fourth edition. The 1977 revision of the International Nomenclature of Constitutional Diseases of Bone, published in 1979 by the March of Dimes Birth Defects Foundation, is the classification used for the plates on dwarfism. For the plates on congenital limb malformations, we have used the 1964 Swanson modification of the Frantz-O'Rahilly classification.

We express our sincere thanks to all the authors who contributed their time and expertise to the development of this book. During the long period of its preparation, we had to ask them to review and rewrite their texts to reflect the advances in the current knowledge of the various disorders and their treatment. This they did with patience and understanding.

We especially thank our consulting editors, Dr. Richard H. Freyberg and Dr. Robert N. Hensinger, for their contributions as medical consultants as well as authors. Dr. Freyberg's involvement in the area of rheumatic diseases dates back to the earliest planning of the book, carried out under the guidance of the late Dr. Charles Frantz. Dr. Hensinger joined the project later and spent many hours with Dr. Netter selecting, from the vast field of congenital and developmental disorders, the topics that comprise Section I as well as the contributors who wrote the accompanying texts.

In addition, we acknowledge and thank a number of experts for their advice and technical assistance in the development of many of the illustrations:

In Section I, Dr. Steven E. Kopits supplied information on the correction of bowleg deformity in achondroplasia, shown in Plate 3, and Dr. John A. Ogden provided the description and demonstration of the points of blood compromise, shown in Plate 56. Dr. Robert E. Eilert collaborated on the development of Plates 68–74.

In Section II, the table on page 149 is adapted from W.F. Enneking, *Musculoskeletal Tumor Surgery*, 1983, Churchill Livingstone.

In Section III, we are grateful to Dr. Morris Ziff for reviewing illustrations and texts on the rheumatic diseases. Dr. John Calabro developed Plates 1–2, 11–13, 17–22; Dr. David Koffler, Plate 8; Dr. Seymour Diamond and Dr. José L. Medina, Plate 37. Dr. Stuart C. Kozinn kindly supplied radiographs included in Plates 4, 24, 31, 35, and 42.

In Section IV, Dr. William Harris supplied the slide on bone ingrowth used in Plate 1; Dr. C. Ranawat provided assistance in the technique for the Triad prosthesis shown in Plate 2. Dr. Ralph W. Coonrad and Mr. J. Wadsworth supplied examples of the elbow prostheses depicted in Plate 28, and the radiographs used in this plate were loaned by Dr. Coonrad and Mr. J. Fairclough.

No acknowledgment is complete without mention of the many people involved in the complicated process of guiding a book from manuscript to printed copy. We extend our thanks to Gamma One Conversions for the fine quality color transparencies of original art. Color separations and films from which the printing plates were made were prepared by Daiichi Seihan, whose president, Tomeji Maruyama, we thank for a pleasant and productive collaboration. We are also indebted to our long-time associate, Jack Cesareo, for preparing the graphic elements—linework and captions—that are an integral part of each illustration.

Within the CIBA-GEIGY organization, we thank the team responsible for guiding this project to completion: Kristine Bean, for editing manuscripts and plate legends and for helping with all stages of proofreading; Don Canter, Clark Carroll, and Scott Lanzner for preparing and supervising the manufacturing process; Nicole Friedman, Sally Chichester, and Jeffie Lemons for their meticulous attention to the preparation of texts and illustrations—in particular, Nicole Friedman is also thanked for maintaining the smooth functioning between the many departments involved; and Gina Dingle, our Managing Editor, for her patient and persistent efforts to keep this project moving in spite of all problems and delays.

Finally, no acknowledgment would be complete without profound thanks to Dr. Netter, whose grasp of the complexities of the subject, uncanny abilities to condense and organize the details, and long-recognized conceptual and artistic talents are the very source of this book and of all its predecessors. That this has been an uplifting and heartwarming experience as well is further tribute to his greatness.

PHILIP B. FLAGLER
DIRECTOR,
MEDICAL EDUCATION DIVISION

Contents

Section I

Congenital and Developmental Disorders

Frank H. Netter, M.D.

in collaboration with

George T. Aitken, M.D. *Plates 46–49*

Crawford J. Campbell, M.D. *Plates 21–23*

Sherman S. Coleman, M.D. *Plates 88–92*

Henry R. Cowell, M.D. *Plates 93–95*

Alvin H. Crawford, M.D. *Plates 17–19, 82–87*

Robert N. Hensinger, M.D. *Plates 20, 24–28, 37–40, 50–56, 76–81, 96*

John E. Herzenberg, M.D. *Plate 36*

Hugo A. Keim, M.D. and Robert N. Hensinger, M.D. *Plates 29–34*

Thomas F. Kling, Jr., M.D. *Plates 35, 41–45, 97–98*

G. Dean MacEwen, M.D. *Plates 66–67*

John A. Ogden, M.D. *Plate 75*

Charles I. Scott, Jr., M.D. *Plates 1–16*

Alfred B. Swanson, M.D. and Genevieve de Groot Swanson, M.D. *Plates 99–111*

George H. Thompson, M.D. and Robert B. Salter, M.D. *Plates 57–65*

Edward M. Wojtys, M.D. *Plates 68–74*

Achondroplasia

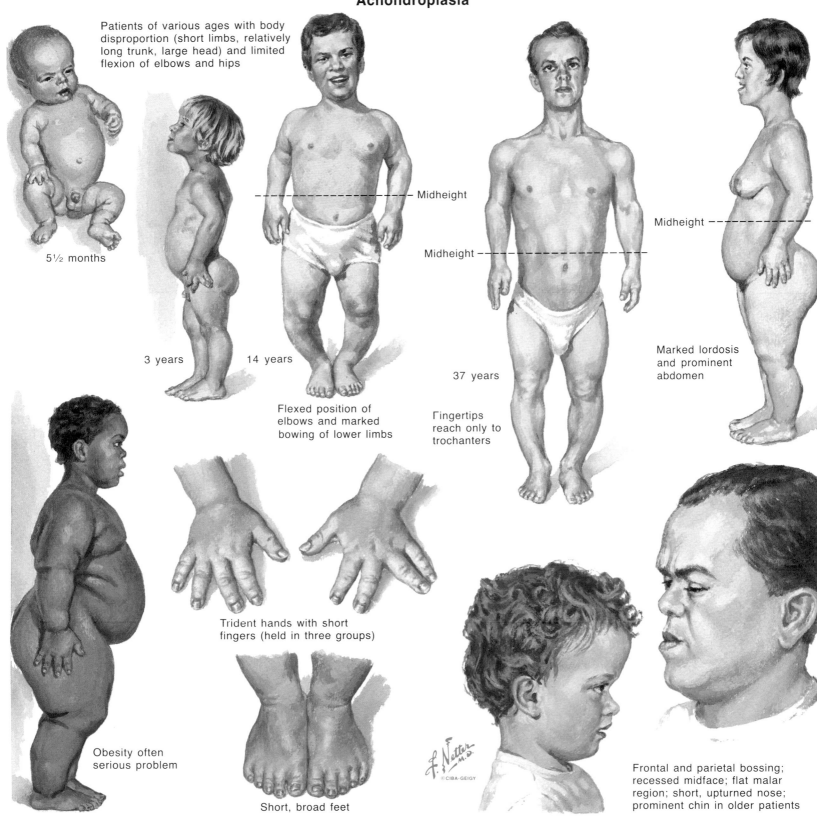

Patients of various ages with body disproportion (short limbs, relatively long trunk, large head) and limited flexion of elbows and hips

5½ months

3 years

14 years

Flexed position of elbows and marked bowing of lower limbs

Midheight

37 years

Fingertips reach only to trochanters

Midheight

Midheight

Marked lordosis and prominent abdomen

Obesity often serious problem

Trident hands with short fingers (held in three groups)

Short, broad feet

Frontal and parietal bossing; recessed midface; flat malar region; short, upturned nose; prominent chin in older patients

Dwarfism

Classification

Although hereditary disorders of the skeleton are relatively rare, they attract a great deal of interest. Many of these disorders are associated with short stature. Most have been known by a variety of names and have frequently been misdiagnosed or misclassified. In the past 25 years, studies and epidemiologic surveys have formu-

lated a classification and improved the understanding of these intrinsic bone disorders.

Skeletal dysplasias, or chondrodystrophies, are a heterogeneous group of disorders resulting in short-limb or short-trunk types of disproportionate short stature. In the types of dwarfism that primarily affect the limbs, the shortening may predominate in the proximal segments (rhizomelia), the middle segments (mesomelia), or the distal segments (acromelia). The term "dwarf" has traditionally been applied to persons of disproportionate short stature, whereas the term "midget" referred to those of proportionate short stature. In clinical practice, the preferred terms are "small," "little," and "short people."

Disproportionate dwarfism is caused by a hereditary intrinsic skeletal dysplasia, whereas proportionate dwarfism results from chromosomal, endocrine, nutritional, or nonosseous abnormalities. Although the mode of inheritance is known for many of these disorders, in most of them, the fundamental biochemical and/or molecular fault is not yet understood. Many cases of dwarfism are the result of a rare genetic event, the spontaneous mutation. Unaffected parents of a child with a mutation are essentially at no risk of having another affected child, and unaffected siblings are not at risk of having children with the disorder. Affected parents may pass the trait on to their children, depending on the mode of

Dwarfism
(Continued)

inheritance—autosomal dominant, autosomal recessive, or X-linked.

Genetic counseling must be based on an accurate diagnosis and on familiarity with the natural history, range of manifestations, severity, and associated findings of the specific disorder.

Diagnosis

Prenatal Testing. Prenatal diagnosis of certain skeletal dysplasias without biochemical markers can be established by radiography, ultrasonography (most widely used), fetoscopy, and amniography. Knowledge of the natural history of intrauterine growth in dwarfing conditions is incomplete. Ossification of the fetal skeleton is not well established until 16 weeks, and it is not known when limb-length discrepancy becomes apparent in the fetus. Serial sonograms are necessary to recognize the decreased growth rate of the femur or to monitor the fetal biparietal diameter, polydactyly, and other skeletal abnormalities.

History. A thorough family history is a particularly important factor in reaching the correct diagnosis. Since disorders with clinically indistinguishable features may have different patterns of inheritance, evaluation of other family members can be very helpful.

Physical Examination. Measurements of head circumference, height, weight, and arm span are taken, and body proportions are evaluated. A careful examination should be done for nonosseous signs such as cleft palate, cataracts, or congenital heart disease that may contribute to the diagnosis. Ophthalmologic examination and evaluation of speech and hearing may also be needed.

Intelligence is normal in nearly all types of dwarfism. Exceptions include, but are not limited to, hypochondroplasia (Plate 4), the rare Dyggve-Melchior-Clausen dysplasia (Plate 14), pycnodysostosis (Plate 11), and Hurler's and Hunter's syndromes (Plate 16). The need for specific intellectual evaluation or treatment is dictated by the diagnosis and the patient's past performance.

Radiographic Evaluation. Radiographs must be taken of the entire skeleton because diagnosis of most bone dysplasias cannot be made on the basis of one or two radiographs of selected body parts. It is particularly important to look for atlantoaxial instability of the cervical spine. Abnormal vertebral movements occur in many bone dysplasias and, unless detected, may lead to acute compressive myelopathy. Since the radiographic characteristics of many dysplasias change with time, review of earlier radiographs is often necessary (eg, in the epiphyseal dysplasias, the growth plates fuse with age, and all evidence of disturbed epiphyseal development is obliterated).

Achondroplasia (continued)

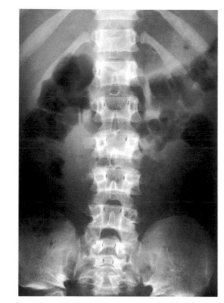

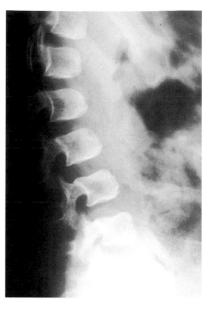

Anteroposterior radiograph shows progressive decrease in interpedicular distance (in caudad direction) in lumbar region, with resultant transverse narrowing of vertebral canal

Lateral radiograph shows scalloped posterior borders of lumbar vertebrae and short pedicles, causing sagittal spinal stenosis

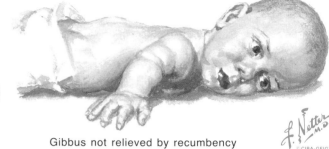

Gibbus not relieved by recumbency

Infant with severe thoracolumbar kyphosis that usually reverses to characteristic lordosis at weight–bearing age. If it does not, true gibbus with cord compression may result. Neurologic signs and vertebral wedging are indications for surgery

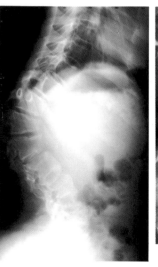

Gibbus with wedging of 2nd lumbar vertebra

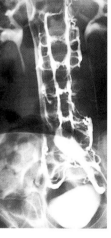

Venogram shows areas of ischemia; supply of blood to lumbar spinal cord impaired

Laboratory Tests. Initial symptoms or the preliminary diagnosis may suggest the need for specific laboratory tests. For example, if Schmid-type metaphyseal chondrodysplasia (Plate 7) is suspected, a complete blood analysis is needed to differentiate this disorder from vitamin D–resistant rickets. The mucopolysaccharidoses, a group of biomechanical storage disorders, also require testing for specific enzymes.

Achondroplasia

Achondroplasia, which occurs in about 1 of 40,000 persons, is the most common and best-known type of short-limb dwarfism (Plates 1–3). It is transmitted by a single autosomal dominant gene. Infants with homozygous achondroplasia generally do not survive for more than a few weeks or months. About 80% of cases result from a spontaneous mutation. The parents are usually average size, and no other family member is affected. Statistical evidence suggests that elevated paternal age (>37 years) may be linked to this type of mutation.

Clinical Manifestations. The characteristic signs of achondroplasia—disproportionate short stature, a comparatively long trunk, and rhizomelic shortening of the limbs—are evident at birth (Plates 1–2). The head is both relatively and absolutely large with a prominent, or bulging, forehead (frontal bossing); parietal bossing

Dwarfism
(Continued)

and flattening of the occiput may also be evident. In infancy, the head increases rapidly in size, and hydrocephalus can occur. It can be recognized early by using established norms for head size in patients with achondroplasia, and appropriate treatment can be instituted.

Midfacial hypoplasia of variable degree is manifested by a flat or depressed nasal bridge, narrow nasal passages, and malar hypoplasia (Plate 1). The nose has a fleshy tip and upturned nostrils. These features result from restricted development of the chondrocranium and the middle third of the face.

Recurrent and chronic middle ear infections (otitis media) are common in infancy and early childhood and, if untreated, may lead to significant hearing loss. Generally, these infections become less frequent by the time the patient is 8 to 10 years of age.

A relative protrusion of the jaw is often mislabeled prognathism. Dental development is normal, but underdevelopment of the maxilla may cause dental crowding and malocclusion. About 70% of patients have tongue thrust or other speech defects that seem to be related to the dysplastic bone structure. These problems usually subside spontaneously by school age.

The root portions of the limbs are shorter than the middle or distal segments. Soft tissues may appear excessive with redundant, partially encircling folds and grooves on the limbs. Because the long bones are shortened, the muscle mass looks bunched up, creating the appearance of great strength.

Initially, the legs appear straight but with ambulation may develop a valgus position, resulting in bowleg (genu varum) with or without back knee (genu recurvatum).

The hands and feet may appear large in relation to the limbs, but the digits are short, broad, and stubby (brachydactyly). The so-called trident hand (Plate 1) is common but becomes less apparent in late childhood and adulthood. The fingertips may reach only to the level of the trochanters or even the iliac crests. Elbow extension is restricted (30°–45°), but this has little functional significance.

Although the trunk is relatively long, deformities contribute to the overall height reduction. The chest tends to be flat and broad and the abdomen and buttocks protuberant. Excessive lumbar lordosis and a tilted pelvis cause a waddling gait, and fixed flexion contractures of the hip appear early.

In a sitting position, infants commonly exhibit thoracolumbar kyphosis (Plate 2). A hump, or

Achondroplasia (continued)

Diagnostic testing

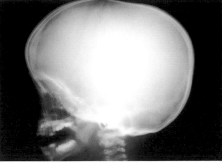

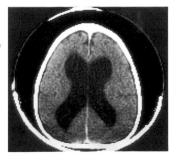

CT scan shows large ventricles but normal thickness of cortical mantle and normal CSF pressure (false hydrocephalus)

Lateral radiograph of large head shows frontal bossing, flattened occiput, open anterior fontanelle, recessed midface, and occipitalization of C1

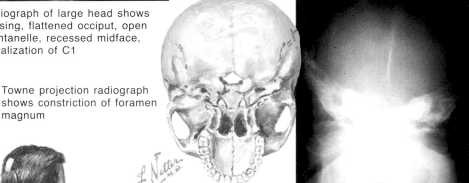

Towne projection radiograph shows constriction of foramen magnum

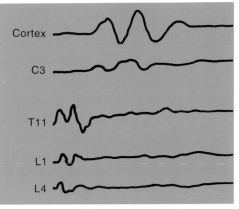

Somatosensory evoked responses (SER) determine delay in neurotransmission and its location on stimulation of peroneal nerve (evidence of cord compression). Ulnar or radial nerve may be similarly tested

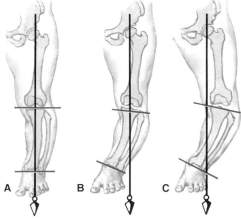

Alignment of lower limb. (A) Good alignment, plumb line centered on hip, knee, and ankle joints; (B) hip and knee aligned but ankle inside plumb line; (C) knee outside and ankle inside plumb line. Malalignment plus pain on walking may indicate need for surgical correction

gibbus, seen in some babies, may be associated with anterior wedging of the first or second lumbar vertebra. The kyphosis is related to a variety of factors, including ligamentous laxity, hypotonia, and immature strength and motor skills. Although it requires monitoring, the kyphosis usually disappears when the child begins to walk.

Neurologic complications are common. Respiratory abnormalities suggest stenosis of the foramen magnum and compression of the normal-sized medulla oblongata and/or cervical spinal cord. This quite frequent complication results in hypoventilation or apnea, paralysis of voluntary respiration, and compressive myelopathy at the level of the foramen magnum

(Plate 3). (Therefore, hyperextension of the neck and sudden, whiplashlike movement should be avoided.) Sudden infant death syndrome has also been reported. Somatosensory evoked responses (SER) and polysomnography coupled with computed tomography (CT) of the foramen magnum can provide valuable information to help avert both short-term and long-term complications.

Stenosis of the lumbar spine, prolapse of intervertebral discs, osteophytes, and deformed vertebral bodies may compress the spinal cord and/or nerve roots, frequently causing neurologic manifestations. Pressure on blood vessels impairs the regional blood supply, producing focal areas of ischemia.

Dwarfism
(Continued)

In the teenage period, slowly progressive symptoms such as paresthesias, weakness, pain, and paraplegia develop and may be aggravated by obesity and prolonged standing or walking. Initially, the patient can quickly relieve these symptoms by flexing the spine and hips forward, squatting, or assuming a nonweight-bearing position. As the condition progresses, pain develops and may be localized to the low back or, more commonly, may radiate into the buttocks, posterior thigh, and calf. Muscle weakness and foot drop may also develop. Although these symptoms are more common in the legs, the arms may also be affected.

Patients with symptomatic spinal stenosis need a physical examination with attention to sensory levels, and a careful neurologic history should also be obtained. Specific laboratory tests such as somatosensory evoked responses, computed tomography, magnetic resonance imaging, thermography, and myelography all have a diagnostic function.

Growth rate is normal in the first year of life, then drops to about the third percentile, where it remains for the first decade; it may increase during puberty. Obesity is a common problem. Adult height ranges from 42 to 56 inches.

Children with achondroplasia should not be evaluated against normal developmental milestones but rather against standards developed for children with the condition. Motor skills are often delayed because of the physical difficulties posed by short limbs and hypotonia (which tends to abate by age 2); cognitive skills are usually attained at the expected ages.

Radiographic Findings. The characteristic features are present at birth and change little throughout life. Although virtually all bones of the body are affected, the abnormal configuration of the skull, lumbar spine, and pelvis are hallmarks of the disease. Typical are a shortened skull base, large cranium with prominent frontal and occipital areas, and superimposition of the sphenooccipital synchondrosis over the mastoid. The angle of the base of the skull is 85° to 120° (110°–145° is normal), and the foramen magnum is small.

The radial heads may be partially or completely dislocated and dysplastic. The phalanges in the hands are short, broad, and conic. The femoral necks are short and the long bones relatively thick and short. Distinctive rectangular or oval radiolucencies in the proximal humerus and femur that are apparent in infancy disappear by age 2. The inverted V-shaped (chevron) growth plate of the distal femur is characteristic, creating a ball-and-socket configuration of the epiphysis

Hypochondroplasia

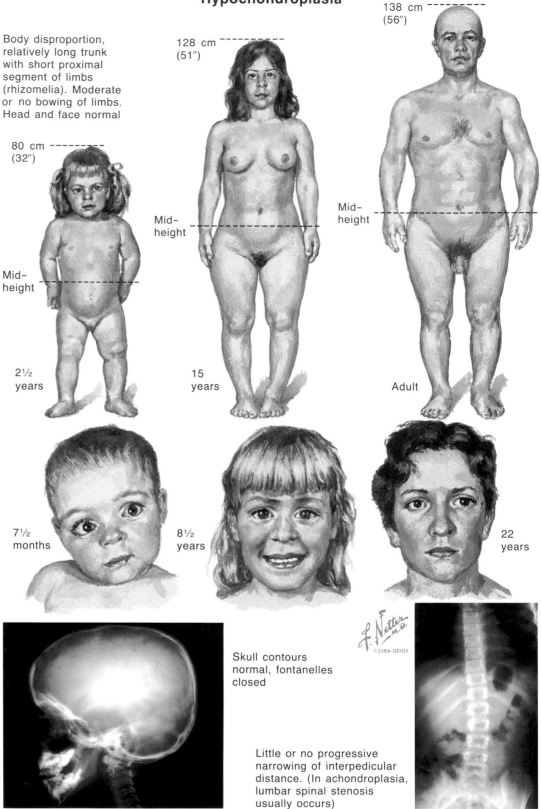

Body disproportion, relatively long trunk with short proximal segment of limbs (rhizomelia). Moderate or no bowing of limbs. Head and face normal

80 cm (32")
Mid-height
2½ years

128 cm (51")
Mid-height
15 years

138 cm (56")
Mid-height
Adult

7½ months

8½ years

22 years

Skull contours normal, fontanelles closed

Little or no progressive narrowing of interpedicular distance. (In achondroplasia, lumbar spinal stenosis usually occurs)

and metaphysis. The fibulas tend to be longer than the tibias, especially at the knees.

A diagnostic feature is a decrease of the interpedicular distance in a caudad direction, primarily in the lumbar spine (in the normal spine, the interpedicular distance increases in the caudad direction). Spinal stenosis, most evident in the lumbosacral region, is more pronounced in adulthood. Lateral radiographs reveal posterior scalloping of the vertebral bodies. Dorsolumbar kyphosis, commonly seen in infancy, disappears with ambulation and is replaced by an exaggerated lumbar lordosis. As the lordosis increases, the plane of the sacrum becomes more horizontal. The pelvis is short and broad with relatively

wide, nonflaring iliac wings, small and deep greater sciatic notches, and horizontal superior margins of the acetabulum.

Hypochondroplasia

For many years, hypochondroplasia was considered a mild or atypical form of achondroplasia, and many cases are probably overlooked or misdiagnosed because the height reduction and body disproportion are often relatively mild (Plate 4).

Hypochondroplasia is inherited as an autosomal dominant trait but most cases appear to be sporadic, presumably the result of a spontaneous mutation. For unknown reasons, about 10% of patients are mentally retarded.

Dwarfism

(Continued)

Clinical Manifestations. Birth weight and length may be low normal, and the short stature may not be recognized until the patient is 2 or 3 years of age. The typical appearance is a thick, stocky physique with a relatively long trunk and disproportionately short limbs, making the upper body segment longer than the lower body segment.

Head circumference is normal, although the forehead may be slightly prominent. The face is also normal with no midfacial hypoplasia or depression of the nasal bridge.

The limbs are short and stocky. Mild bowleg is common but tends to disappear with age. Ligamentous laxity is usually mild, and range of motion in the elbow, especially extension and supination, is often limited. The hands are broad with short fingers but no trident formation.

The trunk commonly shows mildly exaggerated lumbar lordosis with a sacral tilt and a slightly protuberant abdomen. Aching knees, elbows, and ankles and low back pain are common in adulthood. Adult height ranges from 52 to 59 inches.

Neurologic complications, particularly compressive myelopathy or radiculopathy, are much less frequent than in achondroplasia.

Radiographic Findings. Characteristic findings permit differentiation from achondroplasia. The skull is essentially normal, except for a mild bossing of the forehead. Generalized shortening of the long bones with mild metaphyseal flaring is most notable at the knees. In children, the growth plates of the distal femurs may show a shallow, V-shaped indentation, but this is not as pronounced as the chevron-shaped notch seen in achondroplasia. The femoral necks are short and broad. The pelvis may be basically normal or mildly dysplastic (eg, the greater sciatic notches are reduced in width and the ilia are square and shortened). In the lumbar spine, interpedicular distances lack the normal caudad widening, but these alterations are not as profound as in achondroplasia. The height of the vertebral bodies is normal, and the dorsal borders are only mildly scalloped.

Diastrophic Dwarfism

Like so many other bone dysplasias, diastrophic dwarfism, or dysplasia, (Plate 5) was originally mistaken for a variant of achondroplasia with clubfoot or arthrogryposis multiplex congenita. The disorder is transmitted as an autosomal recessive trait, and a lethal variant is characterized by a lower birth weight than in the classic form, radiographic evidence of overlapping joints, dislocation of the cervical spine, and congenital heart disease.

Clinical Manifestations. Clinical findings vary widely. Formerly, patients with similar but less severe signs were thought to have a variant

Diastrophic Dwarfism

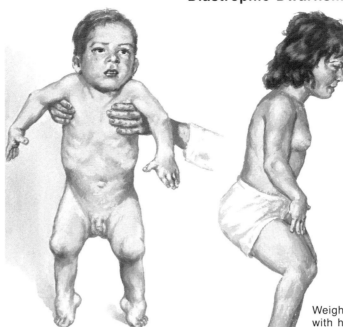

Short-limbed (mesomelic) boy with marked clubfoot, flexion deformities, dislocation of knees and patellae, and broad philtrum

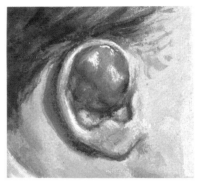

Weight bearing on balls of feet and toes with heels high off floor, compensatory knee and hip flexion, lordosis, and forward position of head

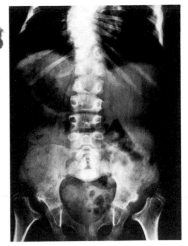

Scoliosis, bilateral hip dislocation, and coxa vara

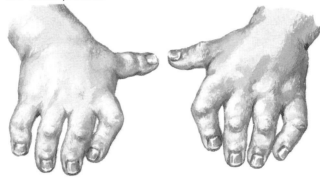

Broad, short hands with characteristic abducted (hitchhiker) thumbs and ankylosed proximal interphalangeal joints

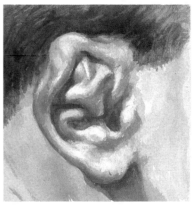

Acute inflammatory swelling of auricle in infancy

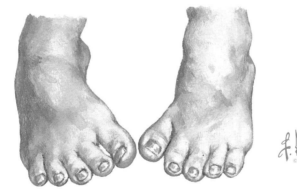

Marked clubfoot resistant to correction

Progression to typical cauliflower deformity

form or a different condition. The differences, more apparent than real, were due to variable phenotypic expression.

A unique group of malformations is evident at birth, with additional characteristics appearing later. In the newborn period, the head appears normal, but many patients develop a characteristic facial appearance with a narrow root and broad midportion of the nose, long and broad lip philtrum, and square jaw. The prominent area around the mouth, coupled with the other characteristic facial features, gave rise to the now obsolete term "cherub dwarf." The face is long and full with a high, broad forehead. Capillary hemangiomas are common in the midforehead

but fade or disappear with age. Abnormalities of the palate are seen in 50% of patients and include complete, partial, or submucous clefts, bifid uvula, or double uvula with a median longitudinal ridge. These palatal abnormalities—and possibly laryngeal defects—produce the characteristic soft rasping or hoarse voice.

In 80% of patients, the ears swell in the first few days or weeks after birth, giving the appearance of acute inflammation. The swelling subsides spontaneously in 4 to 6 weeks, resulting in a cauliflower ear. Calcification and ossification occur later. Hearing is not affected by the small size of the external auditory canals but can be impaired by deformity of the middle ear ossicles.

Dwarfism
(Continued)

Pseudoachondroplasia

Reduced height is primarily due to rhizomelic shortening of the limbs and is further augmented by flexion contractures of the joints, especially the hips and knees. Adult height ranges from 34 to 48 inches.

Partial and complete joint dislocation is also common, particularly in the shoulders, elbows, hips, and patellae. The dysplastic hip changes, coxa vara, and hip dislocation combine to produce a grossly abnormal gait.

Hand malformation is a hallmark of diastrophic dwarfism. The hypermobile thumb and deformed first metacarpal create an abducted hitchhiker position. The fingers are short and broad with ulnar deviation; there is limitation of movement due to ankyloses of the proximal interphalangeal joints (symphalangism). Severe progressive clubfoot is another characteristic.

The trunk is deformed by excessive lumbar lordosis that develops early in life. Scoliosis, which may also begin in infancy, becomes more severe with weight bearing and leads to trunk deformity and barrel chest. Kyphosis of a variable degree accompanies the scoliosis, and the resultant deformity further reduces height. Spinal changes, especially cervical kyphosis, may cause catastrophic neurologic problems.

Radiographic Findings. Characteristic signs are short, broad, long bones with flared metaphyses. Development of the epiphyses is delayed and irregular, and stippling has been observed. The epiphyses of the proximal femurs, absent at birth, are flat and distorted when ossification does occur. The epiphyses of the proximal tibias tend to be triangular and larger than those of the distal femurs. Other findings include cervical kyphosis and dysplasia; thoracolumbar kyphoscoliosis; partial or complete dislocation of the hips; precocious ossification of the costal cartilage; small, oval, or triangular first metacarpals; irregular deformity of the metacarpals, metatarsals, and phalanges; and clubfoot.

Pseudoachondroplasia

For many years, pseudoachondroplasia was confused with achondroplasia (Plates 1–3) and Morquio's syndrome (Plate 16). Pseudoachondroplasia (Plate 6) is most often inherited as an autosomal dominant trait, but a rare autosomal recessive form has also been proposed. Hyaline cartilage, fibrocartilage, and growth plate cartilage are affected. Proteoglycan abnormalities have been identified and are probably related to the core protein or enzymes responsible for the formation of the glycosaminoglycan chains in cartilage.

Clinical Manifestations. Growth retardation is usually not apparent until the child is 1 year old and often not until age 2 or 3. A delay in walking or an abnormal gait is often the first clinical clue. By this time, body measurements clearly reveal the disproportionate short stature.

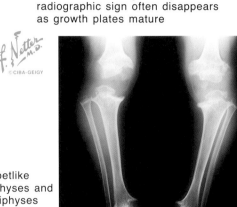

Squared-off, tonguelike projections on anterior borders of lumbar vertebrae due to defects in growth plates. This radiographic sign often disappears as growth plates mature

Sisters with short upper and lower limbs. Girl on left has bilateral bowing of lower limbs; girl on right shows genu valgum on one side and genu varum on the other side, causing pelvic obliquity that may lead to scoliosis

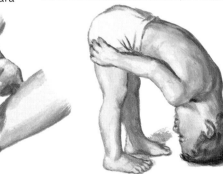

Wide, trumpetlike tibial metaphyses and irregular epiphyses with medial deficit, causing tibia vara

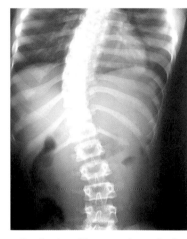

Scoliosis with some irregularity of vertebral growth plates

Wrist and finger hyperextension due to ligamentous laxity. Because of body disproportion, head can touch floor easily

As the growth rate slows, the typical habitus of long trunk, exaggerated lumbar lordosis, prominent abdomen, and rhizomelic shortening of the limbs develops.

Head size and face are normal. By early childhood, the patient has a waddling gait. Malalignment of the knees develops, including bowleg, knock-knee, or windswept deformities (bowleg on one limb, knock-knee on the other). Flexion contractures develop in the hips and knees, with joint pain and precocious osteoarthritis. The hands and feet are short and stubby with considerable ligamentous laxity, particularly at the wrists and fingers. Incomplete elbow extension is typical and is related to the dysplastic bone changes rather than to soft-tissue problems. Adult height ranges from 32 to 51 inches.

Radiographic Findings. The skull and facial bones are normal. The long bones in the hand appear short and stubby, and the carpals are dysplastic, with late ossification. In childhood, the small, irregular epiphyses of the femoral heads may become severely deformed and fragment by early adulthood. The ilia tend to be large and straight sided, while the pubic and ischial bones are short and broad; the greater sciatic notches are smaller than normal.

Spinal changes in childhood include moderate flattening of the vertebral bodies (platyspondyly) with biconvex deformity and irregularity of the

Slide 4443

Metaphyseal Chondrodysplasias

Dwarfism
(Continued)

superior and inferior growth plates, producing a tonguelike projection apparent on the lateral view. By adolescence, most of these characteristic vertebral changes disappear, and only mild platy-spondyly persists. Scoliosis and excessive lumbar lordosis may also be evident.

Metaphyseal Chondrodysplasia, McKusick Type

Commonly known as cartilage-hair hypoplasia, this disorder belongs to a group of intrinsic bone dysplasias characterized by significant changes in the metaphyses of the long bones (Plate 7). It is transmitted as an autosomal recessive trait and is relatively common in Finland and among the Old Order Amish in Pennsylvania.

Clinical Manifestations. At birth, weight is normal but body length is reduced. The config-uration of the head and face is normal. The elbows do not extend fully. The excessive length of the distal fibulas in relation to the short tibias results in ankle deformity, and unilateral bowleg or knock-knee may develop in childhood. The hands and feet are short and pudgy; the fore-shortened nails are normal in width and grow normally. Ligamentous laxity of the fingers and toes permits extraordinary hypermobility in the joints. A prominent sternum and mild flaring of the lower ribs with Harrison's grooves are also typical. In many patients, a distinctive feature is the sparse, fine, light-colored hair, which grows slowly and breaks easily. Cross-sectional micro-scopic examination reveals a reduced, somewhat elliptic hair shaft of small diameter that fre-quently lacks a pigment core. Body hair is simi-larly affected. However, in some patients, the hair is nearly normal.

About 10% of patients with the McKusick-type metaphyseal chondrodysplasia manifest intestinal malabsorption and Hirschsprung's dis-ease. They may be unusually susceptible to chickenpox. Neutropenia, persistent lympho-penia, normal serum immunoglobulins, and diminished delayed skin hypersensitivity may also be present. Adult height ranges from 41 to 57 inches.

Radiographic Findings. Radiographic abnor-malities do not become evident until the patient is 9 to 12 months old. Although changes are seen primarily in the limbs and ribs and around the knees (where they are most severe), subtle changes occur in other bones such as the verte-brae and pelvic bones. The metaphyses are wid-ened and irregular with sclerosis and cystic alterations. Other findings include cupping of the ribs and ankle deformity.

Histologic Findings. Microscopic examination of the metaphysis shows normal ossification but a hypoplastic cartilage. Chondrocytes are decreased in number, and columnization is disorganized. The cartilaginous cores on which bone mineral can deposit appear to be inadequate.

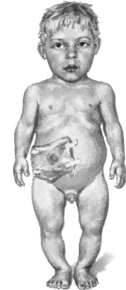

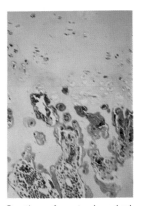

Greatly magnified hairs from six siblings. A, B, D, and F from normal siblings; C and E from siblings with metaphyseal chondrodysplasia

4½-year-old boy with short-limb dwarfism, sparse, fine hair, and Harrison's grooves on chest. Colostomy for megacolon

19-year-old patient with sparse, fine hair, normal face; scars from severe chickenpox

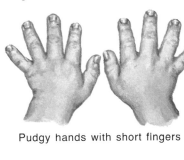

Pudgy hands with short fingers

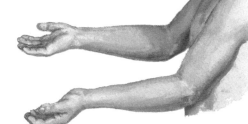

Inability to fully extend elbows

Great hyperextensibility of wrist and fingers

Section of costochondral junction shows paucity of chondrocytes and failure to form columns for calcification and bone formation

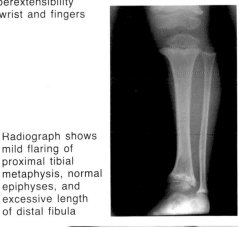

Radiograph shows mild flaring of proximal tibial metaphysis, normal epiphyses, and excessive length of distal fibula

Schmid type

------- 145 cm (58")

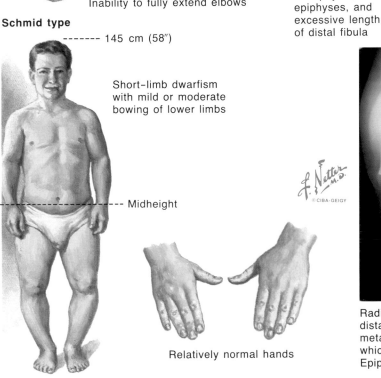

Short-limb dwarfism with mild or moderate bowing of lower limbs

-------- Midheight

Relatively normal hands

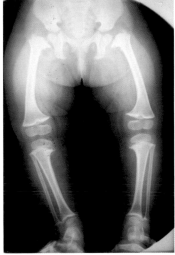

Radiograph shows wide, flaring distal femoral and proximal tibial metaphyses with medial deficit, which contributes to bowing. Epiphyses appear normal

Dwarfism
(Continued)

Metaphyseal Chondrodysplasia, Schmid Type

In 1949, Schmid described a form of metaphyseal chondrodysplasia that has been known by many names, including metaphyseal dysostosis and familial bone disease resembling rickets. The Schmid-type metaphyseal chondrodysplasia (Plate 7) is transmitted as an autosomal dominant trait with variable expressivity; females are usually less severely affected. Sporadic cases may be linked to advanced paternal age.

Clinical Manifestations. The moderately short stature of the short-limb type is evident by 18 to 24 months of age. The head and face are not affected. The wrists are prominent or enlarged, and often the fingers do not extend fully. Bowleg, commonly the first sign, becomes obvious shortly after the child begins to walk; if severe, the bowing produces a waddling gait and contributes to the height reduction. Poor alignment of the lower limbs can lead to symptomatic osteoarthritis in the hips and knees. Flaring of the lower rib cage signals trunk involvement, and the general habitus is stocky or chubby. Adult height is 51 to 63 inches.

Radiographic Findings. Metaphyseal abnormalities vary from mild scalloping to gross irregularities in the ankles, knees, wrists, shoulders, and hips. Although metaphyseal lesions appear to heal with bed rest, they recur once weight bearing is resumed. The epiphyseal lines are wide, and epiphyseal ossification centers appear normal.

Coxa vara and bowleg are common, and the long bones and femoral necks are short. The acetabular portions of the ilia tend to be broad, and the acetabular roof, normally vertical, is horizontal. Long bones in the hand and foot are mildly to moderately shortened, but metaphyseal changes are minor or absent.

Differential Diagnosis. This type of metaphyseal chondrodysplasia has frequently been confused with vitamin D–resistant rickets (see CIBA COLLECTION, Volume 8/I, pages 209-210). Clinical and radiographic findings are quite similar. However, vitamin D–resistant rickets has an X-linked dominant inheritance, whereas the Schmid-type metaphyseal chondrodysplasia is transmitted as an autosomal dominant trait. Unlike vitamin D–resistant rickets, there are no characteristic biochemical changes (serum calcium, phosphate, and alkaline phosphatase levels are normal) and no beneficial response to administration of vitamin D.

Chondrodysplasia Punctata, Conradi-Hünermann Type

Chondrodysplasia punctata (Plate 8) has been known by a bewildering array of names including chondrodystrophia calcificans congenita, Conradi-Hünermann disease, and dysplasia epiphysealis punctata. Although it is commonly considered

Chondrodysplasia Punctata

Conradi-Hünermann type

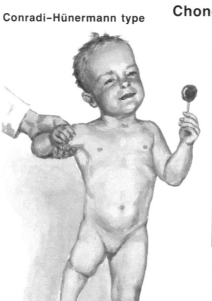

Marked lower limb–length discrepancy and sparse, coarse hair

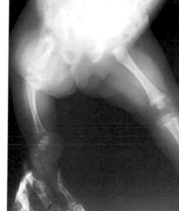

Radiograph shows short right femur with punctate calcifications in and around epiphyses of knee joint

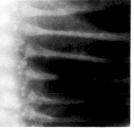

Punctate stippling of costovertebral joints

Scoliosis in older patient; related stippling of facet joints disappears by midchildhood

Linear striation and dry, scaling skin

Rhizomelic type

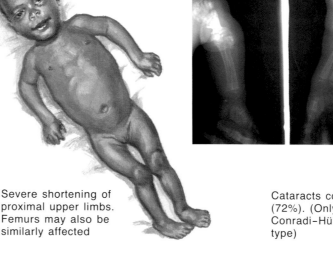

Severe shortening of proximal upper limbs. Femurs may also be similarly affected

Very short, dumbbell-shaped humerus with punctate stippling

Cataracts common (72%). (Only 18% in Conradi-Hünermann type)

a discrete entity characterized by radiographic evidence of punctate epiphyseal and extraepiphyseal calcifications (stippling) in childhood, this form of intrinsic bone dysplasia actually has nonosseous manifestations. To complicate the diagnosis further, epiphyseal stippling is seen in a number of unrelated disorders, including cerebrohepatorenal syndrome, generalized gangliosidosis, cretinism, Smith-Lemli-Opitz syndrome, Down's syndrome (trisomy 21), and anencephaly.

In genetic counseling, it is important to distinguish this autosomal dominant type from the clinically similar X-linked dominant type, which is fatal in hemizygous males. Severely affected infants are either stillborn or die soon after birth.

Prognosis for survival is relatively good for those less severely affected.

Clinical Manifestations. The major signs are usually evident at birth: a head of average circumference with a distinctive flat facies, mildly flattened nasal bridge, relatively short neck, and asymmetric shortening of the limbs. By early childhood, the characteristic facies largely disappears, but the limb asymmetry may need surgical correction. Congenital cataracts are seen in about 18% of cases. Scoliosis is common after age 1; joint contractures occur later. The skin is often dry, scaly, and atrophic. The ichthyosiform skin changes and alopecia usually persist into adulthood. Adult height is 51 to 63 inches.

Dwarfism
(Continued)

Chondroectodermal Dysplasia
Ellis–van Creveld syndrome

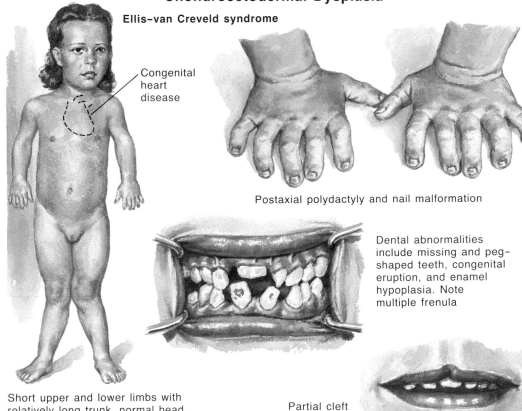

Congenital heart disease

Postaxial polydactyly and nail malformation

Dental abnormalities include missing and peg-shaped teeth, congenital eruption, and enamel hypoplasia. Note multiple frenula

Short upper and lower limbs with relatively long trunk, normal head circumference, and marked knock-knee (genu valgum)

Partial cleft of upper lip

Radiographic Findings. Early signs consist of punctate calcifications in the vertebral column and the epiphyses of the long bones and the carpal, tarsal, and pelvic bones, usually in asymmetric distribution. The metaphyses are intact, but the epiphyses frequently become dysplastic (flattened, small, or irregularly shaped).

Chondrodysplasia Punctata, Rhizomelic Type

Rhizomelic-type chondrodysplasia punctata (Plate 8) has an autosomal recessive inheritance and is more severe than the Conradi-Hünermann or X-linked dominant type. Recurrent infections usually cause death in the first year of life. Survivors have a high incidence of profound psychomotor retardation and other neurologic abnormalities, such as spastic quadriparesis.

Clinical Manifestations. The features of rhizomelic-type chondrodysplasia punctata are the same as those of the Conradi-Hünermann type, but the rhizomelic shortening of the limbs is more severe and congenital cataracts extremely common. Microcephaly, contractures, and postnatal failure to thrive are also typical.

Radiographic Findings. The epiphyseal and extraepiphyseal calcifications are usually severe, with a symmetric distribution sparing the vertebral column. Lateral radiographs reveal vertical coronal clefts of the vertebral bodies. In the humeri and/or femurs, severe shortening, splaying, and metaphyseal cupping are characteristic.

Chondrodysplasia Punctata, X-linked Dominant Type

Approximately 25% of reported cases of chondrodysplasia punctata are probably transmitted as an X-linked dominant trait. Most patients are female, and the disorder is usually fatal in males.

Clinical Manifestations. This disorder shares many features with the Conradi-Hünermann type, with hypoplasia of the distal phalanges a distinctive trait. Pathognomonic cutaneous findings in the first months of life include erythematous skin changes and striated ichthyosiform hyperkeratosis. Patterned ichthyosis, coarse and lusterless hair, and cicatricial alopecia become evident later. A variable severity, marked asymmetry of long bones, and cataracts are thought to be consistent with functional X-chromosome mosaicism in females.

Chondroectodermal Dysplasia (Ellis-van Creveld Syndrome)

This very rare type of short-limb dwarfism has an autosomal recessive mode of inheritance (Plate 9).

Clinical Manifestations. At birth, the head and face are normal, but oral and dental abnormalities are common, including natal teeth, multiple frenula that obliterate the buccolabial

Grebe Chondrodysplasia

Severe distal limb deficit. Fingers typically resemble toes; toes rudimentary, ball-like structures

Acromesomelic Dysplasia

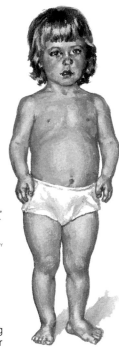

Short limbs, especially forearms and hands; short stature, normal head circumference. Attractive, often doll-like face. Minimal bowing of lower limbs may occur

sulcus, and partial or pseudocleft in the midline of the upper lip. Precocious exfoliation and missing or peg-shaped teeth are evident later. Mesomelic limb shortening is greater in the lower limbs, and with growth, knock-knee becomes serious enough to require surgical treatment. The hands are short and stubby with postaxial polydactyly, which also occurs in the feet in 10% of patients. The fingernails and toenails are hypoplastic or dysplastic. The trunk is not affected. Adult height varies from 42 to 60 inches. Congenital heart disease, typically an atrial septal defect, is seen in more than 50% of patients.

Radiographic Findings. The long bones show a progressive distal shortening with broadened metaphyses. In the hands, the capitate and hamate are fused or deformed. Retarded ossification of the lateral portions of the epiphyses and metaphyses of the proximal tibias results in knock-knee. The pelvis has short iliac crests and, in infancy, spurlike inferior projections from the medial and lateral margins of the acetabula. The configuration of the pelvis becomes normal by late childhood.

Grebe Chondrodysplasia

The rare Grebe chondrodysplasia (Plate 9) is transmitted as an autosomal recessive trait. Mild shortness of the hands and feet may be an indicator of the carrier state (heterozygosity).

    Multiple Epiphyseal Dysplasia

Dwarfism
(Continued)

Although stillbirth is frequent and neonatal mortality high, after infancy, prognosis for survival is good.

Clinical Manifestations. Marked shortening of both upper and lower limbs is apparent at birth. The legs are more affected than the arms, and length reduction of the long bones increases progressively from the proximal to the distal segments. The fingers are extremely short and toe-like. In the short, valgus feet, the toes may be rudimentary, ball-like structures. Polydactyly occurs in 50% of patients. Adult height is only 39 to 41 inches.

Radiographic Findings. The skull and axial skeleton appear essentially normal. The limbs, however, show severe dysplasia or aplasia of all bony elements.

Acromesomelic Dysplasia

Transmitted as an autosomal recessive trait, acromesomelic dysplasia results in severely restricted growth (Plate 9).

Clinical Manifestations. This short-limb form of dwarfism is usually apparent in the first few weeks or months of life. Head size is normal, but the frontal bones may be prominent and the midface mildly hypoplastic and flattened. Limb shortening is greatest in the middle or distal segments. Range of motion of the elbow joints is limited by partial dislocation of the radial heads. The forearms are often bowed. Fingers, toes, and nails are very short. The thorax is small with mild anterior flaring of the lower ribs. Exaggerated lumbar lordosis makes the buttocks prominent; lower thoracic kyphosis is also common. Adult height ranges from 38 to 48 inches.

Radiographic Findings. Radiographs reveal a progressive shortening of the long bones, bowing of the radii, and often subluxation of the radial head. The epiphyses are relatively normal in infancy and become cone shaped later. The hands are unusually squat, and the phalanges appear square or sugarloaf shaped. The height of the vertebral bodies is minimally reduced, primarily in the posterior portions.

Multiple Epiphyseal Dysplasia, Fairbank Type

Multiple epiphyseal dysplasia, Fairbank type, refers to a group of disorders with variable clinical and radiographic signs (Plate 10). Usually an autosomal dominant trait, it can also be transmitted as an autosomal recessive trait.

Clinical Manifestations. Multiple epiphyseal dysplasia usually remains unrecognized until the child is 5 to 10 years of age. The hands sometimes appear short and stubby, especially the thumbs. The shortening in the limbs is variable, and the trunk is normal.

Symptoms include morning stiffness, difficulty in running or climbing stairs, and a waddling

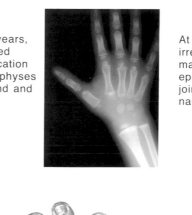

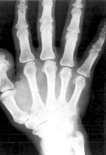

At 5 years, delayed ossification of epiphyses in hand and wrist

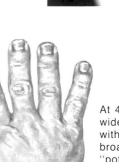

At 42 years, irregular, malformed epiphyses; joint spaces narrowed

At 40 years, wide hands with short, broad, flat "potter's thumbs"

Relatively normal habitus, body proportions, and facies; mildly short stature. Joint stiffness may lead to progressive incapacitation

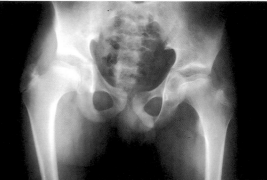

Epiphyses of femoral heads flattened and irregular with narrowed joint spaces. Vigorous physical activity must be avoided to prevent severe disability requiring total hip replacement

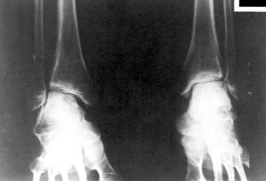

Slanted distal articular surfaces of tibias; usually evident after epiphyseal fusion at puberty

gait. Joint discomfort, pain, and stiffness also develop, especially in the lower limbs. At first, symptoms tend to be episodic, transient, and fluctuating, but the waddling gait becomes more pronounced as the disorder progresses, and increased discomfort and stiffness force patients to limit their activities. Severe osteoarthritis of the hips often develops in older patients. Some affected persons, however, remain asymptomatic. Adult height ranges from 54 to 61 inches.

Radiographic Findings. Accurate diagnosis requires radiographic examination of the entire skeleton. Bilateral epiphyseal abnormalities, primarily in the hips, knees, and ankles, are the chief manifestations. The ossification centers of

the epiphyses appear late, and fusion with the bone shaft is late. The epiphyses are irregular and flattened, and the ossification centers may be mottled with secondary centers, but there is no true stippling.

Mild shortening of the long bones develops, and metaphyseal irregularity is minimal. A deficiency in the lateral portion of the epiphyses of the distal tibias produces a sloping, wedge-shaped distal articular surface, an important diagnostic sign in adults. Bipartite patella is a common finding. Short, stubby phalanges and metacarpals with epiphyseal irregularities are seen. Vertebral changes are minimal, usually manifested as Schmorl's nodules or mild anterior

Dwarfism
(Continued)

wedging of the vertebral bodies in the thoraco-lumbar area.

Differential Diagnosis. Multiple epiphyseal dysplasia is often mistakenly diagnosed as bilateral Legg-Calvé-Perthes disease (Plates 57–64). Family history, bone scans, and a radiographic survey of the entire skeleton help distinguish the two conditions. In patients with multiple epiphyseal dysplasia, the epiphyses of the femoral heads are symmetrically affected, unlike the asymmetric involvement that characterizes Legg-Calvé-Perthes disease; multiple epiphyseal dysplasia is also found in other parts of the skeleton.

Pycnodysostosis

Pycnodysostosis (Plate 11) was once thought to be achondroplasia with cleidocranial dysostosis. Parental consanguinity has been implicated in more than 30% of cases of this autosomal recessive disease. Mental retardation occurs in about one-sixth of patients.

Clinical Manifestations. The major signs are failure to thrive, with resultant short stature in infancy and persistence of an open anterior fontanelle even into adulthood.

The head is large in relation to the body, with protrusion of the frontal and occipital bones. The major cranial sutures and anterior fontanelle often remain open, giving the impression of hydrocephalus. The face is small in proportion to the cranium and is characterized by bulging or prominent eyes, parrotlike nose, receding chin, and an obtuse angle of the jaw. Dental anomalies include premature or delayed eruption of teeth, persistence of the deciduous dentition, malocclusion, and hypoplasia of the enamel. The vault of the palate is highly arched and sometimes deeply grooved. The sclerae may be blue.

Because of increased bone density, even such mild trauma as tooth extraction can cause fractures. Deformities of the long bones, often due to fractures and malunion, may exacerbate the short-limb dwarfism. Arm span tends to be less than normal, and the terminal phalanges of the fingers are short and wide. Kyphosis, scoliosis, and exaggerated lumbar lordosis may develop. In some patients, the thorax is narrow and long. Adult height varies from 51 to 59 inches.

Radiographic Findings. Sclerosis is seen throughout the skeleton. The cranium is large, shortened, and brachycephalic with separation of sutures and an open anterior fontanelle. Multiple sutural (Wormian) bones are often present, and the facial bones, particularly the jaw, are underdeveloped. There is variable cortical thickening of the long bones with moderate metaphyseal undermodeling, with or without evidence of fractures. In the hands and feet, partial aplasia of the tufts and distal portions of the phalanges creates a bizarre drumstick appearance on radiographs. The acromial ends of the clavicles are dysplastic and hypoplastic.

Pycnodysostosis

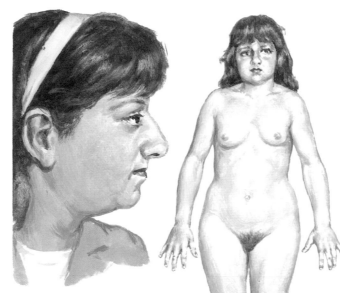

Prominent nose and small facial bones. Prominent eyes due to hypoplastic orbits

Mildly short stature (≤152 cm) with relatively normal body proportion

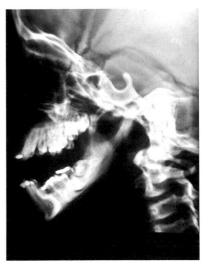

Obtuse, almost flattened angle between ramus and body of mandible

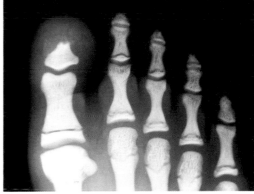

Marked shortening and tapering of distal phalanges without terminal tufts in hands and feet

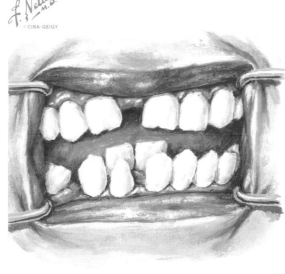

Delayed shedding of deciduous teeth results in double row of teeth, crowding, and malocclusion

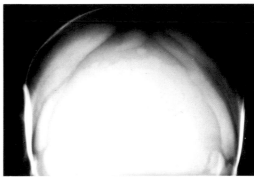

Open fontanelles and wide cranial sutures are characteristic

Differential Diagnosis. Pycnodysostosis is easily distinguished from cleidocranial dysostosis (Plate 40) and osteopetrosis (Plate 22).

Campomelic Dysplasia

A rare form of congenital short-limb dwarfism, campomelic dysplasia (Plate 12) is characterized by prenatal bowing of the long bones of the lower limbs in association with anomalies of other organs. However, although bowing of the limbs is common, it is not always present or pathognomonic.

The disorder is an autosomal recessive trait, although there may be other modes of inheritance. Campomelic dysplasia is in some cases associated with XY sex reversal. The majority of infants born with campomelic dysplasia appear to be female, but genetic studies show that many are actually male with XY gonadal dysgenesis.

In one-third of cases, hydramnios is detected during pregnancy. Stillbirth is common, and many live-born infants die in the neonatal period or live for only several months; many develop severe respiratory distress, in part related to hypoplasia and other abnormalities of the tracheobronchial tree.

Although prognosis is guarded during the first year of life, with medical intervention, more and more children with campomelic dysplasia survive into young adulthood.

Dwarfism

(Continued)

Campomelic Dysplasia

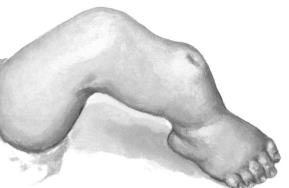

2-year-old child with typical flat facies, depressed nasal bridge, and small chin. Laryngotracheomalacia causes respiratory deficiency with stridor, necessitating tracheostomy

Extreme angulation of tibia with dimple at apex (same infant as on left)

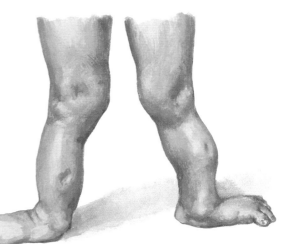

Short legs and saber-shaped, bowed tibias in 5½-year-old girl

6-year-old child with moderate dwarfism, largely due to short, deformed legs. Normal intelligence

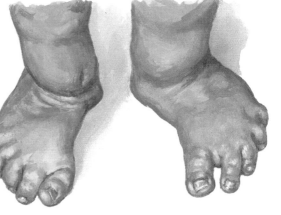

Clubfoot resistant to correction; persistent metatarsus varus

Clinical Manifestations. At birth, infants have a low-normal weight, a relatively large and long (dolichocephalic) head, and disproportionate short length, primarily in the lower limbs.

The prominent forehead, rather flat face, depressed nasal bridge, long philtrum, small mouth, small jaw (micrognathia), and occasionally wide-set eyes and low-set ears produce a characteristic facies. Cleft palate occurs in most patients.

The arms are normal or only slightly shortened and bowed. The tibias are often bent, or boomerang shaped, with a cutaneous dimple over the apex of the bend. The femurs tend to be anterolaterally bowed, and clubfoot is common. The thorax is often small, narrow, and bell shaped. Hypotonia is an additional feature.

Stridor and laryngotracheomalacia are major hazards in infancy, leading to long-term episodes of apnea, pulmonary aspiration, cyanosis, respiratory failure, seizures, and feeding difficulties. Tracheostomy and ventilatory assistance are frequently necessary for long periods of time. Congenital heart disease is found in nearly 25% of patients and hydronephrosis in 38%. Hemorrhagic phenomena in the central nervous system, hydrocephalus, and absence or hypoplasia of olfactory bulbs or tracts occur in 20% of patients.

Radiographic Findings. The typical findings reflect the three phenotypes: (I) classic (long-limb) type, characterized by bowed long bones with normal caliber and moderate shortening; (II) short-limb type, marked by severely shortened and bowed long bones and essentially normal neurocranium; and (III) short-limb type, associated with premature closure of cranial sutures (craniosynostosis).

Common to all three types are a large skullcap (calvaria) in relation to facial size; a small, bell-shaped thorax with thin, wavy ribs; slender clavicles; and small scapulas. The femurs and tibias show variable degrees of bowing, and the fibulas are hypoplastic. Congenital dislocation of the hips is common. The pelvis is narrow with dysplastic pubic rami, and the ischia appear vertical or even divergent. Scoliosis or kyphoscoliosis occurs frequently.

Spondyloepiphyseal Dysplasia Tarda

This group of intrinsic bone dysplasias is characterized by progressive abnormalities of spinal and epiphyseal development (Plate 13). The disorders must be differentiated from spondylometaphyseal and spondyloepimetaphyseal dysplasias, which primarily involve the metaphyses instead of, or in addition to, the epiphyses.

Although most cases of spondyloepiphyseal dysplasia tarda have an X-linked recessive mode of inheritance, both autosomal dominant and autosomal recessive forms are also known.

Clinical Manifestations. Growth failure does not become evident until 5 to 10 years of age. The height reduction, which is primarily due to trunk shortening, becomes quite obvious by adolescence. At this time, patients complain of pain and stiffness in the back or hips. Secondary osteoarthritis of the hip is common and may become disabling. The chest is broad or barrel shaped. Adult height ranges from 52 to 61 inches.

Radiographic Findings. The distinctive configuration of the vertebral bodies is most evident in the adult lumbar spine. Initially, the vertebral bodies are mildly flattened with a hump-shaped accumulation of bone in the posterior and central portions of the cartilage ring apophysis; the disc space appears narrowed. The thoracic cage is broad, while the pelvis is small and deep. The epiphyses of the long bones show variable dysplastic changes, and osteoarthritis of the hips is evident.

Spondyloepiphyseal Dysplasia Congenita

Most cases of spondyloepiphyseal dysplasia congenita are a result of spontaneous mutation (Plate 13). This type of short-trunk dwarfism is typically transmitted as an autosomal dominant trait, although cases of autosomal recessive inheritance are known.

Clinical Manifestations. In the newborn, a broad or barrel chest, deep Harrison's grooves,

Dwarfism
(Continued)

and pigeon chest suggest the diagnosis. Flat, dishlike facies, cleft palate, and wide-set eyes are other early signs. In older children, the short neck makes the normal-sized head appear to rest directly on the shoulders. Myopia and retinal detachment or degeneration are occasionally seen.

The limbs show mild rhizomelic shortening but are long in comparison with the trunk; the hands and feet are essentially normal. Ligamentous laxity is excessive. Marked lumbar lordosis and moderate kyphoscoliosis occur in late childhood or early adulthood. Adults reach a height of only 33 to 52 inches.

Motor development is often delayed. In 50% of patients, hypotonia, ligamentous laxity, and odontoid hypoplasia result in atlantoaxial instability leading to spinal cord compression, which first manifests as overwhelming fatigue and decreased endurance.

Radiographic Findings. Retarded ossification of the pubic bones, femoral heads, and epiphyses of the knees, calcanei, and tali is the major feature in young children. Early in life, the vertebral bodies are ovoid or pear shaped but become flattened and irregular with time, resulting in kyphoscoliosis. Careful radiographic evaluation of the cervical spine is important because of the hazards associated with odontoid hypoplasia. Coxa vara is common, and rhizomelic shortening of the long bones with minimal dysplastic changes in the hands and feet may also be seen.

Spondylocostal Dysostosis

Syndromes that comprise vertebral and thoracic abnormalities have been called by many designations, and more data are needed for a complete understanding of this group of disorders. However, evidence suggests genetic heterogeneity in spondylocostal dysostosis (Plate 14) with at least three phenotypes: (I) autosomal recessive with high mortality in the first 2 years; (II) autosomal recessive with good prognosis for survival; and (III) autosomal dominant with mild-to-moderate clinical manifestations.

Clinical Manifestations. Posterior shortening of the thorax and thoracolumbar lordosis are the major causes of short stature. The neck is short and often nearly immobile, and the head appears to rest on the shoulders. The limbs are long in relation to the trunk. The barrel chest bulges anteriorly, the lower anterior ribs may infringe on the iliac crests, and the abdomen protrudes. Recurrent respiratory infections are common and may be related to the chest deformity, pulmonary hypoplasia, or cor pulmonale. Laryngotracheomalacia is an uncommon feature.

Radiographic Findings. Severe vertebral abnormalities—hemivertebrae, fused (block) vertebrae, absent and butterfly vertebrae—characterize this disorder. The ribs are reduced in number

Spondyloepiphyseal Dysplasia Tarda

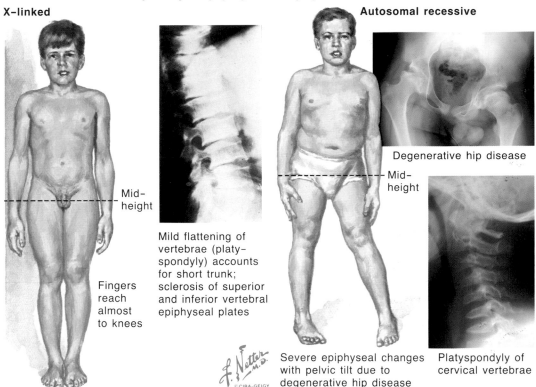

X-linked

— Mid-height

Fingers reach almost to knees

Mild flattening of vertebrae (platy-spondyly) accounts for short trunk; sclerosis of superior and inferior vertebral epiphyseal plates

Autosomal recessive

Degenerative hip disease

— Mid-height

Severe epiphyseal changes with pelvic tilt due to degenerative hip disease

Platyspondyly of cervical vertebrae

Spondyloepiphyseal Dysplasia Congenita

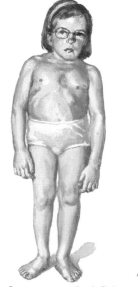

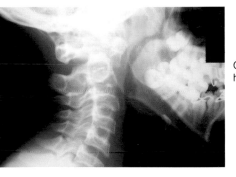

Odontoid hypoplasia

Severe growth deficiency with short trunk, barrel chest, pigeon or funnel chest, short neck, flattened midface, scoliosis, lumbar lordosis, and occasionally cleft palate. Myopia and retinal detachment in about 50% of patients

Late epiphyseal ossification, flat epiphysis of femoral head, coxa vara

and the posterior costovertebral articulations may be bizarrely approximated, producing a fanlike radiation of ribs. The posterior shortening of the spine causes anterior flaring of the chest and deformity of the rib cage. No significant abnormalities are seen in the appendicular skeleton or skull.

Dyggve-Melchior-Clausen Dysplasia

Dyggve-Melchior-Clausen dysplasia is a rare and unusual disorder with an autosomal recessive inheritance (Plate 14).

Clinical Manifestations. Recognizable as early as 6 to 12 months of age, this disorder results in short-trunk dwarfism with a short

neck, exaggerated lumbar lordosis, scoliosis, and prominent interphalangeal joints of the fingers with mild contractures and claw hand. Mental retardation and speech delay are common but not invariable. Adult height is about 52 inches.

Radiographic Findings. Radiographs reveal a generalized platyspondyly that usually persists into adulthood. In childhood, lateral views show anterior pointing of the vertebral bodies, with broad notches in the superior and inferior epiphyseal plates. The dens of the axis (odontoid process) may be hypoplastic. Irregular ossification of the iliac crests creates a characteristic lacelike appearance on radiographs. The ilia are short and broad.

Dwarfism
(Continued)

In young children, the growth plates of the proximal femurs are horizontal, with prominent spurlike projections on the medial side of the femoral necks. Ossification of the femoral epiphyses is delayed, and the long bones are short with irregular epiphyseal and metaphyseal ossification.

Differential Diagnosis. Patients with this condition bear some resemblance to persons with Morquio's syndrome (Plate 16). However, there is no corneal clouding and the urine contains no keratan sulfate. In fact, studies of lysosomal enzymes and histologic examination refute the hypothesis that Dyggve-Melchior-Clausen dysplasia is due to an abnormality of mucopolysaccharide metabolism.

Kniest Dysplasia

Now considered a distinct autosomal dominant entity, Kniest dysplasia (Plate 15) was previously thought to be a variant of metatropic dysplasia and, as a consequence, has been referred to as metatropic dwarfism, type II, and pseudometatropic dwarfism. This confusion occurred because dumbbell-shaped long bones are found in both of these skeletal disorders.

Clinical Manifestations. The condition is usually evident at birth. Although the average birth length is 16½ inches, adult height varies widely depending in part on the degree of contractures and kyphoscoliosis. The characteristic facies is round with midfacial flatness, a depressed and wide nasal bridge, protruding eyes in shallow orbits, and a broad mouth. Myopia occurs in 50% of patients and may become severe; retinal detachment is also common. About 50% of patients have a cleft palate without harelip. Recurrent otitis media and hearing loss, both conductive and neurosensory, are frequent.

At birth, the limbs are short in relation to the trunk, but the proportions change and the trunk becomes comparatively shortened and kyphotic by early childhood. The knee and elbow joints are particularly prominent and enlarged, with limited range of motion; widespread flexion contractures develop. The fingers are relatively long and have bulbous and knobby joints. Stiffness of the metacarpophalangeal and interphalangeal joints prevents the patient from making a complete fist. Precocious osteoarthritis develops and may become incapacitating by late childhood. Lumbar lordosis is pronounced by early childhood, and kyphoscoliosis is common. Adult height ranges from 41 to 57 inches.

Radiographic Findings. Generalized platyspondyly with anterior wedging of the vertebral bodies in the lower thoracic and upper lumbar spine is a major feature. In infancy, coronal clefting may be seen in the lumbar vertebrae. The ilia are broad with hypoplastic basilar portions. Ossification of the femoral head may not be apparent until age 3 or even later. The short femoral necks are extremely broad, and in the newborn period,

the femurs are dumbbell shaped. The epiphyses at the knees are relatively large, and a peculiar flocculent calcification develops in the metaphyses of the long bones. The hands are affected by osteoporosis, large carpal centers, and bulbously enlarged interphalangeal joints with narrowed joint spaces.

Histologic Findings. The histopathology in Kniest dysplasia is unique. The resting cartilage contains large chondrocytes in a loosely woven matrix with numerous empty spaces (like Swiss cheese). In contrast, the growth plate is hypercellular. Electron microscopy reveals these cartilage cells to be filled with dilated cisterns of the rough endoplasmic reticulum.

Differential Diagnosis. Radiographs help to distinguish Kniest dysplasia from similar disorders; in the neonatal period, the ribs are essentially normal, and there is moderately elongated platyspondyly. Metatropic dysplasia is characterized by waferlike vertebral bodies and very short ribs. In spondyloepiphyseal dysplasia congenita (Plate 13), ossification centers are not present in the neonatal period, and the femurs are not dumbbell shaped.

Hurler's Syndrome

The mucopolysaccharidoses (MPS) are a large group of biochemical storage disorders caused by lysosomal enzyme defects. More than eight major

Spondylocostal Dysostosis

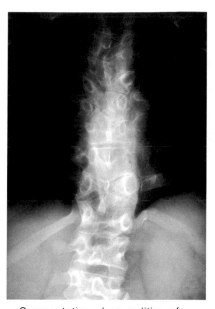

1½-year-old girl with short-trunk dwarfism; short neck and bulging abdomen

Segmentation abnormalities of vertebrae include hemivertebrae, fused vertebrae, and butterfly vertebrae. Scoliosis common

Dyggve-Melchior-Clausen Dysplasia

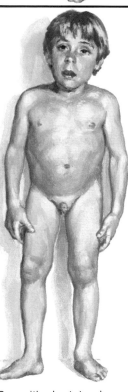

Boy with short-trunk dwarfism; broad chest and mental retardation

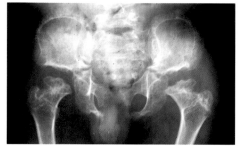

Lacelike appearance of iliac crests due to irregular ossification. Dysplastic pelvic bones and acetabula. Late appearance of femoral epiphyses

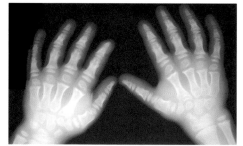

Broad and short metacarpals and phalanges; dysplastic carpals ossify late

Broad notches in superior and inferior epiphyseal plates of vertebrae with anterior spurs

Kniest Dysplasia

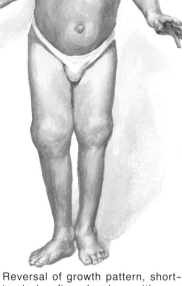

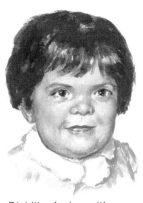

Dwarfism

(Continued)

types and many subtypes have been identified, and all are hereditary and progressive. Hurler's syndrome (MPS I-H) has an autosomal recessive inheritance (Plate 16).

Clinical Manifestations. Affected infants are large at birth, but growth rate decreases in the early months of life. Stature is markedly restricted, and contractures develop, limiting ambulation. Facial features progressively coarsen, and the nasal bridge flattens. Corneal clouding, hepatosplenomegaly, joint stiffness, claw-hand deformity, and thoracolumbar kyphosis develop slowly. Hernias, hirsutism, macrocephaly, macroglossia, noisy respirations, and mucoid rhinorrhea are present by the second year of life.

Mental retardation is severe, with a lag in developmental milestones. Cardiac murmurs, deafness, and poor vision develop with time, and respiratory complications become more frequent. A combination of cardiac and pulmonary problems usually causes death between 6 and 12 years of age.

Radiographic Findings. Common to all the mucopolysaccharidoses are multiple skeletal changes that vary in severity. In patients with Hurler's syndrome, the J-shaped sella turcica is enlarged, the skull is scaphocephalic, and the ribs are splayed. Other major findings include beaking of the lumbar vertebral bodies, kyphosis with gibbus formation in the thoracolumbar area, and abnormally short and broad long bones. Modeling of the metacarpals is poor, and their proximal ends are pointed. Broad, short phalanges contribute to claw-hand deformity.

Laboratory Findings. A high concentration of acid mucopolysaccharides, primarily chondroitin sulfate B and heparitin sulfate, is found in the urine. There is a deficiency of lysosomal enzyme α-L-iduronidase in fibroblasts or leukocytes, and metachromatic granules may be observed in leukocytes.

Hunter's Syndrome

Hunter's syndrome (MPS II) is transmitted as an X-linked recessive trait (Plate 16).

Clinical Manifestations. Clinical signs, present only in males, may not appear until age 2 or 3. The phenotypic presentations develop slowly. Two subtypes are recognizable. The severe form (MPS II-A) is marked by progressive mental retardation, and death occurs before age 15. A mild form (MPS II-B) is compatible with survival to adulthood and reproduction.

Affected persons are generally taller than those with Hurler's syndrome, reaching a height of 47 to 59 inches. Coarse facies, joint stiffness and contractures, claw-hand deformity, hepatomegaly, hernias, cardiac complications, hirsutism, and deafness are major features. Usually, corneal clouding is not clinically evident, although in older patients, slit lamp examination may reveal

Infant with short limbs and hypoplastic midface

Dishlike facies with button nose, prominent eyes. Cleft palate and ear infections with hearing deficits common

Reversal of growth pattern, short–trunk dwarfism develops with age. Knobby joints, characteristic stance, and severe myopia

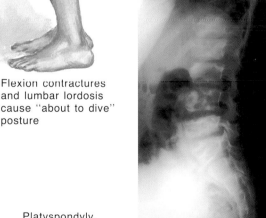

Flexion contractures and lumbar lordosis cause "about to dive" posture

Platyspondyly, characteristic ventral spurs, and clefts in vertebrae

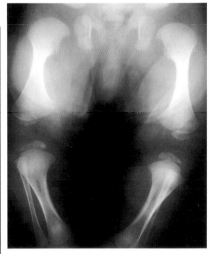

Characteristic dumbbell–shaped femurs and wide metaphyses in 1–month–old child

a light haze. Occasionally, a pebblelike rash is seen in regions of the scapula and upper arm.

Radiographic Findings. Findings of enlarged sella turcica, spatulate ribs, beaking of lumbar vertebrae, kyphosis, and short and broad long bones are less pronounced than those in Hurler's syndrome.

Laboratory Findings. Increased levels of chondroitin sulfate B and heparitin sulfate are seen in the urine. The lysosomal enzyme α-L-iduronidase is deficient in cultured fibroblasts.

Morquio's Syndrome

Clinical Manifestations. Morquio's syndrome (MPS IV) has an autosomal recessive inheritance

(Plate 16). Appearance at birth is normal, but the growth rate is usually restricted by 2 years of age and ceases by age 12. Medical attention is sought for dwarfism, awkward gait, knock-knee, bulging sternum, flaring of the rib cage, flatfoot, prominent joints, or dorsal kyphosis. Corneal clouding develops between 5 and 10 years of age but is not as severe as in Hurler's syndrome. The teeth are discolored and have easily fractured enamel. Ligamentous laxity can be extreme, particularly at the wrists. Severe knock-knee may interfere with ambulation.

Other complications include aortic regurgitation and atlantoaxial instability leading to spinal cord compression, which may in turn lead to

Mucopolysaccharidoses

Dwarfism
(Continued)

quadriparesis. Adult height is less than in Hunter's syndrome, ranging from only 32 to 47 inches.

Radiographic Findings. Flattened vertebrae with central anterior projections in the lumbar spine, odontoid aplasia or hypoplasia, delayed development of ossification centers, wide ribs, pointed proximal metacarpals, and coxa valga are the principal findings.

Laboratory Findings. The presence of keratan sulfate with normal or elevated levels of acid mucopolysaccharides in the urine is typical and is associated with a deficiency of the lysosomal enzyme galactosamine-6-sulfatase in cultured fibroblasts.

Principles of Treatment of Skeletal Dysplasias

Because of the widespread skeletal and nonosseous manifestations in many forms of dwarfism, successful treatment requires a multidisciplinary approach coordinated by the family physician. The child's growth and physical development must be monitored and compared with those of other children with the same disorder. Because eye and ear problems are fairly common in some types of dwarfism, ophthalmologic and hearing examinations should be frequent.

For genetic counseling of the family and patient faced with the choice of reproduction, it is essential to determine the specific diagnosis and mode of inheritance. It is no longer adequate to label a condition a "variant." However, in some cases the diagnosis remains unclear, and reproductive risks cannot be predicted. Psychosocial counseling may therefore be needed to promote a feeling of self-worth in the patient and social adjustment. Parents must encourage age-related—not size-related—behavior, social interaction, and independence in their affected children.

Medical Management. Patients must develop good nutritional habits early in life. Obesity is a serious problem; in a small person, even a minor weight gain is immediately apparent and may contribute to biomechanical imbalances or complications. Particularly common in persons with achondroplasia, overweight must be avoided not only to prevent hypertension and other cardiovascular diseases but also because it can precipitate or aggravate compressive myelopathy. Thus, weight loss often relieves symptoms of spinal cord ischemia. Exercise can help maintain ideal body weight, but in little people, specific skeletal problems obviously impose some limitations, and patients should select activities that do not stress the weight-bearing joints, such as swimming and bicycling.

Custom-made shoes and orthotic devices placed in the shoe help compensate for any limb-

Hurler's syndrome (MPS I–H)
Marked dwarfism with protruding abdomen, hepatosplenomegaly, coarse facies, and umbilical hernia. Joint contractures (hips, knees, elbows), mental retardation, corneal clouding (above), and cardiac anomalies. Usually fatal by ages 6 to 12. Autosomal recessive

Hunter's syndrome (MPS II)
Dwarfism less severe than in Hurler's syndrome; hepatosplenomegaly and umbilical hernia. Corneal clouding can occur late in childhood; intelligence may be normal. Life expectancy, adulthood. X-linked recessive

Morquio's syndrome (MPS IV)
Marked dwarfism with short trunk, severe flexion deformities, knock-knee, corneal clouding (may occur), and normal intelligence. Life expectancy, adulthood. Autosomal recessive

Odontoid hypoplasia, common in Morquio's syndrome, may lead to atlantoaxial subluxation with spinal cord compression injury

length discrepancy, but surgery and/or a limb prosthesis may be needed in severe cases.

Surgical Treatment. Most skeletal limb deformities and malalignment problems are not amenable to conservative measures such as bracing and must eventually be corrected with surgery. Scoliosis and kyphoscoliosis are managed with bracing or spinal fusion. Symmetric extensive limb lengthening is experimental at this time and highly controversial.

Surgical decompression is the usual treatment for spinal stenosis; spinal fusion is occasionally required. Since wide posterior laminectomy may create spinal instability, anterior vertebral body fusion followed by posterior laminectomy is often

performed. Timing for surgical decompression is critical; if performed too late, it will not restore function or prevent progression. Surgery is also associated with significant morbidity.

Whenever a dwarfing condition is suspected, the cervical spine must be examined carefully for atlantoaxial instability. Radiographs should be taken with the neck in flexion, extension, and neutral position. Spinal fusion is often the treatment of choice for this hazardous complication.

Skeletal malalignment, obesity, and participation in proscribed activities may lead to or aggravate early osteoarthritis. Short people are now frequent candidates for total joint replacement, especially of the hip. □

Cutaneous Lesions in Neurofibromatosis

Neurofibromatosis

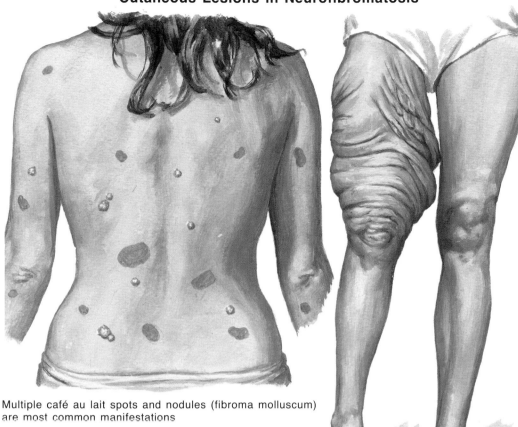

Multiple café au lait spots and nodules (fibroma molluscum) are most common manifestations

Localized elephantiasis of thigh with redundant skin folds

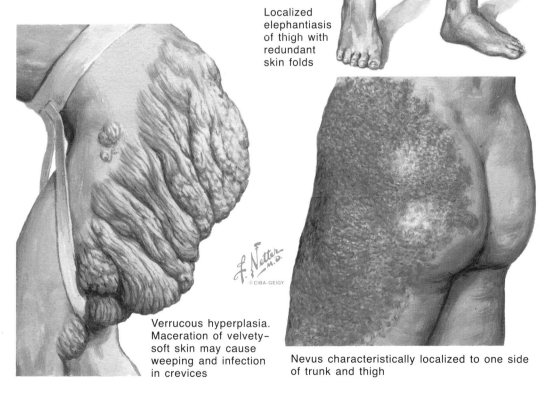

Verrucous hyperplasia. Maceration of velvety-soft skin may cause weeping and infection in crevices

Nevus characteristically localized to one side of trunk and thigh

Neurofibromatosis, first fully described by von Recklinghausen, is a disturbance in the neuroectodermal and mesodermal tissues, the supportive tissue of the nervous system. It is a multisystemic congenital and sometimes familial disorder and is progressive when it involves the central nervous and musculoskeletal systems (see CIBA COLLECTION, Volume 1/II, page 128, for a discussion of neurologic aspects).

Neurofibromatosis occurs in 1 of 2,500 to 3,000 persons. It is transmitted as an autosomal dominant trait with variable penetrance and a very high rate of mutation. The gene for peripheral (von Recklinghausen's) neurofibromatosis (NF 1) is located on chromosome 17; central (bilateral acoustic) neurofibromatosis (NF 2) has its gene locus on chromosome 22. This discussion is limited to von Recklinghausen's neurofibromatosis. Spontaneous mutations may explain why only about 50% of patients have a family history of the disease. However, the heterogeneity of the disorder's presentation and gene linkage studies may disprove the hypothesis of spontaneous mutation.

Diagnostic Criteria

The diagnosis of von Recklinghausen's neurofibromatosis in a child requires a high index of suspicion. The diagnostic criteria are (1) six or more café au lait macules greater than 5 mm in diameter in prepuberal persons (>15 mm in diameter in postpuberal persons); (2) two or more neurofibromas of any type or one plexiform neurofibroma; (3) freckling in the axillary or groin regions; (4) optical glioma; (5) two or more Lisch nodules (iris hamartomas); (6) a distinctive bone lesion such as dysplasia of the sphenoid, anterolateral bowing of the tibia, short-segmented and sharply angulated spinal deformity, and cortical thinning of a long bone without pseudarthrosis; (7) a first-degree relative (parent, sibling, or offspring) with von Recklinghausen's neurofibromatosis identified with the above criteria.

With time, all manifestations of neurofibromatosis increase in number, size, and severity.

The most common musculoskeletal manifestations are spinal deformity, limb-length discrepancy, pseudarthrosis of the tibia, and problems such as pathologic fractures and hemihypertrophy of the foot, face, and hand. Neurologic, visual,

and hearing problems are associated characteristics. In children, the incidence of several manifestations, such as sexual precocity, learning disorders, retarded sexual development, malignant hypertension secondary to diffuse renal artery changes, and mental retardation, is not statistically significant. The often-noted delay of speech and motor development may signify central nervous system involvement.

Cutaneous Lesions

Café au lait spots—the characteristic cutaneous lesions of neurofibromatosis—are present in 90% of patients (Plate 17). These spots are macular and melanotic with smooth edges, in contrast

to the jagged edges seen in lesions of fibrous dysplasia. Café au lait spots have been likened to the coast of California, while lesions of fibrous dysplasia resemble the rugged coast of Maine (see CIBA COLLECTION, Volume 4, page 195).

An adult with more than six café au lait spots with diameters of 15 mm or greater must be presumed to have neurofibromatosis. Results of an evaluation of children under age 5 indicate that two or fewer café au lait spots occur in under 1% of normal children, and that five spots with a diameter of at least 5 mm are pathognomonic. Nodules (fibroma molluscum), pigmented nevi, elephantiasis, and verrucous hyperplasia are other characteristic skin lesions.

Neurofibromatosis
(Continued)

Spinal Deformities in Neurofibromatosis

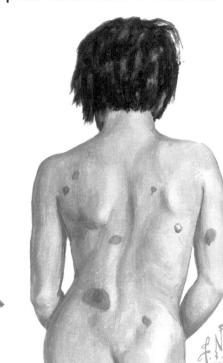

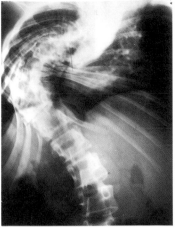

Radiograph shows severe scoliosis with characteristic short–segmented, sharply angulated curve

Girl with moderate scoliosis and café au lait spots

Boy with kyphoscoliosis. Foreshortening of trunk secondary to kyphosis gives appearance of longer upper limbs

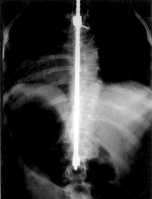
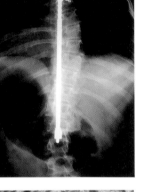

Relatively mild curve largely corrected and stabilized with fusion and Harrington rod

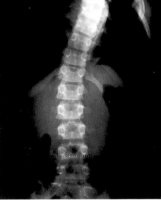

Benign-appearing scoliosis in child with neurofibromatosis

2 years later, progression of curve apparent

Spinal fusion resulted in nonunion. Exploration 3 years later revealed neurofibrosarcoma at fusion site. Section shows whorled, spindle–cell pattern of tumor (H and E stain)

Bone Lesions

Deformity of Spine. Scoliosis is the most common bone lesion in neurofibromatosis, occurring in 60% of patients. The deformity can vary from mild, nonprogressive forms to "grotesque" hairpin curves (Plate 18). Two patterns of deformity have been identified. *Type I spinal deformity*, the characteristic short-segmented, sharply angulated curve, appears to include dysplasia of the vertebral bodies and resembles congenital scoliosis. Computed tomography is needed to rule out congenital deformity and dysplasia. This type of scoliosis tends to be progressive and to resist stabilization of the spine with the usual methods. The classic neurofibromatosis curve is further divided into two subtypes: lateral curve (scoliosis) and anterior curve (kyphoscoliosis), in which the kyphotic element predominates over the scoliotic phase. The kyphotic type of spinal deformity is believed to contribute more to paraplegia than the lateral deformity. Flexion of the spine causes elongation of the vertebral canal and plastic deformation of the spinal cord. Increased spinal flexion due to the kyphotic deformity increases axial tension in the spinal cord parenchyma, resulting in functional neurologic impairment or paraplegia. This type of deformity is not successfully treated with routine posterior spinal fusion as it tends to result in pseudarthrosis. Spinal fusion with both anterior and posterior approaches is needed to prevent progression of the deformity and decrease the risk of pseudarthrosis.

Type II spinal deformity appears to be indistinguishable from idiopathic scoliosis and is an incidental finding in patients with neurofibromatosis. Follow-up studies of patients with type II deformity show less progression of the curve and better response to treatment. The incidence of pseudarthrosis in the spine tends to be higher than in patients with idiopathic scoliosis.

Bone Overgrowth. Disorders of bone growth are fairly common manifestations of neurofibromatosis. They are usually recognized clinically by changes in the overlying soft tissues, for example, hemangioma, lymphangioma, elephantiasis, and occasionally beaded plexiform neurofibroma (Plate 19). The overgrowth in bones and soft tissue is usually unilateral, involving the limbs or the head and neck. Joseph Carey "John" Merrick, who gained fame in the nineteenth century as "The Elephant Man," exemplified the classic case of unilateral bone overgrowth associated with neurofibromatosis. Recently, the diagnosis of neurofibromatosis in The Elephant Man has been challenged, with some authors proposing that he

had Proteus syndrome. Since lesions in the limbs occasionally continue to overgrow even after skeletal maturity, epiphysiodesis to equalize limb length should be performed when the diagnosis is confirmed (Plate 85).

Pseudarthrosis of Tibia. An anterolateral bowing deformity in neurofibromatosis may represent pseudarthrosis of the tibia (Plate 77). Management of a fracture is problematic because of its failure to unite. The bowing always develops before age 2. It is often progressive and should be treated very carefully. Posteromedial bowing, which is not associated with neurofibromatosis, is not progressive and does not present severe management problems.

Bone Overgrowth and Erosion in Neurofibromatosis

Neurofibromatosis
(Continued)

Hemihypertrophy of lower limb in 2½-year-old boy

↓

Same patient at 6 years of age. Marked progression and deformity

Overgrowth of lower limb in 5-year-old child. Limb was so heavy that child was anchored to bed; amputation was necessary

Progression of unilateral facial deformity. Note skin pigmentation. Infancy (left); 2½ years (center); 17 years (right)

Anterolateral bowing of the tibia in neurofibromatosis has been classified into two types according to the intactness of the medullary canal, involvement of the fibula, and risk of fracture (Plate 76). *Type I* is an anterolateral bowing with increased cortical density and a sclerotic medullary canal. *Type IIA* is an anterolateral bowing with failure of tubulation (abnormal medullary canal). *Type IIB* is an anterolateral bowing associated with a cystic lesion, or prefracture. *Type IIC* includes anterolateral bowing and frank fracture with pseudarthrosis of both tibia and fibula.

Type I anterolateral bowing has the best prognosis and may never progress to fracture. Management with bracing is usually unnecessary, unless the bowing starts to increase severely. Corrective osteotomy for the bowing may result in nonunion and pseudarthrosis. Type IIA bowing may lead to fracture, and protective management is essential from the time of diagnosis. Parents should be prepared for surgical intervention. Type IIB bowing deformity is extremely susceptible to fractures, with risk of nonunion. Attempts to obtain osteosynthesis include various bone-grafting techniques such as massive onlay, inlay, delayed autografts, and turnaround grafts; fixation with an intramedullary rod; vascularized bone grafts using microsurgical techniques; and electric stimulation. None of these methods have produced consistent results. Parents should participate in deciding how many surgical procedures should be attempted before resorting to amputation.

Type IIC bowing has the worst prognosis, and amputation should be considered early in treatment. The number of operations attempted and the length of hospitalizations must be carefully considered in light of the course of the disease

Radiographs show enlargement of spinal foramina at C2-3 junction due to erosion by dumbbell tumor. Excised tumor (right)

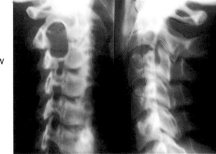

| | | | | | | |
|1|2|3|4|5|6|7|

CENTIMETERS

and the psychologic and financial costs. Recent reports of obtaining successful osteosynthesis of these pseudarthrotic lesions using the Ilizarov technique (Plate 87) have not stood the test of time.

Tumors. Neurologic hamartomatous lesions in neurofibromatosis are uncommon but not rare (Plate 19). A dumbbell tumor is a neurofibroma that arises in the vertebral canal and grows outward through the intervertebral (neural) foramen, its midportion being constricted by the bony foramen. Although only 12% to 16% of these lesions undergo malignant transformation, even a benign lesion has significant consequences; for example, a retroperitoneal mass or a dumbbell

tumor that extends from the vertebral canal may cause intestinal obstruction or neurologic compromise, or both. Some tumors recur and overgrow into a vital area, and repeat excision is not possible. Some benign lesions become life threatening because of their inaccessible location or encroachment on the spinal cord.

Bone Erosion. Erosive defects of bone in neurofibromatosis, which appear on radiographs as cysts, may be secondary to contiguous neurogenic tumors. Increased pressure in the dural sac may give rise to dural ectasia or pseudomeningocele in the vertebral canal. Dumbbell tumors of the spinal cord cause enlargement of the intervertebral foramen as they exit the vertebral canal. □

Arthrogryposis Multiplex Congenita

Arthrogryposis multiplex congenita (multiple congenital curved joints) is a nonprogressive syndrome that probably encompasses several different conditions. Its etiology remains unclear. The classic and most common form is evident at birth and is believed to be caused by an intrauterine infection, probably viral, leading to failure of development or destruction of the anterior horn cells, with resultant loss of muscle tone and mobility or absence of muscles. A primary, myogenic type of arthrogryposis, inherited as an autosomal trait, is a nonprogressive form of congenital muscular dystrophy.

Clinical Manifestations. The newborn displays multiple contractures, dislocated joints, adduction and internal rotation of the upper limbs, and stiff, diamond-shaped lower limbs. These deformities are usually bilateral but not always symmetric and may be limited to the upper or lower limbs or affect all four. Active and passive range of motion is excessively limited, and the limbs also appear featureless because of the scarcity of skin creases at the joints; soft-tissue webbing may also be evident. The skin is thin and smooth, and subcutaneous tissue is scanty. Muscle atrophy proximal and distal to the stiff joints is striking. The bones are thin and spindly, and fractures, particularly in the lower limbs, may occur at delivery.

Children with arthrogryposis have normal sensation and the potential for normal intelligence. They can be expected to have good general health and most will walk and attain bowel and bladder control.

Arthrogryposis has been associated with other conditions such as tuberous sclerosis, neurofibromatosis, myelodysplasia, and lumbosacral agenesis. The differential diagnosis includes Larson's syndrome, congenital contractural arachnodactyly, Marfan's syndrome, and trisomy 18.

Treatment. In the newborn period, the focus of management is on treating both the deformity and the muscle weakness. Vigorous physical therapy and stretching exercises are recommended to correct the rigid deformities, but care should be taken to avoid undue force because the thin bones fracture easily.

Deformities of Upper Limb. In the neonatal period, management of upper limb deformities comprises splinting and vigorous passive range-of-motion exercises. If the elbows are fixed in flexion, early exercises and splinting may be sufficient. More commonly, the elbows are fixed in extension, and surgical release is necessary. Although the wrist and hand are usually severely involved, patients have adequate function.

Deformities of Foot. The foot is nearly always involved in arthrogryposis; most common is rigid clubfoot (equinovarus). Surgical release of the contracted structures is necessary to allow correct positioning of the foot. The surgery, which should be performed in early infancy, often

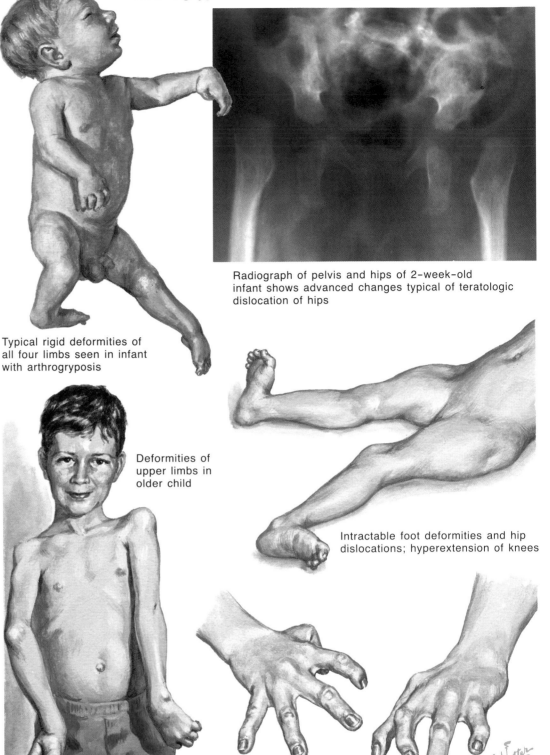

Arthrogryposis Multiplex Congenita

Typical rigid deformities of all four limbs seen in infant with arthrogryposis

Radiograph of pelvis and hips of 2-week-old infant shows advanced changes typical of teratologic dislocation of hips

Deformities of upper limbs in older child

Intractable foot deformities and hip dislocations; hyperextension of knees

Hand deformities

includes removing segments of the calcaneal (Achilles) tendon, long toe flexors, and tibialis posterior tendon. Patients with severely affected feet are treated with bracing and splinting in the growth years to maintain the surgical correction.

Deformities of Knee. The knees are usually held stiffly in extension or, rarely, in flexion. Early passive range-of-motion exercises, supplemented with splints or casts, may be necessary to restore motion. Surgical release or lengthening of the contracted quadriceps muscle may be needed if knee motion fails to improve. Flexion deformity of the knee rarely responds to conservative treatment and often requires early surgical release of the posterior capsule and hamstring muscles.

Deformities of Hip. Hip involvement is of two types—soft-tissue contractures and dislocations. Soft-tissue contractures are evident in the neonatal period. Management includes early passive stretching exercises, splinting or casting, and surgery. In the child with mild involvement, dislocated hips can be managed with the standard techniques used in congenital dislocation of the hip (Plates 54–55). More commonly, however, the hips are both stiff and dislocated, and radiographs reveal advanced and adaptive changes similar to those seen in the older child with classic congenital dislocation of the hip (Plate 53). If surgery is necessary, it is generally performed after the neonatal period but in the first year. □

Myositis Ossificans Progressiva and Progressive Diaphyseal Dysplasia

Myositis Ossificans Progressiva

Myositis ossificans progressiva, also called fibrodysplasia ossificans progressiva, is a syndrome in which the major and most disabling manifestation is an inflammatorylike lesion, and later, ectopic ossification of the voluntary muscles, fascia, and tendons. Skeletal anomalies in the feet are also characteristic.

The syndrome is hereditary and occurs more often in males. Unaffected family members may have the toe deformities without the subsequent ectopic ossification. The name of the disease indicates its histologic resemblance to the ectopic ossification found in other forms of myositis ossificans (see Section II, Plate 25).

Clinical Manifestations. Congenital anomalies of the digits are present at birth, before any other clinical signs appear. Microdactyly of the great toe occurs in 90% of patients and microdactyly of the thumb in 50%. Other digits may also be affected. In the great toe, this deformity is characterized by the presence of only one phalanx or a synostosis of the two phalanges and is associated with a marked hallux valgus.

By age 10, localized swellings arise in the neck, back, and limbs, often accompanied by considerable tenderness, pyrexia, and occasionally ulceration and drainage. The ossification develops somewhat later and may cause ankylosis of the vertebral bodies and joints such as the elbow, knee, hip, and shoulder. Its most debilitating effects occur in the jaw muscles, causing an inability to move the jaw, and in the chest muscles, impairing breathing. Fortunately, the tongue, diaphragm, and sphincters are not involved.

Treatment. There is no known cure for this disease, and excision of the ossifications is followed by massive recurrence. Supportive measures to ensure adequate nutrition and respiration may be needed. Despite a marked disability, many patients with myositis ossificans progressiva survive for many years, even into late adulthood (see CIBA COLLECTION, Volume 8/I, page 239).

Progressive Diaphyseal Dysplasia (Engelmann's Disease)

This hereditary disorder is characterized by a cortical thickening of the diaphysis of the long bones. Inherited as an autosomal dominant trait with variable penetrance, the disease becomes manifest in childhood as neuromuscular dystrophy, which causes the child to walk with a peculiar waddling gait with the legs spread apart; generalized weakness and fatigability are other major symptoms. Growth and sexual development are often retarded. Involvement of the skull may lead to optic and auditory nerve entrapment. The patient appears weak and undernourished.

With progression of the disease, the diameter of the diaphysis enlarges and the medullary canal becomes increasingly narrowed. The lesions

Myositis Ossificans Progressiva

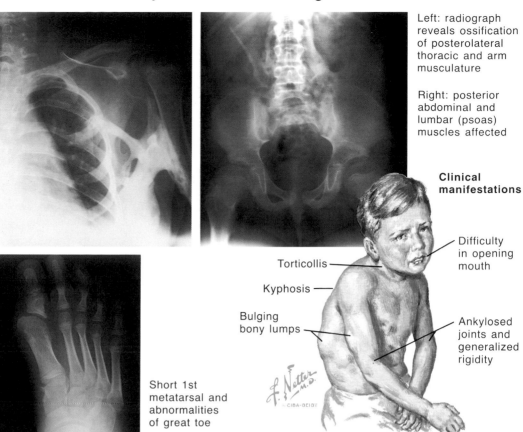

Left: radiograph reveals ossification of posterolateral thoracic and arm musculature

Right: posterior abdominal and lumbar (psoas) muscles affected

Clinical manifestations

Torticollis

Kyphosis

Bulging bony lumps

Short 1st metatarsal and abnormalities of great toe

Difficulty in opening mouth

Ankylosed joints and generalized rigidity

Progressive Diaphyseal Dysplasia (Engelmann's Disease)

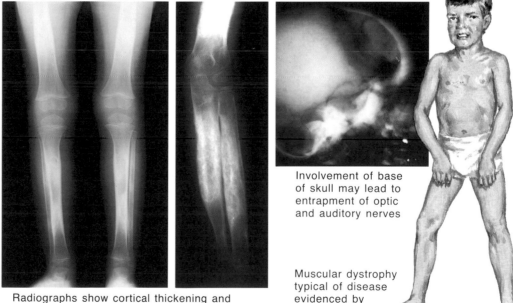

Radiographs show cortical thickening and increased cortical density in diaphysis of long bones of lower and upper limbs

Involvement of base of skull may lead to entrapment of optic and auditory nerves

Muscular dystrophy typical of disease evidenced by waddling gait with feet apart

spread proximally and distally toward the epiphyses. With the near obliteration of the medullary canals, hematopoiesis is diminished, resulting in secondary anemia and hepatomegaly.

Diagnostic Studies. Typical radiographic findings include (1) symmetric skeletal distribution; (2) fusiform enlargement of the diaphysis of the long bones and amorphous increase in density at the base of the skull; (3) thickening of the cortex by both periosteal and endosteal accretion of mottled bone without a recognizable trabecular pattern; (4) abrupt demarcation of the lesion; (5) progression of the lesion proximally and distally along the long axis of the bone, with gradual alteration of the previously normal cortical bone;

(6) relative elongation of the limb; (7) changes in soft tissue associated with underdevelopment and malnutrition; and (8) normal epiphyses and metaphyses.

Histologic examination shows that bone formation is increased on both the periosteal and endosteal surfaces. The increased osteoclastic and osteoblastic activity in the affected area destroys much of the lamellar bone and lays down large amounts of irregularly arranged trabecular bone, making the bone more porous than normal.

Treatment. The only treatment for this disorder is symptomatic care. Good nutrition is essential in the treatment of secondary anemia, and blood transfusions may be needed. □

Osteopetrosis and Osteopoikilosis

Osteopetrosis (Albers-Schönberg's Disease)

Also known as marble bones and chalk bones, osteopetrosis is a dysplastic process in bone characterized by a lack of resorption of the calcified cartilage and new bone and no remodeling in lines of stress, resulting in abnormal bone density. Even the bone formed by intramembranous ossification in the skull and the periosteal surface of the long bones have this abnormal structure.

The disease may be transmitted by either sex. The more severe autosomal recessive form is usually noted shortly after birth; death usually occurs in the first few years. The milder autosomal dominant form may not be evident until adulthood. The extent of bone involvement varies widely. The thickening of the bones at the base of the skull may cause impingement on the foramina at the base of the skull, leading to cranial nerve defects such as entrapment of the optic nerve and blindness.

Pathologic fractures are a significant complication of osteopetrosis because, despite its dense appearance on radiographs, the bone is structurally weak. Normal callus formation occurs in the early stages of fracture healing, but it eventually changes to the abnormal trabeculae typical of osteopetrosis.

Clinical Manifestations. The abnormal bone encroaches on the metaphyses and medullary canals, leaving no space for the hematopoietic marrow and resulting in severe aplastic anemia and secondary enlargement of the liver and spleen.

Radiographic Findings. The most striking characteristic is the extreme density of the bone. On radiographs, the abnormal bone appears amorphous, with no obvious trabecular pattern, cortex, or medullary canal. Occasionally, there may be transverse or longitudinal streaking. The chalklike density is caused by the persistence of irregularly shaped trabeculae of calcified cartilage surrounded by bone.

Treatment. In patients with mild-to-moderate involvement, the focus is on the management of secondary complications with good medical and surgical methods. Fractures should be treated with standard modalities. Severe secondary anemia necessitates blood transfusions, and bone marrow transplantation has been helpful in carefully selected patients with severe forms of the condition. In severe cases, such as threatening or impending blindness, bone marrow transplant has become the treatment of choice with excellent remission of the disease. However, this procedure is risky. Cranial nerve entrapment must be relieved with surgical release of the nerve from the surrounding bone. (For additional information on osteopetrosis, see CIBA COLLECTION, Volume 8/I, pages 234–235.)

Osteopoikilosis

Osteopoikilosis is an asymptomatic dysplasia of bone in which tiny foci of dense bone form in

Osteopetrosis (Albers-Schönberg's Disease)

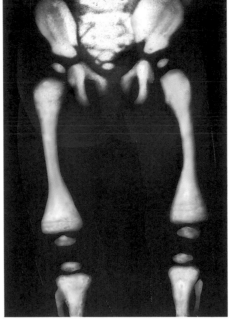

Radiograph shows marked increase in bone density with almost complete obliteration of medullary canals

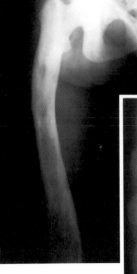

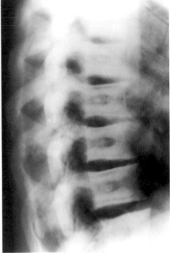

Excessive density of upper femur and pelvis with evidence of healed fracture

Increased density of epiphyseal plates and spinous processes in thoracic spine

Osteopoikilosis

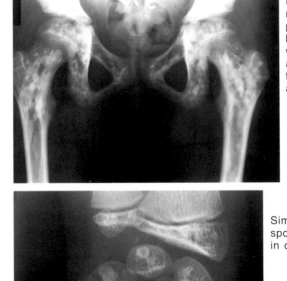

Radiograph reveals spotty patches of dense bone contrasting with radiolucent areas in proximal femur, ischium, and pubis

Similar dense, spotty patches in carpal bones

Characteristic skeletal distribution of spotty lesions

the spongiosa of the epiphyses and metaphyses of the long bones and the small bones of the hands and feet. Although the spine, sacrum, ribs, and sternum can be involved, these occurrences are quite rare.

Dermatofibrosis lenticularis disseminata, a congenital disorder characterized by the small foci of connective tissue hyperplasia, is occasionally associated with osteopoikilosis.

Radiographic Findings. Radiographs reveal small, rounded spots of increased density. The foci consist of rounded areas of normal-appearing, densely compacted bone in the spongiosa. The trabeculae in the bone surrounding the ossification center are decreased in number or are more slender than usual. The pathologic structure of each focus is identical to that of the common hyperostotic lesion called a bone island.

In a closely related dysplasia called osteopathia striata, radiographs show parallel and straight-lined striations that represent slender streaks of normal bone. These striations are most common in the metaphyses of long bones and in the pelvis. The hands are rarely affected, and the clavicle is never involved. It is not unusual for spots resembling those seen in osteopoikilosis to occur in association with the slender striations.

Treatment. Because there are no symptoms or complications of osteopoikilosis, no medical or surgical treatment is indicated. ☐

Melorheostosis

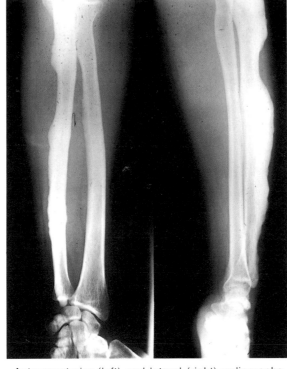

Anteroposterior (left) and lateral (right) radiographs reveal characteristic linear thickening of medial margin of ulna

Characteristic distribution of linear lesions. Often, only one limb involved

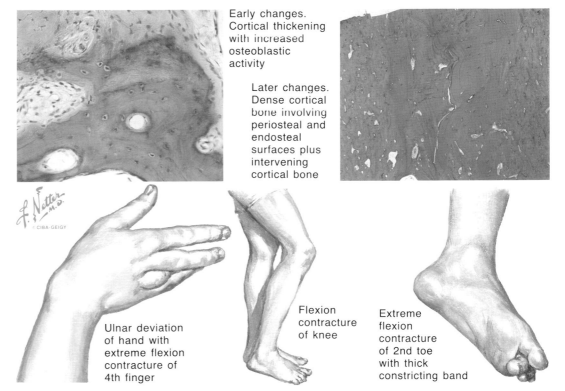

Early changes. Cortical thickening with increased osteoblastic activity

Later changes. Dense cortical bone involving periosteal and endosteal surfaces plus intervening cortical bone

Ulnar deviation of hand with extreme flexion contracture of 4th finger

Flexion contracture of knee

Extreme flexion contracture of 2nd toe with thick constricting band

Melorheostosis is a rare form of hyperostosis characterized by a linear pattern of distribution along the axis of long bones. The name—derived from the Greek words for member and flow—was suggested by the lesion's radiographic appearance, which resembles wax melting down one side of a candle. The characteristic pattern of distribution coupled with the abnormality in other tissues of mesodermal origin overlying the bone suggests an origin from mesodermal cells arising from somites in early embryonic development.

One or more bones of the limbs may be involved, but the spine, ribs, and skull are rarely affected. However, when the disease occurs along the full length of a limb, the hyperostotic process almost always extends to the shoulder girdle or pelvis as well.

Clinical Manifestations. Patients report pain, stiffness, limitation of motion, and deformity. The pain, usually over the affected bones and joints, can radiate along the limb.

When the hyperostosis extends to the growth plate, growth may be altered, resulting in reduced length or angulation of the limb. Involvement of the articular cartilage leads to osteoarthritis.

Hyperostosis affecting the full length of a limb is almost always accompanied by extensive fibromatosis. This soft-tissue manifestation lies close to the affected bones and joints (most often the hands and feet), causing contractures, muscle weakness, and limitation of joint motion. Soft-tissue changes are often the first evidence of this disorder in children.

Diagnostic Studies. Radiographs reveal a broad, irregular linear density along the axis of the long bones. The linear streaks may not be as evident in radiographs taken early in the disease, but they gradually increase in size and density as the child grows. In the epiphyses of the long bones and in the small bones of the hands and feet, the hyperostosis takes the form of spots and patches that resemble osteopoikilosis (Plate 22).

Histologic examination reveals an excessive amount of normal-appearing bone formed by membranous ossification. Thickened, sclerotic, and somewhat irregular laminae surround and almost obliterate the haversian systems (osteons). Ectopic ossification may also occur near the joint or may extend into the soft tissue along the fascial planes.

Treatment. Surgical management of melorheostosis focuses on preventing or correcting deformities. To ameliorate contractures and joint stiffness, excision of the foci, fasciotomy, and capsulotomy are done. For deformities of bone, osteotomy, epiphysiodesis (Plate 85), triple arthrodesis, and occasionally, amputations of deformed digits are performed. Unfortunately, no medical or surgical treatment can eradicate the pain of this disorder. □

Congenital Anomalies of Occipitocervical Junction

The articulation of the atlas and axis (C1–2) is the most mobile part of the vertebral column and consequently the least stable. The dens (odontoid process) of the axis acts as a bony buttress to prevent hyperextension of the neck, but the rest of the normal range of motion—and the protection of the spinal cord in the area—is maintained by the integrity of the surrounding ligaments and capsular structures. Atlantoaxial instability may result from occipitalization of the atlas, basilar impression, odontoid malformations, and laxity of the dens-retaining ligaments. It is often associated with Down's syndrome (trisomy 21) and some of the skeletal dysplasias that cause dwarfism. The most significant risk is compression of the spinal cord.

Occipitalization of Atlas

This condition is characterized by partial or complete fusion of the bony ring of the atlas to the base of the occiput (Plate 24). The clinical signs—torticollis, short neck, a low posterior hairline, and restricted neck motions—are similar to those of Klippel-Feil syndrome (Plate 26). One-fifth of patients have associated congenital abnormalities, including jaw malformations, incomplete cleft of the nasal cartilage, cleft palate, external ear deformities, cervical ribs, hypospadias, and urinary tract anomalies.

Fusion of the atlantooccipital joint may increase the strain on the C1–2 articulation and lead to instability, particularly when a C2–3 fusion is also present. The dens may gradually encroach anteriorly into the spinal cord or medulla, or the posterior ring of C1 may be pulled forward into the spinal cord.

"Relative" basilar impression is seen in about 50% of patients. It is caused by diminished vertical height of the ring of the atlas, which brings the tip of the dens of the axis closer to the foramen magnum and the medulla oblongata. Neurologic symptoms develop if the dens projects into the opening of the foramen magnum.

Congenital Odontoid Anomalies

Odontoid anomalies include agenesis, hypoplasia, and os odontoideum, in which the body of the dens is a free ossicle separated from the axis by a wide gap, suggesting a nonunion (Plate 25). In normal children under age 2, the dens is separated from the body of the axis by a broad cartilaginous band that corresponds to a rudimentary intervertebral disc. Complete fusion occurs after age 5. Abnormalities of the dens are more commonly associated with bone dysplasias and Down's and Klippel-Feil syndromes.

Minor trauma is commonly associated with the onset of symptoms, which may be due to local irritation of the atlantoaxial articulation or neurologic impairment resulting from C1–2 instability, decreased space for the spinal cord, and spinal cord compression. The abnormality is

Congenital Anomalies of Occipitocervical Junction

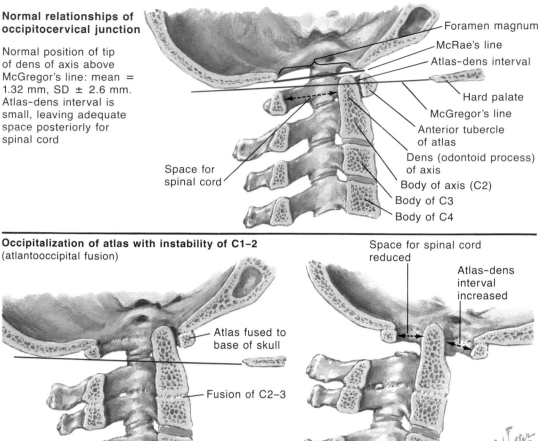

Normal relationships of occipitocervical junction

Normal position of tip of dens of axis above McGregor's line: mean = 1.32 mm, SD ± 2.6 mm. Atlas-dens interval is small, leaving adequate space posteriorly for spinal cord

Foramen magnum
McRae's line
Atlas-dens interval
Hard palate
McGregor's line
Anterior tubercle of atlas
Dens (odontoid process) of axis
Body of axis (C2)
Body of C3
Body of C4
Space for spinal cord

Occipitalization of atlas with instability of C1–2 (atlantooccipital fusion)

Atlas fused to base of skull
Fusion of C2–3

Space for spinal cord reduced
Atlas-dens interval increased

Atlas fused to base of skull. Dens projects into foramen magnum well above McGregor's line. 70% of patients with occipitalization of atlas and fusion of C2–3 develop C1–2 instability

When neck is flexed, space available for spinal cord may be considerably reduced as atlas-dens interval increases. Fusion of C2–3 accentuates instability

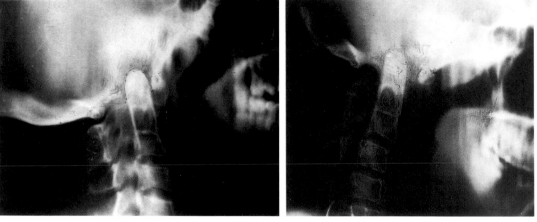

Lateral radiographs in extension (left) and flexion (right) of patient with occipitalization of atlas and hypermobile dens extending well into foramen magnum (basilar impression)

often marked by the insidious onset of slowly progressive neurologic impairment of both posterior and anterior spinal cord structures. In children, presenting symptoms may be subtle and nonspecific, such as generalized weakness, frequent falling, or requests to be carried.

Laxity of Transverse Ligament of Atlas

Laxity of the transverse ligament (Plate 25) may be due to acute or repetitive trauma, or the attachment may be weakened by inflammation from infection or rheumatoid arthritis. In Down's syndrome, the laxity may be due to rupture or attenuation of the transverse ligament and may lead to severe C1–2 instability. Lateral flexion-

extension radiographs are required in children with Down's syndrome who have neurologic problems or plan to participate in sports that may cause trauma to the head and neck.

Pseudosubluxation of C2 on C3

Cervical spine flexibility is greater in children than in adults. A common and normal finding in children is the anterior displacement of C2 on C3 when the neck is flexed (Plate 25). This pseudosubluxation is due to the normal laxity of the intervertebral ligaments, and nearly 50% of children under 8 years of age have anteroposterior movement of 3 mm or more. The straight-line relationship of the posterior elements in flexion

Congenital Anomalies of Occipitocervical Junction
(Continued)

(the posterior cervical line) is helpful in differentiating physiologic from pathologic anterior displacement of C2 on C3. Also common in normal children is overriding of the atlas on the dens with the neck in extension.

Clinical Manifestations

The clinical signs and symptoms of instability of the C1–2 junction are inconsistent. Only a few patients report a trauma or pain of the head or neck or exhibit torticollis, quadriparesis, or signs of high spinal cord compression.

The clinical signs of basilar impression or occipitalization of the atlas suggest that major neurologic damage is occurring as the dens encroaches on the spinal cord (Plate 24). Muscle weakness and wasting, ataxia, spasticity, hyperreflexia, and pathologic reflexes—the signs of pyramidal tract irritation—are common. Posterior impingement from the rim of the foramen magnum or the posterior ring of the atlas is typical of odontoid anomalies; symptoms include alterations of sensation for deep pressure, vibration, and proprioception. Nystagmus, ataxia, and incoordination may be due to an associated cerebellar herniation, and signs and symptoms of vertebral artery compression—dizziness, seizures, mental deterioration, and syncope—may occur alone or in combination with symptoms of spinal cord compression.

Radiographic Evaluation

The atlas-dens interval (Plate 24) is the space between the anterior aspect of the dens of the axis and the posterior aspect of the anterior ring of the atlas. In children, the atlas-dens interval should be no greater than 4.5 mm, particularly on neck flexion. (In adults, the upper limit of normal is <3 mm.) A subtle increase in the atlas-dens interval with the neck in neutral position may indicate disruption of the transverse ligament of the atlas. This is a valuable sign in evaluation of acute injury, when standard flexion-extension views are potentially hazardous.

The atlas-dens interval is of limited value in evaluating chronic atlantoaxial instability resulting from congenital anomalies of the occipitocervical junction, rheumatoid arthritis, and Down's syndrome. In patients with these conditions, the dens is frequently hypermobile, resulting in an increased atlas-dens interval, and measurement of the amount of space available for the spinal cord is more valuable. This is accomplished by measuring the distance from the posterior aspect of the dens to the nearest posterior structure (foramen magnum or posterior ring of the atlas). This measurement is particularly helpful in evaluating a nonunion of the dens or os odontoideum, because in both conditions, the atlas-dens interval may be normal, but on neck flexion or extension, the space available for the spinal cord may be considerably reduced. A reduction of the

Congenital Anomalies of Occipitocervical Junction (continued)

Laxity or tear of dens–retaining ligaments

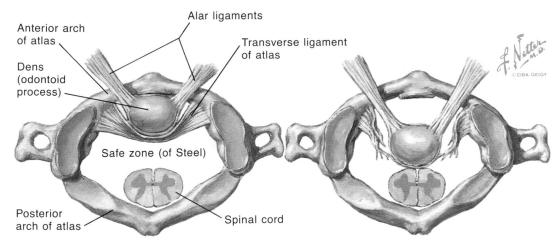

Dens normally held in place by transverse ligament of atlas and by alar ligaments attached to anterior margin of foramen magnum. Dens occupies anterior third of area enclosed by arches of atlas. Spinal cord occupies posterior third. Middle third is safe zone (of Steel)

If transverse ligament is attenuated or torn, dens may drop back into safe zone on neck flexion but alar ligaments act as checkreins and may prevent spinal cord injury. If alar ligaments also give way, spinal cord damage may result. Laxity or tear of retaining ligaments is also factor in odontoid hypermobility in occipitalization of atlas

Os odontoideum

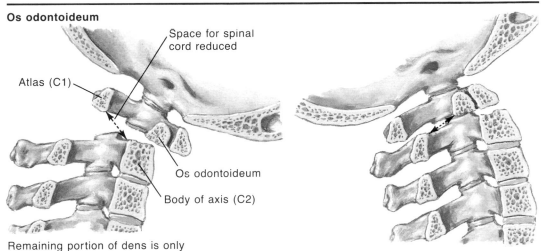

Remaining portion of dens is only a small, free ossicle that cannot stabilize atlantoaxial joint. On neck flexion, atlas slides forward with skull, carrying ossicle with it and reducing space for spinal cord

On neck extension, reverse occurs but space for spinal cord may also be compromised. Os odontoideum is functionally equivalent to odontoid fracture. Odontoid aplasia or hypoplasia has similar effects

lumen of the vertebral canal to 13 mm or less may be associated with neurologic problems.

Obtaining a satisfactory radiograph is often hampered by the patient's limited ability to cooperate, by fixed bony deformity, and by overlapping shadows from the mandible, occiput, and foramen magnum. Directing the x-ray beam 90° to the lateral of the skull usually produces a satisfactory view. Visualization may be enhanced with flexion-extension radiographs or computed tomography, and motion studies are frequently necessary.

Treatment

Effective treatment of atlantoaxial instability can be provided only if the exact cause of the symptoms is determined. Before surgical intervention, reduction of the atlantoaxial articulation should be achieved either by positioning or by traction with the patient awake. Surgical reduction should be avoided, as it has been associated with increased morbidity and mortality. ☐

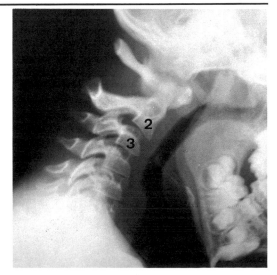

Pseudosubluxation of C2 on C3

In young children, normal laxity of ligaments may allow anterior displacement of C2 on C3. This usually improves with maturation

Synostosis of Cervical Spine (Klippel-Feil Syndrome)

Synostosis of Cervical Spine (Klippel-Feil Syndrome)

Klippel-Feil syndrome refers to the congenital fusion of two or more cervical vertebrae. In some patients, the entire cervical spine is involved. The fusion is a result of failure of segmentation of the cervical somites during the third to eighth weeks of embryonic development. Although the etiology is not yet determined, the developmental defect is not limited to the cervical spine. Unilateral or bilateral elevation of the scapula occurs in 25% to 30% of patients (Plate 40). Other, less apparent defects in the genitourinary, nervous, and cardiopulmonary systems and hearing loss often occur in patients with Klippel-Feil syndrome.

Clinical Manifestations. The classic clinical signs of the syndrome—low posterior hairline, short neck, and limitation of neck motion—are not consistent findings; less than one-half of patients exhibit all three signs. Although the most common finding is limitation of neck motion, many patients with marked cervical involvement maintain a deceptively good range of motion.

Whereas anomalies of the atlantoaxial joint (C1–2) may be symptomatic, fusion of lower cervical vertebrae causes no symptoms. Rather, the problems commonly associated with Klippel-Feil syndrome originate at the open segments adjacent to the area of synostosis, which may become compensatorily hypermobile. As a result of trauma or increased demands placed on these joints, hypermobility can lead to frank instability or degenerative osteoarthritis. Symptoms may be due to mechanical irritation at open articulations, nerve root irritation, or spinal cord compression. The development of symptoms is most likely with fusion of more than four vertebrae; occipitalization of the atlas plus a C2–3 fusion, leading to excessive demands on the atlantoaxial articulation; and an open articulation between two zones of vertebral fusion.

Potentially serious conditions that are associated with Klippel-Feil syndrome include scoliosis or kyphosis (60% of patients); urinary tract abnormalities (33%); congenital heart disease (14%); and deafness (30%). Since the urinary tract problems are often asymptomatic in children, ultrasonography or intravenous pyelography should be performed routinely.

Radiographic Findings. Radiographic examination can be problematic because fixed bony deformities frequently prevent proper positioning of the patient for standard views, and overlapping shadows from the mandible, occiput, and foramen magnum may obscure the upper vertebrae. Standard laminagraphic views of the neck on flexion and extension are therefore helpful,

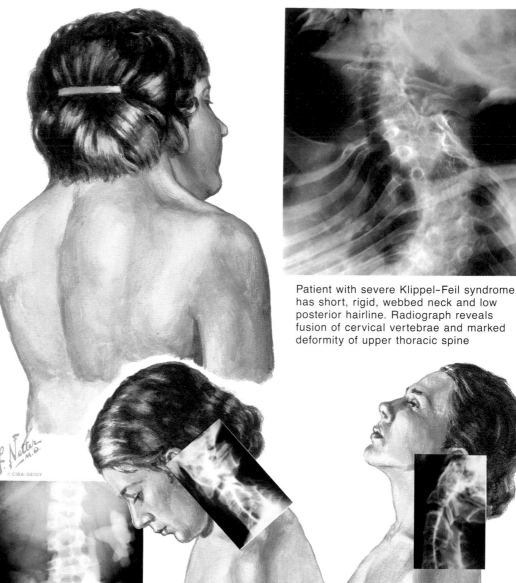

Patient with severe Klippel-Feil syndrome has short, rigid, webbed neck and low posterior hairline. Radiograph reveals fusion of cervical vertebrae and marked deformity of upper thoracic spine

Unilateral absence of kidney with hydronephrosis and hydroureter. Associated anomalies of genitourinary tract or other systems may be less apparent yet more serious than cervical spine fusions

Patient demonstrates relatively normal range of cervical flexion and extension despite fusion of most cervical vertebrae; motion occurs chiefly at one open disc space. No cervical webbing or abnormality of posterior hairline

and computed tomography is also useful in assessing spinal cord problems and nerve root impingement.

Ossification of the vertebral body is not complete until adolescence, and in children, the unossified epiphyseal plates may give the false impression of a normal disc space. Therefore, a suspected fusion in a child should be confirmed with lateral flexion-extension radiographs.

The bony cervical defects may extend to the upper thoracic area, particularly in patients with severe involvement. However, narrowing of the vertebral canal, due to degenerative changes or hypermobility, does not usually occur until adulthood.

Treatment. Children with minimal involvement usually lead a normal, active life with minor or no restrictions or symptoms. Symptoms referable to the cervical spine may occur in adulthood as a result of osteoarthritis or instability of the hypermobile articulations. While conservative treatment is sufficient in most patients, a few require judicious surgical stabilization. Scoliosis must be monitored carefully and treated if necessary. However, the relatively good prognosis of the cervical condition is overshadowed by the hidden or unrecognized associated anomalies. Early recognition and treatment of these problems may spare the patient further deformity or serious illness. □

Congenital Muscular Torticollis (Wryneck)

Congenital muscular torticollis (congenital wryneck) is a common condition, usually discovered in the first 6 to 8 weeks of life. Contracture of the sternocleidomastoid muscle tilts the head toward the involved side, rotating the chin to the contralateral shoulder. The cause is believed to be ischemia of the sternocleidomastoid muscle, particularly the sternal head, due to intrauterine positioning or increased pressure during passage through the birth canal. The contracture usually occurs on the right side, and 20% of children with congenital muscular torticollis also have congenital dysplasia of the hip. These observations support the hypothesis that both problems are related to intrauterine malpositioning or presentation.

Clinical Manifestations

In the first month after delivery, a soft, nontender enlargement, or "tumor," is noted beneath the skin and attached to the body of the sternocleidomastoid muscle (Plate 27). The tumor usually resolves in 6 to 12 weeks, after which contracture, or tightness, of the sternocleidomastoid muscle and the torticollis become apparent. With time, fibrosis of the sternal head of the muscle may entrap and compromise the branch of the accessory nerve to the clavicular head, further increasing the deformity.

If the contracture does not improve, deformities of the face and skull (plagiocephaly) can develop in the first year. The face becomes flattened on the side of the contracted sternocleidomastoid muscle. The deformity is related to the sleeping position. Children who sleep prone are more comfortable with the affected side down; consequently, that side of the face becomes distorted. Children who sleep supine develop flattening of the back of the head.

Treatment

In the first year of life, conservative measures comprising stretching and range-of-motion exercises and positioning produce good results in 85% to 90% of patients. If conservative measures fail, surgical intervention is required. Surgery should be performed in patients 18 months to 2 years of age. Allowing the deformity to persist results in further facial flattening and poor cosmetic result.

Surgery usually consists of resection of a portion of the distal sternocleidomastoid muscle. The incision should be placed transversely in the neck to coincide with the normal skin folds. It should not be placed near the clavicle, as scars in this area tend to spread. Postoperative treatment includes passive stretching exercises and, occasionally, a brace or cast to maintain the corrected position.

Nonmuscular Causes of Torticollis

Torticollis is a common childhood complaint that can be caused by a wide variety of problems,

Congenital Muscular Torticollis (Wryneck)

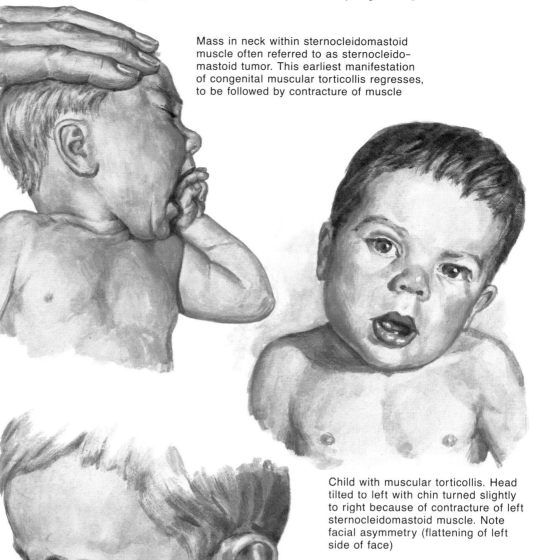

Mass in neck within sternocleidomastoid muscle often referred to as sternocleidomastoid tumor. This earliest manifestation of congenital muscular torticollis regresses, to be followed by contracture of muscle

Child with muscular torticollis. Head tilted to left with chin turned slightly to right because of contracture of left sternocleidomastoid muscle. Note facial asymmetry (flattening of left side of face)

Untreated torticollis in 5-year-old boy. Thick, fibrotic, tendonlike bands have replaced sternocleidomastoid muscle, making head appear tethered to clavicle. Two heads of left sternocleidomastoid muscle prominent

but identifying the cause can be difficult (Plate 28). If the characteristic posture of the head and neck is noted shortly after birth, congenital anomalies of the cervical spine should be considered, particularly those of the occipitocervical junction (Plates 24 25). Torticollis may be a sign of Klippel-Feil syndrome, basilar impression, or occipitalization of the atlas. In these conditions, however, the sternocleidomastoid muscle on the short side is not contracted.

Wryneck that appears several weeks after birth is usually congenital muscular torticollis. Less commonly, soft-tissue problems such as abnormal skin webs or folds (pterygium coli) maintain the neck in a twisted position. Tumors in the region

of the sternocleidomastoid muscle, such as cystic hygroma, branchial cleft cysts, and thyroid teratomas, are rare but must be considered.

Intermittent torticollis can occur in the young child. A seizurelike condition called benign paroxysmal torticollis of infancy can be the result of a variety of neurologic causes, including drug intoxication. Similarly, sudden posturing of the trunk and torticollis associated with gastroesophageal reflux are often reported.

A major cause of torticollis in older children is bacterial or viral pharyngitis with involvement of the cervical nodes. Spontaneous atlantoaxial rotatory subluxation can occur following acute pharyngitis.

Congenital Muscular Torticollis (Wryneck)

(Continued)

Surgery in the upper pharynx, such as a tonsillectomy, may also precipitate rotatory subluxation. Inflammation and local edema in the retropharyngeal region lead to laxity of the ligamentous restraints, allowing greater motion of C1–2. Standard radiographic techniques are inadequate for diagnosis, and special views, including tomography and computed tomography, are often required. Bed rest, aspirin, and use of a soft collar may be sufficient if the diagnosis is made early. A head halter or halo brace may be necessary for long-standing problems or if the simple measures fail. If the torticollis persists beyond 3 weeks, recurs, or becomes subacute, postreduction immobilization in a Minerva cast brace or halo brace is indicated. Surgical stabilization is required for rare neglected cases.

Other inflammatory conditions, such as juvenile arthritis, infection of the cervical spine, and acute calcification of a cervical disc, are also sources of torticollis.

Traumatic causes should be considered and carefully excluded in the diagnosis of torticollis. Unrecognized and untreated injuries may have serious neurologic consequences. Torticollis commonly follows an injury to the C1–2 articulation. It may also be due to fractures and dislocations of the dens, which may not be apparent on initial radiographs. Skeletal dysplasia, Morquio's syndrome, spondyloepiphyseal dysplasia, and Down's syndrome are commonly associated with C1–2 instability and accompanying torticollis.

Torticollis is also a sign of certain neurologic problems, particularly space-occupying lesions of the central nervous system, such as tumors of the posterior cranial fossa or the spinal cord, chordoma, and syringomyelia. Uncommon neurologic causes include dystonia musculorum deformans and hearing and vision problems, which can lead to head tilt. Although hysterical and psychogenic causes have been described, they are very uncommon and can be diagnosed only after careful evaluation has excluded other causes.

Calcification of the vertebral disc, an uncommon problem of childhood, most often involves the cervical vertebrae. The C6–7 disc space is the most frequent site, but any disc space can be involved. In 30% of children, trauma is the apparent cause; 15% of children report an upper respiratory infection. The onset of symptoms is abrupt, with torticollis, neck pain, and limitation of neck motion the usual presenting complaints. Only 25% of patients are febrile on presentation. Rarely, the disc herniates posteriorly, causing spinal cord compression, or anteriorly, causing dysphasia. Typically, the clinical manifestations resolve rapidly and the radiographic signs more gradually. Two-thirds of children are symptom free within 3 weeks and 95%, within 6 months. Resolution of neurologic symptoms occurs in 90% of patients. ☐

Nonmuscular Causes of Torticollis

Atlantoaxial rotatory subluxation and fixation (after Fielding and Hawkins)

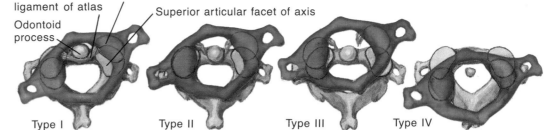

Transverse ligament of atlas
Inferior articular facet of atlas
Superior articular facet of axis
Odontoid process

Type I — Rotatory subluxation of atlas about dens but transverse ligament intact. No anterior displacement

Type II — One articular facet subluxated, other acts as pivot; transverse ligament defective. Anterior displacement of 3–5 mm

Type III — Both articular facets subluxated, transverse ligament defective. Anterior displacement of >5 mm

Type IV — Posterior rotatory subluxation (rare). Os odontoideum or absent or defective dens

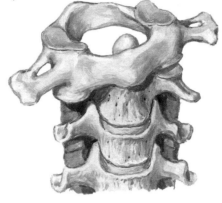

Type I rotatory subluxation

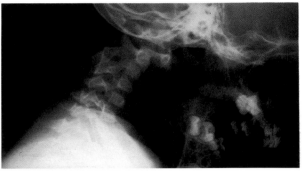

Radiograph shows lateral mass of atlas rotated anteriorly. CT scans helpful in confirming diagnosis

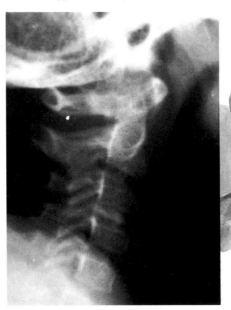

Acute intervertebral disc calcification
7-year-old girl with spontaneous onset of torticollis. Radiograph reveals calcification of C3–4 disc

Cervical adenitis

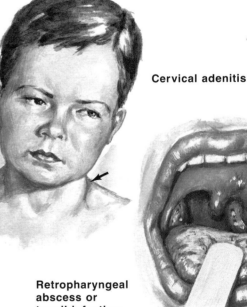

Retropharyngeal abscess or tonsil infection

Juvenile arthritis of cervical spine
Radiographs show progression

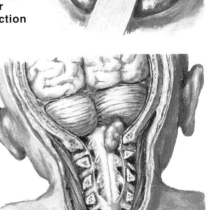

Tumor in region of foramen magnum (rare)

Scoliosis

Scoliosis is a rotational deformity of the spine and ribs. While in most cases the cause of scoliosis is unknown, a genetic factor appears to have a role. Scoliosis may also result from a variety of congenital, neuromuscular, mesenchymal, and traumatic conditions, and it is commonly associated with neurofibromatosis.

Pathology

A complicated deformity, scoliosis is characterized by both lateral curvature and vertebral rotation. As the disease progresses, the vertebrae and spinous processes in the area of the major curve rotate toward the concavity of the curve (Plate 29). The rotating vertebrae push the ribs on the convex side of the curve posteriorly and cause the ribs on the concave side to crowd together. In more advanced cases, the entire thoracic cage becomes ovoid, causing the ribs on the concave side to protrude anteriorly while the ribs on the opposite side are recessed. Kyphosis (hunchback) and lordosis (swayback) often accompany the scoliotic deformity.

In addition to rotation, scoliosis also causes other pathologic changes in the vertebrae and related structures in the area of the curve. The disc spaces become narrower on the concave side of the curve and wider on the convex side. The vertebrae also become wedged (ie, thicker on the convex side). On the concave side of the curve, the pedicles and laminae are shorter and thinner and the vertebral canal is narrower.

The structural changes described are most common in idiopathic forms of scoliosis; the pathology may vary somewhat in paralytic and congenital forms. Generally, in the paralytic curve, which is caused by severe muscle imbalance, the ribs assume an almost vertical position on the convex side.

Classification

Scoliosis is broadly classified into nonstructural and structural types. In *nonstructural scoliosis*, the curve is flexible and corrects on side bending toward the convex side. In contrast, *structural scoliosis* is characterized by a curve that fails to correct on side bending. Early loss of normal flexibility in the spine is the first sign of structural scoliosis. Within the broad categories of nonstructural, transient structural, and structural forms, scoliosis is further classified by etiology. This discussion deals with forms of structural scoliosis.

Idiopathic Scoliosis

About 80% of patients with scoliosis exhibit an idiopathic (genetic) form. It is currently believed that a dysfunction of the brainstem, possibly due to a lesion of the posterior columns or the inner ear, is the primary cause of idiopathic scoliosis. The disease, therefore, is not primarily a problem of bone and joint but a response to a

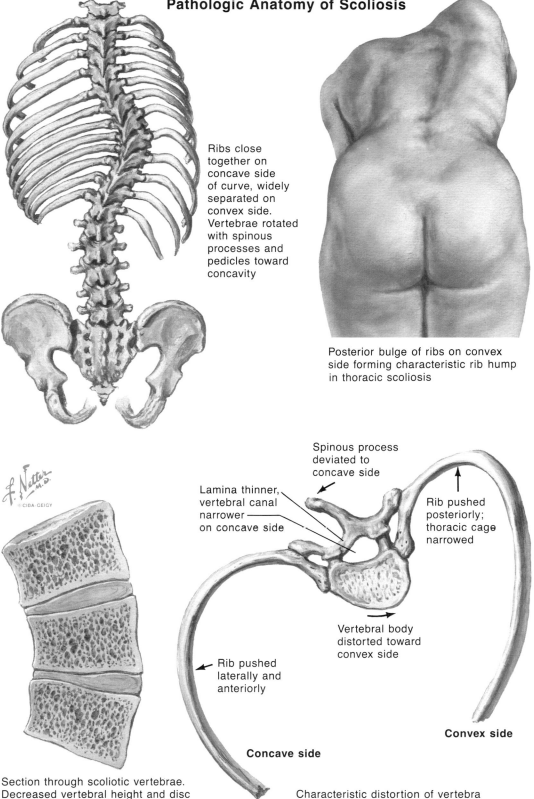

Pathologic Anatomy of Scoliosis

Ribs close together on concave side of curve, widely separated on convex side. Vertebrae rotated with spinous processes and pedicles toward concavity

Posterior bulge of ribs on convex side forming characteristic rib hump in thoracic scoliosis

Spinous process deviated to concave side

Lamina thinner, vertebral canal narrower on concave side

Rib pushed posteriorly; thoracic cage narrowed

Vertebral body distorted toward convex side

Rib pushed laterally and anteriorly

Convex side

Concave side

Section through scoliotic vertebrae. Decreased vertebral height and disc thickness on concave side

Characteristic distortion of vertebra and rib in thoracic scoliosis (inferior view)

disruption in neuromuscular balance. Significant scoliosis (ie, curves severe enough to require treatment) occurs seven times more often in girls than boys, while mild scoliosis affects boys and girls in equal numbers.

About 90% of all idiopathic curves are probably genetic, and thus the two terms are used synonymously. Genetic scoliosis appears to be a sex-linked trait, which can be transmitted by a mother to either a son or daughter but can only be transmitted from a carrier father to his daughter. The scoliotic trait may not pass on to every generation (incomplete penetrance) and may cause a severe curve in a parent and a mild curve in a child, or vice versa (variable expressivity). If

a person with idiopathic scoliosis has children, about one-third of all offspring will have scoliosis; if both parents have genes for scoliosis, even if one parent does not exhibit the disease, the odds that offspring will be afflicted are even greater.

Curve Patterns. Four distinct curve patterns are seen in idiopathic scoliosis (Plate 30).

The *right thoracic curve* is one of the most common patterns. The curve usually extends to and includes T4, T5, or T6 at its upper end and T11, T12, or L1 at its lower limit. Typically, these curves do not correct on side bending. Because of severe vertebral rotation, the ribs on the convex side become badly deformed, resulting in a severe

Scoliosis Curve Patterns

Scoliosis
(Continued)

cosmetic defect and serious impairment of cardio-pulmonary function when the curve exceeds 60°. Right thoracic curves can develop rapidly and therefore must be treated early.

The right thoracic curve is always a *major* curve (ie, the curve is structural and of great significance). There are usually smaller curves in the opposite direction above and below the right thoracic curve. These *secondary* curves are usually referred to as *minor* curves. A minor curve usually forms as a compensatory mechanism to help keep the head aligned over the pelvis.

The *thoracolumbar curve* is a fairly common idiopathic curve pattern. It is longer than the right thoracic curve and may be to either right or left. The upper end of the curve extends to and includes T4, T5, or T6 and the lower end includes L2, L3, or L4, usually with minor upper thoracic and lower lumbar curves. The thoracolumbar curve is usually less cosmetically deforming than the thoracic curve; however, it can cause severe rib and flank distortion due to vertebral rotation.

The *double major curve* consists of two structural curves of almost equal prominence. Double major curves can be any of the following combinations: right thoracic–left lumbar (most common); right thoracic–left thoracolumbar; left thoracolumbar–right lower lumbar; and right thoracic–left thoracic (double thoracic).

The *lumbar major curve* is quite common and usually runs from T11 or T12 to L5. In 65% of cases, the curve is to the left. The thoracic spine above the curve usually does not develop a structural compensatory curve and remains flexible. Lumbar major curves are not very deforming but can become quite rigid, leading to severe arthritic pain in later life and during pregnancy.

The extent of deformity varies with the underlying curve pattern, tending to be most severe with the right thoracic and thoracolumbar curves and less severe with balanced double major curves. Severe right thoracic and thoracolumbar curves often produce a marked overhang of the thorax toward the convexity of the curve and a rib hump, and the torso tilts to the convex side. In contrast, with a balanced double major curve, the shoulders are level over the pelvis, and the rib and lumbar prominences are not too severe. The major deformity with this type of curve is trunk shortening.

Age at Onset. Idiopathic scoliosis is classified into infantile, juvenile, and adolescent types according to peak periods of onset.

Infantile idiopathic scoliosis, which occurs between birth and 3 years of age, is usually noticed in the first year of life. Curiously, it is far more common in England, usually occurs in boys, and generally results in a left thoracic curve. The majority of these curves, thought to

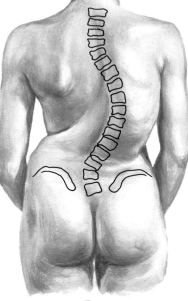

Right thoracic curve of 70°

Right thoraco-lumbar curve of 70°

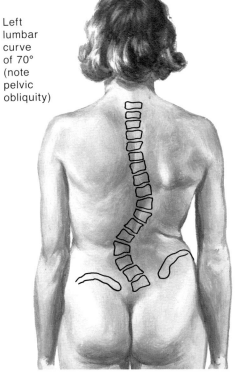

Left lumbar curve of 70° (note pelvic obliquity)

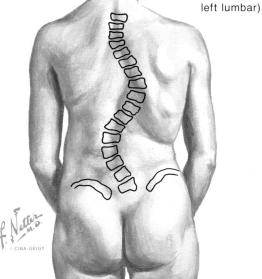

Double major curve of 70° (right thoracic, left lumbar)

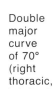

be a result of molding in the uterus, resolve spontaneously, even if untreated. Some, however, progress to severely rigid structural curves unless treated early and aggressively with bracing.

Juvenile idiopathic scoliosis occurs between the ages of 4 and 10 and is most often detected at or after age 6. Both sexes are affected equally. Most curves in this group are right thoracic curves. Unless early standing and side-bending radiographs are available, it is almost impossible to distinguish cases of late infantile onset from those of early juvenile onset.

Adolescent idiopathic scoliosis is diagnosed when the curve is noticed between 10 years of age and skeletal maturity. Many curves first noticed

at this age are probably present before age 10 but are not recognized until the adolescent growth spurt. Although adolescent scoliosis occurs in both boys and girls equally, 70% of cases that progress and need treatment occur in girls. The double major and right thoracic patterns predominate.

Progression. Idiopathic curves may or may not progress during growth. The risk of progression may be linked to various factors such as sex, age at onset, delayed maturation, and vertebral anatomy. Usually, the younger the child is when the structural curve develops, the less favorable the prognosis will be. In general, structural curves have a strong tendency to progress rapidly during

Scoliosis

(Continued)

the adolescent growth spurt, whereas small, non-structural curves may remain flexible for long periods, never becoming severe. Nevertheless, the worst advice a physician can give a patient with scoliosis is "as soon as you finish growing, your curve will stop." In a significant number of adults, scoliosis remains progressive, eventually causing pain and disability.

The curve is most likely to progress 1° to 2° a year during adult life if the curve is greater than 60° at maturity, the curve pattern throws the trunk out of balance, or the patient has extremely poor muscle tone. Generally, a curve that is less than 30° at age 25 is unlikely to progress.

Congenital Scoliosis

Congenital scoliosis is probably the result of some form of trauma to the zygote or embryo in the early embryonic period that causes a vertebral or extravertebral defect. Because many organ systems develop at the same time, children with congenital scoliosis almost always have some urinary tract or cardiac anomaly as well. Children with congenital scoliosis should also be examined for cervical spine anomalies such as Klippel-Feil syndrome (Plate 26) and scapular deformities such as Sprengel's deformity (Plate 40).

Congenital curves must be followed carefully. While most do not progress significantly, some become severe and irreversible. Posterior vertebral defects can be open or closed. The open (dysraphic) defect caused by myelomeningocele can be very severe and is usually associated with partial or complete neurologic deficit with paraplegia and urinary tract problems.

Closed vertebral defects are classified into four types (Plate 31): (1) partial unilateral failure of vertebral formation (wedge vertebra); (2) complete unilateral failure of vertebral formation (hemivertebra); (3) unilateral failure of segmentation (congenital bar); and (4) bilateral failure of segmentation (block vertebra). Other congenital combinations, some of which are extravertebral (eg, rib fusions), are so mixed and bizarre they defy classification.

In hemivertebral conditions, as the anomalous vertebrae grow, they cause the spine to lengthen on the convex side, leading to severe curves. Unilateral bars can also cause severe curvature. The worst possible congenital curve results from hemivertebrae on one side of the spine and several unilateral bars on the opposite side.

The best treatment for a progressive congenital curve is a short, in situ spinal fusion performed as soon as progression is noted.

Neuromuscular Scoliosis

Neuropathic forms of neuromuscular scoliosis are caused by a variety of disorders. Muscle imbalance due to poliomyelitis, a lower motor neuron

Congenital Scoliosis

Closed vertebral types
(MacEwen classification)

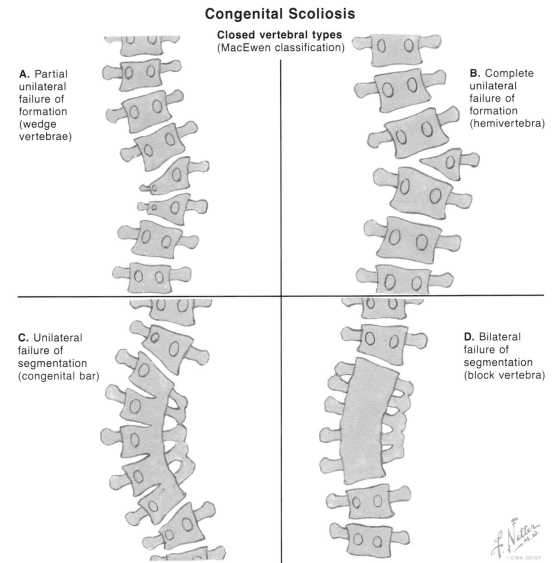

A. Partial unilateral failure of formation (wedge vertebrae)

B. Complete unilateral failure of formation (hemivertebra)

C. Unilateral failure of segmentation (congenital bar)

D. Bilateral failure of segmentation (block vertebra)

disease, and cerebral palsy, an upper motor neuron disease, may lead to severe, long C-shaped curves that may extend from the lower cervical region to the sacrum. Curves caused by syringomyelia also tend to become quite severe, often necessitating surgery. Since many patients with syringomyelia live well beyond their teenage years, treatment is definitely indicated when progression of the curve is noticed. Occasionally, neurosurgical drainage of the syrinx can help control the curve.

Myopathic forms of neuromuscular scoliosis are caused by both progressive and static disorders. The progressive disorders are exemplified by the muscular dystrophies. These disorders cause muscle imbalance, generally producing long C-shaped curves. Some children with scoliosis due to muscular dystrophy are so weak that their spines appear to collapse when they assume the erect posture. Judicious bracing or surgery may be helpful in some patients, but the prognosis is always guarded.

Other neuromuscular forms may be caused by mixed disorders, such as Friedreich's ataxia, in which a muscle imbalance causes muscle weakness plus overpull by the stronger trunk and paraspinal muscles.

Mesenchymal and Traumatic Disorders

Congenital mesenchymal disorders leading to scoliosis can occur with various types of dwarfism (Plates 1–16) and in Marfan's syndrome (see CIBA COLLECTION, Volume 8/I, page 232). Because

patients with Marfan's syndrome are usually very tall, their curves can become quite severe.

In osteogenesis imperfecta, the extreme brittleness of the bones results in hundreds of microfractures of the spine, eventually producing a scoliotic deformity. Scheuermann's disease, if not properly treated, may also lead to a progressive kyphotic deformity in adolescents (Plate 35).

Direct vertebral trauma such as a fracture with wedging or nerve root irritation can cause scoliosis. In some instances, the scoliosis may be secondary to irradiation for cancer treatment which, while saving the child's life, destroys the growth plates of the vertebral body, resulting in unequal growth and causing spinal deformity.

Clinical Evaluation

As part of the thorough physical examination, the development of secondary sexual characteristics should be noted. Their presence or absence, in addition to a height comparison with siblings and parents, can be significant in predicting future growth patterns. The skin is examined for café au lait markings indicative of neurofibromatosis, and the lumbar spine is searched for pigmented areas or patches of hair that can indicate an underlying congenital condition, such as spina bifida or diastematomyelia.

Following the general examination, a more specific examination of the deformity is done, beginning with evaluation of trunk alignment, which is used to gauge balance or displacement of the torso (Plate 32). A tape measure dropped

Scoliosis
(Continued)

as a plumb line from the occiput can show if the head and trunk are aligned. In patients with a very severe double major curve, however, alignment may remain perfect.

The shoulder girdle should be examined for symmetry, and scapular prominence should be noted. The neck-shoulder angle may be distorted by asymmetry of the trapezius muscle caused by cervical or high thoracic curves.

The type of curve is recorded and its flexibility evaluated on side bending and distraction. Lifting the patient gently by the head distracts the curve, allowing the degree of rigidity and flexibility of the spine to be assessed.

Deformities of the thoracic cage are carefully recorded. With the patient bending forward, a scoliometer is used to measure the rib hump (Plate 32). Anterior rib and breast asymmetry should also be noted.

Pelvic obliquity must be carefully assessed. It can be nonstructural, occurring as a result of a habit, or structural, resulting from a lower limb—length discrepancy. Structural pelvic obliquity can also be caused by contractures of muscle groups either above or below the iliac crests.

A brief but thorough neuromuscular examination including evaluation of all reflexes, response to stimuli, and motor capabilities is an important part of the scoliosis work-up. In children with congenital conditions, sensory or motor loss can indicate an internal spinal condition, such as diastematomyelia. Decreased vibratory sensation in the limbs is a consistent sign in idiopathic scoliosis, which is due to a brainstem dysfunction; a more extensive neurologic examination is usually not warranted. The findings of the neuromuscular examination should be carefully correlated with the physical examination of the back. Painful scoliosis is uncommon in children, and its presence suggests the possibility of osteoid osteoma, spinal cord tumors, spondylolysis or spondylolisthesis, or infection.

Radiographic Evaluation

A single erect anteroposterior radiograph from the occiput to the iliac crest is sufficient for the initial examination of a new scoliosis patient. A spot lateral view of the lumbosacral spine is indicated if spondylolisthesis or spondylolysis is suspected (Plate 37). The thyroid, breasts, and gonads should be shielded, and radiation exposure kept to a minimum.

Side-bending radiographs are taken to distinguish structural from nonstructural curves. Right side bending allows a right thoracic curve to uncoil, and the radiograph provides evidence of the suppleness of the ligaments and other soft-tissue structures. Left side bending uncoils a left lumbar curve.

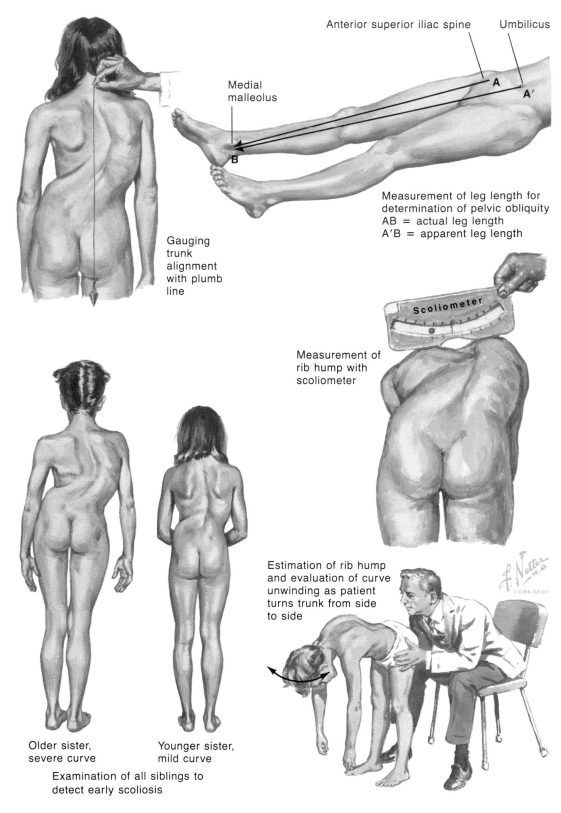

Gauging trunk alignment with plumb line

Measurement of leg length for determination of pelvic obliquity
AB = actual leg length
A'B = apparent leg length

Measurement of rib hump with scoliometer

Estimation of rib hump and evaluation of curve unwinding as patient turns trunk from side to side

Older sister, severe curve

Younger sister, mild curve

Examination of all siblings to detect early scoliosis

The curve is measured on the initial radiograph using the Cobb method, which is preferred by the Scoliosis Research Society (Plate 33). The accuracy of the Cobb method relies on determining the upper and lower end-vertebrae of the curve. The end-vertebrae at both the upper and lower limits are those that tilt most severely *toward* the concavity of the curve. In other words, the superior end-vertebra is the last vertebra whose superior border inclines toward the concavity of the curve to be measured. The inferior end-vertebra is the last one whose inferior border inclines toward the concavity of the curve. Horizontal lines are drawn at the superior border of the superior end-vertebra and the inferior border

of the inferior end-vertebra. Perpendicular lines are then drawn from each of the horizontal lines and the intersecting angles measured. (The broken arrows on the illustration do not converge toward the concavity being measured, indicating that these vertebrae are not end-vertebrae but are in another curve above or below the curve being measured.)

Vertebral rotation is measured most accurately by estimating the amount that the pedicles of the vertebrae have rotated, as seen in the anteroposterior radiograph.

Skeletal maturation must also be determined accurately because scoliosis progression may slow (although it does not always stop) when a patient

Determination of Skeletal Maturation

Measurement of Curvature (Cobb method)

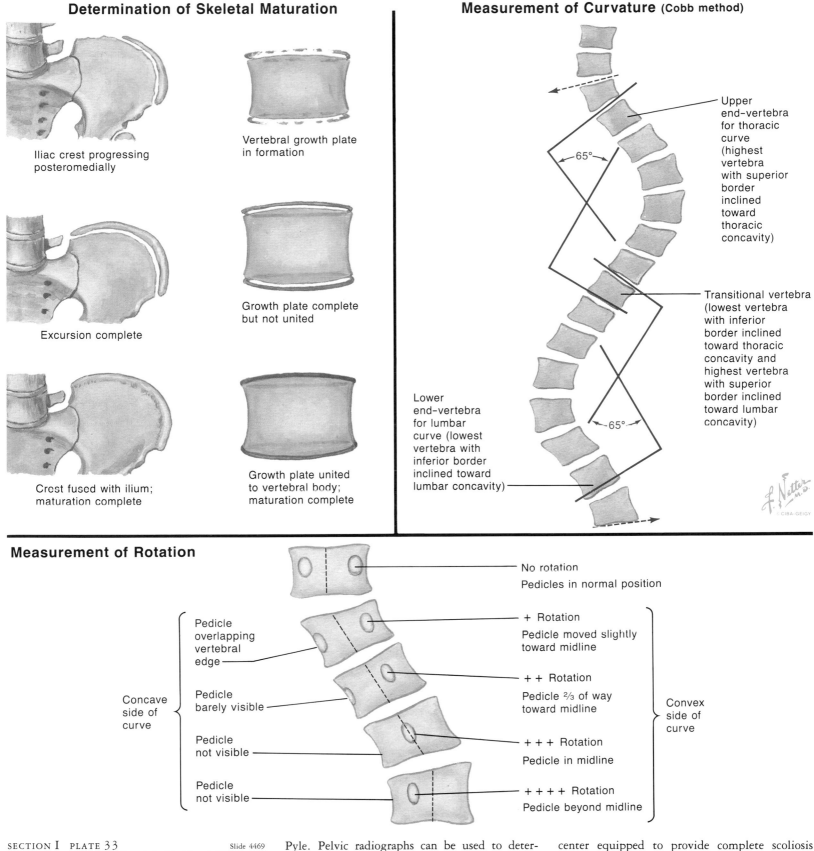

Iliac crest progressing posteromedially

Vertebral growth plate in formation

Excursion complete

Growth plate complete but not united

Crest fused with ilium; maturation complete

Growth plate united to vertebral body; maturation complete

Upper end-vertebra for thoracic curve (highest vertebra with superior border inclined toward thoracic concavity)

65°

Transitional vertebra (lowest vertebra with inferior border inclined toward thoracic concavity and highest vertebra with superior border inclined toward lumbar concavity)

Lower end-vertebra for lumbar curve (lowest vertebra with inferior border inclined toward lumbar concavity)

65°

Measurement of Rotation

No rotation
Pedicles in normal position

Pedicle overlapping vertebral edge

+ Rotation
Pedicle moved slightly toward midline

Concave side of curve

Pedicle barely visible

+ + Rotation
Pedicle 2/3 of way toward midline

Convex side of curve

Pedicle not visible

+ + + Rotation
Pedicle in midline

Pedicle not visible

+ + + + Rotation
Pedicle beyond midline

SECTION I PLATE 33   Slide 4469

Scoliosis
(Continued)

is fully mature. Girls generally cease growing and mature at about 16½ years of age; boys, 15 to 18 months later.

Several methods are used to estimate skeletal age. Radiographs of the left hand and wrist are compared with the *Radiographic Atlas of Skeletal Development of the Hand and Wrist* by Greulich and

Pyle. Pelvic radiographs can be used to determine the degree of iliac crest excursion. When the iliac crest meets the sacroiliac joint and firmly seals to the ilium, maturation is nearly complete. Another technique involves examining the superior and inferior growth plates of the thoracic and lumbar vertebrae on high-quality radiographs. If the growth plates are mottled in appearance, the skeletal growth is not complete. Solid union of the growth plates with the vertebral bodies indicates that maturation is complete.

Treatment

School Screening. The best treatment for scoliosis is early detection and prompt referral to a

center equipped to provide complete scoliosis care. Most curves can be treated without surgery if detected before they become too severe. Scoliosis screening is now being done in schools across the United States and in other countries. A physician or school nurse can screen a hundred children in less than an hour. The screening procedure is simple: the child bends from the waist with the arms hanging freely (Plate 32). This position accentuates even a slight asymmetry in the ribs or lumbar area. School screening should begin in the fifth grade, and boys as well as girls should be examined every 6 to 9 months. If scoliosis or kyphosis is detected in a child, all siblings should be screened.

Scoliosis

(Continued)

Exercises. Exercises are mentioned under treatment only to be strongly condemned as a *sole* cure for scoliosis. Unfortunately, physicians under the mistaken impression that exercises help to improve or eliminate a curve continue to prescribe an exercise program to many patients, who are then lost to follow-up until their curve becomes more severe. Basically, only two treatments effectively correct scoliosis: spinal bracing and surgery.

Braces. With close supervision, a properly constructed, well-fitted brace, such as the Milwaukee brace (Plate 34), can successfully halt progression of a curve in perhaps 70% of patients, if the patient and family are cooperative. Some curves, however, progress to greater deformity no matter what is done. Unfortunately, there is as yet no way to predict if a curve will respond successfully to bracing.

In recent years, several low-profile braces have been designed that do not require a neck ring. They are primarily used in treating lower curves in thoracolumbar and lumbar regions. Patient acceptance is much greater with these braces because they are barely visible under clothing. The inner pad is adjustable to add further pressure on the apex of the curve as the curve improves. The braces can be modified depending on the curve pattern and the presence or absence of kyphosis.

Most braces are generally worn over a long undershirt for 23 hours a day, but some mild curves can be managed with a part-time program. Children can run and play in them relatively freely. Exercises are done daily both in and out of the brace to maintain muscle strength.

Patients using braces are seen every 3 months for brace adjustment. At 6-month intervals, new radiographs are taken with the patient erect and not wearing the brace. When radiographs show that skeletal maturation is nearly complete, the patient is weaned gradually from the brace, eventually wearing it only at night until the spine is absolutely mature.

Electric Stimulation. In recent years, electric stimulation of muscle has gained popularity in the treatment of scoliosis. While it is an enticing alternative to bracing, long-term follow-up of large groups of children has not yet proven its efficacy.

Surgery. The main indications for scoliosis surgery are (1) relentless curve progression, (2) significant curve progression in spite of bracing, (3) inability to wean the patient from a brace, (4) significant thoracic and lumbar pain, (5) progressive thoracic lordosis, (6) progressive loss of

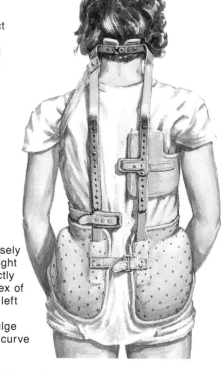

Milwaukee Brace
(fitted to a right thoracic–left lumbar curve)

Throat mold does not distract mandible; left axillary sling counteracts pressure of right thoracic "L" pad and centers neck ring on patient

Occipital pad fits closely to base of occiput; right "L" pad applied directly to ribs leading to apex of right thoracic curve; left lumbar pad applied directly to muscle bulge over apex of lumbar curve

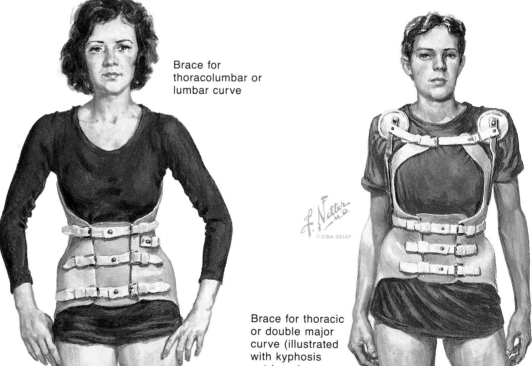

New York Orthopaedic Hospital Low-Profile Brace
(designed by Isidore Zamosky, Inc)

Brace for thoracolumbar or lumbar curve

Brace for thoracic or double major curve (illustrated with kyphosis outrigger)

pulmonary function, (7) emotional or psychiatric problems with bracing, and (8) severe cosmetic changes in the shoulders and trunk. Since the first spinal fusion was performed in 1911, many different surgical techniques and types of instrumentation have been developed, each with its own advantages and risks, including neurologic impairment. Regardless of the method and hardware, the goal of surgery is to produce a solid arthrodesis of a balanced spine in the frontal and sagittal planes over a level pelvis.

Posterior fusion techniques using Harrington rod instrumentation are still most widely used for idiopathic scoliosis. In some patients, a compression rod is added and the rods are attached to the

vertebrae with wires passed through holes drilled in the spinous processes.

In the Luque technique, the spine is straightened with two rods attached with wires. The Cotrel-Dubousset method, employing two rods coupled together with transverse traction rods and hooks, effectively derotates the spine. Anterior fusion techniques, reported by Dwyer, Zeilke, and others, are usually reserved for patients with rigid thoracolumbar or lumbar curves or with posterior spinal defects. Postoperative bracing is not always needed with these new techniques. The technique and approach used should be based primarily on the surgeon's preference and expertise. □

Scheuermann's Disease

Although an exaggerated thoracic kyphosis has been documented for centuries, it was only with the advent of medical radiography that Scheuermann identified the disease. This progressive disorder occurs in patients near puberty, manifested by an increase in the normal kyphosis in the thoracic spine with an abnormal degree of wedging of the vertebrae at the apex of the kyphotic curve. The diagnosis of Scheuermann's disease is limited to patients with a curve greater than 40° (Cobb method, Plate 33) in which at least three adjacent vertebrae are wedged 5° or more. Although irregularity of the vertebral epiphyseal plates, Schmorl's nodules, and narrowing of disc spaces are common radiographic findings, they are not in themselves diagnostic.

The etiology of Scheuermann's disease is not yet understood, but there appears to be a genetic factor. Scheuermann speculated that the disease was caused by avascular necrosis of the anterior portion of the cartilage ring apophysis of the vertebral body, similar to the pathogenesis of Legg-Calvé-Perthes disease. Mechanical factors (particularly heavy labor), contractures of the hamstring and pectoral muscles, and herniation of the intervertebral disc through the anterior portion of the epiphyseal plate have also been suggested as contributing factors. Specimens obtained from patients undergoing anterior spinal fusion for Scheuermann's kyphosis have revealed wedge-shaped vertebral bodies and a contracted, thickened anterior longitudinal ligament that acts as a tether across the kyphosis, maintaining a relatively inflexible deformity. Subsequent histologic studies, while confirming a disruption of the epiphyseal plates and extravasation of disc material into the bony spongiosa of the vertebral body, have revealed no evidence of avascular necrosis or inflammatory changes in bone, disc, or cartilage.

Clinical Manifestations. Characteristic signs of Scheuermann's disease are the exaggerated, rounded appearance of the back, round shoulders, and poor posture; pain and deformity are uncommon. In adolescents, so-called poor posture may be an important clue to significant structural alterations of the vertebral column that can only be identified with radiography. Despite urging by their parents, children with a true structural problem like Scheuermann's disease cannot stand straight. As a result of the exaggerated thoracic kyphosis and lumbar lordosis, affected children typically stand slumped, with the arms folded across a prominent abdomen. The kyphosis is relatively inflexible, is not fully corrected when the patient attempts thoracic hyperextension in the prone position, and is accentuated by forward bending. Mild scoliosis is an associated finding in 20% to 30% of patients, and contracture of the hamstring and pectoral muscles, which leads to forward protrusion of the shoulder girdle, is

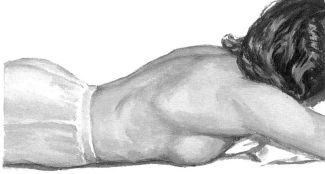

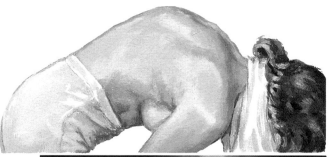

Unlike postural defect, kyphosis of Scheuermann's disease persists when patient is prone and thoracic spine extended or hyperextended (above) and accentuated when patient bends forward (below)

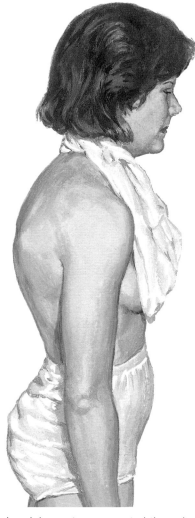

In adolescent, exaggerated thoracic kyphosis and compensatory lumbar lordosis due to Scheuermann's disease may be mistaken for postural defect

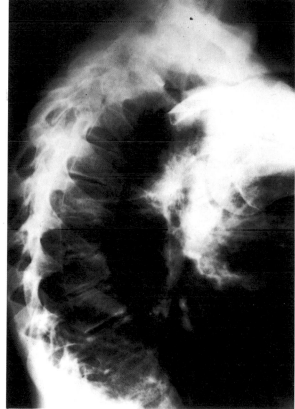

Radiograph shows wedging of several lower thoracic vertebrae, resulting in marked kyphosis. Epiphyseal plates of affected vertebrae are irregular and discontinuous due to herniation of intervertebral disc into bony spongiosa (Schmorl's nodules); disc spaces narrowed

common. Neurologic examination, usually normal, may reveal a more serious condition such as kyphosis secondary to congenital vertebral deformity or trauma.

Scheuermann's disease is often misdiagnosed as postural round-back deformity, which also occurs in preadolescent children. However, this type of kyphosis is supple (ie, it is corrected with prone hyperextension) and is not accompanied by muscle contractures, wedging of the vertebral bodies, or irregularities of the epiphyseal plates. Differential diagnosis includes infectious spondylitis, hypoparathyroidism and hyperparathyroidism, rickets, osteogenesis imperfecta, idiopathic juvenile osteoporosis, neurofibromatosis, tumors,

Morquio's and Hurler's syndromes, and traumatic injuries.

Treatment. In growing children, treatment is instituted to arrest progression of the deformity, improve the cosmetic appearance of the back, and alleviate any pain. The deformity can be corrected as long as there is potential for further vertebral growth. The spine is held in a corrected position with a cast or a Milwaukee brace. The kyphosis will usually correct to a normal curvature in the first year as evidenced by reconstruction of the wedged vertebral bodies and anterior portion of the vertebral apophysis. Untreated, the deformity may progress to a large degree and require surgical correction. ☐

Congenital Kyphosis

Congenital kyphosis is due to the same embryologic failure of segmentation or formation of the vertebrae as congenital scoliosis. The direction of the curve (lateral or posterior) depends on the location of the spinal defect. Anterior defects cause kyphosis and lateral defects cause scoliosis. A combined deformity, kyphoscoliosis, is common. In about 15% of patients, congenital deformities are associated with an anomaly of the neural elements (eg, diastematomyelia, neurenteric cyst).

A kyphotic deformity that is secondary to failure of segmentation (congenital bar or block vertebrae) rarely causes neurologic deficits. However, a progressive kyphosis due to failure of formation may lead to paraplegia. In partial failure of formation (wedge vertebrae or hemivertebrae), neurologic deficits can occur whether the vertebral canal is in good alignment or dislocated.

Symmetric failure of formation (absent vertebrae), a rare defect, causes a pure angular kyphosis with a high risk (25%) of paraparesis. Asymmetric failure of formation commonly leads to formation of hemivertebrae and resultant kyphoscoliosis, most often in the thoracic or thoracolumbar spine. While the alignment of the canal is usually maintained by the strong, intact posterior elements, the kyphoscoliosis may be relentlessly progressive, often increasing 10° per year. The risk of paraplegia is greatest when the apex of the curve is in the upper thoracic spine where there is less room for the spinal cord and the blood supply to the cord is most tenuous.

Partial failure of formation with vertebral canal dislocation (congenital dislocated spine) is characterized by a lack of continuity of the posterior elements of the vertebral canal, leading to instability and the risk of catastrophic neurologic loss from even minor trauma. Even if the injury does not occur, the curve progresses inexorably, producing a gradual loss of neurologic function. In some patients, the neurologic deficit is present at birth, the result of spinal cord compression rather than congenital malformations of the spinal cord.

Neurologic complications are common when the kyphosis or kyphoscoliosis is complicated by rotatory dislocation of the spine, because the spinal cord is twisted over a very short segment. The hump, or kyphos, is abrupt and angular and the cord is fixed at the apex by the roots above and below, which are twisted in opposite directions.

Although functional impairment may be noted at birth or in early childhood, it occurs most commonly at the time of the adolescent growth spurt. Once present, the neurologic deficit gradually worsens. A sudden decline in neurologic function may result from minor trauma. Occurrence or worsening of spasticity in a child with kyphosis is an early sign of myelopathy and

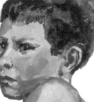

Young child with myelodysplasia and congenital kyphosis (lateral radiograph at right)

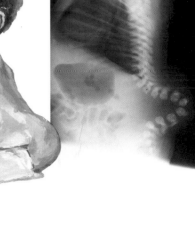

Myelogram of older boy shows congenital kyphosis with closed vertebral canal

Congenital kyphoscoliosis

should prompt an evaluation leading to spinal fusion with anterior decompression of the spinal cord, if necessary. Magnetic resonance imaging has largely replaced computed tomographic myelography as the procedure of choice in the diagnosis of intraspinal defects. In infants and young children whose posterior elements are still cartilaginous, ultrasonography done by an experienced examiner is an excellent screening modality.

Treatment. Bracing and other nonoperative techniques have very limited application in the management of congenital kyphosis. Before significant kyphosis develops, spinal fusion may often be accomplished by the posterior approach alone. In the patient with a neurologic deficit

secondary to either a congenital or a secondary kyphosis and a fixed deformity, anterior decompression of the vertebral canal is essential. If the curve is flexible, gradual traction may improve neurologic function, but traction over a rigid kyphos is contraindicated.

About 10% of children with myelodysplasia have a variant of congenital kyphosis in the lumbar spine. The curves are frequently very large at birth and often lead to chronic ulceration of the gibbus. Kyphectomy at the time of sac closure may be necessary to achieve primary skin closure. In older children, kyphectomy with shortening of the lumbar spine and stabilization with instrumentation are often required. □

Spondylolysis and Spondylolisthesis

Spondylolysis may represent a stress fracture of the pars interarticularis of the fifth lumbar vertebra. When the fracture allows L5 to slip forward on S1, it is called isthmic spondylolisthesis. Dysplastic, or congenital, spondylolisthesis, in contrast, is due to anomalous development of the posterior structures of the lumbosacral junction.

In children, spondylolysis rarely occurs before 5 years of age and is more common at age 7 or 8. Although a history of minor trauma is common, the injury is seldom severe. The onset of symptoms coincides closely with the adolescent growth spurt.

Lumbar lordosis is exacerbated by the normal hip flexion contractures of childhood. This posture focuses the force of weight bearing on the pars interarticularis, gradually leading to disruption. Shear stresses are greater on the pars interarticularis when the spine is extended and are further accentuated by lateral flexion of the extended spine.

Clinical Manifestations. Symptoms are relatively uncommon in children. Pain, when it occurs, is localized to the low back and, to a lesser extent, to the posterior buttocks and thighs. Symptoms are usually initiated and aggravated by repetitive and strenuous activity—particularly the flexion-extension of the spine common in rowing, gymnastics, and diving—and are decreased by rest or limitation of activity.

Palpation may elicit some tenderness in the low back, and there may be some splinting or guarding with restriction of side-to-side motion, particularly in acute conditions. Hamstring tightness and marked restriction of forward hip flexion are seen in 80% of symptomatic patients. Distortion of the pelvis and trunk may be clinically apparent in the late stages of spondylolisthesis.

Children, unlike adults, seldom have objective signs of nerve root compression such as motor weakness, reflex change, or sensory deficit and rarely have an associated disc protrusion. The examination must include a careful search for sacral anesthesia and bladder dysfunction.

Radiographic Findings. Large defects in the pars interarticularis (spondylolysis) are visible on nearly all radiographic views of the lumbar spine. However, if the spondylolysis is unilateral or not accompanied by spondylolisthesis, special techniques and oblique views of the lumbar spine may be needed.

In an acute injury, the gap in the pars interarticularis is narrow with irregular edges, whereas in the long-standing lesion, the edges are smooth and rounded. Bone scans may be needed to detect an early prespondylolytic stage (before fracture) in children. In dysplastic spondylolisthesis, the posterior facets appear to sublux and the pars interarticularis may become attenuated—like pulled taffy (the "greyhound" of Hensinger).

In unilateral spondylolysis, the radiographic appearance of reactive sclerosis and hypertrophy of the contralateral pedicle and lamina may be confused with osteoid osteoma. This is an important concern since excision of a sclerotic pedicle

associated with a contralateral spondylolysis may increase instability, leading to spondylolisthesis. Bone scans are not helpful in differentiating the two conditions.

Treatment. Spondylolysis usually responds well to conservative measures, restriction of some activities, and exercises for the back and abdominal muscles. Asymptomatic spondylolisthesis is more problematic, as the risk of further slippage is difficult to determine. Symptomatic spondylolisthesis may require stabilization of the spine, either with a brace, cast, or surgery. □

Spondylolysis and Spondylolisthesis

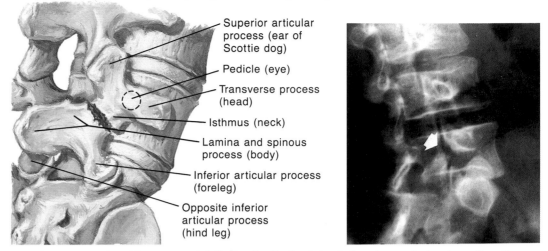

- Superior articular process (ear of Scottie dog)
- Pedicle (eye)
- Transverse process (head)
- Isthmus (neck)
- Lamina and spinous process (body)
- Inferior articular process (foreleg)
- Opposite inferior articular process (hind leg)

Spondylolysis without spondylolisthesis. Posterolateral view demonstrates formation of radiographic Scottie dog. On lateral radiograph, dog appears to be wearing a collar

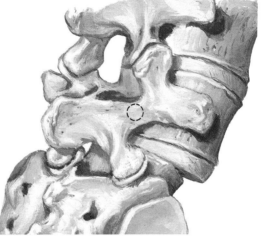

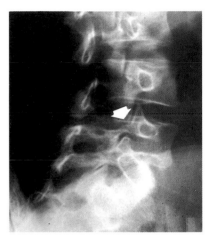

Dysplastic (congenital) spondylolisthesis. Luxation of L5 on sacrum. Dog's neck (isthmus) appears elongated

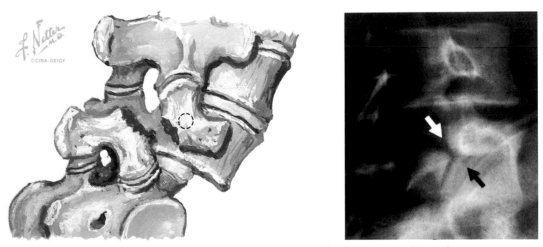

Isthmic type spondylolisthesis. Anterior luxation of L5 on sacrum due to fracture of isthmus. Note that gap is wider and dog appears decapitated

Effects of spondylolisthesis on sacral nerve roots

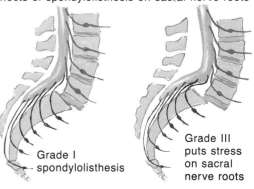

Grade I spondylolisthesis

Grade III puts stress on sacral nerve roots

Myelodysplasia

The number of babies with myelodysplasia who survive infancy has increased dramatically, and as clinical experience with these patients has increased, new principles and techniques of treatment have emerged. (A discussion of myelodysplasia appears in CIBA COLLECTION, Volume 1/II, Section I.)

Management of the patient with myelodysplasia requires a team approach. The team coordinator should visit the patient and family in the first days after birth and discuss the long-term implications of the patient's condition. The urologist, orthopedist, and neurosurgeon should conduct the initial evaluation, and physical therapy to improve and maintain joint motion should be started as soon as possible.

The clinical findings dictate the specific orthopedic procedures employed. The neurologic level of both motor and sensory function should be estimated. However, in newborns, it is often impossible to determine the exact level, and the findings vary depending on the examiner and the child's age. Because there is considerable variation from one side of the body to the other, each limb should be evaluated separately. The effects of muscle imbalance and presence of soft-tissue contractures must be considered in the neurologic examination. Evaluation of the newborn should focus on determining which joints the child can control, and muscle strength can be assessed more accurately later.

The lesion generally follows anatomic lines; thus, even in children with only mild involvement of the foot, there may be significant weakness of the hip and the abductor muscles and increased tendency to late hip dislocation.

Deformities of Hip. In an otherwise normal child, if the hips are dislocated but can be easily reduced, treatment is the same as that for congenital dislocation of the hip (Plates 54–55). If the hip has been dislocated early in fetal life (teratologic dislocation) and there are advanced adaptive changes of bone and soft tissue, reduction is not indicated. The primary goal is to produce a freely movable hip joint.

Contracted and/or spastic adductor muscles in conjunction with weak power of abductor muscles frequently lead to hip dislocation. If this imbalance is discovered early, intervention with physical therapy, bracing, or splinting can help prevent dislocation.

Many patients have contracture of the iliotibial band, which maintains the hip flexed, abducted, and externally rotated. Early and intensive physical therapy should be instituted to avoid a fixed deformity.

Deformities of Knee. The newborn with extension or flexion contractures should be treated with stretching exercises. A major goal of treatment is the ability to extend the knee and take advantage of the normal locking mechanism.

Deformities of Foot and Ankle. Both conservative and surgical management may be necessary

Infant with spina bifida and bilateral clubfoot

Although spinal defect has been corrected surgically, severe, progressive scoliosis has developed

Skin ulceration secondary to sensory loss

Malfunction of sphincter predisposing to urinary tract infection is common and serious complication

to correct the position of deformed feet, increase suppleness, and allow proper shoe fit.

Cavovarus and equinovarus (clubfoot) should be corrected before the child learns to stand—before extensive adaptive and remodeling changes in both bone and soft tissue occur, making surgical intervention necessary. In the newborn period, calcaneovalgus with overpull of the anterior and paralysis of the posterior muscles (S1 distribution) often responds well to exercises, braces, or splints. Deformities such as vertical talus and stiff, rigid feet are less common.

Deformities of Spine. Although common in patients with myelodysplasia, spinal deformities are not usually a problem in the newborn period.

However, congenital anomalies of the vertebrae occur in about 30% of affected children. In addition, 50% of patients eventually develop a curve in the otherwise normal-appearing vertebral bodies (developmental scoliosis).

Congenital kyphosis is unique to myelodysplasia and is of such magnitude that it can be recognized at birth. The kyphosis usually involves the entire lumbar spine from the thoracolumbar junction down, including the sacrum, with its apex at L2 or L3; there is usually complete paralysis below the level of the lesion. In the newborn, the size of the cutaneous defect and the rigidity and magnitude of the curve may make skin closure extremely difficult. □

Lumbosacral Agenesis

Lumbosacral agenesis is a condition in which the sacrum and some of the lumbar vertebrae, or both, fail to develop. Although the etiology is not certain, it has been noted that 14% to 18% of patients have mothers with diabetes or a strong family history of diabetes.

Clinical Manifestations. The patient's appearance varies with the level of the vertebral lesion. Although partial sacral agenesis may not be noticeable, lumbar or complete sacral agenesis is a severe deformity.

The posture of the lower limbs has been likened to that of the "sitting Buddha" and is characterized by flexion-abduction contractures of the hips and severe knee flexion, with popliteal webbing; the feet are in equinovarus and tucked under the buttocks. Inspection of the back reveals a bony prominence, which is the last vertebral segment, and often gross motion between this and the pelvis. Flexion-extension may occur at the junction of the spine and pelvis rather than at the hips. When the patient sits unsupported, the pelvis rolls up under the thorax. Scoliosis, hemivertebrae, spina bifida, and meningocele are common associated spinal anomalies.

With low-level lesions, deformities of the foot and lower limb resemble those of resistant clubfoot (Plate 88) or arthrogryposis (Plate 20). Children may be misdiagnosed for several years or until problems with toilet training call attention to the sacral anomalies. Although the clinical signs resemble those of arthrogryposis, patients with arthrogryposis have full sensation in the lower limbs, bowel and bladder control, and normal vertebral architecture.

The neurologic deficit is one of the most unusual features of this condition. Motor paralysis is profound, with no voluntary or reflex activity, and it corresponds anatomically within one level to what might be expected from the vertebral loss. Even patients with the most severe involvement have sensation to the knees and spotty hypesthesia distally. Trophic ulceration of the feet is quite uncommon, suggesting at least protective sensation.

Bladder dysfunction is a consistent finding in all patients, even those with a relatively minor hemisacral defect, but the patterns of urinary function vary. Patients exhibit individual mixtures of upper and/or lower motor neuron disorders; perineal electromyography is necessary to obtain the correct diagnosis. Severe constipation with absence of the normal sensation of rectal distention is a common bowel abnormality.

The visceral anomalies are usually confined to the anogenital region (imperforate anus is the most common) and urinary tract (eg, bladder dysfunction, hydronephrosis, vesical reflux and diverticulum, fused or absent kidney, exstrophy of the bladder, and hypospadias).

Radiographic Findings. A lesion at the level of the lumbar spine results in the complete absence of all vertebral development below it,

Lumbosacral Agenesis

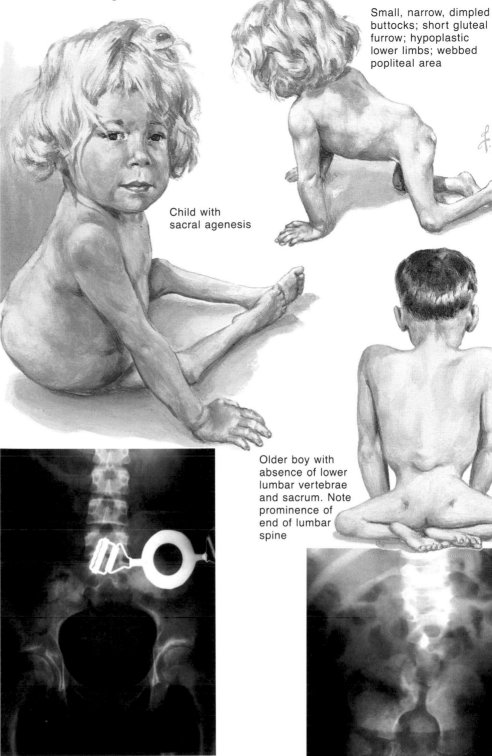

Small, narrow, dimpled buttocks; short gluteal furrow; hypoplastic lower limbs; webbed popliteal area

Child with sacral agenesis

Older boy with absence of lower lumbar vertebrae and sacrum. Note prominence of end of lumbar spine

Anteroposterior radiograph shows total absence of sacrum. Urinary drainage bag visible

Lumbosacral agenesis

including the sacrum and coccyx. However, lesions of the sacrum are less consistent, and in about one-third of patients, the defect occurs on one side only. In lumbar or complete sacral agenesis, there is usually no bony connection of the spine to the pelvis. The spinopelvic articulation should be examined with flexion-extension radiographs because its stability has important implications in treatment and rehabilitation.

Treatment. Treatment measures vary with the level of involvement, and the management plan, based on the following broad concepts, must be highly individualized.

If the sacropelvic ring is intact, the spinopelvic junction is usually stable, and the patient can walk with minimal or no brace support. Patients with significant deformities of only the feet and legs require vigorous correction, begun at birth, including serial plaster casts in conjunction with stretching, and exercises to position the feet plantigrade and the knees in extension. Surgical release may be necessary if conservative measures are inadequate.

Because of the high incidence of associated defects that may lead to serious renal impairment, recognition and treatment of urinary abnormalities are an important part of management. Delay in diagnosis and treatment may lead to upper tract deterioration and severely limit therapeutic options. □

Congenital Elevation of Scapula, Absence of Clavicle, and Pseudarthrosis of Clavicle

Congenital Elevation of Scapula (Sprengel's Deformity)

In patients with this condition, the scapula is elevated and hypoplastic, and the affected side of the neck is fuller and shorter than the uninvolved side, with a decrease in the cervicoscapular line and the appearance of torticollis. The involved shoulder is typically smaller and the distance from the acromion to the spine is shorter than on the normal side. A decrease in scapulocostal motion limits shoulder abduction, but motion of the scapulohumeral joint is usually normal. There is no right or left preponderance, and in one-third of patients, the deformity is bilateral.

Congenital scoliosis is a common associated finding, and renal anomalies occur in one-third of patients. In some patients, an osseous and cartilaginous structure called an omovertebral bone originates in the upper part of the scapula and attaches to the spinous process of a cervical vertebra. This abnormal bar, occasionally in combination with contracture of the levator scapulae muscles, may further limit scapular motion.

If the deformity is severe enough to warrant surgical intervention, surgery provides considerable cosmetic benefit in appropriately selected patients. It restores a more natural contour to the shoulders and neck and also produces an apparent increase in neck length. The affected shoulder, however, remains smaller. Removal of an omovertebral bone may increase neck and shoulder motion. Surgery is usually recommended in patients between 3 and 5 years of age. In the older child, there is an increased risk of injury to the brachial plexus from stretching or compression by the clavicle.

Congenital Absence of Clavicle (Cleidocranial Dysostosis)

This hereditary condition results in incomplete formation of the clavicles, skull, and pubis and, in some patients, involves other skeletal structures as well. The entire clavicle may be absent or simply a small segment of the middle or outer portion may be missing. The defect is bilateral in 82% of patients. Delayed closure of the cranial sutures and fontanelles and incomplete development of the pubis are frequent major manifestations. The defect in the pubis may be quite alarming and has been mistaken for erosion by a tumor.

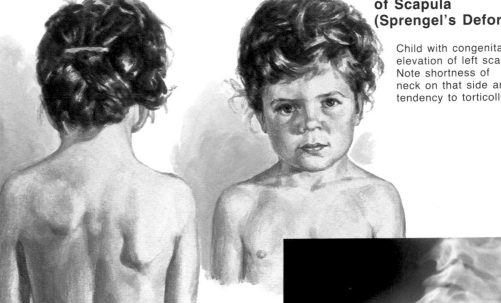

Congenital Elevation of Scapula (Sprengel's Deformity)

Child with congenital elevation of left scapula. Note shortness of neck on that side and tendency to torticollis

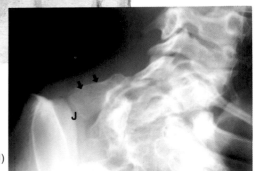

Radiograph shows omovertebral bone (arrows) connecting scapula to spinous processes of cervical vertebrae via osteochondral joint (J)

Congenital Absence of Clavicle (Cleidocranial Dysostosis)

Excessive mobility of shoulders permits patient to bring them forward almost to midline. Radiograph shows total absence of clavicles; vestige present in some patients

Congenital Pseudarthrosis of Clavicle

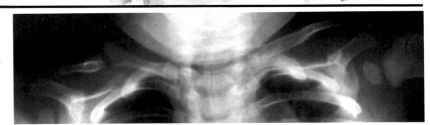

Scoliosis and anomalies of the mandible, teeth, and small bones of the hands and feet occur in severely affected patients. The typical patient has a large head, small face, long neck, drooping shoulders, narrow chest, and short stature. In most patients, the condition is not disabling.

Congenital Pseudarthrosis of Clavicle

A rare condition, congenital pseudarthrosis usually occurs in the middle third of the clavicle. The nonunion is present at birth and does not heal spontaneously. Recent studies indicate that the condition occurs most often on the right side, and the lesion may thus be due to pressure on the developing clavicle by the subclavian artery, which is normally at a higher level on the right side. The deformity may become larger and more obvious as the child grows, with a false joint developing between the enlarged ends of the clavicular fragments. The affected shoulder tends to droop forward and lower nearer the midline than the normal shoulder. The condition may be confused with a simple fracture, cleidocranial dysostosis, or neurofibromatosis (Plates 17–19). The enlarged ends of the clavicular fragments are palpable, and there is a variable degree of painless motion between them. Functional problems are rare, and surgery is recommended only for patients who have pain, an unsightly lump, or shoulder weakness. □

Kienböck's Disease

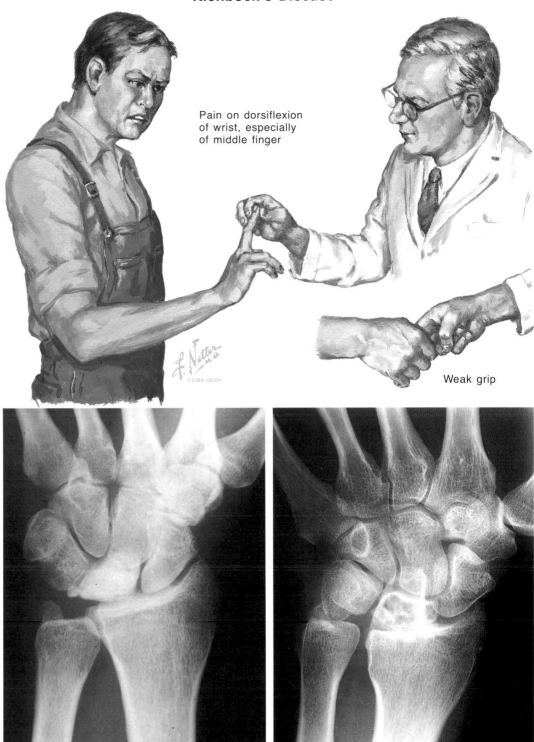

Pain on dorsiflexion of wrist, especially of middle finger

Weak grip

Radiograph of wrist shows characteristic sclerosis of lunate

In more advanced stage, resorptive changes seen as cystic radiolucency and loss of height of lunate

In Kienböck's disease, also known as lunatomalacia, the collapse of the carpal lunate occurs because of avascular necrosis. The disease occurs most often in young adults between 15 and 40 years of age and is usually unilateral. The actual cause of the vascular impairment has not been determined, although several etiologic factors have been proposed: (1) single or repetitive microfractures that result in vascular embarrassment; (2) traumatic disruption of circulation or ligamentous injury with subsequent degeneration; (3) primary circulatory disease; and (4) shortening of the ulna relative to the radius, which decreases the support for the lunate. The current theory is that the disease occurs in persons with a mechanical and/or vascular predisposition, when repetitive compression of the lunate between the capitate and distal radius disrupts the intraosseous structures. Chronic compression of the lunate (which is unavoidable in normal wrist function), effusion, and synovitis may interfere with healing and provide a mechanism for progressive collapse of the bone.

Clinical Manifestations. The primary signs and symptoms of Kienböck's disease are wrist pain that radiates up the forearm and stiffness, tenderness, and swelling over the lunate. Passive dorsiflexion of the middle finger produces the characteristic pain. Physical examination reveals limitation of wrist motion, usually dorsiflexion, and a striking weakness of grip. The pain and weakness increase as the lunate collapses and degenerative changes develop, making the disability both severe and chronic.

Radiographic Findings. The avascular necrosis of the lunate may vary in degree but produces consistent and typical radiographic changes. Initial radiographic findings may be normal except for a short ulna, but sclerosis of the lunate—the radiographic hallmark of the disease—develops with time. The lunate progressively loses height and eventually fragments. Further lunate collapse leads to carpal instability and resultant degenerative joint changes, including the formation of cysts within the lunate. The degenerative changes may ultimately involve the entire wrist.

Treatment. Since the specific etiology of Kienböck's disease is not fully understood, no

reliable treatment has been established, although many have been proposed. Prolonged immobilization relieves symptoms, but the revascularization of the lunate does not occur readily in adults, and a decrease in range of motion in the wrist and grip strength gradually occurs. A simple excision of the lunate produces good results initially, but ultimately, the remaining carpal bones migrate, leading to joint incongruity, limited wrist motion and grip strength, and degenerative osteoarthritis. A lunate-shaped spacer implant made of silicone, Vitallium, or acrylic is inserted into the resulting space to prevent migration of the other carpal bones. However, this procedure requires meticulous reconstruction

of the ligaments and the palmar joint capsule to provide firm support and prevent displacement of the implant.

Limited fusion of the capitate to the hamate has also been used successfully to prevent carpal collapse, but following this procedure, grip strength is slow to return. Joint-leveling procedures (shortening the radius or lengthening the ulna), popular in Europe, have produced excellent long-term results, particularly if performed early in the disease process. Wrist arthrodesis is indicated in persons who use their hands for heavy labor, have severe degenerative changes, or fail to improve following other surgical procedures. □

Panner's Disease

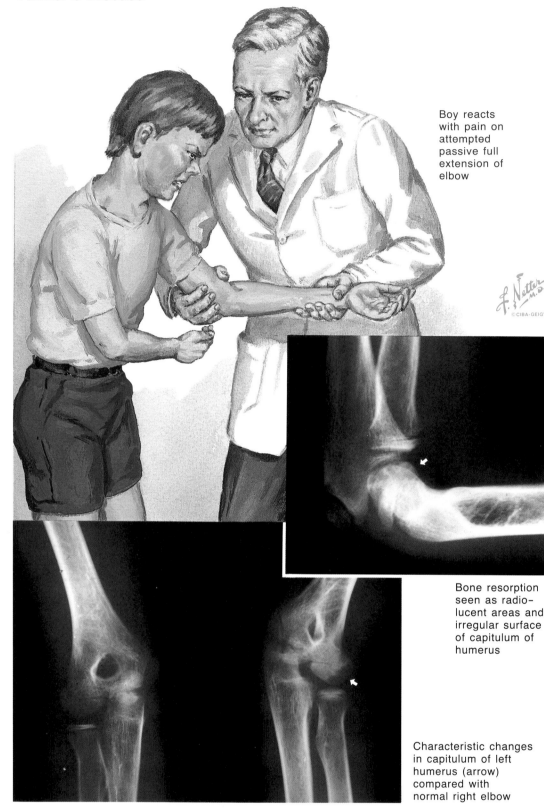

Boy reacts with pain on attempted passive full extension of elbow

Bone resorption seen as radio-lucent areas and irregular surface of capitulum of humerus

Characteristic changes in capitulum of left humerus (arrow) compared with normal right elbow

In 1927, Panner described a disease involving the capitulum of the distal humerus that produced changes similar to those observed in Legg-Calvé-Perthes disease, which affects the hip joint. Panner's disease almost always occurs in the dominant elbow in boys between 4 and 10 years of age.

The pathologic process is believed to be caused by an interference in the blood supply to the growing epiphysis, which results in resorption and eventual repair and replacement of the ossification center. The exact cause of this avascular necrosis, or bone infarct, continues to be debated, with popular theories including chronic repetitive trauma, congenital and hereditary factors, embolism (particularly fat), and endocrine disturbances. Whatever factors are responsible, the end result is avascular necrosis.

Clinical Manifestations. Patients report intermittent pain and stiffness in the affected elbow that last for several months; the symptoms are relieved by rest and aggravated by activity. Usually, there is no history of a specific injury associated with the onset of symptoms. Although some patients report that an injury occurred immediately before the symptoms, radiographs show long-standing changes.

On physical examination, local tenderness over the capitulum, slight effusion, and synovial thickening of the elbow joint are found. Limitation of elbow movement—notably extension—is demonstrable. The elbow typically lacks 20° to 30° of full extension; incomplete terminal flexion is less common. Supination and pronation may be limited slightly and, like the extremes of elbow flexion and extension, produce a grimace of pain in the child.

Radiographic Findings. While the exact etiology and pathogenesis of Panner's disease remain unclear, the radiographic changes are distinctive and progress in a consistent pattern (similar to that seen in Legg-Calvé-Perthes disease, Plates 60–61). Initially, the capitulum appears irregular with areas of radiolucency (indicating resorption), particularly adjacent to the articular surface, and sclerosis. In 3 to 5 months, radiographs show larger radiolucent areas followed by reconstruction of the bony epiphysis. In 1 to 2 years, the epiphysis returns to its normal configuration with no flattening, presumably because the elbow is not a weight-bearing joint. In about 50% of patients, the adjacent radial head shows early maturation compared with the uninvolved elbow.

Panner's disease should be distinguished from the more common osteochondritis dessicans of the capitulum seen in adolescent boys, which is related to throwing activities. Although the initial radiographic appearance of the two conditions may be similar, the progression of changes differs.

Treatment. Symptomatic treatment for Panner's disease is sufficient because the epiphysis becomes revascularized and develops a normal configuration in these young patients. Reducing elbow activities, particularly those that strain the joint, usually relieves the pain and allows gradual return of elbow motion. However, use of a long-arm cast or splint for 3 to 4 weeks may be necessary until pain, swelling, and local tenderness subside. The long-term outlook is excellent, but a slight loss of elbow extension may persist in some patients. □

Madelung's Deformity

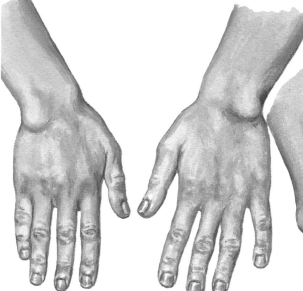

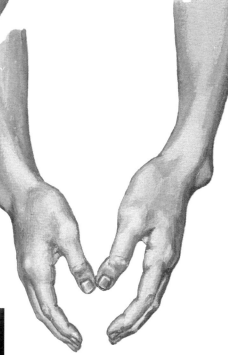

Dorsal view of hands reveals bilateral prominences of ulnar heads

Prominences of ulnar heads, palmar deviation of hands, and bowing of forearms clearly seen on radial view

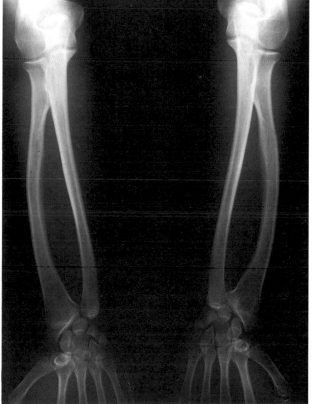

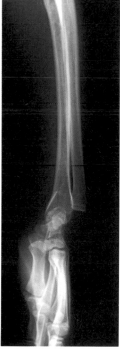

Radiograph shows ulnar inclination of articular surfaces of distal radius, wedging of carpal bones into resulting space, and bowing of radius

Lateral radiograph demonstrates dorsal prominence of ulnar head with palmar deviation of carpal bones

In Madelung's deformity, an increase occurs in the normal palmar and ulnar inclination of the distal radius (in the presence of a normal distal ulna), making the wrist appear subluxed. It is bilateral in two-thirds of patients. Rarely, a reversed Madelung's deformity may occur; the articular surface of the distal radius is angulated dorsally and the distal ulna assumes a relatively palmar position.

Madelung's deformity is caused by an absence or underdevelopment of the ulnar portion of the growth plate of the radius, so that it fails to contribute to the linear growth of the corresponding border of the radial diaphysis. The involved radial and dorsal portions of the growth plate continue to grow. The faster-growing, newly formed bone bends toward the area of slower growth, causing the articular surface of the distal radius to slant in the palmar and ulnar direction. The ulna is unaffected and remains in its usual dorsal position. The exact cause of this localized growth disturbance has not been determined, but hemiatrophy of the epiphysis of the distal radius, abnormal muscle insertions, and dysgenesis of the vascular supply to the epiphysis have been suggested.

Although Madelung's deformity is considered a congenital anomaly, it does not become manifest until late childhood or early adolescence (between 6 and 13 years of age). It is inherited as an autosomal dominant trait with variable expressivity. Females are affected four times as often as males. The moderately short stature of the affected person has led to some confusion as to whether Madelung's deformity is an isolated deformity in the distal radius or a forme fruste of dyschondrosteosis (Léri-Weill syndrome). However, dyschondrosteosis, which is characterized by other associated skeletal deformities, particularly in the tibia, in addition to Madelung's deformity at the wrist, is probably a separate entity. Other bone dysplasias with Madelunglike deformity are achondroplasia (Plates 1–3), multiple osteocartilaginous exostoses (see Section II, Plate 7), multiple epiphyseal dysplasia (Plate 10), and enchondromatosis (Plate 83). This deformity is also seen in Hurler's and Morquio's syndromes (Plate 16) and gonadal dysgenesis (Turner's syndrome), and may develop as a result of trauma or osteomyelitis of the growth plate of the distal radius.

Clinical Manifestations. Madelung's deformity is characterized by an insidious onset of pain in one wrist, then in the other, and increasing prominence of the dorsal ulnar head and bowing of the distal radius; the deformity progresses until the growth plate of the distal radius closes.

The pain usually subsides at maturity, but when the deformity becomes stabilized, the incongruity of the joint surfaces in the wrist may lead to the recurrence of painful symptoms. Wrist motion, particularly extension and supination, is usually limited. The intensity of pain, degree of deformity, and functional disability vary from patient to patient.

Radiographic Findings. The radiographic changes in Madelung's deformity include (1) increased dorsal or radial bowing of the distal radius close to the wrist; (2) exaggerated ulnar or palmar angulation of the articular surface of the distal radius; (3) wide interosseous space between the radius and ulna; (4) carpal bones wedged into the interosseous spaces, forming a triangle with the lunate at the apex; and (5) dorsal subluxation and apparent increased length of the distal ulna. The proximal radius and ulna are normal.

Treatment. Since discomfort usually resolves or remains minimal and function is excellent, surgical treatment is rarely indicated. Madelung advised his patients to avoid forced wrist extension and to use resting wrist splints at night to relieve the pain. Persistent pain, usually due to nerve impingement between the distal ulna and underlying carpal bones, or extreme deformity may require corrective surgery. Limited wrist motion is not an indication for surgery, which does little to improve it. □

Congenital Radioulnar Synostosis

Congenital Radioulnar Synostosis

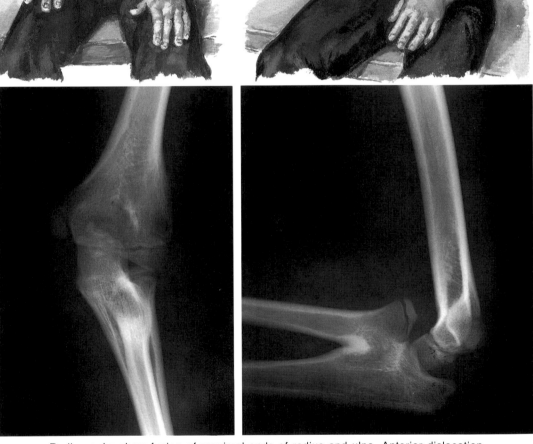

Bilateral radio-ulnar synostosis. Both hands fixed in pronation

Boy exhibits difficulty in drinking from glass due to inability to supinate forearms. Uses scapulohumeral joint and scapular rotation to turn glass

Radiographs show fusion of proximal ends of radius and ulna. Anterior dislocation of radial head apparent in view of flexed elbow (right)

Congenital radioulnar synostosis is an uncommon condition in which the proximal ends of the radius and ulna are joined, fixing the forearm in pronation. The deformity is due to a failure of the developing cartilaginous precursors of the forearm to separate during fetal development. The disorder is believed to be inherited from the father as a dominant trait with varying degrees of expressivity. Chromosomal abnormalities have been reported in some patients with bilateral involvement.

Radioulnar synostosis is bilateral in 60% of patients and is frequently associated with other musculoskeletal abnormalities. Two types of synostosis are seen. In the first, called the headless type, the medullary canals of the radius and ulna are joined and the proximal radius is absent or malformed and fused to the ulna over a distance of several centimeters. The radius is anteriorly bowed and its diaphysis is larger and longer than that of the ulna. In the second type, the fused segment is shorter and the radius is formed normally, but the radial head is dislocated anteriorly or posteriorly and fused to the diaphysis of the proximal ulna. The second type is often unilateral and sometimes associated with deformities such as syndactyly or supernumerary thumbs (Plate 111).

Clinical Manifestations. Radioulnar synostosis is present at birth but is usually not noticed until functional problems arise, most often in patients with bilateral involvement. Commonly, the only clinical finding is lack of rotation between the radius and the ulna, which fixes the forearm in a position of midpronation or hyperpronation. Range of motion in the elbow and wrist joints is usually normal or excessive, although some patients cannot completely extend the elbow.

The degree of functional disability varies with the amount of pronation of the forearm, since the severely pronated hand receives little help from humeral rotation to supinate the palm. Unilateral deformity generally produces no signs except lack of supination, and thus may remain unrecognized for years. However, in patients with bilateral involvement, in which both hands are hyperpronated, the difficulty in turning the palms upward makes many daily activities problematic, especially turning a doorknob, buttoning clothing, drinking from a cup, receiving change, or fielding a baseball bouncing on the ground.

Treatment. Since the disability is so varied, treatment should be specific to the patient. Numerous ingenious operations have been devised to separate the synostosis and permit active forearm rotation. Unfortunately, interposition of a silicone membrane, bone cap, or specially constructed swivel joint between the radius and ulna has not been successful, with new bone often rebridging the gap between the bones. In patients with hyperpronation, particularly if bilateral, rotational osteotomy, either through the distal end of the fused area or through the radius and ulna distal to the fusion, to a position 20° to 35° of supination is indicated in one arm (usually the nondominant one). □

Congenital Dislocation of Radial Head

Congenital Dislocation of Radial Head

Lateral view of arm reveals posterior bulge of head of radius and inability to fully extend elbow

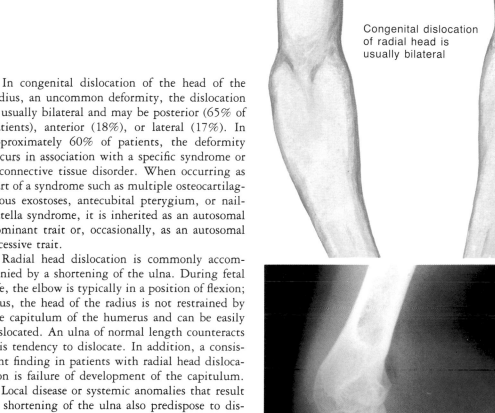

Congenital dislocation of radial head is usually bilateral

Anteroposterior and lateral radiographs reveal posterior dislocation of radial head, most evident on elbow flexion. Note also hypoplastic capitulum of humerus

In congenital dislocation of the head of the radius, an uncommon deformity, the dislocation is usually bilateral and may be posterior (65% of patients), anterior (18%), or lateral (17%). In approximately 60% of patients, the deformity occurs in association with a specific syndrome or a connective tissue disorder. When occurring as part of a syndrome such as multiple osteocartilaginous exostoses, antecubital pterygium, or nail-patella syndrome, it is inherited as an autosomal dominant trait or, occasionally, as an autosomal recessive trait.

Radial head dislocation is commonly accompanied by a shortening of the ulna. During fetal life, the elbow is typically in a position of flexion; thus, the head of the radius is not restrained by the capitulum of the humerus and can be easily dislocated. An ulna of normal length counteracts this tendency to dislocate. In addition, a consistent finding in patients with radial head dislocation is failure of development of the capitulum.

Local disease or systemic anomalies that result in shortening of the ulna also predispose to dislocation of the radial head. Thus, dislocation is commonly associated with multiple exostoses (see Section II, Plate 7), enchondromatosis (Plate 83), and absence and hypoplasia of the ulna. It also occurs with numerous other conditions such as absent thumb ray, acrocephalosyndactylies, ulnar oligodactyly, acroosteolysis congenita, congenital pterygium (epitarsus), auriculoosteodysplasia, chromosomal aberrations of the XXXY or XXXXY type, craniocarpotarsal dystrophy, craniosynostosis, Cornelia de Lange's syndrome, Detenbeck-Abrams syndrome, Ehlers-Danlos syndrome, congenital radioulnar synostosis (Plate 44), König's disease, Larsen's syndrome, mucopolysaccharidosis (Plate 16), multiple epiphyseal dysplasia (Plate 10), nail-patella syndrome, Nievergelt syndrome, oculomelic complex, Taybi syndrome, Rubinstein-Taybi syndrome, Silver-Russell syndrome, and Sprengel's deformity (Plate 40). This long list of regional and systemic associations suggests that a search for other anomalies should be made whenever congenital dislocation of the radial head is diagnosed.

Clinical Manifestations. Congenital dislocation of the radial head is asymptomatic and causes no functional disability. In most patients,

there is little limitation of motion at the elbow. Anterior dislocations cause a slight decrease in flexion and supination, whereas posterior dislocations result in a slight limitation of extension and pronation.

Radiographic Findings. Radiographs reveal an underdevelopment of the humeral capitulum. This finding helps distinguish a congenital dislocation from an acquired postnatal or traumatic dislocation. The radial head is small, with a dome-shaped top (rather than the normal concave cup shape) and a thin, elongated radial neck. Since these changes are also seen in long-standing traumatic dislocations, additional clinical criteria are used to confirm the diagnosis of congenital

dislocation. These include bilateral involvement, familial occurrence, presence of associated congenital anomalies, dislocation at birth, no history of trauma, and dislocation that is irreducible except with surgery and rarely with manipulation.

Treatment. The lack of symptoms and functional limitations make treatment of congenital dislocation of the radial head largely unnecessary. If an unacceptable appearance or pain can be attributed to the dislocation, the radial head can be excised when growth is complete. This procedure effectively relieves pain but does not usually improve range of motion because the many tight and long-standing soft-tissue contractures persist. □

Radiographic Classification of Proximal Femoral Focal Deficiency

Proximal Femoral Focal Deficiency

Type A. Femoral head and adequate acetabulum present. At maturity, ossification centers of femoral head, neck, and trochanter fuse and resulting unit is sharply abducted, causing greater trochanter to impinge on ilium. At junction of this unit with high–riding, short femoral shaft, pseud-arthrosis usually present

Type B. Femoral head and acetabulum present but trochanter never ossifies; no continuity between femoral head and high-riding shaft. Ossific tuft at proximal end of shaft probably represents vestigial trochanter

Type C. Femoral head absent or not ossified; acetabulum dysplastic. Femoral shaft very short and displaced laterally and superiorly

Type D. Acetabulum and femoral head absent. Femoral shortening severe. Proximal end of femoral shaft rides low; no ossific tuft. Often bilateral

Proximal femoral focal deficiency (PFFD) is a randomly occurring congenital abnormality of the proximal femur and hip joint. It is usually unilateral and in 68% of patients is accompanied by fibular hemimelia on the ipsilateral side. About 50% of the patients have skeletal abnormalities of other limbs as well. Based on results of a large radiographic survey, proximal femoral focal deficiency has been classified into four types, according to the type and severity of the femoral and acetabular defects (Plate 46).

Clinical Manifestations

Regardless of the extent of the anatomic defect, the clinical manifestations of proximal femoral focal deficiency are quite consistent (Plates 47–48). The affected limb is held in varying degrees of flexion, abduction, and external rotation at the hip. The femoral segment of the limb is much shorter than the normal femur. In the patient with concomitant fibular hemimelia, the sole of the foot on the affected side is usually level with the knee joint on the unaffected side. Soft-tissue contracture about the hip and some flexion contracture in the knee are also evident.

These deformities result in a number of biomechanical problems: (1) lower limb–length discrepancy, (2) malrotation, (3) inadequacy of the proximal musculature, and (4) instability of the hip joint.

In patients with unilateral involvement, the unequal lower limb lengths obviously hinder bipedal ambulation. In patients with bilateral involvement, symmetric lower limb–length discrepancy results in a striking disproportionate dwarfism (Plate 48).

Radiographic Findings

The radiographic appearance of proximal femoral focal deficiency varies considerably according to the extent of the anatomic defects (Plate 46). The major diagnostic problem is differentiating proximal femoral focal deficiency types A and B from congenital short femur associated with coxa vara (Plate 49). For both conditions, radiographs taken in infancy are difficult to interpret. If the diagnosis is uncertain, treatment should be postponed until the specific deformity is conclusively demonstrated on serial radiographs.

Treatment

In formulating a management plan for this complex deformity, it is important to establish early realistic goals for rehabilitation. The primary aim is to facilitate bipedal ambulation.

Proximal Femoral Focal Deficiency

(Continued)

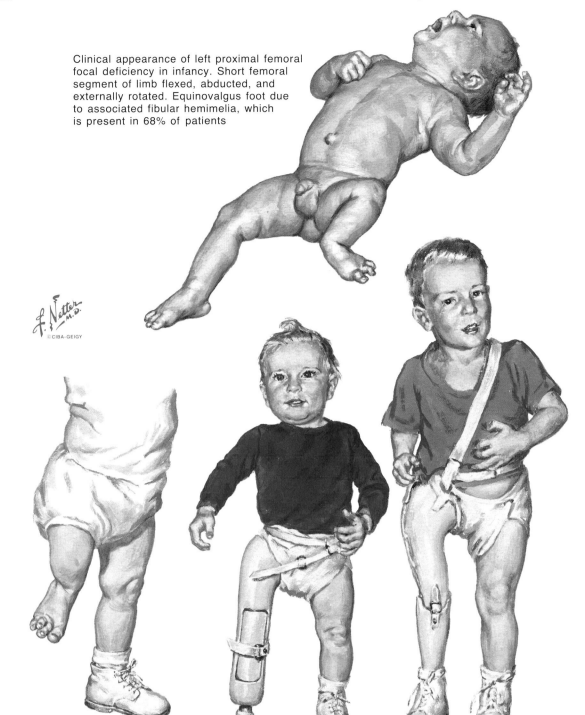

Clinical appearance of left proximal femoral focal deficiency in infancy. Short femoral segment of limb flexed, abducted, and externally rotated. Equinovalgus foot due to associated fibular hemimelia, which is present in 68% of patients

Proximal femoral focal deficiency with fibular hemimelia of right lower limb in toddler

Child initially fitted with prosthetic pylon to enable ambulation. Foot casted in equinus position

Same child after ankle disarticulation with Syme-type heel flap wears nonstandard above-knee prosthesis affixed with straps

Although correction of the flexion, abduction, and external rotation of the hip is desirable, it is not always possible. Several conservative and surgical methods are used to partially compensate for instability of the hip joint and inadequacy of the hip musculature.

In the past, crutches were the only aid for patients with unilateral involvement, and persons with disproportionate dwarfism simply ambulated on their own malformed lower limbs. Later, orthoses such as shoe lifts were devised to compensate for limb-length discrepancy and allow some degree of unassisted ambulation. More recently, nonstandard prostheses have been designed that better equalize limb lengths and improve gait. In some patients, amputation facilitates the application and improves the comfort of prostheses.

Three general treatment options are available for patients with unilateral involvement. The first is to fabricate a prosthesis that fits around the deformity. The design of the device is limited only by the ingenuity of the prosthetist. The second option is to consider the deformity as a homologue of an above-knee amputation and to devise the equivalent of an above-knee prosthesis that accommodates the deformity. The third option is to consider the deformity as the equivalent of a below-knee amputation and to design a suitable prosthesis (Plates 47–48).

Treatment of the deformity as an above-knee amputation is facilitated by removing the foot. The surgical procedure, which comprises ankle disarticulation and Syme-type closure with heel flap, produces a suitable end-bearing stump.

If the deformity is treated as a below-knee amputation, surgical conversion is necessary. A 180° rotational osteotomy of the tibia is performed so that the retained ankle joint functions as a knee joint and the remaining foot becomes the below-knee stump.

The patient with a bilateral condition—whose primary problem is disproportionate dwarfism—should be treated with bilateral prostheses that fit around the deformities. The prostheses, which are lengthened as needed to establish peer height, make the patient a precarious "stilt walker." Many patients learn to ambulate quite competently on these stilts with the assistance of a cane or crutches.

Proximal Femoral Focal Deficiency

(Continued)

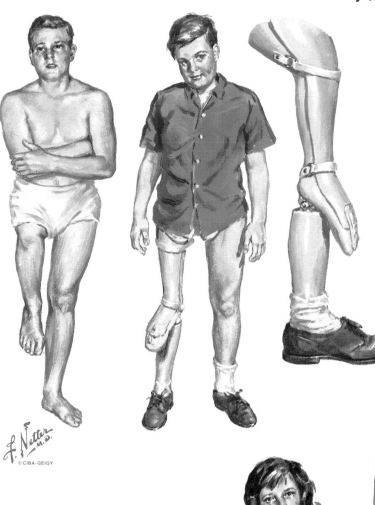

Left: marked shortening of right lower limb in patient with unilateral proximal femoral focal deficiency

Center: patient wears nonstandard above-knee prosthesis fitted around deformity

Right: close-up lateral view of prosthesis shows artificial knee joint mounted under heel

Left: patient with bilateral type D. Many patients become adjusted to their disproportionate dwarfism. They stand and walk well without crutches or prostheses and often prefer to do so at home

Right: patient wears nonstandard above-knee prostheses (which have Velcro straps for ease in application and removal). With prostheses, patient becomes "stilt walker" and achieves peer height. Cosmetic improvement helps psychosocial adjustment

Conversion of bilateral deformities to above-knee or below-knee amputations is not recommended because patients with bilateral involvement can ambulate without assistance. Bilateral Syme amputations and rotational osteotomies may rob the patient of this ability.

When the deformity is treated as a below-knee or above-knee amputation, surgical stabilization of the hip improves gait characteristics. However, establishing a stable valgus relationship between the head of the femur and the diaphysis is possible only in types A and B, which have a competent acetabulum, a femoral head that eventually ossifies, and a congruent relationship between the femoral head and the acetabulum. Thus, hip reconstruction is indicated in types A and B only. Other surgical modalities to promote a more stable hip (such as fusing the femur to the ilium and using the knee joint as a hip joint) have not improved patient rehabilitation.

Arthrodesis of the knee is useful in selected patients. If a unilateral deformity is converted to an end-bearing, above-knee stump, knee arthrodesis overcomes any residual knee flexion deformity. This technique is also beneficial in a unilateral deformity considered as a below-knee amputation. Thus, if the rotational osteotomy is

successful, the child may be fitted with a standard below-knee prosthesis that is secured with a thigh corset (and knee joints), without the need to use other types of auxiliary suspension such as a suction socket.

Congenital Short Femur With Coxa Vara

Congenital short femur is classified into three distinct types: (1) miniaturization of the femur without other deformity, (2) miniaturization of the femur with coxa vara, and (3) miniaturization with lateral bowing or angulation of the femur (Plate 49).

Coxa vara is an abnormality of the proximal femur characterized by a neck-diaphysis angle of

less than 120°. Causes are multiple. Although it is often congenital, it may also result from a metabolic aberration or trauma. Coxa vara is associated with several types of generalized skeletal abnormalities and often accompanies congenital short femur.

Clinical Manifestations. Lower limb–length discrepancy is the major deformity in short femur with coxa vara. Unlike proximal femoral focal deficiency, there is no flexion, abduction, and external rotation deformity of the hip. However, fibular hemimelia with a moderately severe valgus deformity of the ankle may also be present on the affected side, exacerbating the limb-length discrepancy.

Proximal Femoral Focal Deficiency

(Continued)

Congenital Short Femur With Coxa Vara

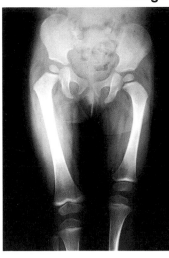

Miniaturization of femur with no deformity

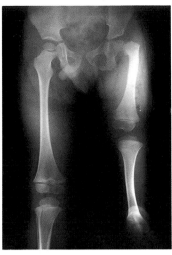

Miniaturization of femur with associated coxa vara

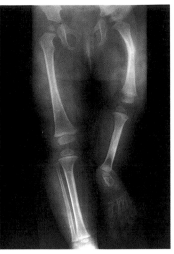

Miniaturization of femur with lateral bowing or angulation

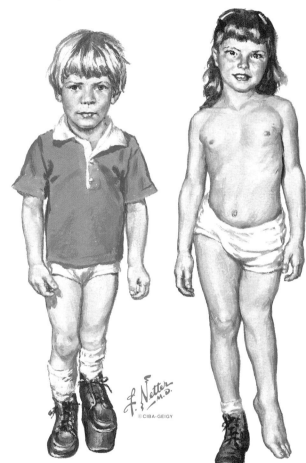

Boy wears built-up boot to compensate for moderate congenital short left femur

Girl with congenital short left femur with associated coxa vara

Radiograph shows congenital coxa vara. Defect in inferior part of femoral neck causes varus deformity to develop between head and neck of femur

Principle of subtrochanteric abduction osteotomy for coxa vara

Radiographic Findings. Radiographs of congenital short femur with associated coxa vara usually show the proximal end of the femoral diaphysis in bony continuity with the femoral head and neck, and the proximal end of the femur does not ride above Hilgenreiner's line. On the other hand, in proximal femoral focal deficiency types A and B, the proximal femur usually rides above the superior rim of the acetabulum; this finding is a useful factor in the differential diagnosis (Plate 46).

Treatment. Management of a deformity of this magnitude requires a team of specialists, including a physician interested in such problems, an experienced prosthetist, and a skilled physical therapist, to evaluate the problem and select the most appropriate treatment modalities. It is most important to describe to the patient and the family the overall management plan that will result in maximal function.

Coxa vara should be treated as soon as the diagnosis is certain. The primary goal is to establish a stable valgus relationship between the diaphysis and the head and neck of the femur.

Subtrochanteric osteotomy is performed to produce a position of maximum valgus, not simply to restore the neck-diaphysis angle to greater than 120°. (This procedure is not appropriate for proximal femoral focal deficiency.) Any incompetence of the acetabulum on the affected side should be treated with appropriate hip reconstruction techniques.

Treatment for the combined deformities of short femur and coxa vara varies. Since the major defect is limb-length discrepancy primarily due to the short femur and concomitant fibular hemimelia, it is usually difficult to equalize the levels of the knees. Shoe lifts to accommodate for the unequal limb lengths are successful in some

patients. The Syme amputation, which produces an end-bearing below-knee stump, permits the use of a below-knee prosthesis; in many patients, this result is both more cosmetic and possibly more functional than a simple shoe lift with or without an orthotic device. Some children may be candidates for limb-lengthening procedures (Plates 86–87).

However, use of shoe lifts and conversion to a below-knee amputation do not equalize the levels of the knees. This can be accomplished by an end-bearing above-knee amputation. In this procedure, a portion of the tibia is fused to the femur and the amputation done at a level that matches the contralateral normal knee joint. ☐

Congenital Dislocation of Hip

Methods for the early detection of congenital dislocation of the hip have been reported for at least 50 years. In 1926, Putti presented results of his program for early screening and treatment of patients. At Babies' Hospital in New York, Howorth in 1932 pioneered the first screening program for infants in the United States. After World War II, extensive screening was begun in the United States, Sweden, and England. Early diagnosis resulted in simple, safe, and effective treatment.

In the United States, 10 of 1,000 infants are born with congenital dislocation of the hip. As a result of early recognition and thus early treatment, 96% of affected children achieve normal hip function. The longer the dislocation remains undiscovered and untreated, the greater are the problems in obtaining a satisfactory end result. Routine screening for congenital dislocation of the hip should be an integral part of the newborn and follow-up examinations.

Etiologic Factors

The etiology of congenital dislocation of the hip is multifactorial, with mechanical and physiologic factors in both mother and fetus and, occasionally, postnatal environmental factors combining to produce hip instability and subsequent dislocation.

The time of onset of the predisposing factors directly influences the degree of hip instability and the severity of the anatomic changes. The typical congenital dislocation occurs just before or just after delivery in an otherwise normal infant. At birth, clinical findings are subtle, and radiographs often appear normal. In contrast, if the dislocation occurs in early fetal life, the clinical and radiographic findings at birth demonstrate more advanced adaptive changes of the pelvis and femoral head. This early type of dislocation (teratologic dislocation) is rare and represents only 2% of congenital hip dislocations. It is usually associated with arthrogryposis multiplex congenita (Plate 20), chromosomal abnormalities, and severe congenital anomalies such as lumbosacral agenesis (Plate 39) and myelodysplasia (Plate 38).

Mechanical Factors. Mechanical factors occur primarily in the last trimester of pregnancy; all have the effect of restricting the space available for the fetus in the uterus. About 60% of children with congenital dislocation of the hip are firstborns, which suggests that the tight, unstretched abdominal and uterine musculature of

Recognition of Congenital Dislocation of Hip

Ortolani's (reduction) test

With baby relaxed and content on firm surface, hips and knees flexed to 90°. Hips examined one at a time. Examiner grasps baby's thigh with middle finger over greater trochanter and lifts thigh to bring femoral head from its dislocated posterior position to opposite the acetabulum.
Simultaneously, thigh gently abducted, reducing femoral head into acetabulum. In positive finding, examiner senses reduction by palpable, nearly audible "clunk"

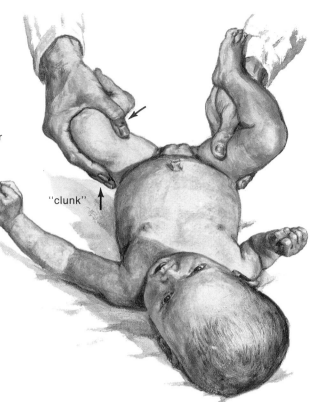

"clunk"

Barlow's (dislocation) test

Reverse of Ortolani's test. If femoral head is in acetabulum at time of examination, Barlow's test is performed to discover any hip instability. Baby's thigh grasped as above and adducted with gentle downward pressure. Dislocation is palpable as femoral head slips out of acetabulum. Diagnosis confirmed with Ortolani's test

the mother inhibits fetal movement. It is believed that the pelvis of the fetus becomes trapped in the maternal pelvis, and the fetus is unable to kick and change position, which prevents the normal flexion of the hip and knee (limb folding).

Breech presentation also plays a significant role in congenital dislocation of the hip: 30% to 50% of affected children are delivered in this presentation. In addition, when the knees are extended in the frank breech position, increased tension in the hamstring muscles further contributes to hip instability. The incidence of dislocation of the hip is also higher in children with congenital genu recurvatum, or dislocation of the knee

(Plate 77) and other conditions caused by intrauterine molding, such as congenital muscular torticollis (Plate 27) and metatarsus adductus (Plate 80).

The left hip is involved more often than the right, possibly because the fetus tends to lie with the left thigh against the mother's sacrum in the breech position. Thus, the fetal pelvis is held securely in the maternal pelvis, with the thigh trapped against the maternal sacrum, which forces the hip into flexion and adduction. In this position, the femoral head is covered more by the joint capsule than by the bony acetabulum. The right hip is dislocated in 20% of patients, and both hips in 25%.

Congenital Dislocation of Hip
(Continued)

Clinical Findings in Congenital Dislocation of Hip
(if untreated, signs become more obvious with growth and weight bearing)

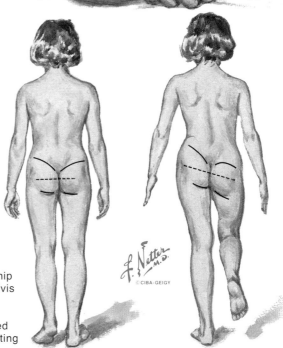

Limitation of abduction due to shortened and contracted adductor muscles of hip

Telescoping, or pistoning, action of thigh can be elicited because femoral head not contained within acetabulum

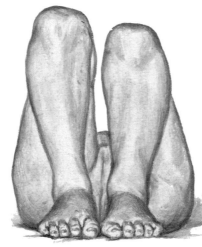

Shortening of thigh with bunching up of soft tissues and accentuation of skin folds

Allis' or Galeazzi's sign
With knees and hips flexed, knee on affected side lower because femoral head lies posterior to acetabulum in this position

Trendelenburg's test
Left: child with congenital dislocation of hip stands on both feet; hips and brim of pelvis are approximately level, except for slight shortening of thigh on affected left side.
Right: child stands with weight on affected side; normal right hip drops down, indicating weakness of abductor muscles of left hip

Hormonal Factors. Maternal estrogens and hormones that effect relaxation of the pelvis immediately before delivery also influence hip instability or dislocation. The pharmacologic effect of these hormones is not limited to the maternal pelvis but also may lead to temporary laxity of the hip joint and capsule in the newborn. Studies suggest that the female infant is particularly affected by these hormonal changes, which may explain the higher incidence of the condition in females (6:1).

The familial tendency to dislocation (20% of cases) may be due to an inborn, possibly inherited, error of estrogen metabolism. Striking clinical examples of this familial tendency are seen in certain Navajo tribes, Lapps of Scandinavia, and Northern Italians.

Postnatal Environmental Factors. In the first months of life, the normal position of the hip is that of flexion and abduction. In societies where infants are customarily wrapped to a cradle board or swaddled to maintain the hip in extension, the incidence of congenital hip dislocation is 10 times greater than normal. Furthermore, the practice of holding the newborn by the feet after delivery, thus forcing the hip into extension, may lead to dislocation and should be avoided.

Pathogenic Factors

The mechanism of a typical congenital dislocation is probably quite simple. Near the time of birth, the joint capsule is distended and elastic. After delivery, the femoral head is loose within the joint and free to "fall out" of the acetabulum. In the newborn period, the femoral head can easily be returned to its normal position, or reduced. At this early stage, the shape of the joint and soft-tissue structures is very close to normal. Thus, for a stable hip to develop, it is only necessary to maintain the normal relationship between the femoral head and the acetabulum for a few weeks while the joint capsule returns to a normal configuration. However, if the dislocation is allowed to persist, the soft tissue and bone adjacent to the joint gradually undergo adaptive changes, the dislocation becomes more difficult to reduce, and the chance of obtaining a successful long-term result diminishes significantly.

Researchers have demonstrated that the stimulus for the normal development of the acetabulum is a normal femoral head contained within it; conversely, a normal femoral head develops if it is contained within a normal acetabulum. The growth rate in the newborn period is rapid, with the infant doubling in size in the first 5 to 6 months and tripling in size in the first year. Thus, if the hip dislocation is recognized early, there is a great potential to obtain successful remodeling of the pathologic changes.

If the dislocation is not treated, the simple problem becomes more complex. The longer the hip stays dislocated, the more the normal muscle action increases the proximal and lateral migration of the femoral head along the pelvis. Because the muscles about the hip—particularly the hamstring, hip adductor, and iliopsoas—are not maintained at their normal resting length, they become contracted. The acetabulum, denied the stimulus of the femoral head, becomes dysplastic—that is, flatter and dish shaped rather than cup shaped. The joint fills with fibrofatty debris known as pulvinar (Plate 53). The capitis femoris ligament (ligamentum teres) is stretched, becoming elongated and redundant. The capsule of the hip joint "balloons" out in front of the femoral head and narrows behind it, flattening against the opening of the acetabulum. The transverse acetabular ligament, which is the inferior continuation of the acetabular labrum, or limbus, is pulled superiorly with the capsule and contracted, blocking the lower portion of the acetabulum. The iliopsoas tendon compresses the

Congenital Dislocation of Hip
(Continued)

trailing capsule, further narrowing the entrance to the acetabulum and resulting in the *hourglass configuration* of the joint space. The femoral head becomes trapped behind the acetabular labrum. Pressure on the labrum causes it to enlarge and in some instances to enfold into the joint, preventing reduction, a condition known as the *inverted limbus*. The femoral head becomes misshapen and flattened as it rubs against the pelvis, blocking the normal rotation of the femoral neck. Thus, the femoral head and neck remain anteverted and in valgus position.

Examination of Newborn and Infant

The examination procedures described by Ortolani and Barlow are the most reliable methods for diagnosing congenital dislocation of the hip in the newborn (Plate 50). *Ortolani's test* is an examination of hip reduction: if the infant's hip is dislocated, the femoral head can be returned into the acetabulum with the Ortolani maneuver. This finding is known as a positive Ortolani. *Barlow's test* demonstrates the reverse: when the infant is examined, the femoral head is located within the acetabulum. However, when the hip is flexed and the thigh adducted, the femoral head "falls," or can be gently pushed posteriorly out of the acetabulum, demonstrating an unstable hip joint. Both parts of the examination are collectively known as Ortolani's test.

Some have erroneously concluded that the primary emphasis of the Ortolani examination is to demonstrate that the infant's hip can be maximally abducted. However, in most infants with hip dislocation, the joint capsule is lax enough to permit full abduction without the femoral head reducing into the acetabulum. In a few weeks, if the hip remains dislocated, limitation of abduction becomes a more consistent clinical finding.

The term "hip instability" is commonly used in the discussion of congenital dislocation of the hip. Instability is classified into three types: type 1, the dislocated hip; type 2, the dislocatable hip; and type 3, the subluxable hip. Type 1 is demonstrated by a positive Ortolani test, and types 2 and 3 are detected with Barlow's test, which can be viewed as a provocative test. If the test is positive, the term "dislocatable hip" is more appropriate. The classification is applicable only during the newborn period.

Clinical Manifestations in Older Children

As the child grows, the clinical findings of an untreated dislocated hip become more obvious

Radiographic Evaluation of Congenital Dislocation of Hip

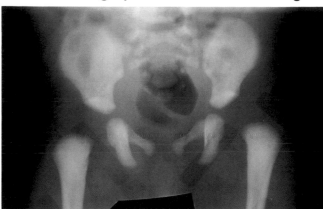

Radiograph of pelvis and hips of 4-day-old infant with congenital dislocation of left hip appears normal. Routine radiographs seldom diagnostic in first month of life

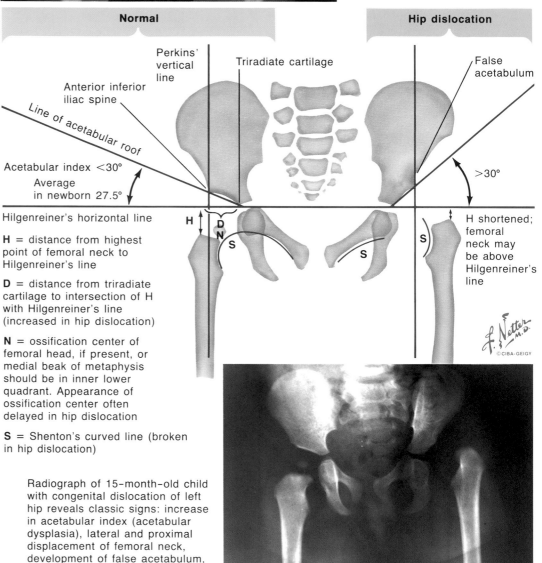

Normal   **Hip dislocation**

Perkins' vertical line

Anterior inferior iliac spine

Line of acetabular roof

Triradiate cartilage

False acetabulum

Acetabular index <30°
Average in newborn 27.5°

>30°

Hilgenreiner's horizontal line

H = distance from highest point of femoral neck to Hilgenreiner's line

D = distance from triradiate cartilage to intersection of H with Hilgenreiner's line (increased in hip dislocation)

N = ossification center of femoral head, if present, or medial beak of metaphysis should be in inner lower quadrant. Appearance of ossification center often delayed in hip dislocation

S = Shenton's curved line (broken in hip dislocation)

H shortened; femoral neck may be above Hilgenreiner's line

Radiograph of 15-month-old child with congenital dislocation of left hip reveals classic signs: increase in acetabular index (acetabular dysplasia), lateral and proximal displacement of femoral neck, development of false acetabulum, broken Shenton's line, and delayed ossification of femoral head

(Plate 51). The surrounding soft tissue and bone gradually adapt to the abnormal position of the femoral head. With time, it becomes more difficult to reduce the femoral head into the acetabulum, and the Ortolani test becomes negative: in other words, the femoral head is trapped outside the acetabulum. All muscle groups about the hip become shortened and contracted. Tightness of the adductor muscles, which is reflected in limited thigh abduction, is most apparent. Since the femoral head is not contained within the acetabulum, the thigh is shortened, the skin and subcutaneous tissue bunch up, and extra skin folds can be observed; with the patient supine and the hips and knees flexed, the knees are not at the

same level (*Allis'* or *Galeazzi's sign*). The femur can be freely moved up and down, which is described as pistoning, or telescoping.

The child walks with a significant limp because of shortening of the limb, telescoping of the femoral head on the pelvis, and a contralateral tilt of the pelvis due to abductor muscle weakness. The *Trendelenburg test* is used to determine abductor muscle strength (Plate 51).

When both hips are dislocated, the perineal space is widened, and the greater trochanters are more prominent than normal. The buttocks are broad and flat, and the lumbar spine is hyperlordotic. The child with bilateral hip dislocation has a waddling gait.

Congenital Dislocation of Hip
(Continued)

Radiographic Evaluation

Routine radiographic evaluation of the newborn to detect a typical congenital dislocation is seldom reliable, because many of the characteristic pathologic changes have not yet developed. Therefore, radiographs are not useful until the infant is at least 6 weeks old. Even if the hip is clinically held in a dislocated position, this may not be apparent on the radiograph because so much of the infant's pelvis is cartilaginous and consequently radiolucent. Thus, *a negative finding on radiographic examination does not rule out the presence of a dislocation.*

As the child grows, the adaptive changes of the hip joint and femur become more evident on routine radiographs (Plates 52–53). Characteristic findings include (1) proximal and lateral migration of the femoral neck adjacent to the ilium; (2) a shallow, incompletely developed acetabulum (acetabular dysplasia); (3) development of a false acetabulum; and (4) delayed ossification of the ossification center of the proximal femur. A useful method for detecting the dislocated hip is a system of lines marked on an anteroposterior radiograph of the pelvis and hips (Plate 52). Accurate positioning of the patient is critical: the hips must be extended and the lower limbs in normal alignment and neutral rotation. These lines are helpful in detecting unilateral hip dislocation because a comparison can be made between the normal and abnormal sides, but they are of limited value in recognizing a bilateral dislocation.

In the older child, an arthrogram may be helpful to visualize intraarticular changes such as the inverted limbus and the hourglass configuration, but routine arthrography is seldom indicated. Arthrography is performed when the usual treatment measures are inadequate or the dislocation recurs following closed reduction.

The goal of treatment is to return the femoral head to its normal position within the acetabulum and to maintain this position until the pathologic changes are reversed. In the newborn and the infant under 6 months of age, closed reduction can usually be accomplished by gently placing the femoral head in the acetabulum. In older children, closed reduction is more difficult, and traction is required before reduction is attempted.

Treatment of Clinically Reducible Hip

Closed Reduction. The hip is flexed, then the thigh is gently lifted and abducted to bring the

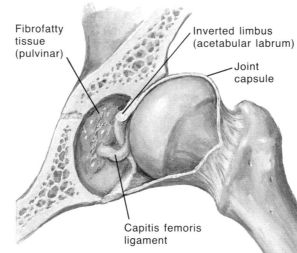

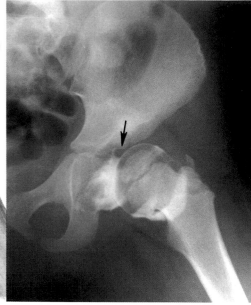

Inverted limbus. Enfolding of labrum prevents femoral head from entering acetabulum. Arthrogram reveals inverted limbus (arrow). Redundant and hypertrophied capitis femoris ligament and contracture of transverse acetabular ligament may also hinder reduction

Fibrofatty tissue (pulvinar)
Inverted limbus (acetabular labrum)
Joint capsule
Capitis femoris ligament

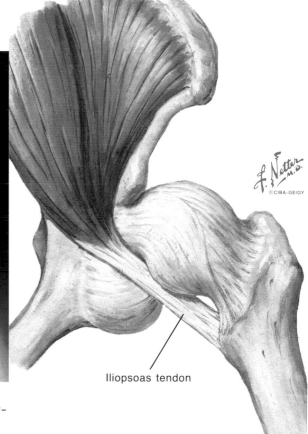

Hourglass configuration of joint space
Arthrogram reveals typical bilocular appearance due to stretching and narrowing of joint capsule. Iliopsoas tendon further constricts isthmus of capsule

Iliopsoas tendon

femoral head into the acetabulum. The reduced hip must be maintained in a comfortable and normal physiologic position of flexion-abduction. The *positioning is critical*: it must avoid excessive stress to the joint yet keep the femoral head from redislocating. The ideal hip position is flexion to approximately 90° and moderate abduction, termed by Salter the "human position" (in contrast to the previously popular "frog position" of extreme abduction). The femoral head must be positioned deep within the acetabulum, and on radiographs, the femoral head and neck should point toward the triradiate cartilage.

In a large number of children, hip instability noted at birth spontaneously resolves in a few

weeks. Simple positioning to maintain the hip flexed and abducted during this time may be sufficient, particularly in children with the dislocatable and subluxable (positive Barlow) types of hip instability. The patient must be observed closely, and more definitive management is required if the instability persists. The newborn with marked instability (positive Ortolani) should be placed in a secure restraint and the reduction maintained for several weeks.

Positioning Devices. Triple diapers are commonly used to maintain abduction of the hip (Plate 54). However, this is a highly unreliable method, and use beyond the first 1 to 2 weeks after delivery is discouraged. Also, triple diapers

Congenital Dislocation of Hip
(Continued)

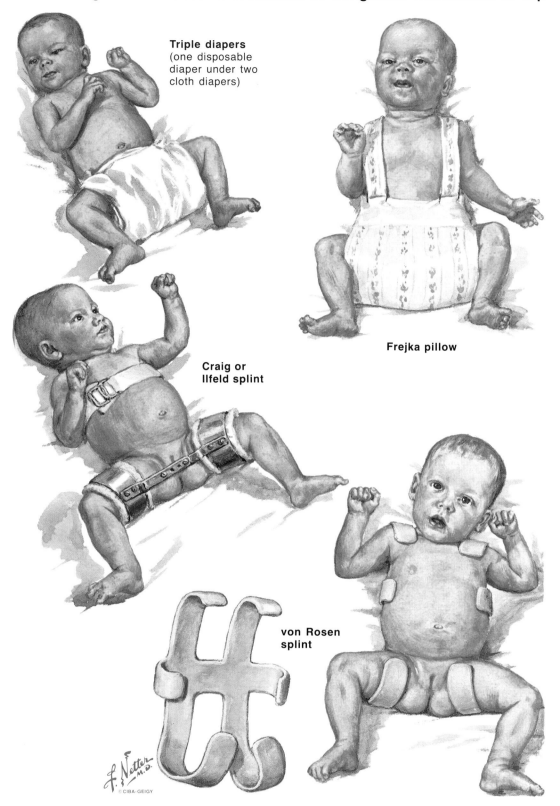

Triple diapers (one disposable diaper under two cloth diapers)

Frejka pillow

Craig or Ilfeld splint

von Rosen splint

cannot be used to treat the highly unstable (positive Ortolani) type of dislocation, since this unstable hip is likely to redislocate. The *Frejka pillow* is a large, bulky device, covered with a plastic or rubberized material to prevent soiling, that is placed in the baby's groin to keep the thighs abducted. Like triple diapers, it has to be reapplied with every diaper change and has the same potential for redislocation.

With the *Craig (Ilfeld) splint*, however, perineal care can be accomplished with the device in place. Unfortunately, it has a tendency to slide down the infant's legs, allowing the hips to become less flexed and more adducted, with the risk of redislocation. The *von Rosen splint*, a molded metal device, does not slide down because it extends over the shoulders and around the thighs. It must be properly bent and molded to the child or it can force the hip into severe abduction, and it must be adjusted frequently to accommodate the child's growth.

To a large degree, the *Pavlik harness* avoids many of the problems mentioned above (Plate 55). This restraint maintains the lower limbs in the proper position with a shoulder harness, foot cuffs, and straps with Velcro closures. The adjustment of the posterior strap is critical. Originally, Pavlik recommended cinching the posterior strap tightly to maintain the hips in maximal abduction (the frog position), a practice that led to a high incidence of avascular necrosis of the femoral head. In its present use, the posterior strap serves only as a checkrein to prevent the thigh from adducting to the point at which the femoral head redislocates. The hips are allowed to fall freely into comfortable abduction.

The harness is applied loosely, and the hip is reduced with the Ortolani maneuver and flexed to 90°. The Barlow maneuver is then used to determine the position of thigh adduction at which the hip dislocates—the *zone of redislocation*. The posterior strap is adjusted to prevent the thigh from entering this zone, while permitting hip motion in the zone of reduction, called the *safe zone of Ramsey*. With the device properly adjusted, radiographs are taken to confirm that the reduction is satisfactory and that the femoral head and neck are directed toward the triradiate cartilage.

The Pavlik harness has several advantages. It allows active hip motion while maintaining the hip reduction within safe limits. Also, it prevents

extension of the hip and knee and tightening of the hamstring muscles, factors known to predispose to continued hip instability. The infant can remain in the restraint during all routine care, nursing, and diaper changes. In addition, the risk of avascular necrosis is diminished because the hip is not maintained in forced abduction.

The duration of treatment is directly related to the age at which treatment is initiated—a good estimate is approximately two times the age of the child when the device is first applied.

Treatment of Clinically Unreducible Hip

The clinically unreducible hip is usually seen in a child over 6 months of age. The hip cannot

be reduced because of soft-tissue contracture about the joint. Since more force is required to reduce the hip with simple measures, there is the increased risk of permanent damage to the hip. *At no time should the hip be reduced with forceful manipulation.* If the hip cannot be reduced easily—that is, the Ortolani examination is negative—or general anesthesia is needed, *traction must be employed* prior to closed reduction to stretch the soft-tissue structures.

Traction. Use of traction prior to reduction of the hip significantly decreases the risk of avascular necrosis. It should be used in every patient who requires cast mobilization to maintain the reduction. The child remains in traction until the

Congenital Dislocation of Hip
(Continued)

Device for Treatment of Clinically Reducible Dislocation of Hip

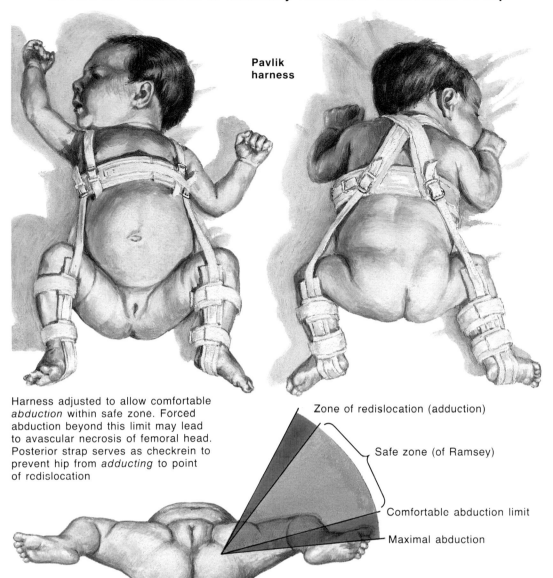

Pavlik harness

Harness adjusted to allow comfortable *abduction* within safe zone. Forced abduction beyond this limit may lead to avascular necrosis of femoral head. Posterior strap serves as checkrein to prevent hip from *adducting* to point of redislocation

Zone of redislocation (adduction)

Safe zone (of Ramsey)

Comfortable abduction limit

Maximal abduction

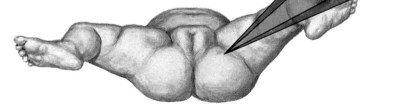

Some infants have adductor tightness that prevents reduction, and safe zone becomes narrower. In many cases, adductor muscles relax and hip spontaneously reduces after 2 weeks of wearing harness. If not, traction, and possibly adductor tenotomy, required prior to reduction under anesthesia

Zone of redislocation (adduction)

Safe zone (of Ramsey)

Comfortable abduction limit

Maximal abduction

femoral head is seen on radiographs to be opposite the triradiate cartilage but not necessarily reduced—usually 2 to 3 weeks.

Cast Immobilization. As soon as the femoral head is positioned opposite the triradiate cartilage, gentle closed reduction is attempted with the child under general anesthesia. If the hip can be reduced easily, radiographs are obtained to document the position of the femoral head within the acetabulum. When the position is satisfactory, the child is immobilized in a plaster cast. Before the cast is applied, the safe zone of Ramsey must be determined; if the safe zone is wide, the hip is positioned in flexion and abduction, avoiding both forced abduction and adduction into the zone of redislocation. If the safe zone is narrow, it may be enlarged with an adductor tenotomy.

Surgical Procedures

After closed reduction, if the position of the femoral head within the acetabulum is not satisfactory, open reduction of the hip should be considered.

Medial (Adductor) Approach. This approach is used in children under 12 months of age. Although age is an important criterion in choosing this approach, the child's size may be a more important one: the larger the child and the more proximal the dislocation, the greater the distance between a medial-based incision and the femoral head.

The medial-based incision allows direct visualization of the area of capsular contracture, but it does not permit exposure of the redundant capsule or any method of plicating the capsule to prevent redislocation. Care should be taken to protect the medial circumflex femoral artery—the primary blood supply to the femoral head—which courses around the iliopsoas tendon a few millimeters proximal to its insertion on the lesser trochanter. Particularly in the infant, this artery can easily be damaged during surgery.

When the capsule is opened, the femoral head can be visualized and returned gently into the acetabulum. In some patients, the acetabulum must be enlarged, which is accomplished by removing the redundant capitis femoris ligament and pulvinar. The inverted limbus, if present, can usually be pushed aside to permit reduction. The transverse acetabular ligament is often contracted and can be incised. Closure of the capsule is not necessary.

After surgery, the child is immobilized in a bilateral hip spica cast. The plaster must be molded carefully over the greater trochanter to prevent the femoral head from redislocating posteriorly into the redundant portion of the capsule.

Anterolateral Approach. In the older or larger child, the femoral head cannot be reached easily from a medial-based incision, and the anterolateral approach to the hip is used. An oblique incision below the iliac crest is preferred, as it leaves a better cosmetic result and the scar is less prone to spread. As in the medial approach, the pulvinar, redundant capitis femoris ligament, and transverse acetabular ligament are excised as

needed to improve the adequacy of the acetabulum. The inverted limbus can usually be repositioned behind the femoral head to help prevent redislocation, or it can be excised if it obstructs the reduction. The redundant portion of the capsule is excised and the capsule repaired to prevent redislocation. The patient is placed in a cast with the hip in slight flexion, abduction, and internal rotation. The position alone should maintain the femoral head in place; if excessive force or an extreme position is required, the adequacy of the reduction should be evaluated.

The child under 2 years of age who has a dysplastic acetabulum can be placed in a brace until acetabular remodeling occurs. In an older child,

Congenital Dislocation of Hip
(Continued)

Blood Supply to Femoral Head in Infancy (after Ogden)

Extracapsular course of medial and lateral circumflex femoral arteries

- Capsule of hip joint
- Medial circumflex femoral a.
- Anastomosis
- Ascending, transverse, and descending branches of lateral circumflex femoral a.
- Iliopsoas m.
- Femoral a.
- Deep femoral a.
- Medial circumflex femoral a.
- Pectineus m.
- Adductor longus m.

Distribution of medial and lateral circumflex femoral arteries

- Acetabular labrum
- Growth plate
- Lateral circumflex femoral a.
- Posterior superior and posterior inferior branches of medial circumflex femoral a. (principal blood supply to femoral head)
- Iliopsoas tendon

Compression of medial circumflex femoral artery in extreme abduction, internal rotation, and flexion

- Posterior superior branch compressed by acetabular labrum in intertrochanteric fossa
- Posterior inferior branch compressed against femoral neck by iliopsoas tendon
- Artery compressed between iliopsoas tendon and acetabular labrum
- Artery compressed between iliopsoas tendon, pectineus muscle, and contracted adductor longus muscle, plus increased tension on vessel

there is less potential for satisfactory remodeling of the acetabulum, and other procedures should be considered. With the Salter *innominate osteotomy*, the acetabulum is rotated to provide additional anterolateral coverage of the femoral head (Plate 64). Severe femoral anteversion requires marked internal rotation and abduction to properly position the femoral head within the acetabulum. This can be accomplished with a *femoral varus derotational osteotomy* (Plate 64). The superiority of either approach is still controversial. However, all authorities agree that alteration of the pelvis, acetabulum, or femoral head is seldom necessary in the management of congenital dislocation of the hip in the young child, as there is a great potential for anatomic remodeling following an adequate reduction.

Complications of Treatment

Avascular Necrosis of Femoral Head. Forcing the hip into an extreme or unusual position during treatment can have serious consequences, the most important being avascular necrosis of the femoral head. Compromise of the blood supply to the femoral head for even a short time results in complete death of the femoral head; even a minor interruption of the circulation significantly increases this risk. Redislocation of the hip can be a problem but can be corrected. It is sometimes tempting to resort to more abduction or internal rotation to maintain the femoral head in the acetabulum, but *extreme positions must be avoided*.

Role of Blood Supply to Femoral Head in Infancy

Ogden has emphasized several important points concerning the blood supply to the femoral head as it applies to the treatment of children with congenital dislocation of the hip (Plate 56). In the newborn, both the lateral and medial circumflex femoral arteries supply the femoral head. At age 5 to 6 months, when the femoral neck begins to develop, the contribution from the lateral circumflex femoral artery to the epiphysis and metaphysis regresses. The medial circumflex femoral artery, on the posterior aspect of the femoral neck, becomes the primary blood supply to the femoral head, as there is very little crossover from the lateral circumflex femoral and anterior vessels. Therefore, interruption of the medial circumflex femoral artery in the first few months of life may affect only a small area, whereas in the slightly older child, occlusion may result in complete death of the femoral head, with a profound

effect on the subsequent development of the proximal femur.

In the past, the incidence of avascular necrosis following hip reduction for congenital dislocation has been unacceptably high—in many series, a 30% to 40% incidence was common. It is postulated that forced abduction is the primary cause of avascular necrosis. When the hip is placed in maximal abduction, the acetabular labrum is brought into the superoposterior intertrochanteric area, placing direct pressure on the medial circumflex femoral artery. If, in addition, the hip is rotated inward, further compression is likely.

Direct pressure on the artery is not the only cause of decreased blood flow. Other potential

sites for occlusion are found along the long and tortuous path of the medial circumflex femoral artery, which renders it vulnerable to stretching and compression external to the hip joint, particularly when the hip is placed in maximal abduction. The artery can be compressed as it passes through the iliopsoas muscle and the pectineus-adductor muscle group or it can be trapped between the iliopsoas tendon and the pubic ramus. The risk of vascular occlusion in the child with congenital dislocation of the hip is high because of contracture of these muscle groups. Traction to stretch the soft tissues and surgical release of the contracture are often successful in reducing the incidence of avascular necrosis. □

Legg-Calvé-Perthes Disease

Legg-Calvé-Perthes disease is defined as idiopathic avascular necrosis of the epiphysis of the femoral head (capital femoral epiphysis) and its associated complications in a growing child. It is a common but poorly understood hip disorder.

The disease develops more often in boys than girls (4 or 5:1). It can occur between 2 and 12 years of age (mean age is 7 years), and when the involvement is bilateral, the changes usually appear in one hip at least 1 year earlier than in the other. If the child is more than 12 years of age at the time of clinical onset, the disorder is not considered true Legg-Calvé-Perthes disease but rather adolescent avascular necrosis, which has a poor prognosis similar to that of the adult form.

Predisposing Factors

Genetic Aspects. The incidence of Legg-Calvé-Perthes disease is 1% to 20% higher in families of involved children, although there is no consistent pattern of inheritance. Studies in England have indicated that affected children are more likely than normal children to have low birth weight, abnormal birth presentation (breech and transverse presentations), and older parents. The disease is also more prevalent in later-born children (particularly the third to the sixth child).

The disorder occurs more frequently in Japanese, mongoloid, Eskimo, and Central European populations, whereas the incidence is decreased in blacks, Australian aborigines, American Indians, and Polynesians.

The English studies have also demonstrated a higher than normal incidence of minor congenital genitourinary anomalies (eg, renal abnormalities, inguinal hernias, and undescended testicles) in affected children as well as in their first-degree relatives.

Abnormal Growth and Development. Legg-Calvé-Perthes disease may be a manifestation of an unknown systemic disorder rather than an isolated abnormality of the hip joint. The bone age of affected children is typically 1 to 3 years lower than their chronologic age. As a consequence, affected children are usually shorter than their peers, and the shortness of stature, although slight, persists into adulthood.

Disproportionate growth, abnormalities in skeletal growth and maturation, and elevated serum levels of somatomedin have been demonstrated. Affected children are typically smaller in all dimensions except head circumference, and their limbs have disproportionately small distal segments. The relationship between growth abnormalities, serum somatomedin, and ischemia of the epiphysis of the femoral head remains obscure. However, these findings support the concept of an underlying systemic disorder.

Pathogenesis of Legg-Calvé-Perthes Disease

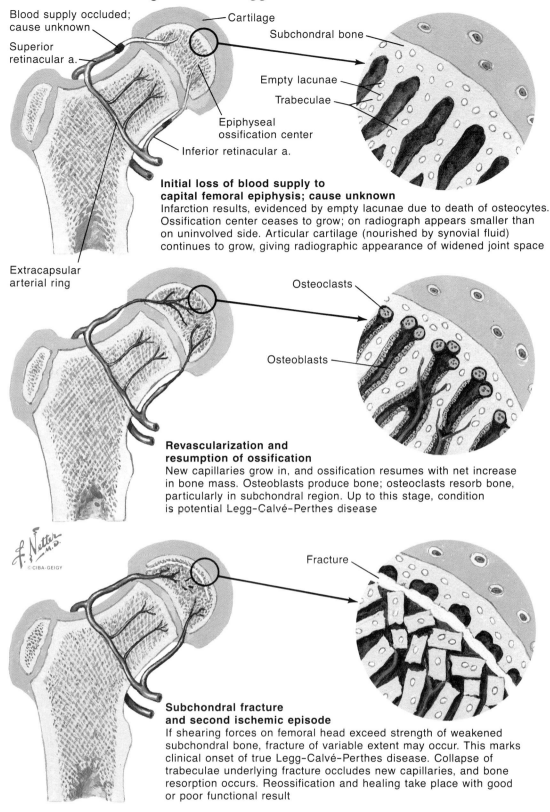

Initial loss of blood supply to capital femoral epiphysis; cause unknown
Infarction results, evidenced by empty lacunae due to death of osteocytes. Ossification center ceases to grow; on radiograph appears smaller than on uninvolved side. Articular cartilage (nourished by synovial fluid) continues to grow, giving radiographic appearance of widened joint space

Revascularization and resumption of ossification
New capillaries grow in, and ossification resumes with net increase in bone mass. Osteoblasts produce bone; osteoclasts resorb bone, particularly in subchondral region. Up to this stage, condition is potential Legg-Calvé-Perthes disease

Subchondral fracture and second ischemic episode
If shearing forces on femoral head exceed strength of weakened subchondral bone, fracture of variable extent may occur. This marks clinical onset of true Legg-Calvé-Perthes disease. Collapse of trabeculae underlying fracture occludes new capillaries, and bone resorption occurs. Reossification and healing take place with good or poor functional result

Environmental Factors. Although the effect of environment on the incidence is not clear, a large number of affected children in England are from lower socioeconomic groups. Whether this reflects dietary or environmental influences or a combination is not clear.

Etiology and Pathogenesis

The etiology of Legg-Calvé-Perthes disease is not yet understood, but it is accepted that the avascular necrosis is due to an interruption of the blood supply to the epiphysis of the femoral head, especially the contributions from the superior and inferior retinacular arteries. Current etiologic theories include trauma to the retinacular vessels, vascular occlusion secondary to increased intracapsular pressure from acute transient synovitis, venous obstruction with secondary intraepiphyseal thrombosis, vascular irregularities (congenital or developmental), and increased blood viscosity resulting in stasis and decreased blood flow.

While the cause remains unclear, numerous studies have delineated the pathogenesis of Legg-Calvé-Perthes disease. Initially, an ischemic episode of unknown etiology occurs, rendering most, if not all, of the epiphysis avascular (Plate 57). Endochondral ossification in the preosseous epiphyseal cartilage and growth plate ceases temporarily, while the articular cartilage,

Physical Examination in Legg-Calvé-Perthes Disease

Legg-Calvé-Perthes Disease
(Continued)

Limitation of internal rotation of left hip. Hip rotation best assessed with patient in prone position because any restriction can be detected and measured easily

15°

Thomas' sign
Hip flexion contracture determined with patient supine. Unaffected hip flexed only until lumbar spine is flat against examining table. Affected hip cannot be fully extended, and angle of flexion is recorded. 15° flexion contracture of hip is typical of Legg-Calvé-Perthes disease

Trendelenburg's test
Left: patient demonstrates negative Trendelenburg's test of normal right hip. Right: positive test of involved left hip. When weight is on affected side, normal hip drops, indicating weakness of left gluteus medius muscle. Trunk shifts left as patient attempts to decrease biomechanical stresses across involved hip and thereby maintain balance

which is nourished by synovial fluid, continues to grow. This results in the radiographic appearance of a widened medial cartilage (joint) space and a smaller ossification center in the involved hip. This is the first radiographic manifestation, and it precedes any change in the density of the epiphysis. At this stage, the marrow space of the epiphysis is necrotic.

Revascularization of the structurally intact but avascular epiphysis occurs from the periphery as new capillaries recanalize the previous vascular channels. Resumption of endochondral ossification within the epiphysis begins peripherally and progresses centrally. With the ingrowth of capillaries, osteoclasts and osteoblasts cover the surface of the avascular subchondral cortical bone and the central trabecular bone. New bone is deposited on the avascular bone, producing a net increase in bone mass per unit area; this accounts for the increased density of the epiphysis that is apparent on radiographs taken in early stages of the disease.

The deposition of new trabecular bone and resorption of avascular bone occur simultaneously. In the subchondral area, bone resorption exceeds new bone formation. A critical point is reached during resorption when the subchondral area becomes biomechanically weak and therefore susceptible to a pathologic fracture. Up to this point, the disease process is clinically silent and asymptomatic. The continuation of this "potential" form of Legg-Calvé-Perthes disease or the development of the "true" form depends on whether or not a subchondral fracture occurs.

In the *potential form* of the disease, a subchondral fracture does not occur because the stresses and shearing forces acting on the revascularized epiphysis of the femoral head do not exceed the strength of the weakened subchondral area. The reossification process continues uninterrupted, with ultimate resumption of normal growth and development. Thus, there is no epiphyseal resorption, no extrusion or subluxation of the femoral head, and no potential for deformity. The child remains asymptomatic and retains a good range of motion in the hip joint. The subchondral area eventually regains its normal strength and stability, and a "head-within-a-head" is visible on radiographs. The head-within-a-head represents a growth arrest line that outlines the ossification center at the time of the initial infarction.

In the *true form* of the disease, the strength of the weakened subchondral area is exceeded, and

a pathologic subchondral fracture occurs (Plate 57). The magnitude of stress or trauma necessary to produce such a fracture is difficult to quantitate and appears to vary both with the degree of preexisting weakness and the applied shearing forces. In most cases, the fracture seems to result from normal vigorous activity rather than from a specific injury. The painful subchondral fracture heralds the clinical onset of true Legg-Calvé-Perthes disease, and only the true form produces the typical clinical and radiographic features and requires 2 to 4 years, or even longer, for complete healing to occur.

Changes in Epiphysis. The subchondral fracture characteristically begins in the anterolateral

aspect of the epiphysis near the growth plate, because this area receives the greatest concentration of stress during weight bearing. The pathologic fracture extends superiorly and posteriorly until it reaches areas where the strength of the remaining subchondral bone exceeds the shearing forces acting on the femoral head. There is minimal, if any, extension of the subchondral fracture after the initial fracture. The reasons for this are not clear, but presumably the resulting pain causes the child to be less active, thereby reducing the stress on the femoral head.

The revascularized trabecular bone beneath the subchondral fracture undergoes a second episode of local ischemia secondary to trabecular collapse

Legg-Calvé-Perthes Disease
(Continued)

"Roll" test for muscle spasm. Patient relaxed and supine on table. Examiner places hands on limb, gently rolls hip into internal and external rotation, noting resistance

and occlusion of the ingrowing capillaries. This second ischemic episode, mechanical in origin, involves either part or all of the epiphysis, depending on the extent of the subchondral fracture. The structural stability of the epiphysis is lost; the ingrowth of new capillaries is impeded by the obliteration of the vascular channels and the presence of fractured bone (both cortical and trabecular) and marrow debris. Consequently, the entire area is slowly revascularized, with resorption of the fibroosseous tissue, by a process termed "creeping substitution." In this reparative process, the avascular bone is slowly resorbed from the periphery of the area of the second infarction and replaced by vascular fibrous tissue that, in turn, is eventually replaced by primary trabecular bone.

During the process of creeping substitution, the femoral head, while not soft in the physical sense, can be molded into a round or flat shape by the forces acting on it. This remodeling property, or biologic plasticity, lasts until subchondral reossification begins. Potential deformities may be caused by the different rates of growth within the femoral head—areas not undergoing resorption grow faster than the involved area. The combined factors of pressure and asymmetric growth result in a potential for extrusion and subluxation of the femoral head and eventual deformity. Thus, true Legg-Calvé-Perthes disease is actually a complication of avascular necrosis.

Secondary alterations in the growth plate and metaphysis also occur and can lead to further disturbances in endochondral ossification and growth in the proximal femur.

Changes in Growth Plate. Since the blood supply to the growth plate comes from the epiphyseal side, the two ischemic episodes also produce ischemic changes in the growth plate. The chondrocyte columns become distorted with some loss of their cellular components; they do not undergo normal ossification, which results in an excess of calcified cartilage in the primary trabecular bone.

Changes in Metaphysis. Four types of metaphyseal changes have been noted: presence of adipose tissue, osteolytic lesions (well-circumscribed areas of fibrocartilage), disorganized ossification, and extrusion of the growth plate. While only adipose tissue changes are detected early in the disease, osteolytic lesions are seen in the later stages. When these fibrocartilaginous lesions are in contact with the growth plate, the normal

Determination of atrophy of proximal thigh. Circumference of each upper thigh measured at most proximal level, and difference noted

Test for limitation of abduction. Patient supine and relaxed on table. Legs gently and passively abducted to determine range of motion of each

architecture of the growth plate is lost, and the lesions appear on radiographs as cysts. In the areas without osteolytic lesions, ossification is disorganized, and bars, or columns, of unossified cartilage appear to "stream" or "flow" down into the metaphysis. Necrosis of bone is not seen in the metaphysis. In some severely deformed femoral heads, the growth plate extrudes down the sides of the femoral neck.

The changes in the growth plate and metaphysis ultimately alter the growth in length of the proximal femur and produce the short, thick femoral neck (coxa vara) and enlarged femoral head (coxa magna) typically seen in Legg-Calvé-Perthes disease. The greater trochanter, being

uninvolved, continues to grow and may eventually rise above the level of the femoral head. The combination of a short femoral neck and a high greater trochanter is considered "functional" coxa vara. The performance of the hip abductor (gluteus medius) muscles is disturbed, with a resultant limp or Trendelenburg gait and a positive Trendelenburg test (Plate 58). The short femoral neck also produces a lower limb–length discrepancy of 1 to 2 cm.

Clinical Manifestations

The pertinent early findings include antalgic gait, muscle spasm and restricted hip motion, atrophy of the proximal thigh, and short stature.

Legg-Calvé-Perthes Disease
(Continued)

A small percentage of children have a history of trauma, usually mild. Nevertheless, such trauma may be sufficient to produce the pathologic subchondral fracture.

Initial symptoms are mild and intermittent pain in the anterior thigh or a limp, or both. Although many children do not complain of pain, on close questioning, most admit to mild pain either in the anterior thigh or the knee. The onset of pain may be acute or insidious. Referred pain from the hip to the anterior thigh or knee must be considered. Because the child's initial symptoms are typically mild, parents frequently do not seek medical attention for several weeks after clinical onset, or longer.

Antalgic gait is noted when the patient shortens the time of weight bearing on the involved limb during walking in order to reduce discomfort. Pain from the irritable hip can also cause reflex inhibition of the hip abductor muscles with a resultant positive Trendelenburg test, a common early sign (Plate 58).

Muscle spasm is best detected by the "roll" test, a painless test that reveals any guarding or muscle spasm (secondary to irritability of the hip joint), especially when the involved limb is rolled inward (Plate 59). Once the child's confidence is gained, the hip can usually be examined more thoroughly to determine the complete range of motion. Mild limitation of motion, particularly abduction and internal rotation, is the typical finding. There may also be limitation of extension, as evidenced by a mild hip flexion contracture (Thomas' sign), as well as deep tenderness over the anterior aspect of the hip.

Disuse atrophy of the proximal thigh muscles is a consequence of prolonged hip irritability and the resultant limitation of motion. The atrophic thigh is usually 2 to 3 cm smaller, especially during the early symptomatic phases. As the symptoms subside, the atrophy resolves.

Short stature due to delayed bone age is another typical finding in affected children. The patient's bone age can be determined with the Greulich and Pyle atlas.

Results of laboratory tests are normal, except for an occasionally abnormal erythrocyte sedimentation rate, which may be slightly elevated (30 to 40 mm/hr).

Radiographic Evaluation

Routine radiographic assessment is essential for diagnosis and for determining progression of

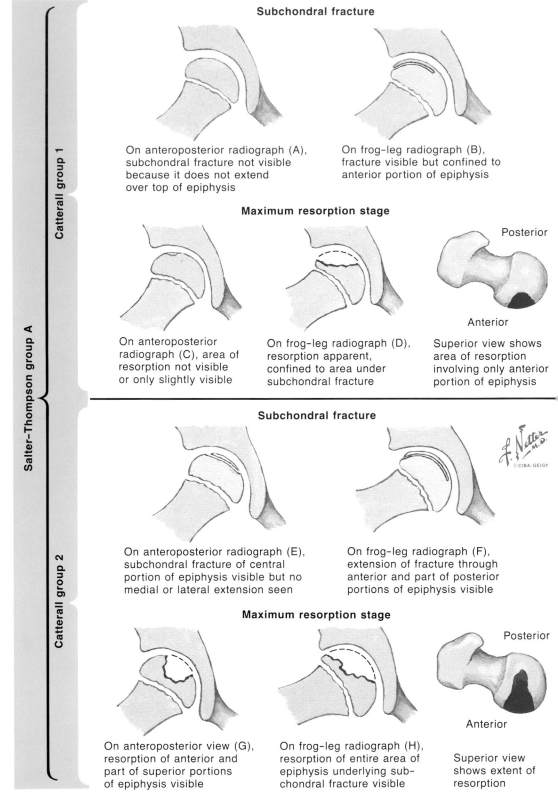

Subchondral fracture

On anteroposterior radiograph (A), subchondral fracture not visible because it does not extend over top of epiphysis

On frog-leg radiograph (B), fracture visible but confined to anterior portion of epiphysis

Maximum resorption stage

On anteroposterior radiograph (C), area of resorption not visible or only slightly visible

On frog-leg radiograph (D), resorption apparent, confined to area under subchondral fracture

Posterior

Anterior

Superior view shows area of resorption involving only anterior portion of epiphysis

Subchondral fracture

On anteroposterior radiograph (E), subchondral fracture of central portion of epiphysis visible but no medial or lateral extension seen

On frog-leg radiograph (F), extension of fracture through anterior and part of posterior portions of epiphysis visible

Maximum resorption stage

On anteroposterior view (G), resorption of anterior and part of superior portions of epiphysis visible

On frog-leg radiograph (H), resorption of entire area of epiphysis underlying subchondral fracture visible

Posterior

Anterior

Superior view shows extent of resorption

Catterall group 1

Salter-Thompson group A

Catterall group 2

the disease, sphericity of the femoral head, possibility of epiphyseal extrusion or collapse, and response to treatment. Useful adjuncts are procedures such as arthrography, radionuclide bone scans, and magnetic resonance imaging (MRI).

The entire disease process can usually be assessed from plain anteroposterior and Lauenstein frog-leg radiographs of the pelvis (both hips). Extrusion and subluxation of the femoral head can be measured on these radiographs using the Wiberg center-edge angle or the Salter extrusion angle. An extrusion index developed by Green and associates has been demonstrated to be prognostically significant. Sphericity of the femoral head in the reossification and healed

stages is currently best determined by the Mose circle criteria. In this technique, a transparent template with concentric circles at 2-mm intervals, placed on both anteroposterior and frog-leg radiographs, is centered over the femoral head to measure both the sphericity and diameter of the femoral head. If the sphericity is equal in both projections, the hip is rated "good." A variance of up to 2 mm is rated "fair," while a variance of 3 mm or more is rated "poor." The good and fair ratings are considered satisfactory results while poor ratings are unsatisfactory. Sphericity may improve with growth and development if the healed femoral head remains well contained in the acetabulum.

and Corresponding Radiographs

Subchondral fracture

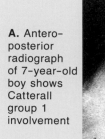
A. Anteroposterior radiograph of 7-year-old boy shows Catterall group 1 involvement

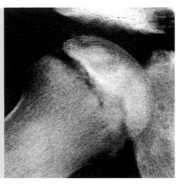
B. Frog-leg radiograph

Maximum resorption stage

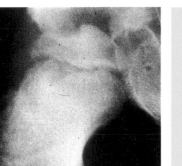
C. Anteroposterior radiograph, 7 months later

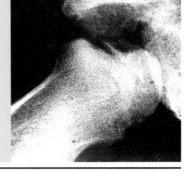
D. Frog-leg radiograph

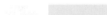
Subchondral fracture

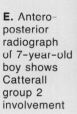
E. Anteroposterior radiograph of 7-year-old boy shows Catterall group 2 involvement

F. Frog leg radiograph

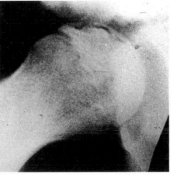

Maximum resorption stage

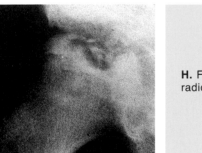
G. Anteroposterior radiograph, 6 months later

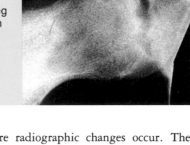
H. Frog-leg radiograph

Computerized methods are currently being investigated to allow better objective quantification of hip joint architecture and for plotting changes in configuration that occur with time.

Early in the resorption stage, arthrography may be required to assess the sphericity of the articular surface of the femoral head. The contour of the partially resorbed ossification center of the epiphysis may not reflect the contour of the articular surface, and range of motion in the hip is usually the best indicator of potential femoral head deformity. Only "questionable" hips require arthrography.

Technetium bone scans are frequently used to detect the potential form of Legg-Calvé-Perthes disease before radiographic changes occur. The absence of radioisotope uptake in the femoral head accurately indicates avascular necrosis, but there is a poor correlation with the extent of epiphyseal involvement.

Magnetic resonance imaging is helpful in defining epiphyseal infarction and the contours of the femoral head, both of which are prognostically significant. Like radionuclide bone scans, MRI does not correlate with the extent of epiphyseal involvement.

Stages of Disease

Radiographic evaluation has determined five distinct stages of Legg-Calvé-Perthes disease, which represent a continuum of the disease process.

Growth Arrest. This stage occurs immediately after the initial ischemic episode in the femoral head, when endochondral ossification of the preosseous cartilage ceases. During this avascular phase, which may last 6 to 12 months, there is a slight but progressive difference in the size (height and width) of the involved epiphysis and that of the opposite normal hip. The joint space also appears to be wider because of the continued growth of the articular cartilage. These relatively small differences (1–3 mm) are visible and measurable on an anteroposterior radiograph of the pelvis. Toward the end of this stage, epiphyseal density increases. During this stage, which is only potential Legg-Calvé-Perthes disease, the disease is clinically silent and asymptomatic.

Subchondral Fracture. The subchondral fracture initiates true Legg-Calvé-Perthes disease. Radiographic visibility of the fracture varies with the age of the patient at clinical onset and the extent of epiphyseal involvement. The duration varies from an average of 3 months in children 4 years of age or younger to 8½ months in children 10 years or older. It also varies from 4 months in Catterall group 1 to almost 6 months in group 4 (Plates 60–61).

Resorption. In this stage, also called fragmentation or necrosis, the necrotic bone beneath the subchondral fracture is gradually and irregularly resorbed. This process produces the radiographic appearance of fragmentation because the bone is resorbed and replaced by vascular fibrous tissue (creeping substitution) and later by primary bone. The resorption phase lasts 6 to 12 months and is longest when there is extensive epiphyseal involvement or when the child is 10 years of age or older at clinical onset. This phase is usually complete 12 to 17 months after clinical onset.

Reossification. During the healing, or reossification, stage, ossification of the primary bone begins irregularly in the subchondral area and progresses centrally. Eventually, the newly formed areas of bone coalesce, and the epiphysis progressively regains its normal strength. Reossification takes 6 to 24 months.

Healed Stage. The healed, or residual, stage signals the complete ossification of the epiphysis of the femoral head, with or without residual deformity.

Legg-Calvé-Perthes Disease
(*Continued*)

Classification

Catterall Classification. In 1971, Catterall described a four-group classification system based on the radiographic appearance of the femoral head at the time of maximum epiphyseal resorption (Plates 60–61). This classification has been extremely helpful in retrospective analyses of the results of treatment or healing. However, its prognostic value is limited because it is difficult to apply in the early stages of the disease.

The major radiographic feature of *Catterall group 1* is the subchondral fracture limited to the anterior portion of the epiphysis (Plate 60). The subchondral fracture is not visible on the anteroposterior radiograph because it does not extend over the superior portion of the epiphysis and therefore is not visualized tangentially. On the anteroposterior radiograph, the epiphysis appears smaller on the involved side; occasionally, slight irregularities of density are also seen in the central portion. The frog-leg radiograph shows the subchondral fracture confined to the anterior portion of the epiphysis.

In the maximum resorption stage, only the portion of the epiphysis beneath the subchondral fracture is resorbed; the medial, lateral, and posterior aspects of the epiphysis are preserved. The prognosis for patients with group 1 involvement is excellent, because healing occurs without loss of femoral head sphericity and with no residual sequelae.

The major radiographic characteristic of *Catterall group 2* is the intact lateral margin of the epiphysis (Plate 60). The subchondral fracture is visible on the anteroposterior radiograph because the disease process extends over the superior portion of the epiphysis and into the posterior aspect. However, the fracture is confined centrally and does not involve the medial or lateral margins of the epiphysis.

The frog-leg radiograph shows the fracture extending through the anterior portion and, to a variable degree, into the posterior aspect. At maximum resorption, the medial and lateral aspects and a portion of the posterior epiphysis are preserved. The prognosis for group 2 involvement remains quite good because the lateral margin of the epiphysis is intact, minimizing the risk of epiphyseal collapse and deformity.

The major radiographic feature of *Catterall group 3* is involvement of the lateral margin of the epiphysis; only the posterior and medial

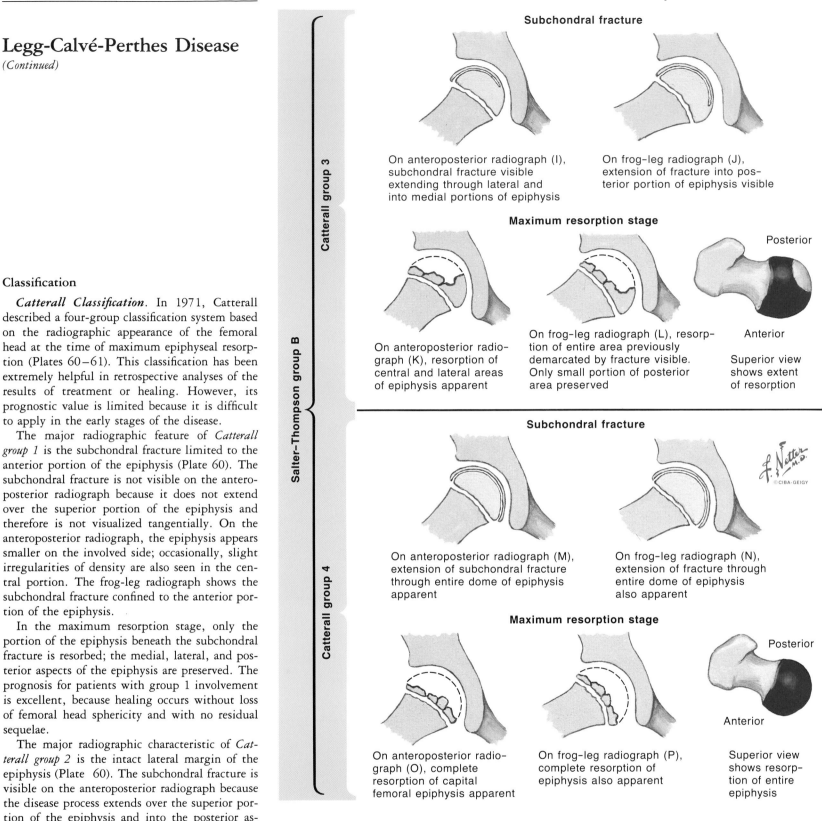

Subchondral fracture

On anteroposterior radiograph (I), subchondral fracture visible extending through lateral and into medial portions of epiphysis

On frog-leg radiograph (J), extension of fracture into posterior portion of epiphysis visible

Maximum resorption stage

On anteroposterior radiograph (K), resorption of central and lateral areas of epiphysis apparent

On frog-leg radiograph (L), resorption of entire area previously demarcated by fracture visible. Only small portion of posterior area preserved

Posterior

Anterior

Superior view shows extent of resorption

Catterall group 3

Salter-Thompson group B

Subchondral fracture

On anteroposterior radiograph (M), extension of subchondral fracture through entire dome of epiphysis apparent

On frog-leg radiograph (N), extension of fracture through entire dome of epiphysis also apparent

Maximum resorption stage

On anteroposterior radiograph (O), complete resorption of capital femoral epiphysis apparent

On frog-leg radiograph (P), complete resorption of epiphysis also apparent

Posterior

Anterior

Superior view shows resorption of entire epiphysis

Catterall group 4

aspects are preserved at maximum resorption (Plate 61). On the anteroposterior view, the subchondral fracture is seen to extend through the lateral portion of the epiphysis and involve a significant portion of the medial aspect. The frog-leg radiograph shows that the anterior and most of the posterior aspects are involved. However, in all cases, a viable posteromedial segment of variable size is preserved at maximum resorption. Loss of the lateral margin increases the risk of collapse and deformity. Consequently, the prognosis is less favorable than for groups 1 and 2.

The major radiographic feature of *Catterall group 4* is "whole head" involvement. Both anteroposterior and frog-leg radiographs show the subchondral fracture extending throughout the entire subchondral area. At maximum resorption, the entire epiphysis is resorbed with no viable portion remaining. Thus, there is a significant risk of epiphyseal collapse and deformity. Frequently, the growth plate is severely damaged, further increasing the risk of significant residual deformity.

Salter-Thompson Classification. In 1984, Salter and Thompson compared the long-term results of three forms of management—observation, noncontainment methods, and containment techniques—reported in other studies of 778 children with Legg-Calvé-Perthes disease. No statistical difference was found between Catterall

Subchondral fracture

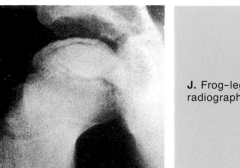
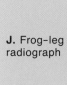

I. Anteroposterior radiograph of 7-year-old boy shows Catterall group 3 involvement

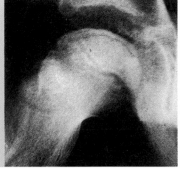

J. Frog-leg radiograph

Maximum resorption stage

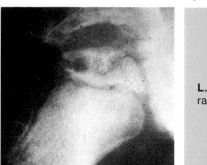

K. Anteroposterior radiograph, 8 months later

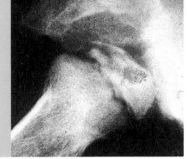

L. Frog-leg radiograph

Subchondral fracture

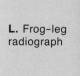

M. Anteroposterior radiograph of 8-year-old boy shows Catterall group 4 involvement

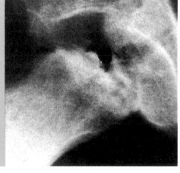

N. Frog-leg radiograph

Maximum resorption stage

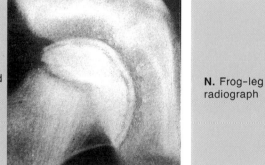

O. Anteroposterior radiograph, 8 months later

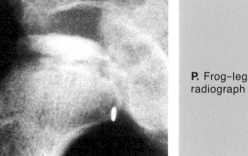

P. Frog-leg radiograph

groups 1 and 2 and only a slight difference was observed between Catterall groups 3 and 4. The greatest statistical correlation was between groups 2 and 3, leading to the development of a simplified, two-group classification. In *Salter-Thompson group A* (Catterall groups 1 and 2), less than one-half of the epiphysis is involved, and in *Salter-Thompson group B* (Catterall groups 3 and 4), more than one-half of the epiphysis is involved (Plates 60–61).

In the Salter-Thompson classification system, the determining factor is the presence (group A) or absence (group B) of an intact and viable lateral margin of the epiphysis. When present, the margin acts as a supporting column that shields

the epiphysis from stress and minimizes the possibility of collapse and subsequent deformity.

The Salter and Thompson analysis revealed that group A involvement rarely required active intervention. With or without treatment, satisfactory results were seen in 96% of patients with group A involvement. In contrast, satisfactory long-term results were seen in only 53% of untreated patients with group B involvement.

The Salter-Thompson classification simplifies the radiographic criteria and permits early diagnosis of the extent of epiphyseal involvement. It provides an accurate method for determining the prognosis and appropriate indications for treatment.

Prognosis

The short-term prognosis for patients with Legg-Calvé-Perthes disease focuses on femoral head deformity at the completion of the healing stage. The long-term prognosis involves the potential for secondary osteoarthritis of the hip in adulthood.

Deformity of Femoral Head. The ultimate goal of treatment is a spheric femoral head at the completion of growth. Six factors determine the potential for femoral head deformity.

(1) Sex of patient. In general, the outcome is less favorable in girls than in boys. Involvement of the femoral head is often more extensive in girls, and because they mature earlier than boys, there is less remaining skeletal growth from the time of clinical onset and consequently less opportunity for epiphyseal remodeling.

(2) Age at clinical onset. The older the child at clinical onset the less favorable the prognosis, particularly in children 10 years of age and older. This may also be related to the reduced remaining skeletal growth and potential for femoral head remodeling in older children.

(3) Extent of epiphyseal involvement. More extensive involvement is correlated with a poorer prognosis.

(4) Containment of femoral head. Extrusion, subluxation, or asymmetric growth of the femoral head increases the stress concentrated on it during weight bearing. The ability to maintain the femoral head well within the acetabulum with appropriate treatment is a significant factor for a favorable prognosis.

(5) Persistent loss of motion. This is usually due to either muscle spasm (adductors or iliopsoas muscle), muscle contractures, anterolateral extrusion or subluxation of the femoral head, or a combination thereof. The loss of motion prevents adequate remodeling of the femoral head by the acetabulum.

(6) Premature closure of the growth plate. When involvement of the epiphysis is extensive (Catterall group 4 or Salter-Thompson group B), the growth plate may be sufficiently damaged to cause premature closure. This can result in asymmetric growth and inadequate remodeling that contributes to femoral head deformity, greater trochanteric overgrowth (functional coxa vara), and a lower limb–length discrepancy.

Late Degenerative Osteoarthritis. The incidence of late degenerative osteoarthritis depends on residual deformity of the femoral head and the patient's age at clinical onset. The risk is directly correlated with the extent of residual deformity.

Conservative Management in Legg-Calvé-Perthes Disease

Legg-Calvé-Perthes Disease
(Continued)

"Slings and springs"
8-year-old girl with Salter-Thompson group A involvement. Following elimination of hip irritability, range-of-motion exercises instituted to restore function

Petrie cast
5-year-old boy with group A involvement. Radiograph of right hip shows adequate coverage of femoral head (lateral margin inside perpendicular line through lateral margin of acetabulum)

Toronto brace
Allows child to sit with knees flexed. However, compliance better with Petrie cast because cast cannot be removed by patient

Three types of congruency between the femoral head and the acetabulum have been classified: spheric congruency, aspheric congruency, and aspheric incongruency. Spheric congruency is not associated with osteoarthritis, whereas aspheric congruency predisposes to mild-to-moderate osteoarthritis in late adulthood. Patients with aspheric incongruency usually develop degenerative osteoarthritis before age 50.

Studies also show that the incidence of osteoarthritis of the hip in adults with deformed femoral heads is negligible in patients 5 years of age or younger at the time of clinical onset, 38% in patients 6 to 9 years of age, and 100% in patients 10 years of age or older. Aspheric incongruency, a predisposing factor for osteoarthritis, is also more likely to develop in children who are older at the time of clinical onset.

Thus, of the two significant factors in the long-term prognosis, only femoral head deformity may be preventable, or at least altered, by appropriate treatment.

Treatment

The only justification for treatment is prevention of femoral head deformity and secondary osteoarthritis. When indicated, treatment should interfere as little as possible with the child's psychologic and physical development.

The four basic goals of treatment are to eliminate hip irritability, restore and maintain a good range of hip motion, prevent femoral head extrusion and subluxation, and attain a spheric femoral head on healing.

Elimination of Hip Irritability. Following the subchondral fracture, the synovium becomes inflamed and the hip irritable. The associated pain and muscle spasm lead to the restriction of motion followed by muscle contractures, especially of the adductor and iliopsoas muscles, and possible anterolateral extrusion or subluxation of the femoral head. Elimination of this irritability is always the first objective and is usually accomplished by strict bed rest for 1 to 2 weeks, usually in the hospital. Balanced suspension with thigh and calf slings supported by springs ("slings and springs") or counterweights may assist mobility in bed (Plate 62).

Restoration and Maintenance of Motion. Generally, satisfactory range of motion in the hip returns as the hip irritability is eliminated, although residual stiffness may persist in some children. Physical therapy with passive and active range-of-motion exercises helps to restore motion, but gentle progressive-abduction traction, especially at night, is occasionally required. To maintain hip motion, a program consisting of abduction exercises may be helpful.

Regardless of the sphericity of the femoral head, almost all children with Catterall groups 3 and 4 (Salter-Thompson group B) involvement show a slight but persistent loss of abduction and internal rotation due to mild coxa magna.

Prevention of Femoral Head Collapse. Extrusion or subluxation of the femoral head increases the risk of epiphyseal collapse and subsequent deformity. Radiographic evidence of extrusion is therefore a prognostic factor and an indication for treatment.

Attainment of Spheric Femoral Head. This goal requires a full understanding of the pathogenesis and prognostic factors associated with deformity of the femoral head as well as the appropriate management techniques.

Concepts of Containment

Until the 1960s, treatment for Legg-Calvé-Perthes disease was complete and prolonged bed

Legg-Calvé-Perthes Disease
(Continued)

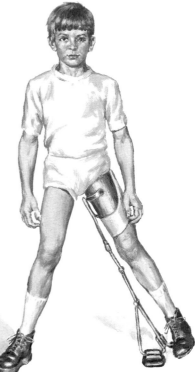

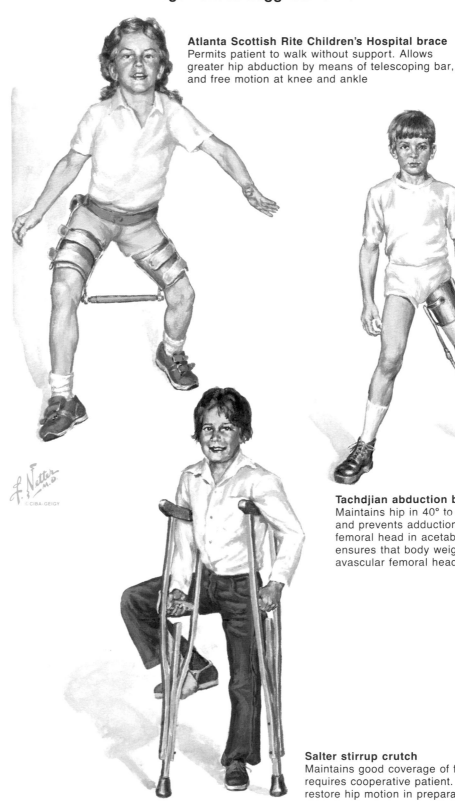

Atlanta Scottish Rite Children's Hospital brace
Permits patient to walk without support. Allows greater hip abduction by means of telescoping bar, and free motion at knee and ankle

Tachdjian abduction brace
Maintains hip in 40° to 45° abduction and prevents adduction, thus keeping femoral head in acetabulum. Also ensures that body weight is kept off avascular femoral head

Salter stirrup crutch
Maintains good coverage of femoral head but requires cooperative patient. Used chiefly to restore hip motion in preparation for surgery

rest—with or without traction or abduction of the involved limb—and the use of so-called weight-relieving devices. All children were treated, and treatment often lasted 2 to 4 years. Containment techniques have been devised to permit weight bearing while redirecting the compressive forces on the femoral head to assist in the healing and remodeling process. The currently accepted forms of management range from observation to surgery.

Observation. Appropriate treatment of all children who are less than 6 years of age at clinical onset regardless of the extent of epiphyseal involvement is by observation only, provided there is no limitation of hip motion and no subluxation. Observation is also appropriate for children 6 years of age or older with Catterall groups 1 and 2 (Salter-Thompson group A) involvement who have a good range of hip motion and no radiographic evidence of femoral head extrusion or collapse.

Intermittent Symptomatic Treatment. Temporary or periodic bed rest and abduction stretching exercises can be used in conjunction with observation. Hip irritability with a temporary decrease in motion often recurs during the subchondral fracture and resorption phases. If these symptoms persist and there is no radiographic evidence of femoral head extrusion, bed rest for 1 to 2 weeks, sometimes with abduction traction, may be necessary. Two or three recurrent episodes of irritability may indicate the need for a short period (2–3 months) of nonsurgical containment to decrease the risk of extrusion. Radiographs should be taken at 2- to 4-month intervals to ensure that the irritability is not due to early deformity of the femoral head.

Definitive Early Treatment. Nonsurgical or surgical containment of the femoral head early in the disease is indicated in children 6 years of age or older at clinical onset—possibly in girls 5 years of age or older—who have Catterall group 3 or 4 (Salter-Thompson group B) involvement, or when femoral head extrusion is seen on the weight-bearing anteroposterior radiograph.

Use of containment techniques requires a good-to-full range of hip motion (especially abduction), no residual irritability, and a round

or almost round femoral head. Containment methods, whether nonsurgical or surgical, appear to increase satisfactory results (Mose good and fair) by approximately 16% to 20% compared to no treatment or natural history.

Nonsurgical containment refers to the use of abduction casts, braces, and the Salter stirrup crutch to abduct the involved limb and redirect the femoral head within the acetabulum (Plates 62–63). This treatment can usually be limited to a period of 18 months or less with no adverse effect on the outcome. Nonsurgical containment for Catterall groups 3 and 4 or Salter-Thompson group B has produced good results in 72% to 90% of patients.

The Petrie cast fixes the lower limbs in 30° to 40° abduction with an approximate 5° internal rotation (Plate 62). The cast provides continuous containment since it cannot be removed by either the child or the parents. Disadvantages include stiffness of the knee and ankle joints with adaptive articular changes, significant restriction in ambulation, frequent need for change and repair, and excessive weight. Petrie casts are now reserved for management following surgical muscle release and capsulotomy.

Abduction braces are lighter and less cumbersome than casts, but they are quite expensive. Also, because they are removable, compliance may not be consistent. The Atlanta Scottish Rite

Legg-Calvé-Perthes Disease
(Continued)

Femoral Varus Derotational Osteotomy

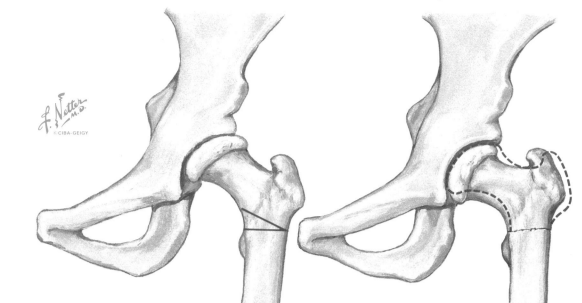

Preoperative view
Femoral head flattened and subluxated, protruding well outside lateral margin of acetabulum. Red lines indicate proposed osteotomy and wedge of bone to be resected

Postoperative view
Resection of bone wedge has abducted neck and head of femur so that epiphysis is well covered within acetabulum. Broken red line indicates original position. Procedure accentuates limb–length discrepancy

Children's Hospital brace provides containment solely by abduction of the hips without internal rotation and is the brace of choice (Plate 63). The child can walk without external support and has a crouched posture with slight flexion at the hips and knees. The hip flexion actually increases coverage over the anterior aspect of the femoral head. This device is well tolerated by patients and parents alike.

The Salter stirrup crutch, a temporary nonsurgical containment device, provides superior, lateral, and anterior coverage of the femoral head and allows the child to sit comfortably at a desk and sleep unencumbered. This device requires extremely cooperative patients and parents and can be used only in patients with unilateral involvement.

Surgical containment has three major advantages: (1) the period of restriction is less than 2 months, after which the child may gradually return to full activity; (2) the femoral head containment is permanent; and (3) the permanent improvement in containment continues to enhance remodeling of the healed femoral head long after the active phase of disease is over. Surgery does not alter the length of the disease process or provide a cure, but it does provide satisfactory results in the great majority of patients.

Treatment with femoral varus derotational osteotomy usually involves a varus angulation of the proximal femur, with or without rotation, to redirect the femoral head into the acetabulum (Plate 64). The varus angulation should be no greater than 110° but should allow containment of the epiphysis of the femoral head within a vertical line drawn on the radiograph at the lateral margin of the acetabulum (Perkins' line); some surgeons also recommend 10° to 15° internal rotation of the proximal segment. The osteotomy is usually held securely with threaded screws and a side plate or blade plate. Femoral osteotomy, while a technically less demanding procedure than innominate osteotomy, produces some inherent problems, mainly the increase in lower limb–length discrepancy, potential coxa vara, and Trendelenburg gait. In addition, the metal fixation device is difficult to remove, and there is a risk of fracture of the proximal femur through the screw holes. The limb shortening associated with femoral osteotomy usually resolves in

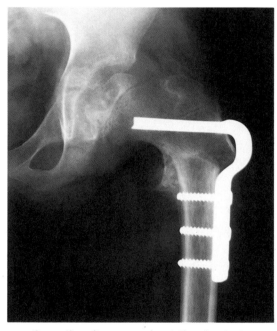

Anteroposterior radiograph of 8-year-old boy shows Catterall group 2 (Salter–Thompson group A) involvement in left hip. Subluxation with lateral margin of acetabulum directly over area of resorption. Lateral margin of femoral head no longer provides support

3 months after varus derotational osteotomy. Anteroposterior radiograph shows subluxation corrected; lateral margin of femoral head within acetabulum and again provides support

younger children and in patients who achieve satisfactory results.

In 1962, Salter began to treat older children with more severe forms of the disease with innominate osteotomy (Plate 65), which is a technically more difficult procedure than femoral osteotomy. However, its advantages include better anterior and lateral coverage of the femoral head, no further shortening of the femoral neck (coxa breva), no increase in limb-length discrepancy (it actually lengthens the lower limb by about 1 cm), and improvement of the Trendelenburg gait. Also, removal of fixation devices is easier, and there is no risk of fracture of the proximal femur.

Late Surgical Management for Deformity. If a significant deformity prevents reduction of the femoral head into the acetabulum or remodeling after treatment with standard containment methods, an alternative must be considered. Several surgical procedures at least partially correct the various existing deformities, thereby alleviating the associated symptoms.

If the healing femoral head is moderately flattened, an anteroposterior radiograph of the hip in extension and abduction reveals an extruded anterolateral portion of the head impinging on the anterolateral margin of the acetabulum. If the femoral head is still in the reossification phase, it is often possible to obtain sufficient abduction

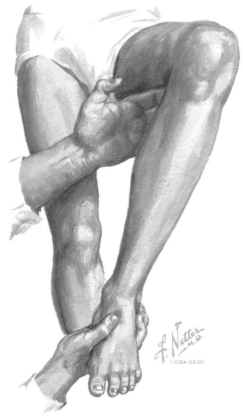

Best diagnostic sign in physical examination. With patient supine, as thigh is flexed it rolls into external rotation and abduction

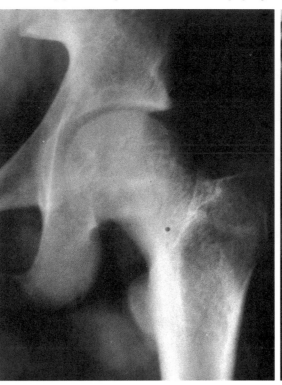

Slipped capital femoral epiphysis not readily apparent on anteroposterior radiograph because slip is usually posterior

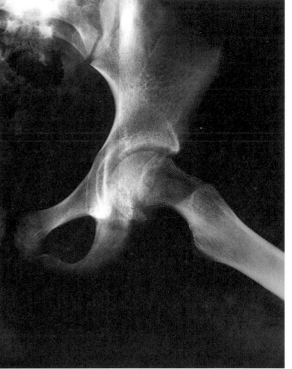

Frog-leg radiograph, which demonstrates slipped epiphysis more clearly, always indicated when disorder is suspected

SECTION I PLATE 66   Slide 4502

Slipped Capital Femoral Epiphysis

Slipped capital femoral epiphysis refers to the displacement of the epiphysis of the femoral head. It occurs most commonly in boys 10 to 17 years of age (average age at onset is 12 years). The initial examination reveals bilateral involvement in about one-third of patients, but patients with unilateral involvement have little risk of a subsequent slip on the contralateral side.

The etiology of slipped capital femoral epiphysis is unclear, although various traumatic, inflammatory, and endocrine factors have been proposed. For example, the position of the growth plate of the proximal femur normally changes from horizontal to oblique during preadolescence and adolescence. Thus, the weight increase that occurs during the adolescent growth spurt puts extra strain on the growth plate.

The disorder is often accompanied by rapid growth and is often associated with adiposogenital dystrophy, a condition characterized by obesity and deficient gonadal development. These findings suggest an endocrine basis for the skeletal problem. The major complications of slipped capital femoral epiphysis are avascular necrosis, chondrolysis, and later, degenerative osteoarthritis.

Clinical Manifestations

The severity and onset of symptoms reflect the three categories of slipped capital femoral epiphysis. Most common is the *chronic slip* (60% of cases), which causes persistent pain referable to the hip or distal medial thigh, and often as far as

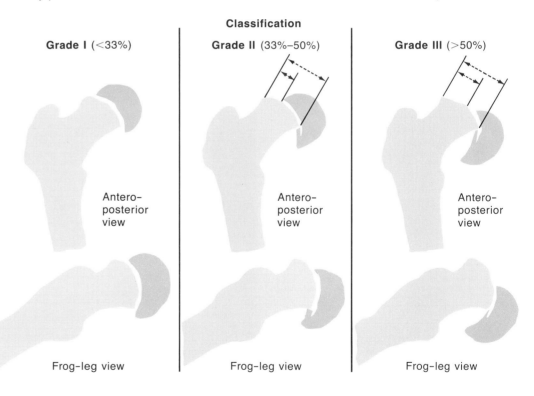

Classification

Grade I (<33%)

Anteroposterior view

Frog-leg view

Grade II (33%–50%)

Anteroposterior view

Frog-leg view

Grade III (>50%)

Anteroposterior view

Frog-leg view

the knee. In some patients, the pain is restricted to the area of the vastus medialis muscle, and the slip itself is overlooked. Limp, pain, and loss of hip motion are the other usual presenting manifestations. The most important diagnostic finding is the loss of internal rotation (Plate 66). This is easily detected on examination because, as the hip is flexed, it rolls into external rotation and abduction; restricted abduction becomes more pronounced as the slip increases.

An *acute slip* (11% of patients), which occurs following significant trauma, produces the sudden onset of pain severe enough to prevent weight bearing. Patients usually report minimal or no previous symptoms.

Patients with the third type, an *acute-on-chronic slip*, first experience a persistent aching in the hip, thigh, or knee and sometimes a limp that is the result of a chronic slip. Subsequent trauma—even a minor accident—causes an acute slip superimposed on the chronic slip. The acute slip is heralded by sudden, severe pain.

Chondrolysis, in which the articular cartilage degenerates and erodes and the capsule and synovial membrane become inflamed and fibrotic, usually develops during or after treatment. It may progress relentlessly until the joint space is nearly obliterated. This problematic complication is heralded by severe, continuous pain on hip motion and weight bearing.

Slipped Capital Femoral Epiphysis
(Continued)

Radiographic Findings

Slipped capital femoral epiphysis produces classic radiographic features. In the earliest stages, there is a widening of the epiphyseal line (representing the growth plate). An anteroposterior radiograph of a normal hip shows the epiphysis of the femoral head projecting above and lateral to the superior border of the femoral neck. A slip must be suspected if a straight line drawn up the lateral surface of the femoral neck does not touch the femoral head. Because the anteroposterior view does not always reveal the initial slip, which is usually posterior, a frog-leg radiograph is essential for the diagnosis.

A three-grade classification of slipped capital femoral epiphysis is helpful in the radiographic evaluation (Plate 66). Grade I refers to displacement of the epiphysis up to one-third the width of the femoral neck. Grade II represents a slip greater than one-third but less than one-half the width of the neck. Grade III includes slips of greater than one-half the width of the neck.

On radiographs, chondrolysis is seen as a progressive irregularity of the subchondral bone and rarefaction of both the acetabulum and the femoral head.

Treatment

The primary goals of treatment are to keep displacement to a minimum while maintaining a close-to-normal range of hip motion and to delay the onset of osteoarthritis.

Acute Slip. Gentle repositioning can reduce the deformity of an acute slip. Gradual reduction—preferably with hand traction—appears to be safer than acute manipulative reduction. Since full reduction may lead to avascular necrosis of the femoral head, which is a greater threat to the hip than incomplete reduction, the goal is to produce less than full correction. This is especially true if even part of the slip is chronic. In this case, the repositioning should reduce only the acute component. Manipulation should not be attempted for an acute slip that has been present for more than 2 weeks. Two or three threaded pins are inserted across the epiphyseal line to secure the reduction.

Chronic Slip. To stabilize the femoral head and maintain hip movement in patients with a chronic slip, bed rest and traction should be maintained before definitive treatment. These measures help reduce the risk of cartilage necrosis. If surgery is indicated, two pins are placed in the femoral neck and head via a lateral approach.

Incorrect placement of pins is the most common error in surgical management. Because of the minor but real risk of segmented avascular necrosis, the pins are placed to avoid the weight-bearing area of the femoral head. In a grade III slip, visible on both anteroposterior and frog-leg radiographs, the epiphysis and metaphysis overlap only 25% of the width of the femoral neck, leaving very little room for the pins to cross from the femoral neck to the head. Placement of the pins

Pin Fixation in Slipped Capital Femoral Epiphysis

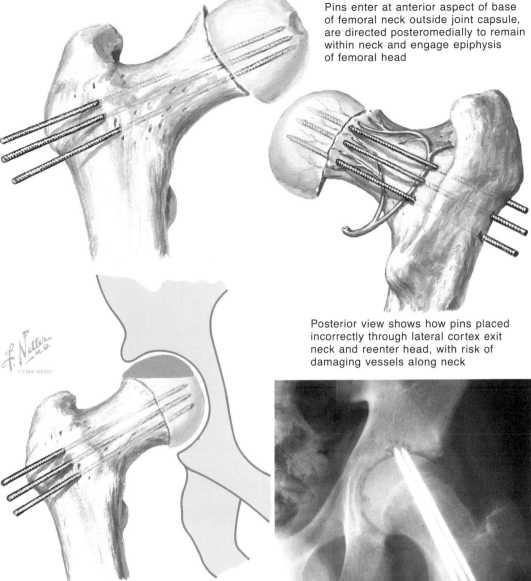

Pins enter at anterior aspect of base of femoral neck outside joint capsule, are directed posteromedially to remain within neck and engage epiphysis of femoral head

Posterior view shows how pins placed incorrectly through lateral cortex exit neck and reenter head, with risk of damaging vessels along neck

Pins must avoid weight-bearing area of femoral head (shown in darker blue shading)

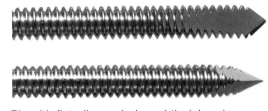

Pin with flat, diamond-shaped tip (above) difficult to remove after bone growth. Trocar-pointed pin (below) easier to remove

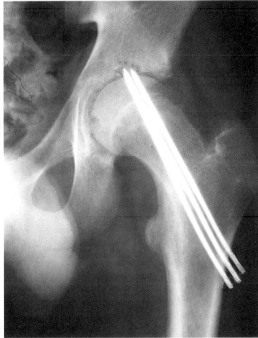

Radiograph shows pins crossing joint space, which may damage surface of acetabulum. Pin position must be checked on both anteroposterior and frog-leg radiographs

through the anterior aspect of the base of the neck and directing them posteromedially allows them to engage the head without leaving the bone (Plate 67). This technique is applicable to slips of any grade.

In an alternative method developed by Howorth, the hip joint is opened, a window is made in the femoral neck, and iliac bone grafts are placed across the epiphyseal line. This method (epiphysiodesis) stimulates early closure of the growth plate and eliminates the need for pin removal. If, after closure of the growth plate, a mechanical block to hip motion is noted, resection of the protruding anterosuperior aspect of the neck improves both abduction and internal rotation.

Pinning is the initial treatment of choice for all grades of slip. After closure of the growth plate, an intertrochanteric osteotomy may be performed if needed. Osteotomy of the femoral neck is never indicated, as it often leads to avascular necrosis.

Chondrolysis. Treatment comprises traction, range-of-motion exercises, and use of salicylates, which help decrease joint reaction and increase hip motion. After resolution, range-of-motion exercises and walking with a crutch should be continued for a prolonged period. After the initial loss of articular cartilage, there may be a gradual improvement in the joint space, and hip movement may improve slightly. □

Disorders of Patella

Bipartite Patella

Congenital fragmentation of the patella is relatively common. One type, bipartite patella, occurs in approximately 1% of the population (Plate 68). This anatomic variant represents a true synchondrosis (a joint whose surfaces are connected by a cartilaginous plate). Most fragmented patellae remain asymptomatic, but occasionally, direct trauma to the patella disrupts the synchondroses, causing symptoms that mimic those of a fracture.

A true fracture is differentiated from congenital bipartite patella on the basis of a history of significant trauma to the patella, hemarthrosis of the knee, point tenderness over the defect, and a sharply outlined fragment seen on the radiograph. In the absence of trauma and hemarthrosis, radiographic evidence of sclerotic smooth borders on the patellar fragments, especially if the lesions are bilateral, suggests the diagnosis of a congenital bipartite patella.

Conservative treatment, including immobilization followed by stretching and strengthening exercises for the quadriceps and hamstring muscles, is usually sufficient. If the fragment remains symptomatic, excision along with lateral retinacular release is appropriate treatment.

Patella Alta and Infera

The position of the patella can best be determined on the lateral radiograph with the knee flexed 30°. The length of the patellar ligament is usually equal to the diagonal length of the patella. Variations of more than 20% are considered abnormal.

Patella alta refers to an abnormally high patella in relation to the femur (Plate 68). Patella alta predisposes to patellar subluxation and dislocation with resultant inflammation of the patellofemoral joint (patellofemoral chondrosis).

Patella infera indicates an abnormally low patella. While it occurs most often secondary to soft-tissue contracture and hypotonia of the quadriceps muscle following surgery or trauma to the knee, it may also represent a congenital variant.

Congenital patella infera is frequently asymptomatic and requires no treatment. If this condition develops after injury or surgery, it can be catastrophic. Prompt recognition of the condition is of utmost importance because treatment in the early stages can reverse it. Vigorous rehabilitation of the quadriceps muscles and mobilization of soft-tissue structures around the knee should be instituted as soon as the complication is recognized. Lack of treatment can lead to significant long-term pain and stiffness around the knee.

Subluxation and Dislocation of Patella

The patella depends on both dynamic and static stabilizers to maintain its proper position in the intercondylar groove. While the entire quadriceps muscle contributes to the dynamic stability of the patella, the contribution of the vastus medialis muscle is critical. The distal oblique portion of this muscle resists lateral migration of the patella. The static patellar restraints, which include the

Disorders of Patella

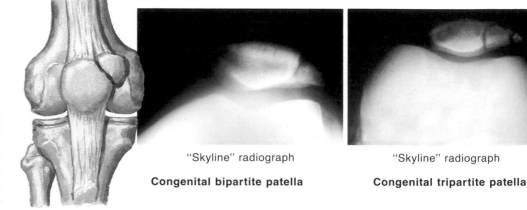

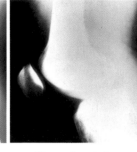
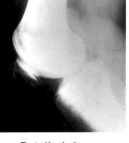

"Skyline" radiograph   "Skyline" radiograph
Congenital bipartite patella   **Congenital tripartite patella**

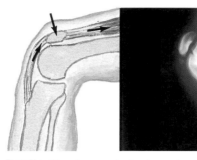
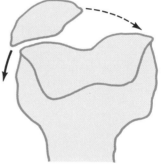
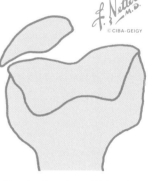

Patella alta. Arrows indicate vectors of force with resultant compression of patella against femoral condyles

Normal patella   **Patella infera**

Subluxation and dislocation of patella

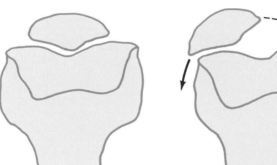

Patella normally glides in groove between femoral condyles (patellar surface)

Tension of lateral muscles and/or retinaculum plus weak vastus medialis muscle causes patella to deviate laterally

Poorly developed lateral condyle permits patella to move laterally ("tabletop" femur)

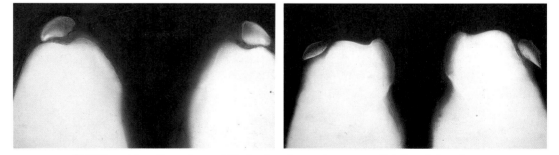

Patellar subluxation ◀── "Skyline" radiographs ──▶ Patellar dislocation

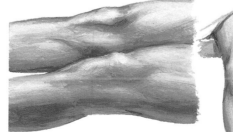
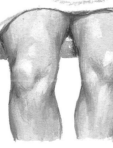

Deficiency of oblique portion of vastus medialis muscle evidenced by depression on medial side of right patella

"Owl-eye" (squinting) patellae face laterally

Fairbank's sign
Patella can be manually displaced laterally out of its groove

Disorders of Patella
(Continued)

bony contour of the distal femur, the joint capsule, the medial and lateral retinacula, and the medial patellofemoral ligament, are equally important. A flat lateral femoral condyle ("tabletop" femur) allows the patella to slide laterally quite easily, whereas a deep intercondylar groove generally keeps the triangular-shaped patella well located.

The medial patellofemoral ligament, a condensation of capsular fibers originating at the medial epicondyle, inserts on the superomedial aspect of the patella and helps resist lateral migration of the patella. The substance of this ligament varies from quite substantial (constituting a formidable checkrein to lateral displacement) to barely discernible.

Other factors affecting patellofemoral stability include the alignment of the femur and tibia in the frontal plane and rotation of the tibia in the axial plane. Increased valgus position of the limb or external rotation of the tibia enhances the lateral displacement forces on the patella.

Patellar subluxation is the partial loss of contact between the articular surfaces of the patella and femur (Plate 68). It is most common when the ligamentous support is loose and when the vastus medialis muscles are poorly developed or atrophied. Just as a weak medial quadriceps muscle permits lateral subluxation, tightness in the lateral peripatellar tissues can pull the patella laterally.

Patellar dislocation is the complete loss of contact between the articular surfaces of the patella and femur. Congenital dislocations are rare; most dislocations are traumatic. The degree of deficiency of the patellar stabilizers determines how much force is needed to cause the dislocation. Underdeveloped femoral condyles, insufficient soft-tissue restraints, and a weak vastus medialis muscle all predispose to patellar dislocation.

Clinical Manifestations. Persons at risk for patellar instability usually exhibit generalized ligamentous laxity and a poorly developed vastus medialis muscle. When these patients are sitting or standing erect in a relaxed position, the patellae often face laterally ("owl-eye" patellae). On physical examination, the patella can normally be manually displaced both medially and laterally between 25% and 50% of the width of the patella. Greater movement indicates loose patellar restraints, a finding frequently seen in adolescent females.

Rupture of the medial patellofemoral ligament after lateral dislocation of the patella causes pain and tenderness along the medial retinaculum. Sometimes, the vastus medialis muscle is avulsed from the medial intermuscular septum, causing pain in the medial region of the knee. However, patellar dislocation should not be confused with a sprain of the medial collateral ligament. After an acute dislocation of the patella, gentle manual lateral subluxation of the patella produces discomfort, a finding not seen with injury to the medial collateral ligaments.

Treatment. With acute dislocations, a period of immobilization may be needed to allow the

Disorders of Patella (continued)

Chondromalacia

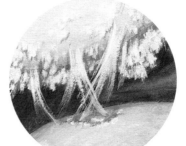

Arthroscopic view shows fragmented patellar cartilage. Bits of cartilage may come free in joint, which may cause synovial effusion

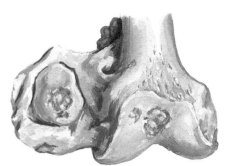

Chondromalacia of patella with "kissing" lesion on femoral condyle

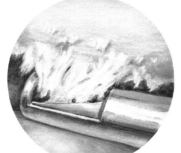

Arthroscopic shaving of patella using motorized instrument

Appearance immediately after shaving

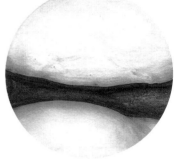

After 15 months, fibrocartilage may fill defect if subchondral bone is perforated and motion is instituted, but is not as durable as normal articular cartilage

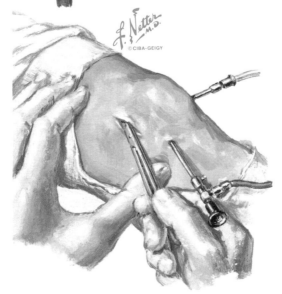

Quadriceps and hamstring muscles simultaneously contracted with knee slightly flexed to improve muscle function

Isometric contraction exercise to strengthen vastus medialis muscle

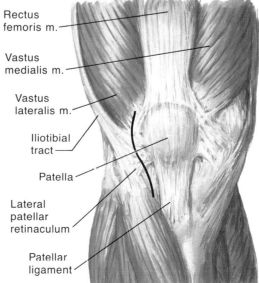

Percutaneous lateral release of patella. Scissors introduced through small lateral skin incision and guided by external palpation and arthroscopic observation

Rectus femoris m.

Vastus medialis m.

Vastus lateralis m.

Iliotibial tract

Patella

Lateral patellar retinaculum

Patellar ligament

Line indicates extent of release

Disorders of Patella

(Continued)

medial restraints to heal. With patellar subluxation, treatment is with muscle-strengthening exercises for the entire quadriceps muscle, particularly the vastus medialis muscle (Plate 68). Patellar knee sleeves may help to maintain the patella in a good position while muscle strengthening continues.

A lateral release for patellar instability, commonly an arthroscopic procedure, should be considered only when extensive muscle strengthening has failed. A lateral release detaches the patella from the lateral soft-tissue structures, including the lateral retinaculum, fibers from the tensor fasciae latae muscle, and joint capsule. After the release, rapid mobilization of the joint is very important to prevent scarring and tightening along the released lateral structures. Intense rehabilitation of the vastus medialis muscle is required.

Pain and effusion in the knee can inhibit the quadriceps muscle through a local spinal reflex. Thus, after injury or surgery to the knee, controlling both pain and swelling improves quadriceps muscle function and hastens recovery.

Patella Overload Syndrome

Patella overload syndrome is a common and painful condition seen in rapidly growing adolescents whose bones appear to be growing faster than the attached soft tissues (Plate 70). This rapid growth results in tightness of the quadriceps and hamstring muscles. Tightness in the quadriceps muscle and patellar retinaculum can increase the compression forces between the patella and femur during knee flexion, causing irritation. Trauma can also contribute to the development of this condition, particularly if followed by immobilization or disuse. These may lead to soft-tissue contracture, resulting in a tight patellofemoral joint.

Patients complain of a toothachelike pain over the anterior surface of the knee, especially along the lateral border of the patella. Conservative management with muscle and soft-tissue stretching and strengthening is sufficient, but the patella must be protected from further irritation. If exercise causes pain, the routine must be carefully evaluated.

Chondromalacia

The term "chondromalacia" describes the softening and fissuring of the articular hyaline cartilage (Plate 69). It frequently refers to the undersurface of the patella. Chondromalacia may result from an excessive load on the patellofemoral joint, but disuse may be a contributing factor.

In clinical practice, chondromalacia is used to describe inflammation of the articular surface of the patellofemoral joint (patellofemoral chondrosis) or degeneration of this joint (patellofemoral arthrosis). Patellofemoral chondrosis is most common in young women. Contributing factors include weakness and tightness in the quadriceps muscle, abnormalities of lower limb alignment (knock-knee, bowleg, an abnormally positioned patella), and obesity. Patellofemoral

Disorders of Patella (continued)

Patella overload syndrome

Rapid growth evidenced by "high-water pants." Muscles, which have not kept pace with bone growth, are tight

Boy runs with short stride and slightly flexed knees because of muscle tightness

Poor flexibility of extensor mechanism can increase patellofemoral contact pressure

Straight-leg–raising test. On passive elevation of leg, patient feels pain behind knee due to tightness of hamstring muscles

Quadriceps femoris m.

Gastrocnemius m.

Hamstring mm.

Straight-leg stretch for hamstring muscles

Wall-leaning exercise to stretch soleus and gastrocnemius muscles

Riding bicycle with elevated seat stretches and strengthens flexor muscles of knee

arthrosis usually occurs with aging. The relationship between chondrosis and the subsequent development of arthrosis is unclear.

Clinical Manifestations. Patients often report pain in the anterior knee while climbing stairs or sitting for long periods. On examination, compression of the patella may cause pain along the medial and lateral retinacula and the patellar ligament. Compression of the patella during flexion and extension of the knee usually elicits crepitation and discomfort; swelling may also be present.

Treatment. Strenuous activities should be reduced until symptoms subside. Athletic activities can continue, with care to reduce stress on the knee joint. Exercises to stretch and strengthen

the quadriceps muscle, especially the vastus medialis muscle, should be initiated immediately. The patient must understand that exercises that cause pain are counterproductive and must be done without aggravating the patellar pain; this may mean avoiding the last 25° to 30° of extension while performing exercises. A few patients benefit from arthroscopic shaving of loose articular fragments or lateral release of the patella, or both. Although removal of the degenerated tissue usually does little to alleviate the symptoms or to improve the long-term prognosis, it can decrease crepitation and synovial effusion. A lateral release may relieve excess patellofemoral contact pressure or denervate a sensitive region. □

Meniscal Variations and Tears

Congenital Meniscal Variations

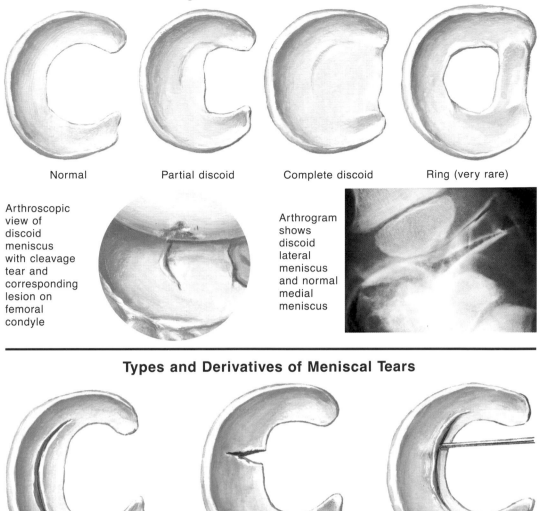

Normal   Partial discoid   Complete discoid   Ring (very rare)

Arthroscopic view of discoid meniscus with cleavage tear and corresponding lesion on femoral condyle

Arthrogram shows discoid lateral meniscus and normal medial meniscus

Types and Derivatives of Meniscal Tears

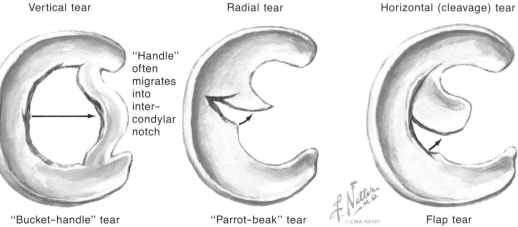

Vertical tear   Radial tear   Horizontal (cleavage) tear

"Handle" often migrates into intercondylar notch

"Bucket-handle" tear   "Parrot-beak" tear   Flap tear

Discoid Meniscus

The meniscus (semilunar cartilage) is normally a crescentic structure, although several forms of discoid lateral menisci have been described. These range from a complete disc to a very rare ring-shaped meniscus with abnormal thickness. The common explanation for these variant discoid forms assumes that the normal meniscus is formed from an original discoid shape and that the discoid lateral meniscus is a congenital variant in which the central portion does not degenerate with time. This theory would explain the variously shaped menisci found at surgery. However, no discoid menisci have been found in fetuses, and a review of comparative anatomy shows no mammal with such a pattern of formation.

A second theory is a developmental one. Discoid lateral menisci have abnormal attachments to the tibia. While the attachment to the posterior tibial plateau is deficient, there is a strong attachment to the medial femoral condyle by the meniscofemoral ligament (Wrisberg's ligament). This pattern of attachment may allow abnormal movement of the lateral meniscus: the posterior horn of the lateral meniscus moves into the center of the lateral compartment during full extension of the knee. With time, scarring and fibrosis of the lateral meniscus occur, with resultant thickening. These changes may account for the popping on flexion and extension that is usually noticed during childhood or early adolescence.

Treatment. Many discoid menisci are asymptomatic, and the mere presence of one is not an indication for treatment. The popping itself is not harmful unless it is accompanied by pain or swelling of the knee. Pain, swelling, and a history of trauma are relative indications for arthroscopy. Tears of the meniscus or degenerative changes on the articular surfaces may necessitate resection. Arthroscopic techniques allow for partial resection of the discoid lateral meniscus, leaving a peripheral rim that may function properly. Resection is often difficult because of the increased thickness in such menisci.

Prognosis for patients with discoid menisci is good. Discoid menisci without degenerative changes have been found in the joints of elderly persons. Therefore, every attempt should be made to salvage function of the meniscus by avoiding complete excision simply to eliminate the snapping, clicking sensation.

Meniscal Tears

The meniscus of the knee joint is very important to normal knee function, and every attempt should be made to preserve meniscal tissue when tears occur, particularly in young patients. When repair is not possible, resection is indicated, but only the unstable, nonfunctioning region should be removed.

The meniscus functions by resisting peripheral displacement, thus providing a larger area of contact between the femur and tibia. When the meniscus is removed, the size of the area through which force is transmitted between the femur and tibia decreases. This concentration of force may cause premature degeneration of the hyaline cartilage. A torn meniscus that cannot resist peripheral displacement does not provide a protective function.

In young, active persons, arthroscopic repair of torn menisci should always be considered. Indeed, the younger the patient, the stronger the consideration should be—the loss of a large portion of a meniscus can be devastating.

Repairs in the peripheral third of the medial and lateral menisci have been quite successful. With proper technique and stabilization of the knee joint with ligament repair where necessary, repair of the meniscus can be successful in 90% of cases. Current research will establish which tears outside the vascular peripheral third can be repaired. Although these tears have less chance of healing, repair may well be indicated in younger patients. □

Synovial Plica

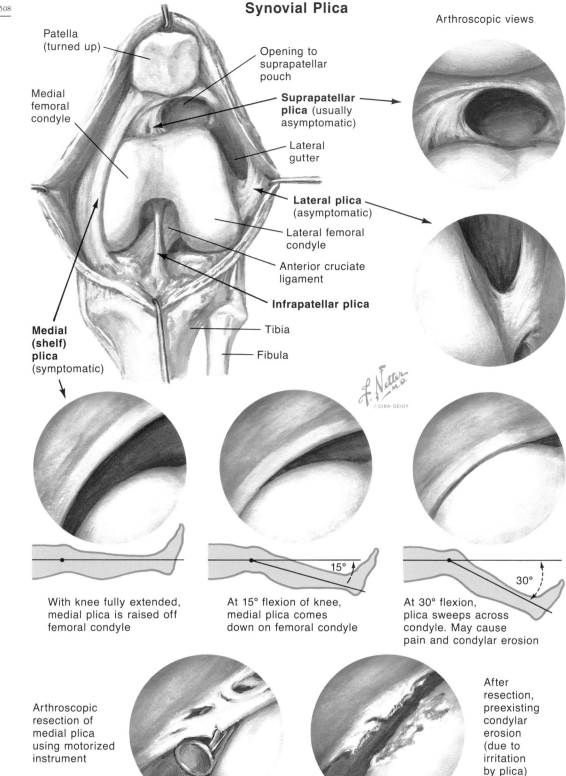

Synovial Plica

Arthroscopic views

Patella (turned up)

Opening to suprapatellar pouch

Medial femoral condyle

Suprapatellar plica (usually asymptomatic)

Lateral gutter

Lateral plica (asymptomatic)

Lateral femoral condyle

Anterior cruciate ligament

Infrapatellar plica

Medial (shelf) plica (symptomatic)

Tibia

Fibula

With knee fully extended, medial plica is raised off femoral condyle

At 15° flexion of knee, medial plica comes down on femoral condyle

15°

At 30° flexion, plica sweeps across condyle. May cause pain and condylar erosion

30°

Arthroscopic resection of medial plica using motorized instrument

After resection, preexisting condylar erosion (due to irritation by plica) can be seen

Synovial plicae are folds of embryonic remnants of the synovial membrane. In the fetus, thin synovial membranes divide the knee joint into three compartments (medial, lateral, and patellar). In the fifth month of fetal development, these partitions usually degenerate, and the knee joint becomes one cavity. Incomplete degeneration of one or more of the membranes can result in the formation of plicae. Most synovial folds contain a considerable amount of elastin and areolar tissue and are thus extensible and asymptomatic. Many are detected during routine arthroscopic procedures performed for other reasons.

Plicae can be found anywhere in the knee joint, but the most common location is over the medial femoral condyle. Folds in this location are called medial, or shelf, plicae. This is the area most susceptible to trauma and subsequent irritation. When the knee is extended, the patella protects the anterior aspect of the femoral condyles, but when the knee is flexed, the medial condyle is more vulnerable. Multiple trauma, even minor, that involves the condyle, repeated flexion-extension activities, or direct contusions can lead to inflammation of the plica with subsequent thickening. The thickened plica may cause local irritation and erosion of the underlying hyaline cartilage on the condyle.

Clinical Manifestations. The symptoms of a pathologic plica may mimic those of a torn meniscus. Patients may complain of mechanical symptoms (snapping or clicking), together with pain along the medial joint line. Medial plicae can be palpated, and some are tender: they are located above the joint line. Palpation of the condyle next to the patella while the patient is flexing and extending the knee may produce a snap or click. Diagnosis can be confirmed by double-contrast arthrography of the knee joint.

Treatment. Symptomatic plicae should be managed with rest from activities that irritate the knee, use of nonsteroidal antiinflammatory drugs (NSAIDs), and application of ice. Excision, while rarely indicated, is very effective when necessary. □

Osteochondritis Dissecans

Osteochondritis Dissecans

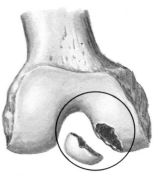

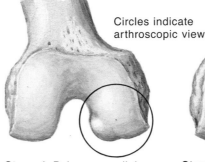

Circles indicate arthroscopic view

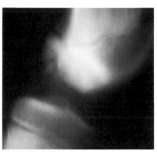

Stage 1. Bulge on medial femoral condyle due to partial separation of bone fragment. Articular cartilage intact, but defect evident on radiographs

Stage 2. Fragment demarcated by separation of articular cartilage

Stage 3. Fragment of cartilage and bone completely separated as loose body. This often migrates to medial or lateral gutter

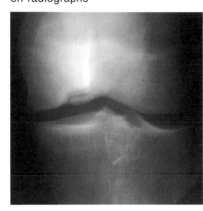

Osteochondritis dissecans evidenced by radiolucent line demarcating fragment on medial femoral condyle

Blumenstat's line (represents roof of inter-condylar notch)

Zone of posterior ossification defects

Zone of osteochondritis dissecans

Tomogram shows posterior ossification defect

Posterior ossification defect, a self-limiting lesion, is differentiated from osteochondritis dissecans by its more posterior location

Radiographs of child treated with conservative measures (splinting and restriction of vigorous exercise) show healing over 4 months

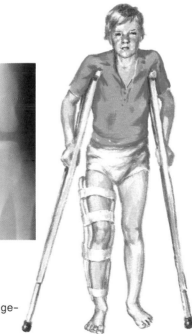

Splint provides symptomatic relief. Velcro straps allow removal for range-of-motion exercises to prevent muscle atrophy and stiffness

Osteochondritis dissecans is a defect in the subchondral region of the apophysis or the epiphysis of a bone, often with partial or complete separation of the bone fragment (Plate 73). When this occurs in the distal femur, it is a common source of loose bodies in the knee. While osteochondritis dissecans most often affects the medial femoral condyle, it can also occur in the shoulder, elbow, and foot.

Trauma is the most likely cause of osteochondritis dissecans, but a single event is probably not responsible: this would cause a true fracture if the force is large enough. Repetitive overloading is thought to affect the local blood supply, making a region more susceptible to fragmentation and separation. Trauma is believed to damage the delicate blood supply to the affected bone in a process similar to Legg-Calvé-Perthes disease of the hip (Plate 57). Obese children are more prone to this problem because of increased load on their joints. Normally, the knee joints are subjected to forces up to six times body weight. Thus, an additional 30 lbs of body weight can add about 180 lbs in forces to the joint. It is no wonder that knee problems arise under such conditions. Fragments may separate from the bone and become loose bodies in the joint. If the defect is large, the joint may become incongruous, leading to mechanical signs and symptoms. While the bony lesion is often the center of attention because of its visibility on radiographs, maintenance of a smooth overlying articular surface in the weight-bearing region is the most important prognostic factor.

Clinical Manifestations

The onset of osteochondritis dissecans is frequently insidious, with patients reporting vague complaints, for example, intermittent, poorly localized aching. Generally, the pain intensifies with exercise but may persist even at rest. The knee may feel stiff, and floating fragments of bone and cartilage can cause the knee to catch or lock. If a sufficiently large fragment becomes loose in the joint and trapped between the condyle and tibia, the patient may feel sudden pain and the knee may "give way." These episodes may produce synovial effusions.

On physical examination, forcible compression of the affected side of the knee joint elicits crepitation during knee flexion and extension. In addition, the affected femoral condyle is tender on palpation.

Radiographic Findings

Radiographs are necessary for diagnosis, and the notch view (anteroposterior view with the knee flexed 90°) or lateral view best reveals the defect. Bone scans can help differentiate acute processes from chronic ones. Computed tomography or magnetic resonance imaging is occasionally needed to define the extent of the defect.

Treatment

The goal of treatment is to maintain a smooth articular surface and remove loose fragments. Conservative measures suffice in the early stages. If the fragment has not separated from the femoral

Pins introduced under arthroscopic control; drill attached to pins

Simple drilling of fragment to promote revascularization. Broken arrows indicate course of drill holes

Loose body in lateral gutter grasped with arthroscopic forceps and removed percutaneously

Pins drilled through fragment and medial femoral condyle, brought out through skin, pulled through until ends are just under surface of fragment. Pins left in place until healing occurs

Healing fragment on femoral condyle

Radiograph shows pins in place

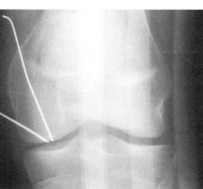

Osteochondritis Dissecans

(Continued)

condyle, the lesion should be considered a healing fracture and protected appropriately. When defects involve the weight-bearing region of the femur, walking with crutches to avoid placing weight on the affected limb is the most important treatment while symptoms persist (Plate 73). Immobilization is rarely needed and should be avoided whenever possible, since knee motion is beneficial to the jeopardized region of the articular cartilage.

A loose or detached fragment is removed with arthroscopy (Plate 74). At the same time, drilling through areas of poorly vascularized bone into regions of good vascularity may induce a vascular healing response. When the fragment represents a large part of the weight-bearing region, internal fixation should be considered if the fragment can be reduced and held in place. The presence of multiple fragments lessens the chances of obtaining a congruous surface. These fragments should be removed and the base of the lesion drilled.

The prognosis for osteochondritis dissecans of the knee depends on the age at which it occurs and the extent of involvement of the weight-bearing region. In short, any process such as this that causes an incongruity in the very delicate surface of the knee joint predisposes to the development of osteoarthritis.

Defects that occur in children before the closure of the growth plate frequently heal well with conservative treatment if the fragment has not detached; in fact, many cases probably go undetected. When radiographs are taken for other reasons, these defects are not unusual findings. Prognosis is guarded if the fragment detaches, leaving a defect in the weight-bearing region. Lesions that occur after closure of the growth plate are less likely to heal. □

Osgood-Schlatter Lesion

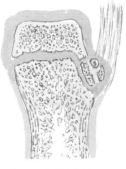

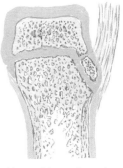

Normal insertion of patellar ligament to ossifying tibial tuberosity

In Osgood–Schlatter lesion, superficial portion of tuberosity pulled away, forming separate bone fragments

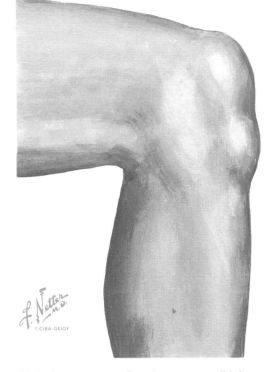

Clinical appearance. Prominence over tibial tuberosity partly due to soft-tissue swelling and partly to avulsed fragments

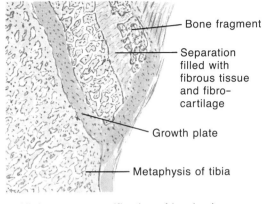

Bone fragment

Separation filled with fibrous tissue and fibro-cartilage

Growth plate

Metaphysis of tibia

High-power magnification of involved area

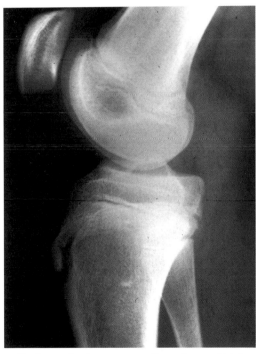

Radiograph shows separation of superficial portion of tibial tuberosity

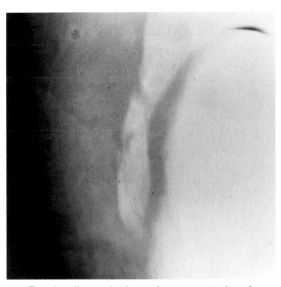

Focal radiograph shows fragment at site of insertion of patellar ligament

The Osgood-Schlatter lesion refers to the partial avulsion of the tibial tuberosity. It usually occurs in late childhood or early adolescence and is more common in boys, possibly because boys often engage in more vigorous activities than girls.

During fetal development, the tibial tuberosity develops as a discrete anterior extension of the epiphysis of the proximal tibia. After birth, it moves distally and develops its own growth plate, which is composed largely of fibrocartilage rather than the columnar-celled hyaline cartilage typical of most growth plates. Since fibrocartilage is better able than hyaline cartilage to withstand tensile stress, this fibrous composition appears to be a structural adaptation to the tension placed on the tuberosity by the patellar ligament.

By 7 to 9 years of age, the tuberosity develops its own center, or several centers, of ossification. Normally, the ossification center of the tuberosity expands and eventually unites with that of the tibial epiphysis. Major or repetitive tensile stress on the tuberosity may cause the developing bone or its overlying hyaline cartilage, or both, to fail, resulting in avulsion of its superficial portion.

The avulsed fragment (or fragments) and the intact portion of the tuberosity continue to grow.

The intervening area usually fills in with bone, leading to overgrowth of the tuberosity at skeletal maturity. This is manifested as a bony prominence over the anterior aspect of the proximal tibia. In some patients, the space between the fragment and the tuberosity becomes filled with fibrous material, creating a painful nonunion or even a pathologic joint.

Clinical Manifestations. The Osgood-Schlatter lesion is manifested by local swelling and tenderness. The pain is aggravated by direct pressure, as in kneeling, and by traction, as in running, jumping, and forced flexion. On physical examination, extension of the knee against resistance and palpation of the prominence are also painful.

Radiographic Findings. The avulsion may occur while the cartilage is still in the preossification phase and thus is not radiographically evident. In this case, diagnosis is difficult. The avulsed cartilage eventually ossifies and becomes visible on radiographs as small fragments of bone that are completely separated from the rest of the tibial tuberosity.

Treatment. The condition is usually self-limiting, and avoidance of strenuous exercise involving the knee is often the only treatment necessary. Some patients may require bracing or a sleeve cast. Surgery should be considered only in rare, resistant cases, after conservative treatment has failed. □

Congenital Bowing of Tibia

Congenital Bowing of Tibia

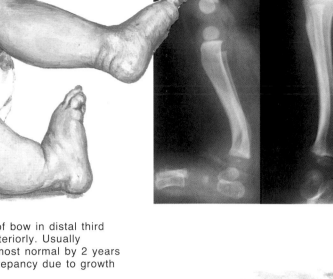

Posterior bowing. Convexity of bow in distal third of tibia and fibula directed posteriorly. Usually regresses spontaneously to almost normal by 2 years of age; lower limb–length discrepancy due to growth inhibition may persist

Posterior Bowing. In this condition, the apex of the bow is at the junction of the lower and middle thirds of the tibia and is directed posteriorly or posteromedially. Usually, the fibula is similarly bowed. The foot is in calcaneovalgus position and can be dorsiflexed to the shin; tightness of the anterior musculature limits plantar flexion. Although the etiology is not yet understood, the condition is believed to represent an intrauterine fracture or the consequence of molding due to entwining of the legs.

Posterior bowing spontaneously corrects by the time the child is 2 to 4 years of age, and correction of the angulation is not necessary. The fact that complications have been reported only in patients who have had an osteotomy suggests that surgical correction is not indicated. Growth of the tibia and fibula will be inhibited, and at maturity, the limb-length discrepancy may be 3 to 7 cm. Epiphysiodesis of the contralateral tibia may be required before growth ceases.

Anterior Bowing. Anterior bowing of the tibia (the high-risk tibia) has been classified into three types: (1) simple anterior bow, (2) anterior bow with cyst at the apex, and (3) pseudarthrosis (false joint) of the tibia (Plate 77). Although the radiographic findings of the three types overlap, in general, the classification represents an increasing risk of fracture in the infant.

Simple anterior or *anterolateral bowing* of the tibia is the most common type. The bowing generally occurs in the middiaphysis. The anterior cortex is thickened and the medullary canal appears normal. The fibula is also bowed at the same level. This is also called prepseudarthrosis, and in the newborn period, it may be difficult to predict if the bowing will correct spontaneously or fracture and develop pseudarthrosis. In most patients with anterolateral bowing of the tibia and a normal medullary canal, protective treatment to prevent fracture is not necessary and the bone spontaneously straightens. Occasionally, surgical alignment may be needed to produce a more acceptable cosmetic appearance.

Anterior bowing with cyst is a more severe form. Although the medullary canal is present, it is narrowed and exhibits sclerotic changes. A cyst is apparent at the apex of the bow. Since fractures often occur in patients less than 1 to 2 years of age, prophylactic treatment should be instituted in the newborn period. □

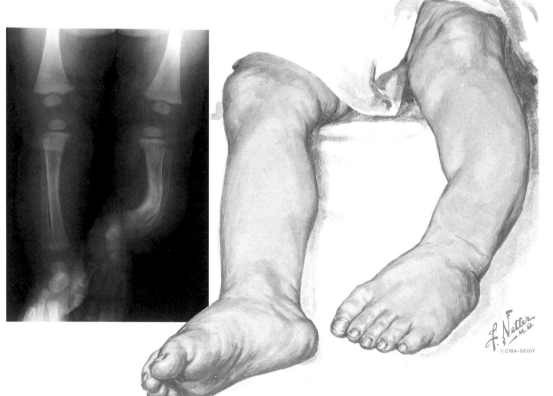

Anterolateral bowing. In infancy, it may be difficult to predict if bowing will correct spontaneously or if bone will fracture and develop pseudarthrosis. Presence of good medullary canal, seen in radiograph, suggests better prognosis

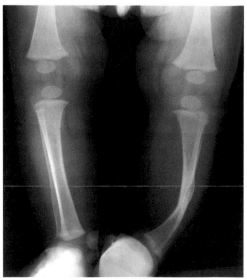

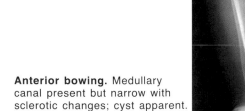

Anterior bowing. Medullary canal present but narrow with sclerotic changes; cyst apparent. Prone to spontaneous fracture and pseudarthrosis

Congenital Pseudarthrosis of Tibia and Dislocation of Knee

Congenital Pseudarthrosis of Tibia

Congenital pseudarthrosis of the tibia results when a tibial fracture fails to heal. A tibia that has an anterolateral bow, usually noted at birth, and a narrow, sclerotic medullary canal (hourglass constriction) is at greatest risk of fracture. In some patients, the fracture is present at birth; 50% of fractures occur in the first year, and 25% in the second year. The fibula is similarly involved. The fractured tibia and fibula fail to unite and a pseud-arthrosis forms at the fracture site.

The etiology of pseudarthrosis of the tibia is unclear, but approximately 70% of affected children subsequently develop clinical findings of neurofibromatosis. In these patients, the lesion is believed to be the result of a neurofibroma. While one description of the pseudarthrosis states it is a hamartomatous proliferation of fibrous tissue, another likens it to a constrictive band.

Treatment. In newborns, anterolateral bowing of the tibia with a narrow, sclerotic medullary canal or cystic changes is an urgent problem that requires immediate treatment, as fracture and pseudarthrosis often develop soon after birth. Treatment of the newborn focuses on preventing a fracture. A custom-made plastic orthosis should be used to protect the limb until the child is ready for a standard orthosis or surgery.

Despite the most intensive conservative management, fractures occur quite frequently, and extensive surgery is required to promote healing. Fracture prophylaxis with bone grafting of the nar-rowed area or curettage and grafting of the cystic lesion prior to fracture may be considered, fol-lowed by bracing. Unfortunately, in many chil-dren with high-risk tibia, healing does not occur, and a significant number of patients ultimately need limb amputation and a prosthesis.

Congenital Dislocation of Knee

Congenital dislocation of the knee is an uncom-mon neonatal problem but an orthopedic emer-gency when it occurs. At birth, the knee may be simply hyperextended (genu recurvatum) or, in the severe form, completely dislocated, with the tibia displaced anterior and lateral to the femur. The dislocation is usually bilateral, but one side may be more severely affected. A mild hereditary or familial tendency has been reported. An asso-ciated congenital abnormality such as torticollis (Plate 27) or dislocation of the elbow is found in 60% of affected children, and in 50%, the ipsi-lateral hip is also dislocated.

Dislocation of the knee is common in patients with arthrogryposis and myelodysplasia; it is related to muscle imbalance, usually contracture of the quadriceps femoris muscle in combination with weak or absent hamstring muscles. In an otherwise normal child, the dislocation is believed to result from an intrauterine position (frank breech presentation), in which the feet of the fetus are locked beneath the mandible or in the axillae.

Clinical Manifestations. The knee appears hyperextended or may be further extended until

Congenital Pseudarthrosis of Tibia

Angulation of right leg. Café au lait spots on thigh and abdomen suggest relationship to neurofibromatosis

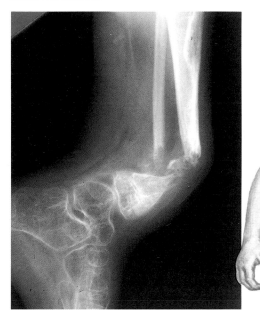

Congenital Dislocation of Knee

Infant with characteristic hyper-extension deformity of both legs. Radiograph shows similar deformity in another patient

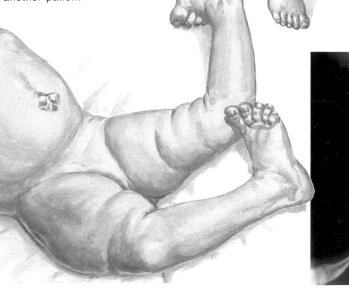

the leg nearly touches the chest. The medial hamstring muscles are often displaced forward, anterior to the axis of the knee, and may function as extensors. The patella may be displaced lat-erally, and the femoral condyles are prominent posteriorly. Circulation below the knee is usually intact.

Radiographic Findings. Radiographs reveal severe genu recurvatum with malalignment of the tibia and femur. Three types of deformity can be recognized: (1) simple genu recurvatum, (2) ante-rior subluxation, and (3) complete anterior dis-location. Deformity of the epiphyses of the distal femur and proximal tibia is not seen in newborns but is found in untreated older children.

Treatment. Dislocation and subluxation both require immediate treatment. Within a few hours after birth, the limb must be passively stretched to bring the knee gradually into a flexed position. In most patients, the knee can be manipulated into slight flexion and splinted in this position. The splint should be changed daily and stretching and passive range-of-motion exercises continued until the knee can be flexed approximately 90°. Then the knee is immobilized for 6 weeks or until there is no indication that it will return to a posi-tion of extension. If manipulative reduction is not possible immediately after birth, surgical correc-tion with open reduction and lengthening of the extensor muscles is required. □

Bowleg and Knock-knee

Bowleg (genu varum) and knock-knee (genu valgum) are angular deformities commonly seen in growing children. While these conditions represent normal development (physiologic bowleg or knock-knee) in the majority of patients and resolve in time without treatment, it is important to differentiate between physiologic angular deformities and the variety of pathologic conditions that require special evaluation and treatment.

Clinical evaluation of the patient with angular deformities includes obtaining a family history and a description of the deformity, its onset, and its progression. The child should be observed ambulating, with particular attention paid to the stance phase of gait to determine if a lateral thrust (bowleg) or a medial thrust (knock-knee) occurs immediately on weight bearing. A thrust indicates that restraint of the knee by the medial or lateral ligaments is not adequate to resist the deformity. In children with physiologic bowleg or knock-knee, a thrust is not present. However, a thrust is seen in patients with most of the pathologic conditions that cause varus or valgus deformities, indicating an incompetence of the knee ligaments and, most likely, a progressive deformity.

Physiologic Bowleg and Knock-knee

The natural history of physiologic bowleg and knock-knee was defined by Salenius and Vankka, who studied the development of the tibiofemoral angle, measured clinically and radiographically, in 1,480 normal children (Plate 78). In the newborn, the tibiofemoral angle is 15° varus. When the child is 18 months of age, the limbs appear to straighten, and between 2 and 4 years of age, the tibiofemoral angle changes to marked valgus (12°) and subsequently reduces to the normal, slightly valgus alignment seen in adults.

Clinical Manifestations. The normal infant usually stands with the legs apart, and early physiologic varus bowing of the lower limbs may be masked by fat. Internal tibial torsion often accompanies physiologic bowleg, accentuating the bowing when the child stands or walks. Physiologic knock-knee usually becomes evident at 2½ to 3 years of age. Flatfoot (pes planus) and external tibial torsion may also be present and accentuate the knock-knee appearance.

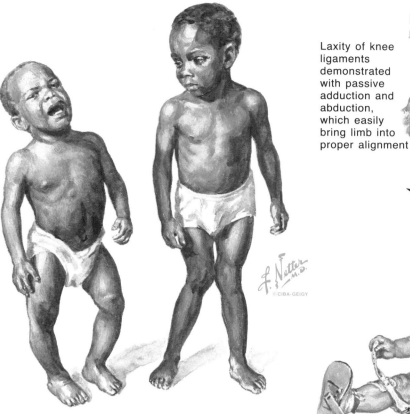

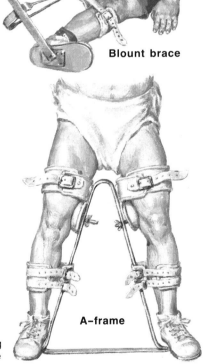

Laxity of knee ligaments demonstrated with passive adduction and abduction, which easily bring limb into proper alignment

Two brothers, younger (left) with bowleg, older (right) with knock-knee. In both children, limbs eventually became normally aligned without corrective treatment

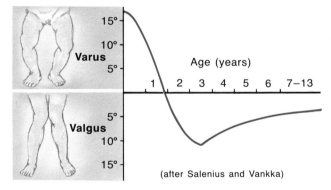

Blount brace

Graph depicts normal developmental changes in tibio-femoral angle. Substantial deviation suggests pathologic cause such as rickets, Blount's disease, or other disorders requiring specific treatment

A-frame

A-frame useful for resistant bowleg and early stage of Blount's disease

Treatment. Reassurance and observation are sufficient treatment for patients with physiologic bowing of the lower limb. Use of sleeping splints, corrective shoes, and active and passive exercises effect no apparent changes in the lower limbs that would not occur with normal growth and development. In children less than 7 years of age, knock-knee may be safely ignored, unless it is excessive (tibiofemoral angle >15° valgus) or asymmetric.

Pathologic Bowleg and Knock-knee

Blount's Disease. The most common cause of pathologic bowleg, or tibia vara, is Blount's disease (Plate 79). The etiology remains unclear. Early studies suggested that the pathologic bowing was caused by a primary disturbance in the growth and ossification of the medial part of the epiphysis and metaphysis of the proximal tibia. Results of more recent studies indicate that the condition is secondary to the mechanical stress of weight bearing on the medial tibiofemoral compartment, delaying the growth of the medial tibial growth plate.

Blount's disease is divided into two types, the infantile and juvenile forms. The *infantile form*, which is usually bilateral and progressive, is associated with significant internal tibial torsion. The *juvenile form* is less common. It becomes apparent between 6 and 14 years of age and usually is unilateral. The resulting deformity is less severe, and there is no associated internal tibial torsion.

Bowleg and Knock-knee
(Continued)

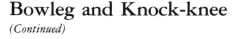

Blount's Disease

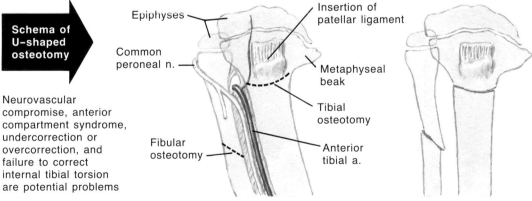

Radiographs demonstrate stages of Blount's disease: progressive deformity of medial side of proximal tibial epiphysis and development of metaphyseal beak

Schema of U-shaped osteotomy

Neurovascular compromise, anterior compartment syndrome, undercorrection or overcorrection, and failure to correct internal tibial torsion are potential problems

Epiphyses

Common peroneal n.

Fibular osteotomy

Insertion of patellar ligament

Metaphyseal beak

Tibial osteotomy

Anterior tibial a.

Plate 79 shows six stages of Blount's disease based on radiographic evidence of the degree of epiphyseal depression and metaphyseal fragmentation of the medial proximal tibia. It is difficult to distinguish between the initial stage of infantile Blount's disease and severe physiologic bowleg, and it is possible that the extreme variation of physiologic bowleg represents the initial stages of Blount's disease. The metaphyseal-diaphyseal angle may be used to predict which cases of physiologic bowleg will progress to Blount's disease. On the anteroposterior radiograph, a horizontal line is drawn through the widest portion of the tibial metaphysis, and an intersecting vertical line is drawn parallel to the lateral border of the tibia. A third line is drawn perpendicular to the line on the metaphysis, and the angle between the perpendicular line and the vertical line on the lateral border of the tibia is measured. When the angle is less than 11°, the bowleg deformity tends to resolve; an angle greater than 11° is predictive of progression to Blount's disease. In addition, if a child with bowleg exhibits a lateral thrust on weight bearing, the prognosis is poor.

Treatment. The degree of deformity and the patient's age determine the treatment plan for Blount's disease. In the infantile form, progression is usually rapid in the first 4 years and then slows for the remainder of the growth period. Observation is usually sufficient until the patient is 18 months of age. If the varus deformity does not improve by the time the child is 18 to 24 months of age, it is treated with an orthosis, such as the Blount brace or an A-frame, until the child is 3 years of age (Plate 78).

Persistent bowleg and a tibiofemoral angle greater than 15° varus and stage III to IV Blount's disease cannot be successfully treated with bracing, and a proximal tibial osteotomy is required (Plate 79). In the young patient with mild-to-moderate bowing, the osteotomy usually corrects the deformity permanently and completely; if surgery is postponed, recurrence is more likely. This is particularly true if the medial portion of the growth plate is closed (stage IV).

A child who undergoes a tibial osteotomy is at risk for serious sequelae and should be observed carefully in the postoperative period for signs of compromise in the neurovascular or motor status of the lower limb.

Other Causes of Pathologic Bowleg and Knock-knee. Rickets can cause bowleg or knock-knee (see CIBA COLLECTION, Volume 8/I, pages 205–214). Vitamin D–dependent and vitamin D–resistant rickets, generally occurring in early childhood when the lower limb is in varus position, lead to bowleg. Conversely, rickets due to chronic renal insufficiency (renal osteodystrophy), which has a later onset, is now a common cause of knock-knee. Treatment with renal dialysis and kidney

transplantation has improved the life expectancy of patients with this disorder, and surgical correction of severe valgus deformities is more often required. It is important that children with rickets who undergo osteotomy receive proper medical management to ensure proper healing.

Unilateral bowleg or knock-knee may be associated with trauma, surgery, tumors, congenital knee deformity, metaphyseal chondrodysplasia (Plate 7), osteocartilaginous exostosis (see Section II, Plate 7), hemihypertrophy (Plate 82), paraxial fibular hemimelia, multiple epiphyseal dysplasia (Plate 10), Morquio's syndrome (Plate 16), rickets, and fibrous dysplasia (see Section II, Plate 9). □

Rotational Deformities of Lower Limb

Rotational abnormalities in the lower limbs are common, particularly in the child's first 2 years. The abnormality may be at one level in the lower limb—the femur, tibia, or foot—or at several levels. Since the position of the feet is the most obvious clinical manifestation, these rotational problems are commonly referred to as toeing in and toeing out.

All rotational abnormalities in children should be evaluated to rule out a pathologic condition such as cerebral palsy, myelodysplasia (Plate 38), diastematomyelia, or subtle onset of a neurologic problem such as peroneal muscular atrophy (Charcot-Marie-Tooth disease, see CIBA COLLECTION, Volume 1/II, pages 220–221). Asymmetric findings and a history of progression, which are not characteristic of the usual rotational problem, strongly suggest a pathologic cause.

To obtain a proper and thorough evaluation, the child must be cooperative. First, the lower limb is examined in a sequential fashion, with the foot, tibia, and femur isolated in turn. Ambulatory children are observed standing and walking, both with and without shoes, to evaluate the coordination of walking, gait, and stance.

Abnormalities of Foot

Metatarsus Adductus. In the newborn, the forefoot may turn in as a result of intrauterine positioning. Diagnosis is best made by inspecting the sole of the foot (Plate 80); a footprint is made for documentation. The lateral border of a normal foot is straight, but in the patient with metatarsus adductus, the border of the forefoot is convex, with the curve beginning at the base of the fifth metatarsal.

When metatarsus adductus is suspected, the foot is tested for stiffness or suppleness by holding the heel firmly and attempting to push the foot laterally into an overcorrected position. In many children, the inward-turning foot can be corrected with the simple passive stretching exercise shown on Plate 80. Parents should perform the exercise 10 times with every diaper change. An out-flaring shoe is sometimes used at this stage to keep the foot in an overcorrected position between exercises.

If no improvement is seen in a few months or if the foot is rigid and resistant to passive correction, serial stretching casts are usually prescribed with the goal of increasing suppleness so that the foot can be passively overcorrected. Treatment initiated before the child is 8 or 10 months old usually produces a satisfactory result; if treatment is delayed past 1 year of age, the bone and soft-tissue changes may not be reversible, and the foot assumes an unusual appearance (ie, adducted forefoot and prominent base of the fifth metatarsal), necessitating use of a wider-than-normal shoe. In older children, the appearance of the foot can be improved with a metatarsal osteotomy.

Calcaneovalgus. In the child with this common neonatal condition, the foot and ankle seem unusually lax and dorsiflex nearly to the shin (Plate 92). Plantar flexion is restricted, and the heel is in valgus position.

Simple calcaneovalgus usually responds quickly to passive stretching exercises. Taping or casting of the foot in inversion and plantar flexion is effective for resistant deformities.

Abnormalities of Tibia

Internal Tibial Torsion. In this condition, the tibia is internally rotated on its long axis, causing the foot to point inward (Plate 80). Internal tibial torsion is usually first noticed when the child is between 6 and 18 months of age and begins to walk.

Tibial torsion is best assessed with the child seated. The femurs are placed in neutral position, the thighs directly in front of the hip joint, and the heels against the flat surface of the examining table. The feet are held in neutral position. Many examiners use the position of the medial malleolus relative to the lateral malleolus to determine the transmalleolar axis and its relationship to the long axis of the tibia or to a specific protuberance of the tibia, such as the tibial tuberosity. The malleoli are usually grasped by the examiner's fingers at the joint line either in the midportion or on the anterior aspect. The transmalleolar axis is then determined by observation or with a simple measuring device.

An alternative method is to use the thigh-foot angle, which reflects the difference in the angle between the axis of the thigh and that of the foot. With the patient prone and the knees flexed to 90°, the foot and thigh are viewed from directly above.

The transmalleolar axis is normally in slight external rotation: about 5° in the normal infant, increasing with growth to an average of 22° in the adult. The greatest increase occurs in the first 18 months. Lateral bowing of the tibia, a common finding in children less than 18 months of age, can accentuate internal tibial torsion.

Some controversy exists regarding the need for treatment. Internal tibial torsion often improves spontaneously, and in most children and adults, toeing in due to internal tibial torsion is seldom a significant handicap.

If the physician chooses to treat internal tibial torsion, the best time is when the child is between 6 and 18 months of age. Younger infants are generally too small for bracing to be effective, and older children are often reluctant to wear a device and have the manual skills to remove it.

The most popular treatment is with the Denis Browne splint or one of several variations. The shoes are adjusted so that the lower limb is in 20° to 30° of external rotation. Forced rotation to any degree should be avoided. The brace is worn only at night and during naps, allowing the child to be free during the rest of the day for crawling, sitting, and walking.

Other general treatment measures include encouraging patients to sit cross-legged (tailor or Indian position) when sitting on the floor or to sit on a chair with hips flexed and legs extended (Plate 81). Sitting or sleeping with the feet tucked under the buttocks is discouraged.

External Tibial Torsion. Less common than internal rotation, external tibial torsion is seldom a clinical problem in the child's first few years (Plate 81). The majority of children whose lower limbs appear to be externally rotated are found to have external rotation of the femur and therefore of the entire limb. If treatment is indicated, the Denis Browne splint can be used with the feet set in neutral position or in slight internal rotation.

Abnormalities of Femur

Internal Femoral Torsion (Anteversion). This condition is the most common cause of toeing in in children 3 to 12 years of age (Plate 80) and is due to an abnormal relationship of the femoral diaphysis and condyles to the femoral head and neck (femoral anteversion). The thighs can be rotated internally to a marked degree, but external rotation is quite limited. In severely affected patients, internal rotation may be as great as 90°, while external rotation is absent or very slight.

Although this condition is often referred to as a problem in hip rotation, the cause lies in the orientation of the femur itself. It is important to reassure parents that there is nothing wrong with the child's hip joint.

Femoral rotation is best assessed with the child recumbent, either supine or prone, and the hips in extension. With the patient supine, the physician rotates the entire limb. The position of the legs is observed in both internal rotation and external rotation. Marked internal rotation and limited external rotation of the femur strongly suggest internal femoral torsion.

Alternatively, with the patient prone, the pelvis is maintained level and the knees are flexed. Medial rotation refers to the angle between vertical and the axis of the tibia when the hips are maximally rotated inward. The internal hip rotation is accomplished by allowing the legs to fall outward by gravity alone. External rotation is also measured, with the patient in the same position, by allowing the legs to cross.

Rotational Deformities of Lower Limb: Toeing In

Metatarsus adductus

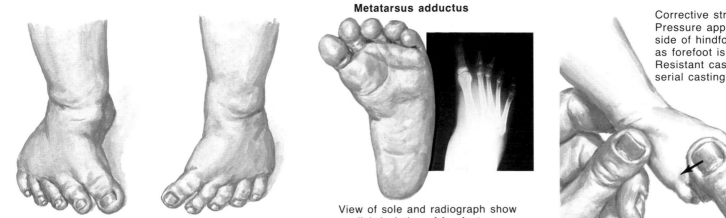

Bilateral metatarsus adductus

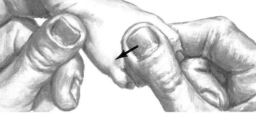

View of sole and radiograph show medial deviation of forefoot

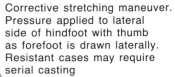

Corrective stretching maneuver. Pressure applied to lateral side of hindfoot with thumb as forefoot is drawn laterally. Resistant cases may require serial casting

Internal tibial torsion

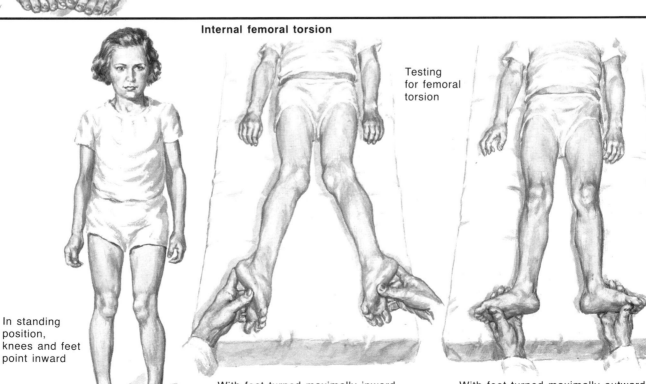

Evaluating patient for internal tibial torsion. Child seated with knees flexed 90°, heels against flat, vertical surface. Patellae point directly forward, indicating that femurs are in neutral position, but feet point inward, indicating internal tibial torsion

Sleeping with feet turned in under buttocks may exacerbate problem or hinder spontaneous correction

Denis Browne splint, worn only at night, maintains lower limbs in external rotation to encourage correction of internal tibial torsion

Internal femoral torsion

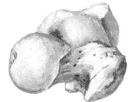

Femoral retroversion (external torsion)

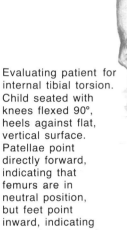

Neutral position

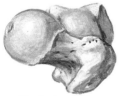

Femoral anteversion (internal torsion)

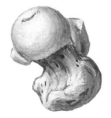

In standing position, knees and feet point inward

Testing for femoral torsion

With feet turned maximally inward, knees point directly medially so that they face each other

With feet turned maximally outward, knees rotate only slightly beyond neutral position

Rotational Deformities of Lower Limb
(Continued)

Rotational Deformities of Lower Limb: Toeing Out

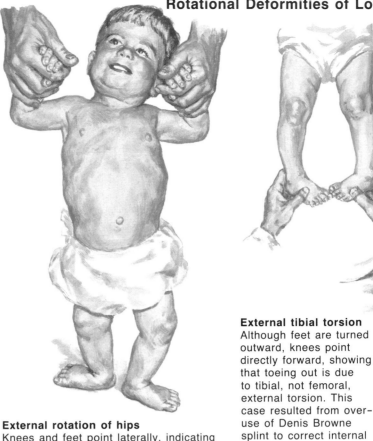

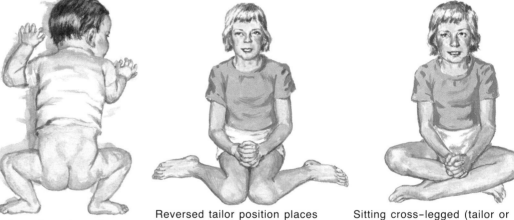

In external rotation of hips, when feet are turned maximally inward, knees are in neutral position or, at most, in slight internal rotation

External tibial torsion
Although feet are turned outward, knees point directly forward, showing that toeing out is due to tibial, not femoral, external torsion. This case resulted from over-use of Denis Browne splint to correct internal femoral torsion

External rotation of hips
Knees and feet point laterally, indicating femoral origin of toeing-out deformity. Common in newborns but usually corrects spontaneously when child begins to walk

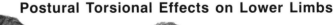

Postural Torsional Effects on Lower Limbs

Spread-eagle or frog sleeping position may contribute to external rotation of hips

Reversed tailor position places internal torsional stress on femurs and external torsion on tibias. May retard correction of torsional deformities

Sitting cross-legged (tailor or Indian position) applies external torsion on femurs and internal torsion to tibias. May help correct external tibial torsion

While it may be tempting to do this type of examination with the patient sitting, the patient *must* be examined with the hips in extension, as this position tightens the anterior joint capsule. When the hips are flexed, these ligaments are relaxed, thus permitting a greater range of external rotation and resulting in an inaccurate evaluation.

Internal femoral torsion may also be measured using biplane radiography, axial tomography, fluoroscopy, or computed tomography. Radiography is only appropriate if surgical correction is contemplated.

In the newborn, internal femoral torsion is at most 40°. This usually decreases rapidly in the child's first 2 years, then continues to decrease more slowly, reaching a plateau at about age 8 to 9 and decreasing to about 16° in adulthood.

Until the child is 2 years of age, the total range of rotation in the hip is about 120°; thereafter, it is about 90° to 110°. Ideally, the ranges of internal rotation and external rotation are about equal (45°–50°).

No conservative treatment has been found to correct internal femoral torsion. Twister cables, braces, and orthopedic shoes have no effect and may produce abnormal external tibial torsion (Plate 81) and a knock-kneed gait.

Fortunately, internal femoral torsion tends to improve with normal growth. However, many affected children prefer to sit in the reversed tailor position, which may prevent spontaneous correction of the problem. This sitting position should be discouraged, and the child should be taught to sit cross-legged.

In their teens, many children no longer toe in, although the degree of internal femoral torsion has not changed. This suggests an adaptive process in the lower limbs, most likely in the joint capsule and soft tissues about the joint. Occasionally, a child is seen with severe internal femoral torsion associated with little or no external rotation. The patient has trouble walking and

running or is clumsy. In these patients, derotational femoral osteotomy should be considered.

External Rotatory Contracture of Hips. This condition is a common finding in children in the first few months of life and seldom represents true external femoral rotation (retroversion). Rather, it is related to the changes in the joint capsule and soft-tissue structures about the hip that are in part due to the position of the fetus. In these patients, treatment with simple internal rotation stretching exercises is sufficient. The condition usually resolves by the time the child begins to walk. If not, use of a Denis Browne splint with the feet set in neutral position or in slight internal rotation is the treatment of choice. □

Limb-Length Discrepancy

Hemihypertrophy

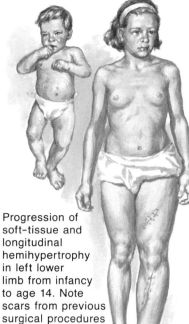

Hemihypertrophy of right side and length discrepancy in upper and lower limbs

‡4 cm

Progression of soft-tissue and longitudinal hemihypertrophy in left lower limb from infancy to age 14. Note scars from previous surgical procedures

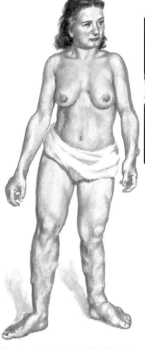

Young adult with Maffucci's syndrome and hemihypertrophy of right upper and lower limbs

Maffucci's syndrome

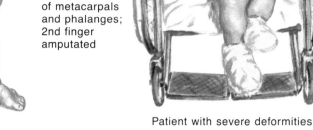

Radiograph reveals multiple enchondromas of metacarpals and phalanges; 2nd finger amputated

Patient with severe deformities

Klippel–Trénaunay–Weber syndrome

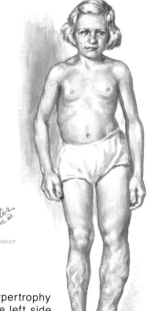

Hemihypertrophy of entire left side with vascular lesions in both lower limbs

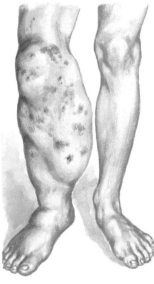

Hemihypertrophy of right lower limb associated with cavernous hemangiomas

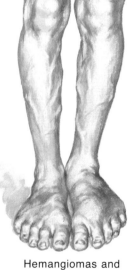

Hemangiomas and varicosities and hypertrophy of both feet in 9-year-old boy

Congenital short femur

Young child with congenital short left femur

Lower Limb–Length Discrepancy

Lower limb–length discrepancies include any inequality in length from the level of the pelvis to, and including, the foot. The numerous causes of the inequality include the following.

Congenital and developmental anomalies with terminal limb deficiencies: hemihypertrophy or hemiatrophy, Klippel–Trénaunay–Weber syndrome,

Maffucci's syndrome, posterior bowing of the tibia, proximal femoral focal deficiency, congenital short femur, enchondromatosis.

Paralytic disorders: poliomyelitis, encephalopathy (eg, cerebral palsy), myelopathy (eg, myelomeningocele).

Infections of bone and joint that retard or arrest bone growth: osteomyelitis (may accelerate or inhibit growth), pyarthrosis (may lead to avascular necrosis with partial or complete growth arrest).

Trauma to bone and joint: injuries to the growth plate (may arrest growth); fractures of the metaphysis or diaphysis (may accelerate growth); malunion, excessive overriding, or angulation due to fracture (may result in limb shortening).

Tumorous conditions that produce bone overgrowth: fibrous dysplasia, enchondromatosis, osteoid osteoma, hemangioma, neurofibromatosis.

Tumors that produce growth retardation: solitary enchondroma of growth plate, simple bone cyst with repeated fractures through growth plate.

Irradiation of malignant tumors of long bones that arrest growth: Ewing's sarcoma, neuroblastoma.

Maffucci's syndrome and enchondromatosis are presented here as exemplary diseases that cause lower limb–length discrepancy.

Maffucci's Syndrome

In 1881, Maffucci described a syndrome comprising subcutaneous cavernous hemangiomas,

---

Lower Limb–Length Discrepancy

(Continued)

phlebectasia, and a dyschondroplasia that was identical to enchondromatosis. Maffucci's syndrome is a congenital, but not familial, disorder characterized by disturbance of bone formation and cartilage, particularly at the ends of long bones. The disease appears to originate from mesodermal dysplasia. The enchondromatosis is bilateral in 60% of patients, and although the enchondromas are often localized to either a hand or a foot, in over 40% of patients, they are extensive and involve multiple bones. Some degree of deformity develops in most patients. Shortening and bowing of the limb differentiate this syndrome from Klippel-Trénaunay-Weber syndrome (Plate 82), which is characterized by bony hypertrophy in association with telangiectasis.

Clinical Manifestations. At birth, patients usually appear normal, but the disease can become evident at any time before puberty.

Islands of cartilage persist in the diaphysis of long bones and may grow to form enchondromas that expand and deform the bone. Enchondromas may also form near the growth plate and interfere with longitudinal growth. Involvement of the long bones and phalanges is common, while the carpal and tarsal bones and the base of the skull are rarely affected.

As in enchondromatosis (Plate 83), the lesions may undergo malignant transformation, and the closer the lesions are to the axial skeleton, the more likely they are to become malignant.

The vascular abnormalities, which appear as firm, dark blue nodules or patches, may be simple cavernous or capillary hemangiomas in the deep layers of the cutis or in the subcutaneous layers. Thrombosis develops in the dilated vessels and vascular spaces. Phleboliths form as the thrombi calcify.

Enchondromatosis (Ollier's Disease)

In this rare, nonhereditary, congenital dyschondroplasia, enchondromas develop in a linear arrangement in the interior of bones (Plate 83). The changes appear to be related to failure of the endochondral ossification sequence. The term "Ollier's disease" refers to the condition in which distribution of the enchondromas is predominantly unilateral. When associated with hemangiomas of the overlying soft tissues, the disease is known as Maffucci's syndrome (Plate 82). The pathologic findings in Ollier's disease are similar to those of enchondromas, although they are often more bizarre (see Section II, Plate 5). The tumors develop in the epiphysis and adjacent areas of the metaphysis and diaphysis in a few or many bones. The resulting deformities include shortening due to retarded growth, broadening of the metaphyses, and bowing of the long bones. Lesions in the axial skeleton and pelvis appear to have a greater tendency toward malignant transformation than enchondromas in the limbs.

Enchondromatosis (Ollier's Disease)

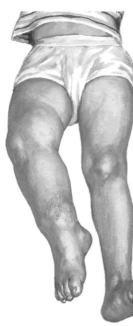 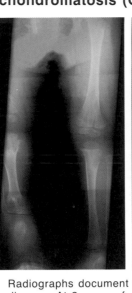 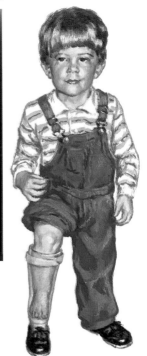

Lower limbs of 3½-year-old boy show inequality of length (9 cm) and girth. Some increased vascular markings also apparent but not severe enough to represent Maffucci's or Klippel–Trénaunay–Weber syndrome

Radiographs document progression of disease. At 2 years of age (left), severe involvement of right lower limb and subtle involvement on left side, with limb-length discrepancy of 6 cm. At 3½ years of age (right), limb-length discrepancy is 9 cm. Spotty longitudinal densities in metaphyses of femur and tibia due to deposits of calcified cartilage. Flaring of metaphyses also evident

Same child wears non-standard prosthesis that equalizes limb length (leg and foot shown in phantom through prosthesis). Discrepancy was so progressive that usual methods of equalization could not be used

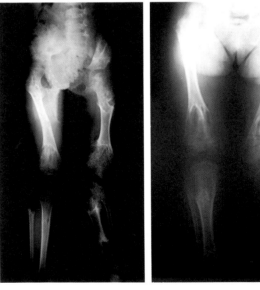

Radiograph of another child with severe involvement of both lower limbs (more severe on left) and limb-length discrepancy of 7 cm. Bilateral lesions of iliac wings also visible

In this patient, bilateral metaphyseal-diaphyseal involvement almost equal and limb-length discrepancy much less than in other case shown

Clinical Manifestations. The first sign is often lower limb–length discrepancy noted at about 4 to 5 months of age. There appears to be a progressive shortening of the limbs and a broadening of the metaphysis and diaphysis on the side of the body that is most affected. The limb-length discrepancy can be as great as 20 to 25 cm at skeletal maturity. Coxa valga and genu valgum also occur in most patients.

Radiographic Findings. Elongated and longitudinal radiolucent streaks involve the metaphysis and extend down the diaphysis. The bone structure of the middiaphysis is invariably normal; however, enchondromatous or osteochondromatous lesions may be present at the junction between the metaphysis and diaphysis, indicating that the enchondromas originate not only from the epiphysis but also from the inner (cambium) layer of the periosteum.

Treatment

The many factors to be considered in the treatment plan for limb-length discrepancy include (1) etiology; (2) degree of the discrepancy; (3) skeletal age and sex; (4) progression of the discrepancy; (5) anticipated adult height (provided the parents' heights are known); (6) strength and balance of the musculature of the limb, especially in neurologic disorders; (7) status of the foot and ankle (eg, availability of muscles in the foot and

Limb-Length Discrepancy

Hemihypertrophy

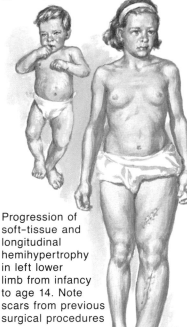

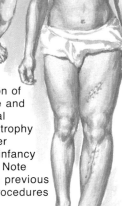

Progression of soft-tissue and longitudinal hemihypertrophy in left lower limb from infancy to age 14. Note scars from previous surgical procedures

⊥4 cm

Hemihypertrophy of right side and length discrepancy in upper and lower limbs

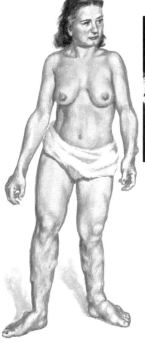

Young adult with Maffucci's syndrome and hemihypertrophy of right upper and lower limbs

Maffucci's syndrome

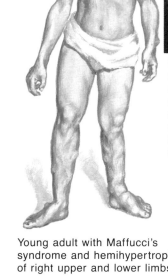

Radiograph reveals multiple enchondromas of metacarpals and phalanges; 2nd finger amputated

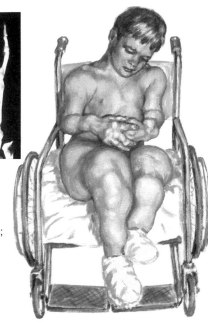

Patient with severe deformities

Klippel–Trénaunay–Weber syndrome

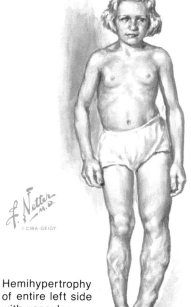

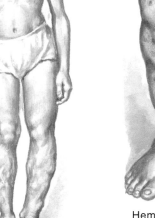

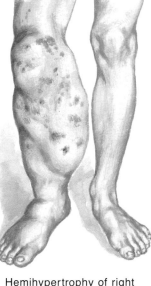

Hemihypertrophy of entire left side with vascular lesions in both lower limbs

Hemihypertrophy of right lower limb associated with cavernous hemangiomas

Hemangiomas and varicosities and hypertrophy of both feet in 9-year-old boy

Congenital short femur

Young child with congenital short left femur

Slide 4518

Lower Limb–Length Discrepancy

Lower limb–length discrepancies include any inequality in length from the level of the pelvis to, and including, the foot. The numerous causes of the inequality include the following.

Congenital and developmental anomalies with terminal limb deficiencies: hemihypertrophy or hemiatrophy, Klippel-Trénaunay-Weber syndrome,

Maffucci's syndrome, posterior bowing of the tibia, proximal femoral focal deficiency, congenital short femur, enchondromatosis.

Paralytic disorders: poliomyelitis, encephalopathy (eg, cerebral palsy), myelopathy (eg, myelomeningocele).

Infections of bone and joint that retard or arrest bone growth: osteomyelitis (may accelerate or inhibit growth), pyarthrosis (may lead to avascular necrosis with partial or complete growth arrest).

Trauma to bone and joint: injuries to the growth plate (may arrest growth); fractures of the metaphysis or diaphysis (may accelerate growth); malunion, excessive overriding, or angulation due to fracture (may result in limb shortening).

Tumorous conditions that produce bone overgrowth: fibrous dysplasia, enchondromatosis, osteoid osteoma, hemangioma, neurofibromatosis.

Tumors that produce growth retardation: solitary enchondroma of growth plate, simple bone cyst with repeated fractures through growth plate.

Irradiation of malignant tumors of long bones that arrest growth: Ewing's sarcoma, neuroblastoma.

Maffucci's syndrome and enchondromatosis are presented here as exemplary diseases that cause lower limb–length discrepancy.

Maffucci's Syndrome

In 1881, Maffucci described a syndrome comprising subcutaneous cavernous hemangiomas,

---

Lower Limb–Length Discrepancy

(Continued)

phlebectasia, and a dyschondroplasia that was identical to enchondromatosis. Maffucci's syndrome is a congenital, but not familial, disorder characterized by disturbance of bone formation and cartilage, particularly at the ends of long bones. The disease appears to originate from mesodermal dysplasia. The enchondromatosis is bilateral in 60% of patients, and although the enchondromas are often localized to either a hand or a foot, in over 40% of patients, they are extensive and involve multiple bones. Some degree of deformity develops in most patients. Shortening and bowing of the limb differentiate this syndrome from Klippel-Trénaunay-Weber syndrome (Plate 82), which is characterized by bony hypertrophy in association with telangiectasis.

Clinical Manifestations. At birth, patients usually appear normal, but the disease can become evident at any time before puberty.

Islands of cartilage persist in the diaphysis of long bones and may grow to form enchondromas that expand and deform the bone. Enchondromas may also form near the growth plate and interfere with longitudinal growth. Involvement of the long bones and phalanges is common, while the carpal and tarsal bones and the base of the skull are rarely affected.

As in enchondromatosis (Plate 83), the lesions may undergo malignant transformation, and the closer the lesions are to the axial skeleton, the more likely they are to become malignant.

The vascular abnormalities, which appear as firm, dark blue nodules or patches, may be simple cavernous or capillary hemangiomas in the deep layers of the cutis or in the subcutaneous layers. Thrombosis develops in the dilated vessels and vascular spaces. Phleboliths form as the thrombi calcify.

Enchondromatosis (Ollier's Disease)

In this rare, nonhereditary, congenital dyschondroplasia, enchondromas develop in a linear arrangement in the interior of bones (Plate 83). The changes appear to be related to failure of the endochondral ossification sequence. The term "Ollier's disease" refers to the condition in which distribution of the enchondromas is predominantly unilateral. When associated with hemangiomas of the overlying soft tissues, the disease is known as Maffucci's syndrome (Plate 82). The pathologic findings in Ollier's disease are similar to those of enchondromas, although they are often more bizarre (see Section II, Plate 5). The tumors develop in the epiphysis and adjacent areas of the metaphysis and diaphysis in a few or many bones. The resulting deformities include shortening due to retarded growth, broadening of the metaphyses, and bowing of the long bones. Lesions in the axial skeleton and pelvis appear to have a greater tendency toward malignant transformation than enchondromas in the limbs.

Enchondromatosis (Ollier's Disease)

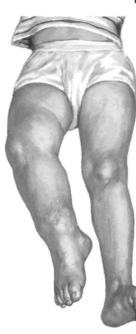

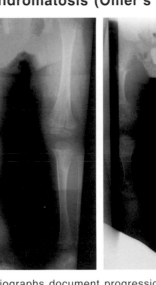

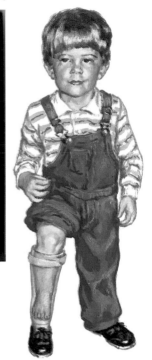

Lower limbs of 3½-year-old boy show inequality of length (9 cm) and girth. Some increased vascular markings also apparent but not severe enough to represent Maffucci's or Klippel-Trénaunay-Weber syndrome

Radiographs document progression of disease. At 2 years of age (left), severe involvement of right lower limb and subtle involvement on left side, with limb-length discrepancy of 6 cm. At 3½ years of age (right), limb-length discrepancy is 9 cm. Spotty longitudinal densities in metaphyses of femur and tibia due to deposits of calcified cartilage. Flaring of metaphyses also evident

Same child wears nonstandard prosthesis that equalizes limb length (leg and foot shown in phantom through prosthesis). Discrepancy was so progressive that usual methods of equalization could not be used

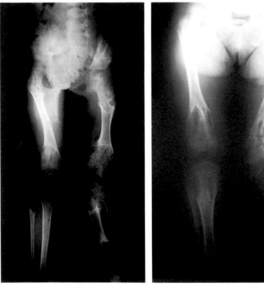

Radiograph of another child with severe involvement of both lower limbs (more severe on left) and limb-length discrepancy of 7 cm. Bilateral lesions of iliac wings also visible

In this patient, bilateral metaphyseal-diaphyseal involvement almost equal and limb-length discrepancy much less than in other case shown

Clinical Manifestations. The first sign is often lower limb–length discrepancy noted at about 4 to 5 months of age. There appears to be a progressive shortening of the limbs and a broadening of the metaphysis and diaphysis on the side of the body that is most affected. The limb-length discrepancy can be as great as 20 to 25 cm at skeletal maturity. Coxa valga and genu valgum also occur in most patients.

Radiographic Findings. Elongated and longitudinal radiolucent streaks involve the metaphysis and extend down the diaphysis. The bone structure of the middiaphysis is invariably normal; however, enchondromatous or osteochondromatous lesions may be present at the junction between the metaphysis and diaphysis, indicating that the enchondromas originate not only from the epiphysis but also from the inner (cambium) layer of the periosteum.

Treatment

The many factors to be considered in the treatment plan for limb-length discrepancy include (1) etiology; (2) degree of the discrepancy; (3) skeletal age and sex; (4) progression of the discrepancy; (5) anticipated adult height (provided the parents' heights are known); (6) strength and balance of the musculature of the limb, especially in neurologic disorders; (7) status of the foot and ankle (eg, availability of muscles in the foot and

Lower Limb–Length Discrepancy

(Continued)

ankle, presence of an equinus contracture of the short limb that allows the child to walk on tiptoe on the short side to balance the pelvis); (8) predominant site of the inequality (ie, femur or tibia); (9) general or extenuating health factors; and (10) needs and desires of the patient and parents.

Evaluation. The limb-length discrepancy can be measured in several ways. A common method is to use a tape measure or place standing blocks beneath the short side to level the pelvis. The limb is measured to the sole of the foot under the lateral malleolus rather than just to the medial malleolus, because of the differences in foot height found so often in children with neurologic and congenital deformities. Radiographic techniques, using a metal ruler on the film, include a one-exposure technique (teleradiography), in which a single exposure is made of both entire lower limbs, or a two-exposure technique with separate exposures for the femurs and the tibias. The one-exposure technique, however, may produce magnification. A more accurate method involves three successive exposures of the hips, knees, and ankles on one long film. Unfortunately, none of the radiographic measurement techniques accurately depicts pelvic asymmetry, differences in pelvic height, or height of the feet. Some physicians prefer to determine the degree of the problem by taking sequential photographs of the child standing in front of a measured wall with and without blocks placed under the short limb to level the pelvis.

Management of a lower limb–length discrepancy may depend more on the predicted difference at skeletal maturity than on the current degree of inequality. A discrepancy less than 3 cm is considered mild; one 3 to 6 cm is considered moderate. The amount of growth remaining is calculated with the chart devised by Green and Anderson or the Moseley straight-line graph (Plate 84).

The Green and Anderson growth-remaining chart is used to estimate the effects of an epiphyseal arrest procedure on the distal femur and proximal tibia at various skeletal ages. The Moseley straight-line graph helps determine the estimated lengths of the long and short bones at maturity, the discrepancy at maturity, and when the best equalization procedure should be performed. While the Moseley graph is felt to be much more accurate in cases of significant growth inhibition, it is simply a logarithmic representation of the Green and Anderson chart. The child's skeletal age, which is determined by comparing the left hand to the Greulich and Pyle *Radiographic Atlas*, is used to determine the appropriate time for equalization procedures.

Regular follow-up is necessary to determine if the discrepancy is progressive and whether conservative measures (eg, orthoses, prostheses) or surgery are the best methods of correction.

Charts for Timing Growth Arrest and Determining Amount of Limb Lengthening to Achieve Limb-Length Equality at Maturity

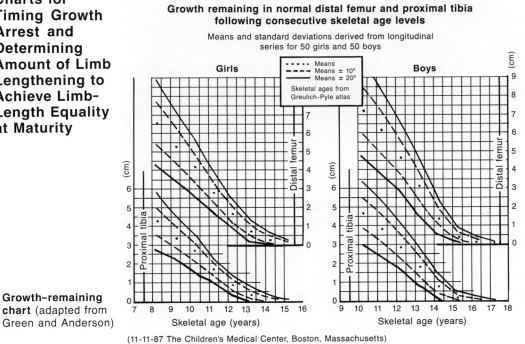

Growth remaining in normal distal femur and proximal tibia following consecutive skeletal age levels

Means and standard deviations derived from longitudinal series for 50 girls and 50 boys

Growth-remaining chart (adapted from Green and Anderson)

(11-11-87 The Children's Medical Center, Boston, Massachusetts)

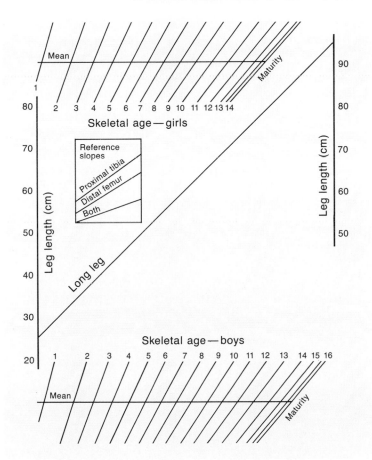

Straight-line graph for leg-length discrepancy (adapted from Moseley)

© CIBA-GEIGY

Surgical procedures for lower limb–length discrepancy include (1) conversion of the short side to an amputation, which is fitted with a prosthesis; (2) shortening of the long side by arresting or retarding epiphyseal growth or resecting a segment of the femur or the tibia and fibula; (3) direct femoral, tibial, or transiliac lengthening; and (4) combined shortening and lengthening.

Growth Arrest and Growth Retardation. *Epiphysiodesis* is the destruction of the growth plate by means of an open or closed surgical technique (Plate 85). The open technique involves removing a rectangular block of bone at the medial and lateral borders of the growth plate. The growth plate is then curetted from both sides

under direct vision. The rectangular blocks are turned upside down and replaced.

The advent of improved clarity of intraoperative radiographic image intensification has facilitated the use of a closed technique, percutaneous epiphysiodesis. A very small incision is made over a Steinmann pin placed medially to laterally in the plane of the growth plate. A cannulated reamer is placed over the pin and used to begin removal of the growth plate; power drilling or curettage, or both, completes the removal. Viscous lidocaine and a radiographic contrast medium are injected into the defect, and the limb is rotated under the image intensifier to determine the adequacy of the procedure. Morbidity

Lower Limb–Length Discrepancy
(Continued)

is quite low, and the scar is much more acceptable to patients than that of open epiphysiodesis.

Epiphyseal stapling retards, but does not stop, growth (Plate 85). Unlike epiphysiodesis, the procedure must be performed on a younger patient in order to achieve the same growth retardation, but it should not be done before the child reaches the skeletal age of 8 years. If growth is to be resumed, the staples must be removed before growth of the epiphysis has ceased.

After the staples are removed, a rebound phenomenon, or initial growth spurt, may occur, followed by continuation of growth at the normal rate. A previously stapled epiphysis usually closes a few months prematurely, which tends to compensate for the spurt in growth. Although there are many technical problems associated with the stapling procedure, the theoretical advantages of stapling—such as the ability to control angular and length deformities—make it a worthwhile alternative to epiphysiodesis.

Resection of the longer limb may be performed to correct limb-length discrepancy in skeletally mature patients. Bone resection also corrects angular and rotational deformities. In some patients, resection of the longer limb is combined with lengthening of the shorter one.

Limb-Lengthening Procedures. Mechanical procedures include (1) osteotomy and gradual distraction; (2) corticotomy and gradual distraction (callotasis); (3) lengthening through the growth plate (chondrodiastasis); (4) osteotomy and sudden distraction; (5) transiliac lengthening; and (6) lengthening and shortening in a one-stage procedure, using the bone fragment from the long side to lengthen the short side.

Lengthening is appropriate in children 8 to 12 years of age who have a predicted limb-length discrepancy of 4 cm or more. The discrepancy in a skeletally immature child should be greater than can be corrected with epiphysiodesis of the long limb. Muscle weakness should be sufficient so that little power is lost by lengthening. However, gradual lengthening causes several systemic complications, such as transient hypertension, anorexia and weight loss, and emotional lability. Lengthening the bone more than 15% increases the complication rate.

Femoral lengthening, first performed in 1905, was originally associated with many serious complications and few good results. In 1971, Wagner described a technique for femoral lengthening with osteotomy and bone grafting using a device of his design (Plate 86). The Wagner device is used in patients between 4 and 20 years of age with a lower limb–length discrepancy of 4 to 10 cm. Prerequisites for its use include a stable hip joint, normal knee function and alignment, pliable soft tissue and muscle, absence of systemic hypertension, and absence of neurovascular

Growth Arrest
Percutaneous epiphysiodesis

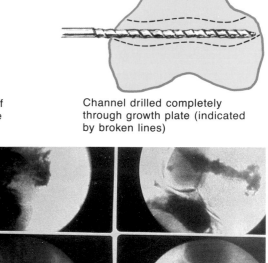

Drill introduced transversely through growth plate of distal femur along tract determined with test needle under image-intensification visualization

Channel drilled completely through growth plate (indicated by broken lines)

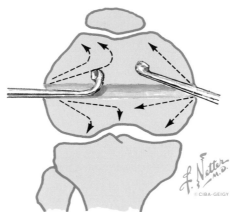

Straight- and right-angled curets of various sizes used for complete removal of peripheries of growth plate (anterior view with knee and hip in flexion)

After injection of viscous contrast medium, radiographs are taken of leg rotated in different planes to verify complete ablation of growth plate

Open epiphysiodesis

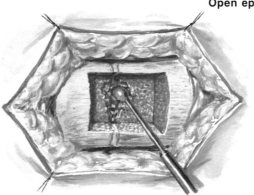

Rectangular bone plug incorporating growth plate resected from each side of distal femur. Growth plate drilled and curetted and gap filled with cancellous bone from above and below

Bone plug reversed and impacted into its bed. Cartilaginous growth plate line on plug now more proximal

Growth Retardation
Epiphyseal stapling

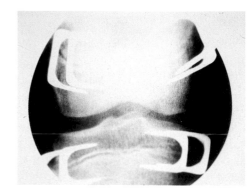

Staples placed across growth plate of distal femur. Broken line indicates incision for stapling growth plate of proximal tibia

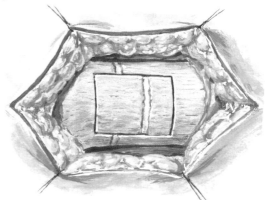

Image-intensification radiograph shows staples in place in femur and tibia

Wagner Technique for Limb Lengthening

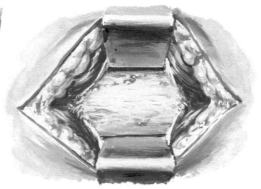

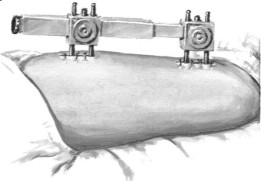

1. Parallel Schanz screws placed in metaphyses of proximal and distal femur in true lateral plane

2. Femur exposed and periosteum reflected via posterolateral incision and approach between hamstring and vastus lateralis muscles (for later osteotomy)

3. Wagner lengthening device attached to Schanz screws. Osteotomy performed through posterolateral incision

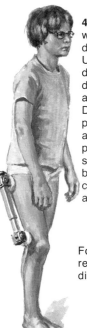

4. Child ambulatory with lengthening device in place. Up to 1.5 mm of distraction applied daily by turning knob at top of device. Dorsiflexion and plantar flexion of ankle, dorsalis pedis pulse, knee motion, sensation, and blood pressure carefully monitored and recorded

Follow-up radiograph reveals about 1 cm of distraction

5. After planned lengthening attained, postero-lateral incision again made to expose osteotomy. Slight additional distraction applied under anesthesia as indicated, and ASIF compression plate applied to femur. Gap filled with bone graft from ilium

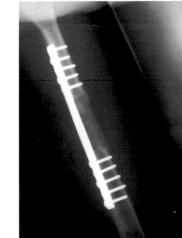

Radiograph shows ASIF compression plate in place and osteosynthesis from bone graft

Patient before (left) and after (right) limb-lengthening procedure. Complete correction of 5-cm discrepancy in limb length

Radiograph shows Anderson limb-lengthening device, which applies distraction to both sides of tibia. Pin affixes distal fibula to tibia to prevent upward migration from talar mortise

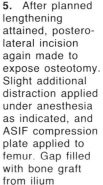

Lower Limb–Length Discrepancy

(Continued)

problems in the limb. The amount of lengthening should never exceed 20% to 25% of bone length or 9 cm. The technique achieves the best results in acquired shortening due to trauma, epiphyseal injury, poliomyelitis, and neonatal osteomyelitis. Congenital deformities are much more difficult to correct because of the presence of soft-tissue contractures.

Complications associated with the Wagner technique are significant. They include minor pin tract infections and skin slough, loosening of Schanz screws, fracture of the lengthened segment, plate failure, osteomyelitis, malalignment, neurovascular injury, hip dislocation, and thrombophlebitis.

Tibial lengthening can be carried out with a similar distraction device designed by Anderson, which is attached to both sides of the metaphyses of the proximal and distal tibia with "through-and-through" pins (Plate 86). The complications associated with the Anderson limb-lengthening technique, however, far exceed those seen with the Wagner procedure.

A technique of limb lengthening known as callus distraction, or callotasis, was introduced by Ilizarov in 1951 (Plate 87). Following sub-periosteal division of the bone at the diaphysis (corticotomy) or metaphysis (compactotomy), without disturbing the medullary canal, the bone fragments are fixed above and below with a fixator device. The Ilizarov device incorporates metal rings that encircle the limb and attach to the bone with metal wires or pins. Telescoping rods connect the rings and provide the distraction capability. The De Bastiani device, called a dynamic axial fixator, is a rigid telescoping bar

Ilizarov and De Bastiani Techniques for Limb Lengthening

Ilizarov technique

After percutaneous or open corticotomy, Ilizarov device secured with wires or pins passing through bone. After 7 days, device extended 0.25 mm four times a day (1 mm/day) until desired limb length attained. Cortical bone grows in to fill distraction gap

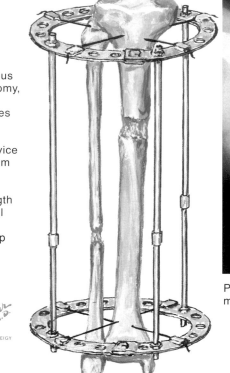

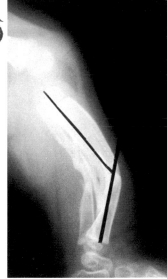

Preoperative radiograph documents short, angulated tibia

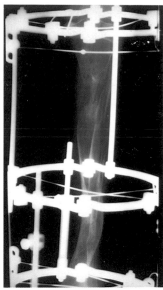

Corticotomy of tibia and fibula carried out, device in place, and distraction begun (additional corticotomy done in this patient to correct angulation)

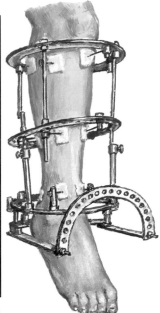

Clinical view with device in place and wires through tibia

De Bastiani technique

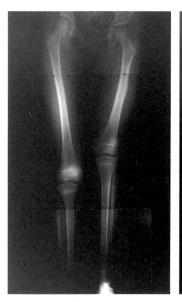

Preoperative radiograph shows unilateral congenital short femur and tibias of equal length

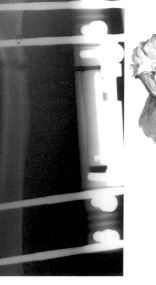

Radiograph shows corticotomy of femur with dynamic axial fixator in place

Child wears De Bastiani device

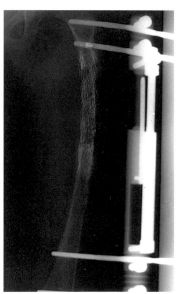

Radiograph taken after 8 cm of lengthening, with new bone growth filling femoral defect. Device still in place

De Bastiani device applied to ulna for lengthening

Lower Limb–Length Discrepancy

(Continued)

that attaches to one side of the limb with screws (Plate 87).

About 2 to 3 mm of lengthening is carried out at the time of the corticotomy. After 10 to 14 days (7 days in the Ilizarov technique), when callus is seen on radiographs, distraction is begun at a rate of 0.25 mm four times a day. Radiographic monitoring is critical because distraction started before callus formation may delay union; if started too late, distraction may not be possible because of early union. Several variations in this technique are being investigated, including bone transport, in which a segment of bone is removed and moved distally to fill another defect while callotasis is occurring at its former site, and bifocal corticotomy, in which the bone is divided at both proximal and distal ends, allowing callotasis to occur twice as fast at both sites.

Chondrodiastasis, or symmetric distraction of the growth plate, is used when the limb-length discrepancy is small. Since the procedure stimulates closure of the growth plate, its use is limited to adolescents nearing completion of growth.

Transiliac lengthening permanently corrects a static limb-length discrepancy less than 3 cm, especially when epiphysiodesis and use of a shoe lift are unacceptable. The procedure is most effective in patients with a postural imbalance in the transverse plane. The technique is similar to the Salter innominate osteotomy for congenital hip dislocation, except that the pelvic fragments are distracted and held open anteriorly and posteriorly with a quadrilateral bone graft. Unlike epiphysiodesis and epiphyseal stapling, transiliac lengthening balances the limbs directly without shortening the overall height. □

Congenital Clubfoot

Clinical appearance
of bilateral clubfoot
in infant

Anteroposterior (above)
and lateral (below)
radiographs
show congenital
clubfoot in newborn

Plantar flexion (equinus)
at ankle joint

Deformity of talus

Tightness of
tibionavicular ligament and
extensor digitorum longus,
tibialis anterior, and
extensor hallucis longus
tendons

Extreme varus position of forefoot bones

Inversion of calcaneus

Pathologic changes in congenital clubfoot

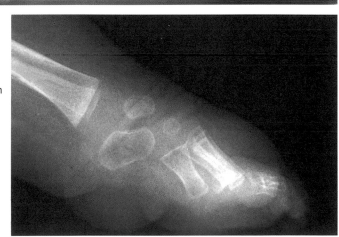

Lateral radiograph
demonstrates
severe clubfoot
complicated by
extreme plantar
flexion of forefoot
in newborn

Slide 4524

Congenital Clubfoot

Congenital clubfoot (congenital equinovarus) is a structural foot deformity that is present at birth (Plate 88). The entire foot is plantar flexed (equinus), and both forefoot and hindfoot are inverted (varus). The deformity, which may be unilateral or bilateral, occurs in about 1 of 800 births and is more common in males than in females. There is a strong genetic tendency, as seen in the increased incidence in the children and grandchildren of affected persons.

Three categories of congenital clubfoot have been described. *Postural clubfoot* is not a true structural abnormality and usually responds rapidly to conservative management. In the so-called *true clubfoot*, the degree of severity varies widely. *Arthrogrypotic*, or *teratologic, clubfoot* is a severe deformity that nearly always requires early, radical surgery to achieve correction.

Etiology and Pathology

The etiology of congenital clubfoot is not known, but a genetic mode of inheritance is well established. Although females are less often affected than males, their deformity is often more severe and more difficult to treat, especially if bilateral.

Congenital clubfoot is characterized by bones that are abnormal not only in their relationship to each other but also in shape and size. Thus, even after correction, the true clubfoot is smaller than normal, and some signs of the deformity persist. In addition, the ligaments connecting the bones and the musculotendinous structures acting on the bones and joints are contracted and foreshortened.

One of the most consistent and important pathologic manifestations is a pronounced medial angulation of the head and neck of the talus, a

Congenital Clubfoot
(*Continued*)

deformity that persists to some degree even after acceptable correction has been achieved. The ossification centers of the tarsal bones demonstrate varying degrees of abnormal endochondral growth and development.

Treatment

Because the pathologic features of congenital clubfoot vary in severity, the types and results of treatment also vary substantially. In some patients, correction can be achieved and maintained with simple surgical methods, whereas in other patients, complex and sophisticated surgery is required, followed by postoperative bracing.

Corrective Manipulation. Treatment for congenital clubfoot should be started as soon as possible after birth. In all patients, the first procedure should be gentle corrective manipulation and casting to maintain the correction (Plate 89). The manipulation technique and the care with which casts are applied are extremely important. Weekly or twice-weekly manipulations should be carried out for a minimum of 10 to 12 weeks or until it is determined that correction is occurring or that the deformity is resistant to conservative measures and thus requires surgery.

Surgical Procedures. The age at which surgery should be performed is somewhat controversial. The minimum age is 3 or 4 months, but some surgeons prefer to wait until the patient is at least 1 year of age. Surgery revises the bone and joint relationships by elongating the contracted ligaments and tendons. A variety of techniques and surgical approaches are used, but the type of procedure is not so important as the principles. It is important to emphasize that the type and amount of surgical correction required vary with the degree of resistance to manipulation and the severity of the deformity.

In the foot, the structures that most commonly require elongation are the tibionavicular portion of the deltoid ligament, the tibialis posterior tendon, the talonavicular joint capsule, and the talocalcaneal joint capsule and interosseous ligament. The long toe flexors may also require elongation. The procedure to lengthen these structures is called a medial release. If the foot has a significant cavus deformity as well, the contracted plantar muscles may also require release; this combined operation is called a plantar medial release.

Corrective Manipulation for Congenital Clubfoot

Manipulation of foot in step–by–step correction of varus deformity. (Excessive force must be avoided)

Manipulation of ankle in progressive correction of equinus deformity

After each stage of manipulation, plaster cast applied to maintain correction

A posterior release is performed to correct the equinus deformity at the ankle: the calcaneal (Achilles) tendon is lengthened; the ankle joint capsule and all posterior tibiotalar, talofibular, and calcaneofibular ligaments are severed; and the tibiofibular syndesmosis is released posteriorly. It is often necessary to combine posterior and medial release procedures in what is called a posteromedial release.

Following surgical correction, the foot and ankle are immobilized in a well-padded above-knee cast. The casts are changed 1 week and 2 weeks after surgery to allow inspection of the wound and verification of the correction. Then, a more snug, well-molded cast with very little padding is applied. After 6 to 12 weeks, casts are replaced with retentive splints and braces, which are required for several months (years for resistant cases, especially the arthrogrypotic clubfoot). All patients must be followed throughout their growth period to assess and ensure that the correction is maintained.

In some patients, the deformity tends to release or recur. Recurrent clubfoot must be corrected with whatever means are appropriate; after correction is achieved, some patients require tendon transfers to prevent recurrence. One recommended procedure involves transferring the tibialis anterior tendon, either whole or in part, to the medial cuneiform. □

Congenital Vertical Talus

Although congenital vertical talus is a deformity present at birth, often the diagnosis is not made because of its superficial resemblance to infantile calcaneovalgus. The heel is in valgus position and the sole of the foot is convex, a clinical appearance that led to the synonyms "congenital convex pes valgus" and "rocker-bottom" foot. True congenital vertical talus is much less common than clubfoot, and there is almost always a coexisting congenital abnormality such as clubfoot, syndactyly, neuromuscular syndrome, or lumbosacral agenesis.

The etiology of the deformity is not yet understood, but because it is a structural congenital deformity, some genetic abnormality must exist.

Clinical Manifestations. As in congenital clubfoot, the bones not only have an abnormal relationship with one another but are abnormal in size and configuration, with abnormal articulating surfaces. The ligamentous and musculotendinous structures about the foot and ankle are contracted and rigidly hold the bones in position.

This paradoxical deformity comprises plantar flexion (equinus) of the hindfoot and ankle and dorsiflexion of the midfoot and forefoot. The navicular is held in fixed dorsal subluxation or dislocation on the top of the head and neck of the talus. This abnormal position of the navicular can be identified readily in a lateral radiograph of the foot because there is an area of increased density in the superior aspect of the talar neck that corresponds to the location of the talonavicular articulation.

Treatment. The unique combination of forefoot dorsiflexion and hindfoot plantar flexion in congenital vertical talus almost always requires surgical correction. The paradoxical nature of the deformity explains the need for lengthening and sectioning of the posterior, as well as the anterior, ligaments and tendons (extensors and dorsiflexors).

Corrective measures should be started as soon as the diagnosis is made. Although surgical correction is usually required, it *may* be possible to correct the deformity with a program of manipulation and casting of the foot. Perhaps more importantly, these conservative measures stretch the skin on the dorsum of the foot and passively lengthen the tendons that dorsiflex the forefoot and toes. Therefore, if surgery is subsequently needed, the skin incision will be easier to close

Congenital Vertical Talus

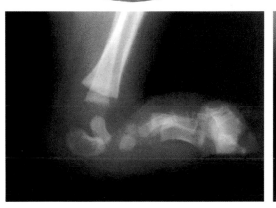

Clinical appearance of infant's foot. Plantar flexion of hindfoot and dorsiflexion of forefoot with resultant "rocker bottom." Valgus position of heel clearly seen in posterior view

Lateral radiograph shows vertical position of talus, plantar flexion of hindfoot, and dorsiflexion of forefoot

Radiograph demonstrates that forced plantar flexion of forefoot fails to correct abnormal position of hindfoot

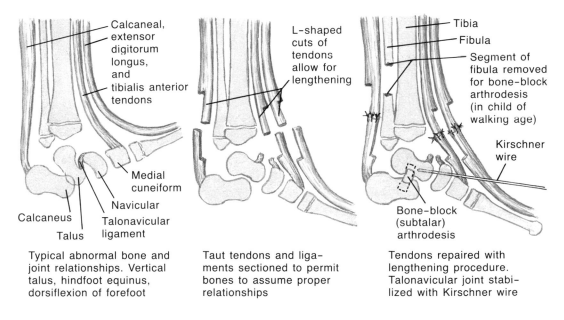

Typical abnormal bone and joint relationships. Vertical talus, hindfoot equinus, dorsiflexion of forefoot

Calcaneal, extensor digitorum longus, and tibialis anterior tendons
Medial cuneiform
Navicular
Talonavicular ligament
Talus
Calcaneus

Taut tendons and ligaments sectioned to permit bones to assume proper relationships

L-shaped cuts of tendons allow for lengthening

Tendons repaired with lengthening procedure. Talonavicular joint stabilized with Kirschner wire

Tibia
Fibula
Segment of fibula removed for bone-block arthrodesis (in child of walking age)
Kirschner wire
Bone-block (subtalar) arthrodesis

and the extensor tendons may not require lengthening.

The aim of manipulation is to achieve plantar flexion of the foot. Every week, the foot is manipulated gently into plantar flexion and a cast applied until maximum plantar flexion has been achieved. Surgery should be planned as soon as the manipulation program has been completed and the child is at least 3 months of age. Surgical correction should be done before walking age because the procedure is much less complex and the results much better in children of this age.

Surgery to correct congenital vertical talus may be done in one or two stages. The sequence of procedures is less important than the concepts of

correction. The forefoot must be aligned with the hindfoot, which means that the talonavicular and subtalar (talocalcaneal) joints must be reduced and stabilized. The posterior structures of the ankle are released to bring the entire foot out of the equinus position.

In children of walking age, it is often necessary to perform a subtalar extraarticular (bone-block) arthrodesis to achieve and maintain stability of the talocalcaneal joint. Bone-block arthrodesis is rarely needed in patients too young to walk.

After surgery, the foot is immobilized in a cast for 3 months, after which it is protectively splinted in a well-molded ankle-foot orthosis for several months. □

Cavovarus

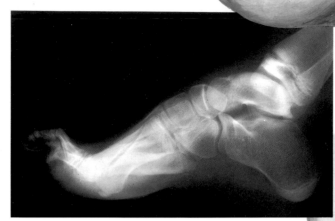

Cavovarus foot with characteristic high arch extending upward from ball of foot and cock–up deformity of toes

Radiograph of foot shown above reveals fixed bony configuration, dorsiflexion of hindfoot, and sharp plantar flexion of forefoot

Right cavovarus foot. When patient stands, weight is on ball of foot and heel is elevated

Posterior view clearly shows varus deformity of affected right foot

The cavovarus foot deformity is unique, largely because it has a variety of causes. While it is not rare, the incidence is not well established. Seldom present at birth, the deformity gradually becomes apparent as the child's foot grows and matures.

Etiology and Pathology. Three distinct etiologic categories have been identified: (1) paralytic muscle imbalance, (2) residuals of congenital clubfoot, and (3) unknown, or idiopathic. Whenever possible, it is important to identify the exact cause, so that proper treatment can be administered. In this regard, the diagnosis of cavovarus, especially in a previously normal foot, necessitates a thorough search for an underlying neurologic cause. If a neurologic problem is suspected, an electromyographic examination should be done, and a radiograph of the lumbosacral spine should be taken. Myelography, computed tomography, or magnetic resonance imaging of the lumbosacral spine may also be necessary.

Clinical Manifestations. The term "cavovarus" refers to the two distinguishing clinical features: a varus hindfoot and a heightened longitudinal arch (cavus). The forefoot—particularly the first metatarsal—is excessively plantar flexed. In fact, in children and young adolescents, the plantar-flexed first metatarsal is the most significant feature, not only because it is responsible for the cavus appearance of the foot but also because on weight bearing it forces the heel into varus position, and weight is thus transferred primarily onto the lateral border of the foot. Cock-up deformity of the toes is another characteristic feature.

Radiographic Findings. The weight-bearing radiograph reflects some of the same clinical manifestations seen on physical examination. The metatarsals are excessively plantar flexed, the midfoot is elevated, and the hindfoot is in varus position (seen in the reduced plantar flexion of the talus). Dorsiflexion of the metatarsophalangeal joints is also apparent.

Treatment. If the deformity results from an underlying neurologic problem that is amenable to surgery, this should be treated before the foot deformity is corrected. Cavovarus always requires surgery. Casts and orthoses are not effective for correcting or preventing the progression of the deformity.

Before surgical correction, the flexibility of the forefoot and hindfoot must be assessed, which can be done in several ways. The technique that provides the best documentation is to have the patient stand on a block of wood about 1 to 1½ inches high. The heel and fifth metatarsal are placed on the block, and the first metatarsal is allowed to "fall" to the floor. This eliminates the effect of fixed forefoot pronation on the hindfoot (tripod effect). If the heel goes into valgus position, the hindfoot is supple; if the heel remains in varus, the hindfoot is considered rigid. In most children and young adolescents, the hindfoot is flexible, and thus forefoot pronation is the principal problem.

In younger children, cavovarus requires a radical plantar release. Deformity due to residual clubfoot is treated with a plantar medial release. These procedures are followed by sequential manipulations and cast applications. Tendon transfers are indicated for deformity due to an identified neurologic disorder with demonstrable muscle imbalance. In most cases, the long toe extensors are moved to the metatarsals (Jones technique) or to the tarsals (Hibbs technique). In some situations, the best balancing procedure includes transfer of the posterior lateral tendon to the dorsolateral aspect of the foot.

In older children and adolescents, simple soft-tissue releases are usually inadequate because adaptive bony changes have occurred. In the child with a flexible hindfoot, soft-tissue release must be accompanied by osteotomy of either the first metatarsal or the medial cuneiform. Older adolescents with rigid hindfoot require a triple arthrodesis, in rare instances coupled with osteotomy of the forefoot. □

Calcaneovalgus and Planovalgus

Calcaneovalgus and Planovalgus

Calcaneovalgus in 2-year-old child. Right foot more severely affected. Condition more apparent when patient stands

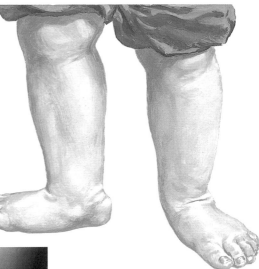

Flexible plastic orthotic device worn inside shoe is helpful in symptomatic cases

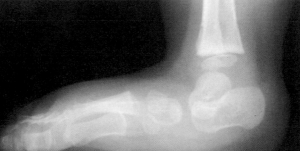

Lateral radiograph of right foot shown above

Lateral radiograph of left foot shown below

Anterior and posterior views of bilateral planovalgus in adolescent boy. Valgus position of heels most apparent in posterior view

The major distinguishing feature of these two foot deformities is the age of onset. Calcaneovalgus (congenital calcaneovalgus) refers to a flexible flatfoot in infants and young children, whereas planovalgus is a similar deformity that occurs in older children and adolescents. Both are nonstructural, flexible, and postural abnormalities of unknown etiology and prevalence. Although by definition the abnormality consists of a flatfoot, the clinical criteria used in diagnosis are highly subjective.

Clinical Manifestations. The physical findings are distinctive in very young infants and children. When the foot and ankle are dorsiflexed, the dorsal aspect of the foot can be opposed to the anterior aspect of the tibia. The plantar surface of the foot is flat, the hindfoot is in valgus position, and the forefoot is abducted. Superficially, this deformity strongly resembles congenital vertical talus (Plate 90). The flexibility of the calcaneovalgus foot is one of several features that allow differentiation of the two disorders. However, some cases require radiographic evaluation for definitive diagnosis.

During weight bearing, the planovalgus foot is characterized by a flattened longitudinal arch, valgus hindfoot, and plantar flexion and medial rotation of the talus on the calcaneus. The midfoot and forefoot are abducted and, in some patients, the calcaneal (Achilles) tendon is contracted. However, in a nonweight-bearing position, the foot assumes a normal configuration. Also, when the patient walks on the toes or on the ball of the foot, the longitudinal arch appears normal.

Radiographic Findings. In both calcaneovalgus and planovalgus, the ossification centers of the foot bones are normal. The only radiographic abnormalities are in the relationships of the bones, and even these can be easily reduced by positioning or nonweight bearing. Lateral radiographs reveal a substantial divergence in the long axes of the talus and calcaneus; a similar decrease in these axes is seen in anteroposterior radiographs of the weight-bearing foot.

Treatment. In most patients, flexible flatfeet are asymptomatic, and it is impossible to predict

which calcaneovalgus or planovalgus feet will become painful in adulthood. A small number of truly flexible flatfeet become substantially rigid if the feet do not correct with growth and permanent adaptive changes occur.

Treatment of calcaneovalgus and planovalgus is controversial for the following reasons: (1) it is impossible to *quantitate* what constitutes a flexible flatfoot; (2) no device has been developed that predictably alters the growth, development, or final adult configuration of a flexible flatfoot; (3) it is difficult to determine how much pain or excessive shoe wear should be tolerated; (4) the results of surgery in the treatment of flexible flatfoot are extremely difficult to assess; and (5) it

has not been proven that the mere presence of a flexible flatfoot requires any form of treatment.

In a few patients, excessive shoe wear, symptoms, or severe deformity justifies the use of a supportive device. The best is a durable plastic foot orthosis that can be used with any shoe.

Surgery is never justified for asymptomatic, *flexible* calcaneovalgus or planovalgus deformity in a young child. A few procedures have been helpful in adolescents with persistent, symptomatic flatfeet who have a substantial problem with wearing shoes. The rare, painfully symptomatic, *rigid* flatfoot, however, requires more aggressive treatment, usually a triple arthrodesis, which corrects the deformity and eliminates pain. ☐

Tarsal Coalition

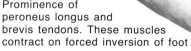

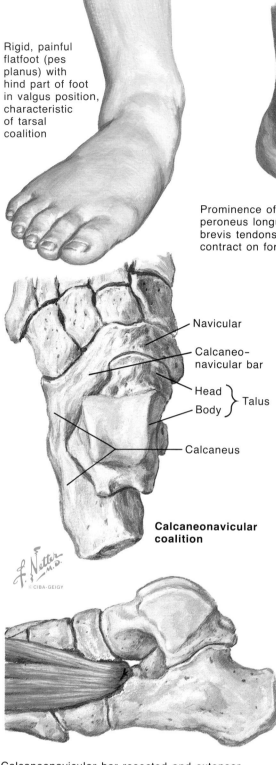

Rigid, painful flatfoot (pes planus) with hind part of foot in valgus position, characteristic of tarsal coalition

Prominence of peroneus longus and brevis tendons. These muscles contract on forced inversion of foot

Navicular

Calcaneo-navicular bar

Head ⎫
Body ⎭ Talus

Calcaneus

Calcaneonavicular coalition

f. Netter
©CIBA-GEIGY

Calcaneonavicular bar resected and extensor digitorum brevis muscle interposed to prevent reformation of coalition

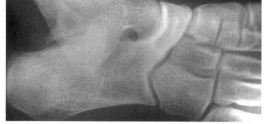

Solid, bony calcaneonavicular coalition evident on oblique radiograph

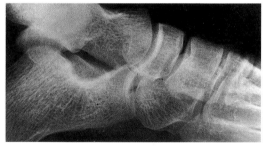

Cartilaginous calcaneonavicular coalition visible but poorly defined on lateral radiograph

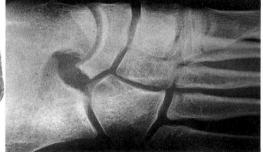

Postoperative radiograph

Coalition between the tarsal bones is a frequent cause of painful flatfoot (pes planus) in the older child or adolescent. Rigid flatfoot, a valgus heel with limited subtalar motion, and pain in the subtalar area are the major clinical findings. Coalition may develop between any of the tarsal bones, but the most common coalitions are between the calcaneus and the navicular and the talus and the calcaneus. While a single coalition is most common, more than one are occasionally found in the same foot.

Calcaneonavicular Coalition

Clinical Manifestations. Coalition between the calcaneus and the navicular usually becomes apparent in patients between 8 and 12 years of age when the cartilaginous coalition that results from an embryologic failure of tarsal segmentation undergoes ossification (Plate 93). Symptoms occur because the ossification limits subtalar motion, which is required for normal walking. When the foot is placed on the ground in normal gait, the subtalar joint rotates externally to compensate for internal rotation of the tibia on the femur with full extension at the knee. If subtalar motion is restricted, the navicular is displaced dorsally on the talus and the calcaneus is forced into valgus position with each step. The peroneus longus and peroneus brevis tendons adaptively shorten. The limited subtalar motion and tendon shortening create the clinical picture of the rigid flatfoot. When inversion of the foot is attempted, the shortened peroneal tendons contract, pulling the foot into eversion. This contraction of the tendons also protects the subtalar area when it is painful.

Radiographic Findings. Calcaneonavicular coalition is most clearly seen on the oblique radiograph (described by Slomann in 1921). Although visible on both anteroposterior and lateral views, the coalition is much more difficult to recognize in these projections.

Treatment. Asymptomatic coalition does not require surgical treatment. Painful flatfoot, limited subtalar movement, and the presence of a cartilaginous bar are the usual indications for an operation. For symptomatic coalition before degenerative changes have occurred (usually seen in patients under age 14), resection is the usual treatment. This procedure is not appropriate if the cartilaginous bar is completely ossified and

degenerative changes have occurred or if coalition between the talus and calcaneus is also present.

The resection is performed through a lateral incision. The extensor digitorum brevis muscle is freed from its insertion and reflected distally, with care to preserve the nerve supply. The coalition is located and the talocalcaneal, talonavicular, calcaneocuboid, and cuneonavicular joints are identified. A rectangular section of the coalition is removed. To prevent recurrence, all cartilage must be removed from both the calcaneus and the navicular; the extensor digitorum brevis muscle is then placed into the defect.

The patient wears a below-knee cast for 7 to 10 days, after which subtalar motion is begun.

Tarsal Coalition
(Continued)

Tarsal Coalition (continued)

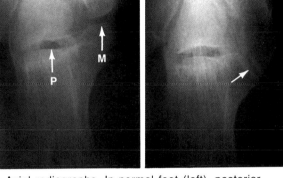

Posterior and middle facets of calca-neus, which articulate with talus, are normally in parallel planes and are usually best visualized on axial radiograph at 45°. In talocalcaneal coalition, angle of middle facet may vary. Additional axial view taken at angle of sustentaculum tali (deter-mined with lateral view). Anterior facet is in a different plane and cannot be seen on axial view because it is obscured by head of talus

Axial (Harris) technique. Patient stands on cassette; x-rays projected at 45° angle

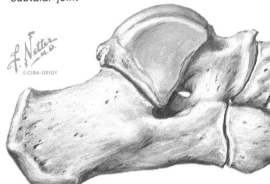

Secondary signs of talocalcaneal coalition. A = beaking of talus; B = broadening of lateral process of talus; C = narrowing of subtalar joint

Axial radiographs. In normal foot (left), posterior (P) and middle (M) facets are open and in parallel planes. Cartilaginous coalition of middle facet (right), which is angled in relation to posterior facet. When coalition ossifies, joint line is obliterated by bone

Bony coalition of anterior facet

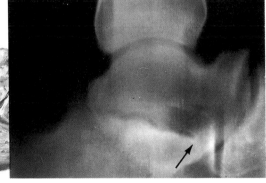

Tomogram reveals bony coalition of anterior facet. Beaking of talus also evident

Weight bearing is not allowed until the amount of subtalar motion reaches that obtained during the operation (3–4 weeks).

In patients over 14 years of age who have degenerative changes, a below-knee, weight-bearing cast, a plastizoate insert for the shoe, or an ankle-foot orthosis may relieve the pain. Fail-ure to respond to these conservative measures and the presence of degenerative changes indicate the need for triple arthrodesis.

Talocalcaneal Coalition

Clinical Manifestations. Although coalition between the calcaneus and the talus may occur in any of the three facets, the middle facet is the one most commonly involved (Plate 94). The anatomic configuration of the middle and ante-rior facets varies from person to person. At least four different patterns are seen: (1) a single, small middle facet; (2) a single middle facet that extends posteriorly and is almost as large as the posterior facet; (3) a middle facet that extends anteriorly; and (4) two facets—the middle and anterior facets—in the medial compartment. Coalition may be seen in any of these facets.

Talocalcaneal coalition generally becomes symptomatic in the early teenage years when the preexisting cartilaginous coalition ossifies.

Radiographic Findings. Coalition between the talus and calcaneus may be difficult to detect on radiographs. Since the normal posterior and middle facets are in parallel planes at approxi-mately 45° to the sole of the foot, these two areas can be identified on an axial (Harris, or ski-jump) radiograph (described by Korvin in 1933). The radiographic appearance of the two facets either

in the same plane or at an angle greater than 20° to each other suggests coalition. Cartilaginous coalition between the talus and calcaneus in the area of the middle facet may also be detected by an irregularity of the joint surfaces of the talus and calcaneus. However, the anterior facet is not seen on the axial radiograph, and tomography is required to visualize it properly.

Treatment. Conservative measures are usually effective for most patients with talocalcaneal coalition. Use of a below-knee, weight-bearing cast for 3 weeks frequently relieves symptoms; thereafter, a plastizoate insert or an ankle-foot orthosis is prescribed. Recurrent symptoms are managed similarly.

Resection is the treatment of choice in the patient under 16 years of age if no degenerative changes are present. Triple arthrodesis may be indicated when symptoms are severe and degen-erative changes are present.

Symptoms often abate when the facet ossifies completely, particularly if the heel remains in a neutral position. In a few patients with a large middle facet, tarsal tunnel syndrome develops from pressure on the median plantar nerve; a large middle facet may also prevent full plantar flexion of the ankle, since it abuts the posterior portion of the ankle joint. In these patients, resection is performed although subtalar motion is not improved. □

Accessory Navicular

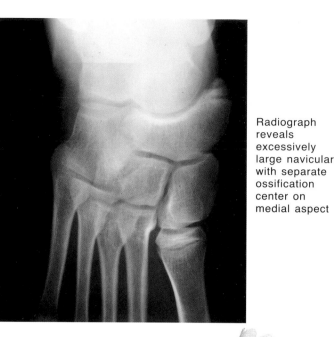

Accessory Navicular

Radiograph reveals excessively large navicular with separate ossification center on medial aspect

Tender, inflamed bony prominence on medial aspect of foot over navicular

Kidner operation. Incision from below medial malleolus to base of 1st metatarsal. Fascia incised and elevated, exposing insertion of tibialis posterior tendon and accessory navicular

Tibialis posterior tendon

Insertion of tibialis posterior tendon into navicular transposed to plantar surface of navicular; its attachment to cuneiforms not disturbed. Accessory navicular and prominent portion of navicular resected

The accessory navicular is located on the medial side of the foot, proximal to the navicular and in continuity with the tibialis posterior tendon. Although the accessory bone appears distinct from the navicular on radiographs, it is actually attached by fibrous tissue or cartilage. A study of 14 patients followed to maturity found that the accessory bone fused to the navicular in five patients, partially fused in three, and failed to fuse in six.

Clinical Manifestations. The accessory navicular is frequently seen in conjunction with flatfoot. A possible cause is that the insertion of the major portion of the tibialis posterior tendon into the accessory bone displaces the tendon, allowing the foot to deviate into valgus position. This results in flatfoot with prominences of the accessory bone and the navicular. Pressure from the shoe on the prominence may cause pain, but the subtalar motion is adequate and the peroneus longus and peroneus brevis tendons do not become shortened.

Treatment. Pain and tenderness over the prominence can be relieved by altering the shoe or by placing a doughnut-shaped piece of moleskin on the skin around the prominence. If symptoms are not relieved with conservative measures or if they recur after conservative measures are discontinued, excision of the accessory navicular may be indicated.

The Kidner operation is used to remove the prominence of the accessory navicular; improvement of associated flatfoot is an ancillary benefit. Asymptomatic flatfoot with an accessory navicular is not an indication for surgery. The incision is placed on the medial side of the foot dorsal to the prominence of the navicular, because a painful scar may result if the incision is placed over the prominence. The tibialis posterior tendon is stripped away from the accessory navicular, leaving a wafer of bone attached to the tendon. The entire accessory navicular and the prominent portion of the navicular are removed so that no prominence remains on the medial side of the foot. The tibialis posterior tendon is attached to the plantar surface of the navicular by suturing the remaining wafer of bone to the undersurface of the navicular, with part of the forefoot in inversion. □

Congenital Toe Deformities

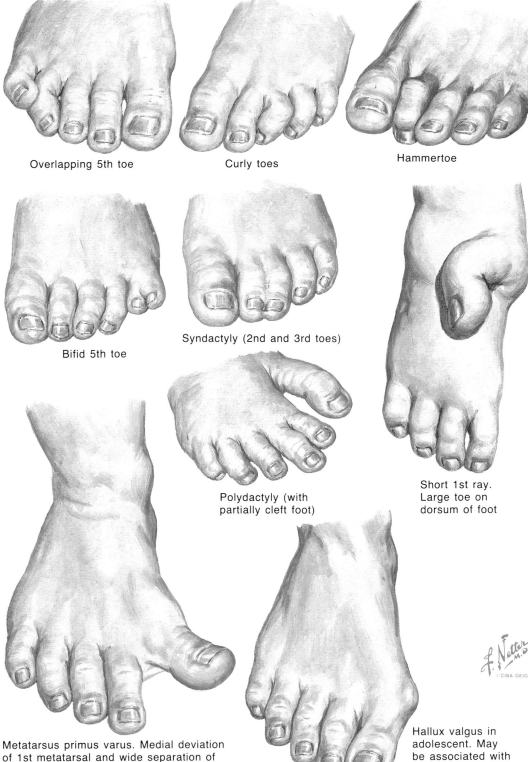

Congenital Toe Deformities

Overlapping 5th toe

Curly toes

Hammertoe

Bifid 5th toe

Syndactyly (2nd and 3rd toes)

Polydactyly (with partially cleft foot)

Short 1st ray. Large toe on dorsum of foot

Metatarsus primus varus. Medial deviation of 1st metatarsal and wide separation of great toe, often called "smart toe" because of unusual prehensility

Hallux valgus in adolescent. May be associated with metatarsus primus varus

Polydactyly (Duplication of Parts). As in the hand, additional or malformed digits are common, often familial, deformities. The primary goal of treatment is to produce a narrow foot and ensure satisfactory shoe fit. The decision as to which toe to remove is based primarily on which procedure will result in the best appearance; the most lateral or the most medial toe is usually the one removed.

Sophisticated surgical procedures used in the hand are not applicable in the foot, as they seldom result in good function. Simple removal of redundant skin and loosely attached toes to restore a satisfactory foot contour can be done in the newborn nursery with the patient under local anesthesia. The traditional method of ligating the base of the toe is discouraged because it may leave an unsightly dimple and is upsetting to the parents. Surgical removal of redundant soft tissue is a less complicated procedure than circumcision.

More extensive procedures requiring use of a general anesthetic and a tourniquet should be delayed until the child is 12 to 18 months of age. For duplicated toes with deformed or duplicated metatarsals, complete removal of the ray is needed. Duplication of the great toe coupled with a deformed and shortened first metatarsal is a special problem because it is often associated with hallux varus. A more extensive procedure that involves lengthening of the abductor hallucis tendon and plication of the adductor and medial soft tissues is required to realign the toe and prevent recurrence of the deformity.

Occasionally, the digit is bifid and shares a common phalanx or base of a phalanx. In this case, the base should be retained because it serves as the attachment for the collateral ligaments and its removal may lead to an unstable joint and progressive malalignment of the remaining toe, or both.

Gigantism (Overgrowth). Enlargement of the toes or the foot is not an uncommon deformity, and sometimes the entire lower limb is enlarged as well. While usually idiopathic, gigantism is frequently associated with neurofibromatosis (Plate 19).

Treatment is usually not necessary in the newborn, but later, cosmetic problems related to poor shoe fit may require surgical procedures such as narrowing the foot by removing a ray, epiphysiodesis, or amputation of the large toe or the distal phalanx.

Curly Toes. In this common deformity, one or more toes are bent or curled downward and overlap one another. The condition, which appears to have a high familial incidence, is believed to be due to congenital hypoplasia or absence of the intrinsic muscles of the affected toes. In some patients, the deformity improves with growth. If improvement does not occur, pressure from the shoe or weight bearing may cause pain.

Conservative management such as strapping or taping is not effective. If surgical correction is necessary in a young child, simple flexor tenotomy usually suffices. In older children whose deformity has become more rigid, more extensive procedures such as surgical syndactyly and resection of the phalanx may be needed.

Overlapping Fifth Toe. A common familial deformity, the overlapping fifth toe is characterized by a contraction of both the skin over the dorsum of the toe and the dorsal capsule of the metatarsophalangeal joint. This makes the fifth toe excessively prominent and thus prone to irritation from the shoe. While conservative measures such as passive stretching and strapping have traditionally been recommended for infants, these procedures are not very successful. If a significant malalignment persists in an older child, surgical correction may be necessary.

Syndactyly. This webbing deformity, which also occurs in the hand (Plate 111), requires treatment only if it leads to angular deformity.

Cleft Foot. The deformity, which is transmitted as an autosomal dominant trait, is usually bilateral. It is often associated with a cleft hand and other anomalies such as urinary tract abnormalities, deafness, and cleft lip and palate. Since foot function remains good, treatment consists of surgery to narrow the foot and produce a better appearance. □

Freiberg's Disease

Freiberg's Disease

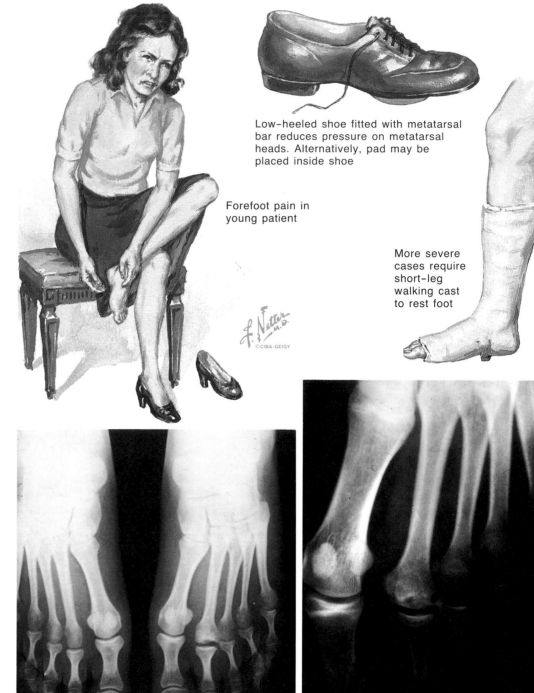

Low-heeled shoe fitted with metatarsal bar reduces pressure on metatarsal heads. Alternatively, pad may be placed inside shoe

Forefoot pain in young patient

More severe cases require short-leg walking cast to rest foot

Radiograph of adult patient shows normal right foot and affected left foot with late degenerative changes. 2nd metatarsal head appears widened and irregular with flattened articular surface

Radiograph of child's foot reveals early avascular cystic changes but normal contour in 2nd metatarsal head

In 1914, Freiberg described an anterior metatarsalgia that usually involved the head of the second metatarsal. Freiberg's disease occurs in adolescents during the growth spurt at puberty; approximately 75% of patients are girls. It is caused by avascular necrosis of the metatarsal head, and the etiology of the vascular insufficiency is not fully understood. It appears that repetitive trauma from the stress of weight bearing causes microfractures at the junction of the metaphysis and the growth plate; these fractures deprive the epiphysis of adequate circulation. This view is supported by the finding that the disease is more common in persons whose first metatarsal is shorter than the second metatarsal, a condition that increases the weight on the second metatarsal head. Freiberg's disease is also known as Köhler's disease II, distinguishing it from Köhler's disease I, which is a similar process in the navicular (Plate 98).

Clinical Manifestations. Freiberg's disease is marked by an insidious onset of pain in the forefoot, usually localized to the head of the second metatarsal. The discomfort is aggravated by athletic activity, toe movement, and wearing high-heeled shoes, and it is relieved by rest. Localized swelling and limitation of motion in the metatarsophalangeal joint are common associated findings.

Radiographic Findings. Following the loss of blood supply, the metatarsal head regenerates slowly as the blood supply is reestablished. This process produces the typical sequential radiographic changes. Initially, the epiphysis becomes sclerotic; radiographs then demonstrate a fragmented appearance followed by osteolysis and,

eventually, reconstitution of the bony architecture. During the fragmentation and osteolytic phases, the metatarsal head becomes irregular, widened, and flattened at its articular surface, presumably from the continued stress of weight bearing on the soft, healing bone; the radiographic appearance is similar to that of the femoral head in Legg-Calvé-Perthes disease (Plates 60–61). Early in the disease, the joint space is widened; much later, it narrows and the irregular bony surfaces, the sclerosis, and the bone spurs at its margins give the appearance of osteoarthritis.

Treatment. Initial management of the pain consists of wearing low-heeled shoes fitted with a metatarsal bar or pad placed beneath the involved

bone and limiting activity for 4 to 6 weeks. Severe or persistent symptoms necessitate immobilizing the foot in a short-leg walking cast until they subside, usually in 3 to 4 weeks, followed by use of the above shoe modifications. Painful activities should be avoided for a year or more after the bone heals. Symptoms may recur in adulthood if osteoarthritis develops in the metatarsophalangeal joint. If symptoms of osteoarthritis persist and are not relieved by conservative measures, surgery may be warranted to remove the metatarsal head and a portion of the metatarsal shaft or to resect the proximal half of the adjoining proximal phalanx and reshape the metatarsal head. □

Köhler's Disease I

Köhler's Disease I

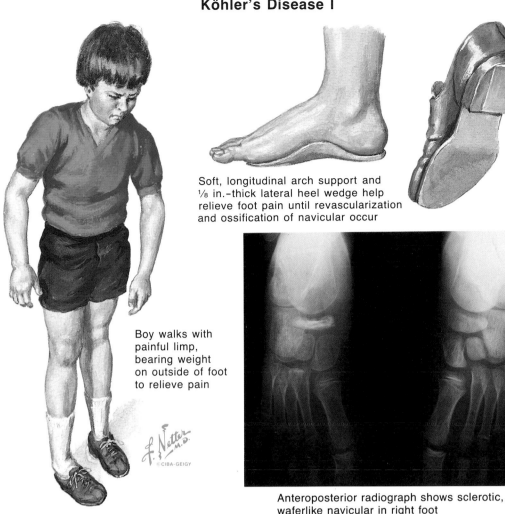

Soft, longitudinal arch support and ⅛ in.-thick lateral heel wedge help relieve foot pain until revascularization and ossification of navicular occur

Boy walks with painful limp, bearing weight on outside of foot to relieve pain

Anteroposterior radiograph shows sclerotic, waferlike navicular in right foot

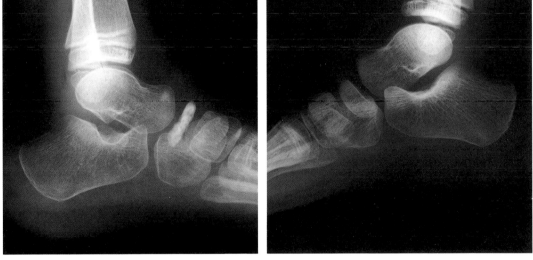

Radiographs reveal characteristic changes in navicular of involved right foot (left) compared with normal left foot (right)

Köhler's disease I is a self-limiting avascular necrosis of the navicular. It is usually unilateral and affects children, most often boys; onset is at age 4 in boys and at age 5 in girls. Although the exact cause of the avascular necrosis is unknown, there is evidence of a mechanical basis. The navicular is located at the apex of the longitudinal arch of the foot, where it is subjected to repetitive compressive forces during weight bearing. Normally, the navicular is the last bone in the foot to ossify, and irregular ossification is not uncommon, especially in boys. The navicular ossifies later in boys than in girls, and delayed ossification appears to make the navicular more vulnerable to compressive damage.

Waught believed that compression of the spongy ossification center of the navicular at a critical phase in its growth caused the irregular ossification. The compressive forces can occlude the vessels of the soft ossification center, rendering it avascular. Histologic studies show the typical changes of avascular necrosis: areas of necrosis, resorption of dead bone, and formation of new bone.

Clinical Manifestations. The child with Köhler's disease I walks with a painful limp, shifting weight to the lateral edge of the foot to relieve pressure on the longitudinal arch. Pain, tenderness, and swelling develop in the region of the navicular; at times, the pain occurs with contrac-

tion of the tibialis posterior muscle. Occasionally, minor trauma precedes the onset of symptoms.

Radiographic Findings. In most patients, the navicular appears on radiographs as a thin wafer of bone with patchy areas of sclerosis and rarefaction and loss of its normal trabecular pattern; these findings produce the appearance of navicular collapse. In some patients, the navicular maintains its normal shape, with a uniform increase in density and minimal fragmentation. This may represent a normal, sometimes familial, variant of ossification that appears irregular; it is occasionally seen on the opposite, asymptomatic foot in children with Köhler's disease I as well as in asymptomatic persons.

Treatment and Prognosis. Because the disease is self-limiting, prognosis is excellent and no long-term disability or deformity results. The vascularity of the navicular is adequately supplied by a circumferential leash of vessels, allowing rapid revascularization. The affected navicular regains its normal shape before the foot completes growth, and normal ossification is usually completed in 2 years. Symptomatic treatment is needed for the pain and swelling. Soft, longitudinal arch supports, a medial heel wedge, and limitation of strenuous activity usually relieve the symptoms. If the pain is severe or persists, a short-leg walking cast may be used for 4 to 6 weeks, followed by use of shoe modifications. □

Congenital Limb Malformation

Etiology and Pathogenesis

Limb malformations are caused by genetic or environmental factors or a combination of both.

A malformation presumably arises at the time of conception if genetic in origin and during the second 25-day period if caused by environmental factors. Fortunately, the incidence of major birth defects is low, and few are due to environmental pollutants. It has been estimated that 10% of malformations are due to chromosomal aberrations, 20% to single-gene (Mendelian) disorders, 60% to multiple-gene disorders (polygenic inheritance), and 10% to environmental factors such as anoxia, irradiation, antivitamins, hormones, chemicals, and some viral infections. Other potentially teratogenic substances continue to be identified. The mother's ability to metabolize or combat these agents and the embryo's genetic pattern may be important factors in modifying the final configuration of the deformity.

Limb differentiation in the human embryo occurs in a definite, sequential order (see CIBA COLLECTION, Volume 8/I, Section II). Small buds of tissue, representing the upper and lower limbs, first appear on the lateral body wall at about the twenty-sixth day. At this stage, the embryo is about 4 mm long. In the ensuing 4 weeks, the limb buds grow and differentiate rapidly in a proximodistal sequence (ie, the arm and forearm appear before the hand).

By the forty-eighth day, the shape of the hand is well defined, and the skeleton is cartilaginous except for the distal phalanges, which have not yet chondrified. No further differentiation occurs after about the fiftieth day. Later changes are essentially related only to increase in size and to the relative position and proportion of the parts.

Most limb malformations develop during the embryonic phase (approximately the third to eighth weeks). During this period, teratogenic factors inhibit the rate of orderly differentiation of the part that is changing most rapidly and whose cellular components are highly sensitive at that moment. The type of deformity is determined by the stage in limb development at which the insult occurs and the location of the destructive process. The severity of the deformity reflects the degree of destruction within the limb mesenchyme.

The insult to an evolving limb bud that causes deformity can be compared to abscess formation in adult tissues. In an abscess, an area of cellular infiltration surrounds a central area of destruction, resulting in formation of scar tissue and structural deformity. If the same destructive process occurs in the embryo before limb formation is complete, the developing tissue of the limb

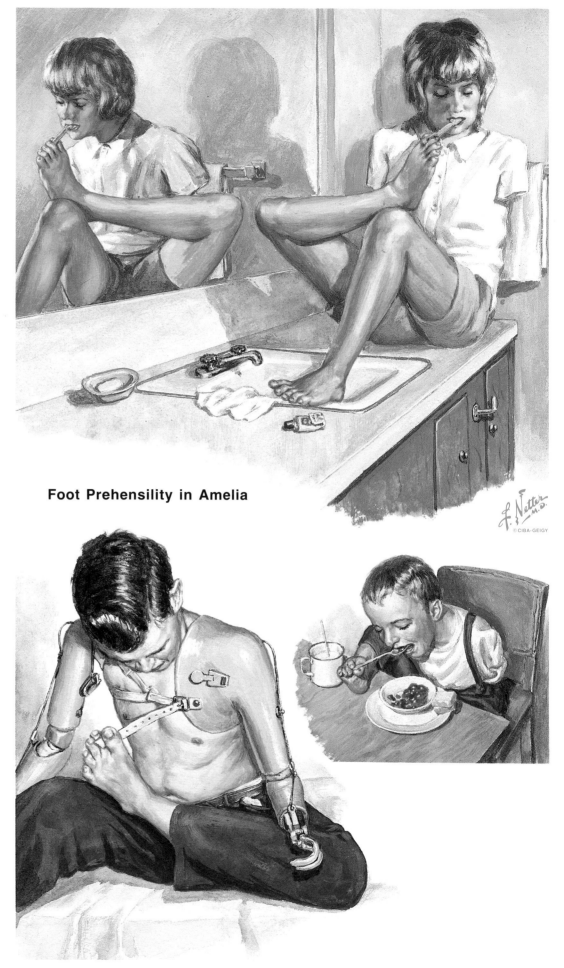

Foot Prehensility in Amelia

mesenchyme around the area of destruction is disturbed.

Classification of Congenital Limb Defects

In the past, Greek and Latin names were used to describe common limb deficits, resulting in much semantic confusion. A workable classification to identify, categorize, and readily retrieve the specific diagnosis of congenital malformations had long been needed, and in 1961, Frantz and O'Rahilly published just such a practical classification.

Congenital Limb Malformation

(Continued)

The method of grouping cases according to the parts that have been primarily affected by certain embryologic failures was first proposed by Swanson in 1964. Committees of the American Society for Surgery of the Hand and the International Federation of Societies for Surgery of the Hand further developed this classification, which was published in 1968 by Swanson, Barsky, and Entin. This classification, used in this discussion, has been accepted by both these societies, as well as the International Society of Prosthetics and Orthotics.

Although the embryologic insult to a limb usually cannot be sharply demarcated, certain similar patterns of deficit do exist. Defects may involve only the dermomyofascial structures or all or part of both the skeletal and associated soft-tissue elements of the limb. Subclassification within the major categories indicates the specific type and severity of the malformation. Deformities involving only the soft tissues are considered milder manifestations of a general deficiency pattern. The seven major categories in the classification are:

    I Failure of formation of parts
    II Failure of differentiation of parts
    III Duplication
    IV Overgrowth
    V Undergrowth
    VI Congenital constriction band syndrome
    VII Generalized skeletal abnormalities

I. Failure of Formation of Parts: Transverse Arrest

Category I comprises congenital deficits characterized by either partial or complete failure of limb formation. This category is further subdivided into transverse arrest and longitudinal arrest.

Transverse arrest deficits include all congenital amputation-type malformations and are classified by the level at which the existing portion of the limb terminates; all elements distal to that level are absent. Deficits in this group range from aphalangia to amelia and are sometimes referred to as congenital amputations, which should not be confused with intrauterine amputations. The transverse stump represents an arrest of formation in the limb anlage. It is usually well padded with soft tissue, and rudimentary digits or dimpling may be present.

Phalangeal Deficiency. One or more digits may be involved, and this defect may occur at

Failure of Formation of Parts: Transverse Arrest
Transmetacarpal amputation type (aphalangia)

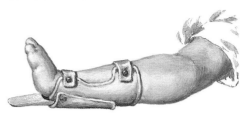

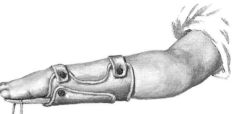

Opposition post applied, permitting child to scoop up and hold object

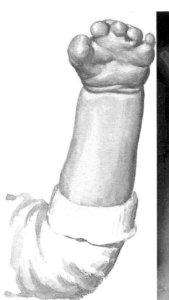

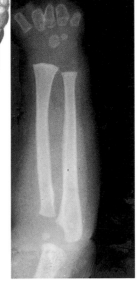

Absence of all fingers. Rudimentary digits represented by skin nubbins with or without fingernails

Radiograph shows absence of phalanges. Metacarpals present but short and osteoporotic

Transtarsal amputation type (adactyly)

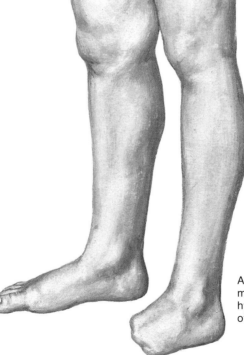

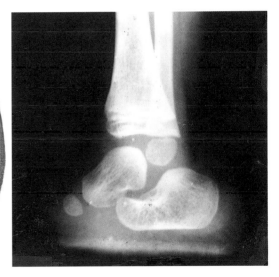

Absence of forefoot. Gastrocnemius and soleus muscles somewhat atrophied; knee tends to hyperextend. Radiograph shows complete deficit of metatarsals, phalanges, cuneiforms, and cuboid

any level of the digit. The mildest forms require no treatment. In patients with severe deficits and functional impairment, a cosmetic prosthesis or surgical reconstruction (eg, bone lengthening, digital transposition, or transplantation) may be indicated. Phalangeal deficiencies in the foot usually require shoe correction only.

Transmetacarpal Amputation Type. This defect is relatively rare, usually unilateral, and often accompanied by a transtarsal amputation-type defect. The hand is short and wide, and skin nubbins may be present (Plate 100). Bone mass insufficiency rules out phalangization (surgical formation of a finger or thumb from a metacarpal). Children with these defects are fitted with

an opposition palmar pad prosthesis secured to the distal forearm with a Velcro strap. Wrist flexion opposes the hand remnant to the prosthesis and provides a crude type of palmar prehension with sensation.

Transcarpal Amputation Type. In this rare defect, the phalanges and metacarpals are totally absent. In some patients, five skin nubbins are present. The wrist joint is normal, and the epiphyses of the distal radius and ulna appear normal on radiographs. The carpal bones are often fused to some degree. Since the limb is usually too long for a wrist disarticulation prosthesis, an opposition palmar pad prosthesis is used to provide prehension with sensation.

Congenital Limb Malformation
(Continued)

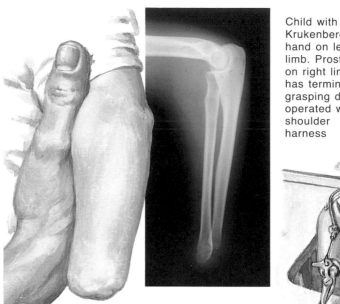

Absence of hand. Radiograph shows radius and ulna with relatively normal distal epiphyses

Child with Krukenberg hand on left limb. Prosthesis on right limb has terminal grasping device operated with shoulder harness

Transtarsal Amputation Type. Absence of the phalanges and metatarsals, and usually the cuneiforms and cuboid, characterizes this rare deficit (Plate 100). The foot is in equinus, although the tibialis anterior tendon prevents an excessive degree of deformity. Transtarsal defects are similar to Lisfranc amputations. The gastrocnemius and soleus muscles (triceps surae) are underdeveloped, and the knee tends to hyperextend. Without the forefoot, normal push off in gait is impossible. Use of a high shoe with a reinforced steel shank and a felt foot or a foam-rubber shoe filler compensates for the defect.

Wrist Disarticulation Type. This apparently autosomal recessive trait is more common in females and is seldom bilateral. Typically, the stump is long, and skin nubbins represent failure of digit development. The epiphyses of the distal radius and ulna are present, but all skeletal elements distal to them are absent (Plate 101). Pronation and supination capabilities usually exist, but a cartilaginous bar bridging the radius and ulna is occasionally present.

In patients with unilateral involvement, a forearm socket is molded to the dorsopalmar diameter of the stump to take advantage of pronation and supination capabilities. The terminal grasping device is activated by contralateral scapular abduction through a shoulder harness and cable-linkage system. With appropriate training, even young patients soon become proficient in the use of the prosthesis.

Patients with congenital bilateral absence of hands present a greater rehabilitation challenge because they lack tactile gnosis when wearing artificial limbs. The Krukenberg procedure splits the forearm stump into a prehensile forceps (Plate 101). Providing the forearm stump is sufficiently long, the procedure can be used in blind patients with bilateral hand loss, patients living in areas where prosthetic services are not available, and any patients with bilateral hand loss. Using the simple mechanical principle of chopsticks, patients with a Krukenberg hand can function with amazing dexterity. The advantages of readily available prehension with sensation are significant, especially in dressing, bathing, eating, and toilet activities.

An artificial limb is usually recommended as an assisting hand for the opposite limb. If the patient desires to wear an artificial limb over the Krukenberg hand, a standard prosthesis can be fitted without difficulty. However, patients often use their Krukenberg hand as the dominant hand and show no desire to wear an artificial limb.

Krukenberg hand

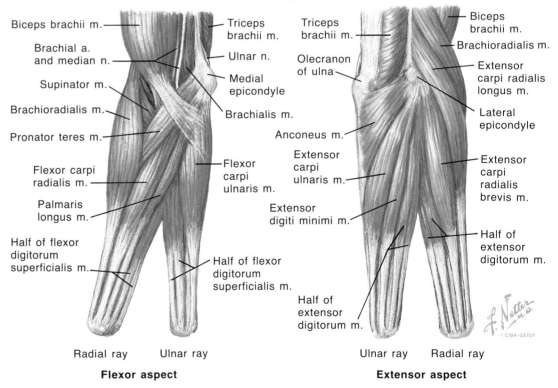

Flexor aspect

Biceps brachii m. — Brachial a. and median n. — Supinator m. — Brachioradialis m. — Pronator teres m. — Flexor carpi radialis m. — Palmaris longus m. — Half of flexor digitorum superficialis m. — Triceps brachii m. — Ulnar n. — Medial epicondyle — Brachialis m. — Flexor carpi ulnaris m. — Half of flexor digitorum superficialis m. — Radial ray — Ulnar ray

Extensor aspect

Triceps brachii m. — Olecranon of ulna — Anconeus m. — Extensor carpi ulnaris m. — Extensor digiti minimi m. — Half of extensor digitorum m. — Biceps brachii m. — Brachioradialis m. — Extensor carpi radialis longus m. — Lateral epicondyle — Extensor carpi radialis brevis m. — Half of extensor digitorum m. — Ulnar ray — Radial ray

In children, the Krukenberg procedure should be performed as soon as feasible. By the time the child is 2 years of age, the parts are usually large enough for easy handling, surgery is well tolerated, and the functional patterns of prehension develop rapidly. If the procedure is done carefully, the epiphyses are not disturbed and future growth is not affected.

The goal of the procedure is to convert the forearm into a strong, active forceps with the radial ray opposing the ulnar ray. The muscles and tendons are divided between the radial and ulnar rays. The interosseous membrane is divided at the ulnar periosteal attachment, preserving the interosseous nerve and vessels. Tactile sensation

should be present between the tips. Any digits present, with their associated vessels and tendons, are retained. The forceps should spread wide enough to accommodate ordinary objects, such as a drinking glass, and should be strong enough to hold common objects securely. If the forceps is too long, it may lack strength; if it is too short, distal spread may be insufficient. The pronator teres muscle limits the proximal depth of the forceps.

Patients with a Krukenberg hand begin a training program 2 to 3 weeks after surgery. They learn how to grasp and release rapidly. Pronation and supination are strong, natural movements, but patients must learn to abduct and adduct the

Failure of Formation of Parts: Transverse Arrest
Forearm amputation type (partial hemimelia)

Congenital Limb Malformation
(Continued)

forceps rays for best function. Moving the radius toward or away from the relatively fixed ulna provides the principal abduction-adduction motion. In strong gripping, however, ulnar adduction is also important. The therapist plays an essential role in teaching patients to use standard implements and perform two-handed activities, using a hook on the contralateral limb.

Forearm Amputation Type. One of the most common transverse arrest deficiencies is the below-elbow defect (Plate 102). Occasionally, rudimentary digits with fingernails are present at the end of the stump. The radius may also be slightly longer than the ulna. The olecranon and trochlea are usually well developed. The radial head may articulate with the capitulum or project lateroproximally beyond it. The elbow joint has lateral stability, hyperextensibility, and excellent flexion.

The length of the stump and the patient's age determine the type of prosthesis used. The infant with a very short below-elbow stump is fitted with a preflexed arm. As the skeleton matures, the child can wear a preflexed socket with rigid elbow hinges. Children younger than 10 months are fitted with a passive mitten (smooth, stuffed plastic prosthesis) or, preferably, with a size 12P hook that is not connected to a cable system. The hook is activated when the child is 1 year of age. If the length of the elbow stump is adequate, the child can be fitted in infancy with a standard socket with flexible elbow hinges. At about age 9, a Munster-type socket, which is closely fitted around the humeral condyles, is substituted.

Elbow Disarticulation Type. The epiphysis of the distal humerus is present, but there are no bony elements distal to it. A standard elbow disarticulation prosthesis is prescribed for this type of defect. The dual-control prosthesis has a prehensile hook and an elbow lock that allows variable positioning of the forearm.

Above-Elbow Amputation Type. In this type of defect, the epiphysis of the distal humerus is absent, and the standard above-elbow prosthesis is usually appropriate (Plate 103). A turntable above the elbow lock allows manual rotation of the forearm piece, providing optimal function.

Shoulder Disarticulation Type. Total absence of an upper limb deprives patients of half of their prehensile power. Children with bilateral deficits present a formidable rehabilitation challenge (Plate 104). These children usually develop compensatory skills at a very early age and they frequently become very adept at using their feet for prehension (Plate 99). Most patients request prostheses for the upper limbs to broaden their

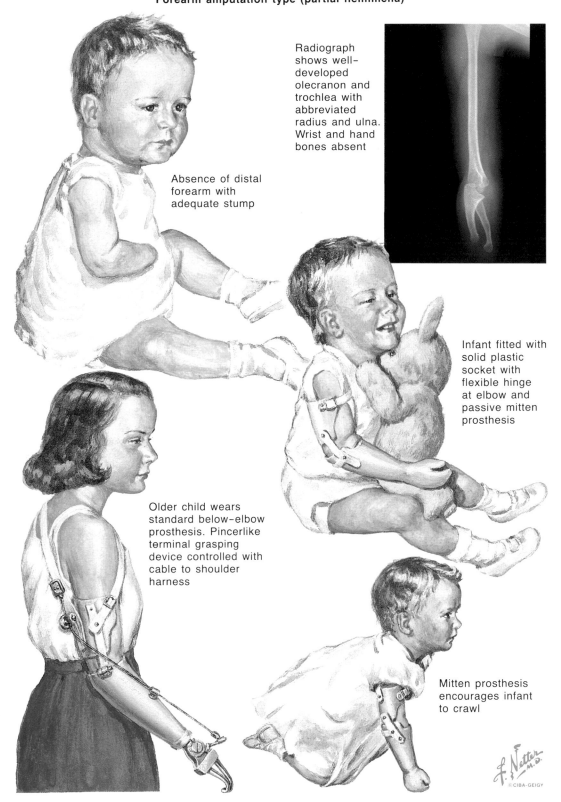

Absence of distal forearm with adequate stump

Radiograph shows well-developed olecranon and trochlea with abbreviated radius and ulna. Wrist and hand bones absent

Infant fitted with solid plastic socket with flexible hinge at elbow and passive mitten prosthesis

Older child wears standard below-elbow prosthesis. Pincerlike terminal grasping device controlled with cable to shoulder harness

Mitten prosthesis encourages infant to crawl

prehensile skills and provide a more acceptable appearance. Because motors are necessary to control the prosthetic shoulder, elbow, and terminal device, fitting these patients is extremely difficult. Fitting prostheses for lower-level amputations is much simpler.

Children with a unilateral shoulder defect should begin wearing a body-powered shoulder disarticulation prosthesis during the third or fourth year. In bilateral amputations, the complexity of the harness and body movements necessary to accomplish simple tasks make the shoulder disarticulation prosthesis impractical. Therefore, patients with bilateral defects are ideal candidates for electrically powered prostheses. In

the electric Michigan Feeder Arm, a rechargeable battery pack is housed in the opposite shoulder cap (Plate 104). A small motor turns a plastic screw that raises and lowers the forearm. For up-and-down movements, a two-way microswitch located in the shoulder cap is activated by movement of the scapula. A special linkage allows pronation and supination. Abduction of the scapula activates the terminal hook device through a cable linkage. The prosthesis can be programmed with a feeding pattern that even a 4-year-old child can learn to use. The prosthesis on one side is programmed for use in the head and neck area and one on the other side for use at a greater distance, such as in toilet care. However, even

Congenital Limb Malformation

(Continued)

children who have been fitted with these devices continue to use their feet for most activities.

Ankle Disarticulation Type. This is a sporadic, nonhereditary, and usually unilateral deficit. The stump is similar to a Syme amputation. The epiphyses of the distal tibia and fibula are present and the limb is weight bearing, but because the talus and calcaneus are absent, it is shorter than the normal one. Use of a standard below-knee socket with a solid ankle-cushioned heel (SACH) foot compensates for the difference in length.

Below-Knee Amputation Type. The proximal half of the tibia is usually present and the fibula is slightly shorter; distally, both bones taper to a point (Plate 105). The proximal epiphyses are present; the stump is usually symmetric but may curve inward.

Children with this deformity are fitted with a below-knee prosthesis that has a plastic socket, condylar cuff, and SACH foot. In some patients, use of rigid knee joints and a leather thigh corset is necessary. The below-knee prosthesis requires little training and allows excellent function, including participation in sports.

Knee Disarticulation Type. In this deficit, the stump is symmetric without distal tapering. The entire femur, including its condyles and lower epiphysis, is present. Toddlers with unilateral defects are fitted with the simplest prosthesis so that they can learn to walk with it. The prosthesis consists of a plastic socket with two aluminum uprights that taper to a crutch tip; a SACH foot is substituted later. Initially, there is no articulated knee hinge. An over-the-shoulder harness helps to hold the prosthesis in place.

When the child is older, a knee disarticulation prosthesis is used. The knee joint is locked with an anterior strap until the child learns to stand independently in the prosthesis. When the child begins to learn thigh lifting and knee swinging, the locking strap is disengaged and later discarded. Some children can be fitted with a suction socket prosthesis as early as 5 years of age.

Above-Knee Amputation Type. In this defect, the epiphysis of the distal femur is absent (Plate 105). Treatment is the same as for a knee disarticulation–type defect.

Hip Disarticulation Type. The femur is totally absent, and there is no acetabular development (Plate 106). In patients with bilateral defects, pelvic contour is wide because fat accumulates over the pelvis. These patients are initially fitted with a pelvic bucket mounted on a board with casters and later with a bilateral hip disarticulation prosthesis with Canadian hip joints. Locking knee straps are used until the

patient can stand alone and disengaged when training for ambulation using parallel bars begins. The upper limbs must have sufficient muscle power for these patients to lift themselves for a swing-to type of progression. Ultimately, they learn to ambulate with crutches.

In unilateral cases, toddlers are first fitted with the simple crutch tip prosthesis, which is later replaced with a hip disarticulation prosthesis. The prosthesis is lengthened as needed.

I. Failure of Formation of Parts: Longitudinal Arrest

All failures of formation of the limbs other than the transverse arrest type are arbitrarily clas-

sified as longitudinal arrests. The deficiencies in this group reflect the separation of the preaxial (radial or tibial) and postaxial (ulnar or fibular) divisions in the limbs and include longitudinal failure of formation of all limb segments (phocomelia) or failure of either the radial, ulnar, or central components.

Radial Deficiency. Preaxial deformities in the upper limb may involve the radius and thumb, radius only, or thumb only. Malformations include deficient thenar muscles; short, floating thumb; deficient carpals, metacarpals, and radius; and classic radial clubhand. Radial deficiencies are often associated with other congenital anomalies and a number of syndromes such as

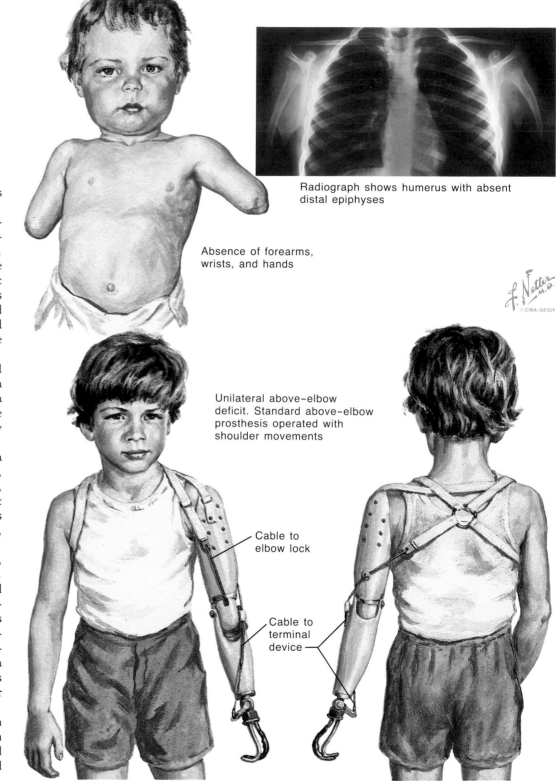

Failure of Formation of Parts: Transverse Arrest
Above-elbow amputation type (hemimelia)

Radiograph shows humerus with absent distal epiphyses

Absence of forearms, wrists, and hands

Unilateral above-elbow deficit. Standard above-elbow prosthesis operated with shoulder movements

Cable to elbow lock

Cable to terminal device

Congenital Limb Malformation
(Continued)

Holt-Oram syndrome, congenital aplastic anemia (Fanconi's anemia), and thrombocytopenia-absent radius (TAR).

In the *radial clubhand*, the forearm is short, the hand deviates radially, and the thumb is absent (Plate 107). Radiographs typically show that the radius and usually the scaphoid and trapezium are absent. The ulna is short and usually bowed, and radial deficiencies are often bilateral and rarely partial. In a partial deficiency, radiographs reveal a very short radius distal to the capitulum.

Treatment is identical for both partial and complete radial deficits. In the first few months after birth, the dislocated hand is treated with corrective plaster casts in an approach similar to that used for clubfoot (Plate 89). Although it is usually impossible to relocate the hand with conservative measures, immobilization in a cast keeps the radial soft-tissue structures stretched. Day and night bracing can be used to assist this correction.

Surgical centralization of the hand over the ulna improves both appearance and finger function. A careful evaluation of hand function, especially of the effects of wrist fixation on hand activity patterns, should always precede surgery. The length of the limb, elbow flexion, and the effect of the malformation on the patient's ability to reach should be noted. Flexion in the radial digits is usually inadequate, and patients tend to favor the often normal ulnar digits. In unilateral defects, wrist flexion is not essential and the advantages of surgery outweigh the disadvantage of a fixed wrist. In bilateral defects, however, fixation of both wrists, while improving finger function, can compromise relatively good patterns of function. This is especially likely if elbow and shoulder movements are insufficient to allow functional positioning of the hands.

Surgery can be done in the patient's first or second year if great care is taken to preserve the ulnar growth plate. In the centralization procedure, the curved ulna is straightened with multiple osteotomies, and the hand is centered over the ulna and held in position with an intramedullary wire extending into the metacarpal of the index, middle, or ring finger (Plate 107). The ulnar growth plate will continue to grow if it is not injured and if the intramedullary wire is placed through its central portion. Pollicization of the index finger to replace the thumb on one hand is occasionally done if the defect is bilateral.

After surgery, the limb is immobilized in a plaster cast for 3 months. Day and night bracing continues for 3 more months, and continued night bracing may be necessary throughout the

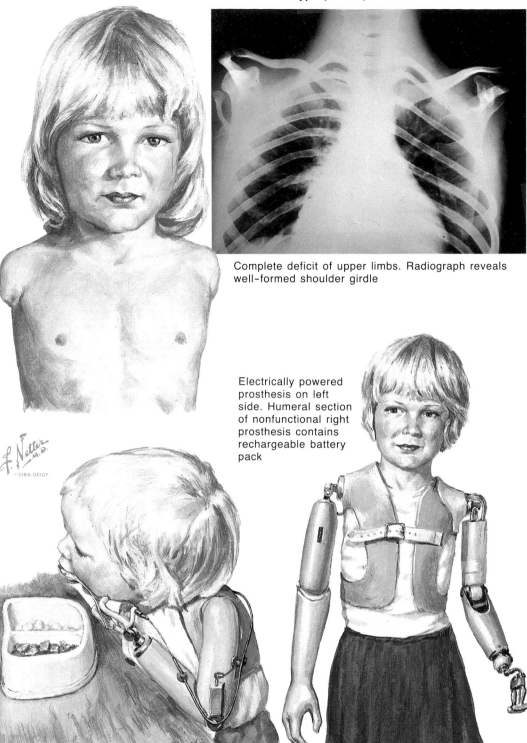

Failure of Formation of Parts: Transverse Arrest
Shoulder disarticulation type (amelia)

Complete deficit of upper limbs. Radiograph reveals well-formed shoulder girdle

Electrically powered prosthesis on left side. Humeral section of nonfunctional right prosthesis contains rechargeable battery pack

Small child effectively uses body-powered prosthesis

growing years. As the child grows, the intramedullary wire is replaced or advanced distally into the metacarpal. If the wire fixation technique is not used or if night bracing is not continued, the hand tends to resubluxate on the ulna.

Thumb defects. If the thumb is absent, the index finger can be pollicized. A floating thumb can be amputated and the index finger pollicized, or the thumb can be lengthened by metacarpal osteotomy, distraction, and bone graft. A hypoplastic thumb may be treated with metacarpal distraction and bone graft, and tendon transfer to compensate for the hypoplastic thenar muscle. Rotational osteotomy may be indicated for the nonopposed thumb.

Tibial Deficiency. Complete tibial deficiency is a serious defect; the affected leg is short, the foot is in varus position, the great toe is absent, and the knee is unstable. The tibia is absent, while the fibula is present but may be bowed. Because the fibula is completely unstable, the limb cannot bear weight. Treatment with surgery and prostheses is not always successful. The recommended treatment is knee disarticulation amputation and fitting with an end-bearing socket prosthesis.

Incomplete tibial deficiency is equally disabling. If the defect is bilateral, ambulation is impossible. Only the proximal third of the tibial shaft or only the tibial condyles are present. The tibia may be

Congenital Limb Malformation
(Continued)

a rectangularly outlined bone with no evident epiphysis; in some cases, only a small bone cap represents the proximal epiphysis. The fibula is positioned normally or rests superiorly and posteriorly in the popliteal space. The feet are usually vertical and may have to be sacrificed. Children with this deficit are fitted with a below-knee prosthesis with metal knee hinges and a thigh cuff.

Ulnar Deficiency. Longitudinal deformities of the ulnar ray (Plate 108) are sporadic and non-hereditary and are among the rarest congenital anomalies of the upper limb. Ulnar ray defects are frequently associated with malformations of the radial ray (most common) or of the central rays as well. Associated deformities in the shoulder girdle, proximal humerus, or both, may also be present. (Involvement of a part proximal to the principal deformity occurs only in ulnar deficiencies, phocomelia, and Poland's syndrome.) Malformations at the level of the elbow, wrist, hand, and digits vary greatly in type and severity. They include radiohumeral dislocation or synostosis, hypoplasia, partial or total absence of the ulna, curvature of the radius, ulnar deviation of the hand, fusion of carpal bones, congenital amputation at the wrist, and oligodactyly with or without syndactyly. In addition, there is a high incidence of associated anomalies in the opposite hand, lower limb, and other parts of the musculoskeletal system.

Management of ulnar ray defects is complex. Functional testing of limb position, power, and stability helps to determine the best treatment. Some patients with total ulnar deficiency and acute flexion contracture of the elbow can wear an elbow disarticulation prosthesis with a terminal device. Other patients with acute elbow flexion can be fitted with an above-elbow amputation prosthesis that has a fenestration in the humeral socket to allow the residual digit to operate the elbow-locking mechanism. In general, surgical treatment is not indicated. However, in partial ulnar defects, the ulnar remnant can sometimes be fused to the radius to provide stability at the elbow.

Fibular Deficiency. Total fibular deficiency is very common and is bilateral in about 25% of patients. In patients with unilateral defects, the limb-length discrepancy is considerable. The lower part of the leg bows anteriorly, with a depressed dimple at its apex; the foot is in valgus position, as there is no ankle mortise; there are usually only three or four toes; and the distal tibial epiphysis is absent or minimal. Treatment

Failure of Formation of Parts: Transverse Arrest
Below-knee amputation type (partial hemimelia)

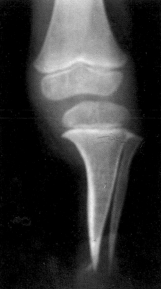

Absence of midportion of leg, ankle, and foot

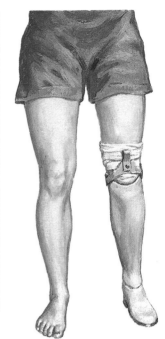

Radiograph shows incomplete tibia and fibula, each tapering to a point

Standard below-knee prosthesis permits ambulation

Above-knee amputation type (hemimelia)

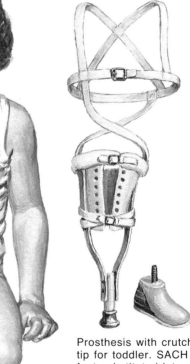

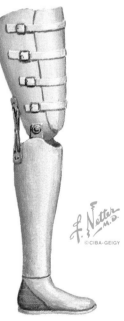

Prosthesis with crutch tip for toddler. SACH foot substituted later

Strap-type prosthesis for older child (some children prefer suction-socket prosthesis)

consists of an ankle disarticulation amputation and use of an end-bearing ankle prosthesis.

Partial fibular deficiencies are quite rare. The tibia is only minimally shortened and the fibula is either shortened or its distal portion appears normal. Treatment is with a shoe lift, but surgical epiphyseal stapling to arrest growth may be necessary (Plate 85).

Central Ray Deficiency. Deficiencies also occur in the second, third, or fourth ray of the hand—the so-called central rays—which do not differentiate at the same time as the radial and ulnar rays.

Central ray deficiencies are further classified into typical and atypical subgroups. Typical

malformations range in severity from a partial or total deficit of a phalanx, metacarpal, or carpal bone of the central rays to a monodigital hand. Atypical central ray deficiencies may be syndactylous or polydactylous. In the syndactylous type, which may be partial or complete, the elements of the third ray are fused to either the second or fourth digital ray, resembling an osseous syndactyly. The hand has a central cleft of soft tissue and the appearance of a lobster claw (Plate 109). In the polydactylous deficiency, supernumerary bony elements are present in the hand, creating a cleft of soft tissue and the appearance of a lobster claw. Similar deformities may also occur in the foot.

Congenital Limb Malformation
(Continued)

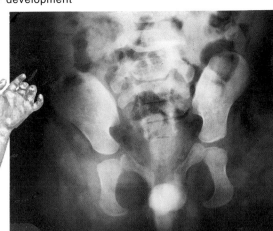

Infant with bilateral absence of lower limbs. Radiograph shows absence of femurs and lack of acetabular development

Wide pelvic contour results from fat accumulation over pelvis

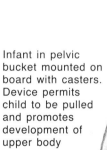

Infant in pelvic bucket mounted on board with casters. Device permits child to be pulled and promotes development of upper body

Child fitted with bilateral hip disarticulation prosthesis with pelvic bucket, Canadian hip joints, and knee joints

In determining treatment for the cleft hand, existing function must be considered. The two opposing digital units are often stable, mobile, and quite functional although not cosmetically attractive. If function (including prehension with sensation) is adequate, the appearance of the hand is of secondary importance, and surgical reconstruction to improve function and appearance is not always indicated. Closure of the cleft includes reconstruction of the deep transverse metacarpal ligament. Rotational osteotomies help correct rotatory deformity of adjacent fingers. The function of a monodigital hand can be improved with rotational osteotomy, opponensplasty, use of a simple opposition post, or a combination of all three.

Intersegmental Deficiency (Phocomelia). The most profound longitudinal arrest is phocomelia (Plate 110), a failure of proximodistal development. Phocomelia may be total (the hand or foot is attached directly to the trunk) or partial (the hand or foot is attached to a deficient, severely shortened limb).

The patient with *bilateral upper limb phocomelia* is unable to position the hands for feeding and toilet activities. Frequently, the problem is further compounded by associated deformities of the lower limbs that prevent good foot prehension.

The joints in phocomelia are usually unstable and hyperextensible because of ligament laxity, and muscle power is decreased. Digits may be missing or have motor deficits. As a rule, patients require a nonstandard prosthesis with external power. Many patients can use the affected limb to control the terminal device or elbow lock in a nonstandard prosthesis, which must be kept as simple as possible to be accepted by the patient.

Patients with *total upper limb phocomelia* are trained to use the lower limbs for many functions and are fitted with a shoulder disarticulation prosthesis or a myoelectric arm. In *partial phocomelia*, treatment may not be necessary, or one of the following alternatives may be indicated: clavicular transfer to replace the missing humerus, use of a nonstandard shoulder disarticulation prosthesis, hand reconstruction to improve grip or pinch, or therapy to improve function with the existing structures.

In *total lower limb phocomelia*, the foot articulates with the pelvis. Treatment in the young child is a nonstandard hip disarticulation prosthesis with a fenestration for the foot, a Canadian

hip joint held in place with shoulder straps, and a SACH foot without a knee hinge. The hinge is added when the child is older.

In *proximal lower limb phocomelia*, the ligaments are extremely lax and the tibia slides up and down in the pelvis. Motor power in the upper limb is often deficient.

In *distal lower limb phocomelia*, the foot articulates with the distal femur and is often monodigital. The pelvic joint is unstable.

II. Failure of Differentiation of Parts

Failure of differentiation (separation) of parts refers to all deficits in which the basic anatomic units are present but development is incomplete.

The homogeneous anlage, or primordium, differentiates into the skeletal, dermomyofascial, and neurovascular elements found in a normal limb, but differentiation, or separation, is incomplete. Therefore, this category includes soft-tissue involvement, skeletal involvement, and congenital tumors (eg, hemangiomas, lymphomas, neuromas, connective tissue tumors, and skeletal tumors—see Section II). Upper limb defects are more disabling than those of the lower limb.

Shoulder Defects. Congenital elevation of the scapula (Plate 40) and absence of the pectoral muscles are the two types of failure of differentiation in the shoulder. Skeletal involvement at this level can result in congenital humerus varus.

Congenital Limb Malformation

(Continued)

Elbow and Forearm Defects. Soft-tissue involvement may be manifested by aberrations of the long flexor, extensor, or intrinsic muscles in the upper limb. Failure of skeletal differentiation can result in either dislocation or synostosis of the humeroradial, humeroulnar, proximal, or distal radioulnar joint (Plate 44). Synostosis of the proximal radioulnar joint, the most severe elbow deformity in this category, is genetically determined and often associated with synostosis elsewhere in the body. Surgical correction may be indicated if flexion/extension or pronation/supination deformities that interfere with function are present.

Wrist and Hand Defects. Failure of differentiation can occur in either the skeletal or soft-tissue elements of the carpus, metacarpals, or fingers.

In *symphalangism*, an intermediary joint in the digit is missing, most commonly the proximal interphalangeal joint. This bilateral malformation most frequently involves the ring and little fingers. Symphalangism of the distal interphalangeal joint is rare and almost never seen in the thumb. The affected joint is immobile, and its flexion and extension folds are absent. Radiographs taken after closure of the epiphysis show bony ankylosis. If ankylosis is established, the deformity can be treated with implant arthroplasty or with osteotomy and fusion of the joint in a functional position.

Syndactyly, one of the two most common malformations in the hand, is often bilateral and can involve two or more digits, usually the middle and ring fingers (Plate 111). In some patients, only the soft tissues are fused (cutaneous syndactyly); in other patients, the nails and bones are joined as well (osseous syndactyly). Syndactyly often occurs in association with webbing of the toes (usually between the second and third toes) and is frequently associated with other deformities in the same hand or elsewhere in the body, such as Poland's syndrome, Apert's syndrome, or craniofacial dysostosis (Crouzon's disease). Syndactyly is occasionally hereditary, and this type affects males more often than females and is rare in blacks. It is believed to arise during the fetal period and must be differentiated from acrosyndactyly secondary to congenital constriction band syndrome (Plate 111).

If the syndactyly does not interfere with alignment of the digits, growth, or hand function, surgical repair can be postponed until the child

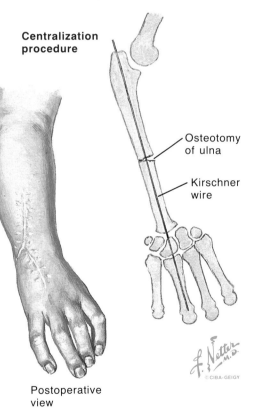

Short, bowed forearm with marked radial deviation of hand. Thumb absent. Radiograph shows partial deficit of radial ray (vestige of radius present). Scaphoid, trapezium, and metacarpal and phalanges of thumb absent

Centralization procedure

Osteotomy of ulna

Kirschner wire

Postoperative view

Radiograph shows double osteotomy to straighten curved ulna. Stabilized with intramedullary wire

Partial carpal resection. Hand centralized and maintained with wire into metacarpal

is 2 or 3 years of age. However, syndactyly in digits of unequal length (eg, ring and little fingers or, more commonly, the thumb and index finger) requires early surgical correction to avoid permanent deformity. In osseous syndactyly, the nails of the joined digits are usually fused, and the nail and bony bridge must be divided and resurfaced with a graft. If more than two digits are affected, adjacent pairs are separated at different times to avoid compromising the blood supply. Pairs of unequal length are divided first.

Congenital Flexion Deformities. These deformities are caused by inadequate extensor tendons, flexor tendon nodules, or arthrogryposis multiplex congenita (Plate 20).

Camptodactyly refers to congenital flexion contracture of the proximal interphalangeal joint of the little finger, a condition that is often hereditary and can be bilateral. Although it usually requires no treatment, surgery may be indicated if the flexion contracture is disabling or associated with deformity of the ring finger. Moderate defects are improved by release of the flexor digitorum superficialis tendon and lengthening of the palmar skin, followed by postoperative splinting. More severe cases may require release of the palmar ligament, reconstruction of the extensor tendon, and arthroplasty or arthrodesis.

In the thumb, the absence of one or all of the extrinsic abductor or extensor pollicis tendons

Failure of Formation of Parts: Longitudinal Arrest
Ulnar deficiency (paraxial ulnar hemimelia)

Congenital Limb Malformation
(Continued)

produces isolated postural deformities related to the missing structures. *Thumb flexion deformities* are usually bilateral and symmetric and are frequently hereditary. They must be differentiated from conditions such as trigger thumb, arthrogryposis multiplex congenita, and upper motor neuron disease (spasticity). If a thumb flexion deformity is recognized in infancy, splinting and daily manipulation can prevent soft-tissue contractures. Surgery should be postponed until the child has developed more complex grasping movements, which usually occurs by 3 years of age. Surgical correction may require tendon transfers and release of skin contracture, as well as release of contracted adductor or short flexor muscles.

Trigger thumb deformity, which is characterized by flexion of both the metacarpophalangeal and interphalangeal joints, is caused by a nodule on the flexor pollicis longus tendon that interferes with tendon excursion. The condition is rare in the other digits. Surgery is indicated to release the flexor pollicis longus tendon longitudinally and to shave the nodule.

Occasionally, anomalous anchorage of the deep transverse metacarpal ligament to the first metacarpal or proximal phalanx of the thumb causes *adduction contracture of the thumb* with narrowing of the first web space. The narrowed web space and deep transverse ligament are released surgically.

Clinodactyly refers to a digit curving medially or laterally in the radioulnar plane. The deformity is due to a failure of skeletal differentiation in a phalanx and is most common in the middle phalanx; the little finger is most often affected. The angulation can begin at the level of the joint or the diaphysis or may result from a delta-shaped phalanx. Relatively severe deformities require surgical treatment.

Arthrogryposis Multiplex Congenita. This deformity is caused by a disseminated failure of differentiation of the soft tissue of the limbs. Isolated muscles or groups of muscles are absent, and the joints they control may become stiff and fuse spontaneously. One or all four limbs may be affected, and usually spinal anomalies are present as well (see Plate 20 for a complete discussion).

III. Duplication of Parts

Duplication of parts is believed to be caused by a specific insult that causes the limb bud, or ectodermal cap, to split very early in development. Defects in the hand range from polydactyly to twinning (mirror hands) and can involve

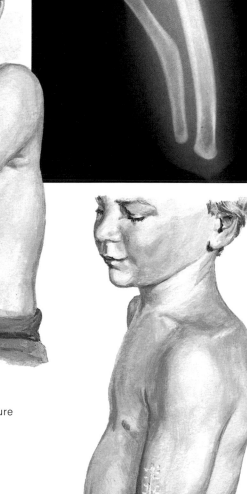

Monodigital hands and acute flexion contracture of elbow with antecubital web. Radiograph shows absence of ulnar ray and presence of single digital ray

Web released and opposition post applied, permitting grasping function

the skin and nails, the soft tissues, or both, plus the skeletal structures. A single bone or an entire limb may be duplicated.

Polydactyly. Along with syndactyly, duplication of a digit, or polydactyly, is one of the most common malformations of the hand (Plate 111), but it may also occur in the feet (Plate 96). Polydactyly has an autosomal dominant inheritance with variable expressivity. Unlike syndactyly, it is more prevalent in blacks.

Duplication of the little finger is most common, followed by the thumb (Plate 111). Polydactyly may be associated with a variety of syndromes, the best known being Laurence-Moon-Biedl syndrome. When the malformation

is part of a syndrome, the postaxial (ulnar) digits are usually duplicated.

Surgical treatment is usually performed to improve appearance. Early amputation is indicated when the polydactylous finger is a flail, poorly attached appendage; when the attachment of the extra digit is more complex, the digit to be sacrificed should be selected carefully. Bony architecture and tendon function and distribution must be considered. The marginal digit or the one that appears most normal is not necessarily the most functional one. In some patients, usable structures from the amputated digit should be preserved for transfer to the digit to be preserved. For example, if one of the two adjoining digits

Congenital Limb Malformation
(Continued)

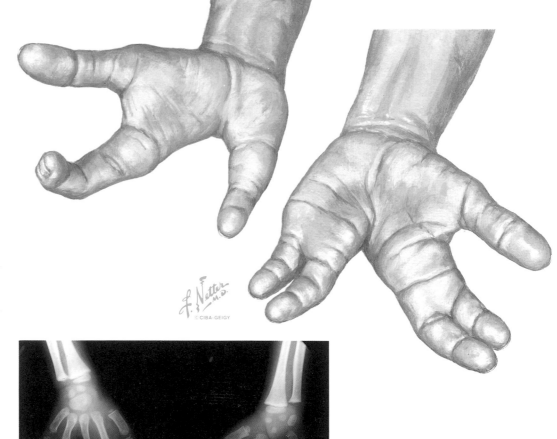

Right hand shows typical deficit with absence of 3rd and 4th central rays. Left hand shows atypical syndactylous deficit with fusion of proximal phalanges of digits II and III. Deep soft–tissue clefts in both hands

has greater flexor power while the other has greater extensor power, the latter is amputated and its extensor mechanism is transferred.

Duplication of the thumb can be partial or complete; partial forms include the bifid and bifurcated thumb. The thumb may be split at the interphalangeal or metacarpophalangeal joint, or the split may stem from the metacarpal diaphysis. When a polydactylous thumb is amputated, tendons should be regrouped to reinforce the power of the thumb or the part to be spared. Treatment of duplication distal to the interphalangeal joint consists of resection of a V-shaped segment of skin, nail, and bone. This principle can be adapted to the treatment of duplications proximal to the interphalangeal joint, although in children, the final correction may be delayed to avoid injury to the growth plates. When a twin digit is divided, the collateral ligaments must be reconstructed at the amputation site.

A triphalangeal thumb is another expression of thumb duplication. If the thumb can be positioned in opposition, treatment is optional. There may be a progressive recurvature deformity caused by a wedge-shaped ossicle interposed between the distal and proximal phalanges; this ossicle can be removed in childhood. If the thumb cannot be opposed and resembles an index finger, surgical treatment may include creation of a first web space, rotational osteotomy, and tendon transfer. In complex preaxial (radial) polydactyly, the thumb is duplicated with triphalangism of one or both of the extra digits.

IV. Overgrowth

The terms "overgrowth" and "gigantism" describe conditions in which either part or all of the limb is disproportionately large. This may occur in the digit (macrodactyly), hand, forearm, or entire limb; similar defects may occur in the lower limb. The condition is seldom bilateral and usually not hereditary.

Macrodactyly. Two types of macrodactyly have been described. In the first type, all the elements of the digit, including the bones, tendons, and neurovascular structures, are enlarged proportionately. In the second type, excess fibrolipomatous and lymphatic tissue is present along with neurofibromas, lymphangiomas, and hemangiomas. Nerve territory—oriented macrodactyly, an example of the second type, occurs with or without localized nerve tumefaction and is often seen in the distribution of the median nerve in the hand and the medial plantar nerve in the foot.

Macrodactyly is often associated with lateral deviation of the digit and excessive formation of bone. In one form, distal gigantism, the abnormality is usually greatest at the periphery. Deformities may increase secondarily as a result of asymmetric growth of the part. The thumb and the second and third fingers are most often affected.

Surgical treatment may include total or partial amputation or reduction in size. If the deformity is unsightly, amputation may be indicated. While surgical reduction of an enlarged digit is possible, the procedure is difficult because of the need to preserve the neurovascular supply and joint function while reducing both the length and width of the digit. Reduction procedures can include epiphyseal arrest (Plate 85) and progressive excision of bone and soft tissue.

V. Undergrowth

Undergrowth, or hypoplasia, denotes defective or incomplete development of the entire limb or its parts. In some classifications, the term "hypoplasia" was used to describe the condition of skeletal elements that persist after some failures of formation of parts (category I defects). However, because of their prevalence, hypoplastic defects are represented separately in the classification used here. Hypoplasia may occur in either the

upper or the lower limb. In the upper limb, it may affect the arm, forearm, hand, or parts of the hand. Only the skin and nails may be involved, or the musculotendinous structures, the neurovascular structures, or both, may be affected as well.

Brachydactyly. Shortening of the digits is the most common hand malformation seen in association with syndromes and systemic disorders. It is usually transmitted as a part of an autosomal dominant phenotype with slight variation. The middle phalanges of the index through little fingers, and especially those of the index and little fingers, are most commonly affected because they develop later than the thumb. The metacarpals are involved less frequently, and the deformity is rare in the distal phalanx of the thumb. Surgical lengthening of the shortened digits is usually not necessary, although osteotomy through the anomalous or proximal phalanx can sometimes correct a deviated finger.

Brachysyndactyly. Shortening of the digits plus syndactyly could be classified in category I (failure of formation of parts) or category II (failure of differentiation of parts) because some of its features are intersegmental failure of development as well as failure of separation of parts. However, the most obvious failure, hypoplasia, explains the reason for inclusion in this category.

Failure of Formation of Parts: Longitudinal Arrest
Intersegmental deficiency (phocomelia of upper limb)

Congenital Limb Malformation
(Continued)

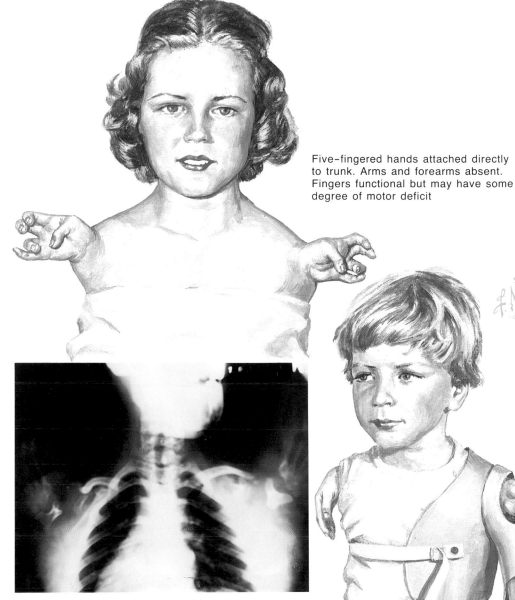

Five-fingered hands attached directly to trunk. Arms and forearms absent. Fingers functional but may have some degree of motor deficit

Radiograph shows absence of humerus, radius, and ulna. Rudimentary bone proximal to metacarpals cannot be identified

Standard shoulder disarticulation prosthesis, fenestrated at shoulder. Hand operates cable that locks and unlocks elbow and opens terminal hook device. Rubber band closes device

VI. Congenital Constriction Band Syndrome

Constriction bands are the result of focal necrosis along the course of the limb during the fetal stage of development. An area of necrosis involving the superficial tissues heals as a circular scar, creating the band. Whether constriction bands are intrinsic or extrinsic defects has not yet been fully determined. Amniotic bands have been implicated as a mechanical cause but may actually be secondary to a healing limb injury. The malformation is probably caused by a focal tissue defect that allows hemorrhage within the limb, with resulting tissue necrosis. The defect can be expressed as a constriction band, congenital amputation, or acrosyndactyly (Plate 111). When the constriction band is severe, intrauterine gangrene may develop and a true fetal amputation occurs.

In *acrosyndactyly*, the syndactylous digits and confused arrangement of anatomic parts sometimes seen may be the result of a healed necrotic infarct that occurred during the stage of separation of parts. The tissue necrosis and the resulting fusion of parts resemble those seen in an untreated third-degree burn with bridges of scar. Unlike syndactyly, acrosyndactyly is characterized by annular grooves, transverse amputations of distal parts, and the presence of a web space or fenestration between the fused digits.

Constriction bands are more likely to involve the distal part of the limb, especially the hand and foot. The central digits are usually affected; severe acrosyndactyly is rare in the thumb. A paralytic clubfoot deformity due to compression neuropathy of the peroneal nerve caused by a deep, below-knee constriction band has been described. Deformities associated with constriction band syndrome include cleft lip and cleft palate, heart anomalies, meningocele, hemangioma, and congenital clubfoot.

Annular grooves caused by constriction bands are released by Z-plasties. If parts are missing, the surgical or prosthetic treatment depends on the level of the amputation.

VII. Generalized Skeletal Abnormalities

Hand defects may be manifestations of a generalized skeletal defect, such as dyschondroplasia, achondroplasia (Plates 1–3), Marfan's syndrome (with arachnodactyly, see CIBA COLLECTION, Volume 8/I, page 232), and diastrophic dwarfism (Plate 5). In this category, the hand deformities are unique to each syndrome.

Improving Function in Patients

Although a malformed limb may not look normal, with proper rehabilitation it can sometimes achieve almost normal function in certain prehensile patterns. Prehension requires two mobile opposing parts that either diametrically oppose each other or can be adducted parallel to each other. If these parts have normal sensation and if the proximal joints can place the hand or foot in the desired position, functional activities can be carried out with some skill.

Foot Prehension in Amelia. In children with bilateral absence of the upper limbs and functional lower limbs, a bilateral upper limb pros-

thesis allows prehension and is useful in social situations. However, prehension with it lacks sensory feedback and is awkward and imprecise, and foot function should be encouraged. Young children with amelia become amazingly adept at using their feet, learning early to explore their environment by touching and manipulating objects (Plate 99). In early childhood, they begin to use their feet for prehension with sensation. They develop extraordinary flexibility in the hips and legs that allows them to position their feet for functions around the head. Eventually, even small objects may be handled with precision. Some older patients learn to put on their prosthesis, take care of personal hygiene, eat, and

Congenital Limb Malformation
(Continued)

Failure of Differentiation of Parts
(syndactyly)

Duplication of Parts
(polydactyly)

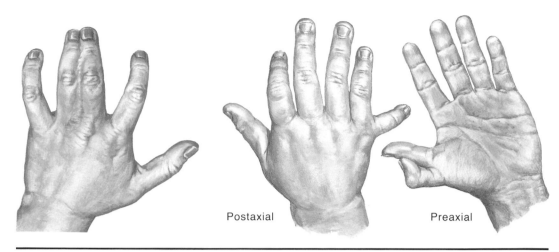

Postaxial   Preaxial

Overgrowth
(macrodactyly)

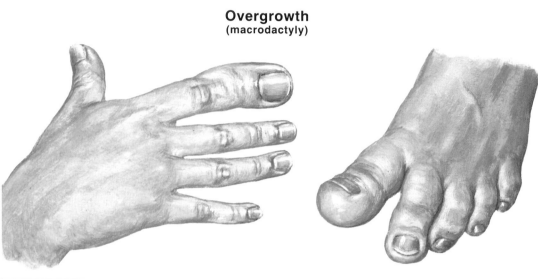

Congenital Constriction Band Syndrome

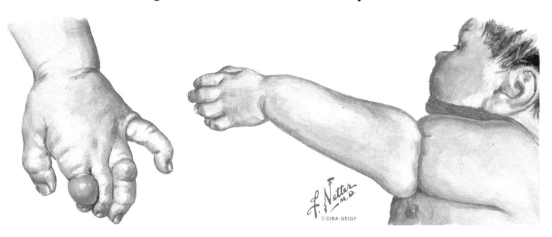

even drive a car with their feet. Special devices extend their skills in dressing, toilet care, and other activities.

Rehabilitation in Upper Limb Defects. In patients with an upper limb defect, the capacity for prehension after treatment is determined by the type of deformity and the patient's ability to respond to training. If strong prehension with sensation can be achieved with training, no further treatment is required. Children can develop skills that will make them independent.

Surgical reconstruction is indicated if it can improve function (and possibly yield cosmetic benefit) without subjecting the patient to many operations. Surgery should be undertaken as early as possible. The goal is to obtain a good grasp-and-release mechanism, preserve good sensation, and facilitate positioning of the hand for optimal function. A very young patient should have frequent postoperative evaluations, especially during the growth period, to avoid recurrence of the deformity due to imbalance or unequal growth.

During surgery, small skin nubbins or rudimentary digits at the distal portions of the limb should be preserved, since even a small nubbin can provide excellent sensation. Amputation should be considered only if there is neurovascular insufficiency, loss of skin cover, or infection, and never if there is good skin cover with sensation. Before undertaking any surgical procedure, whether an amputation or a reconstruction, the surgeon must carefully evaluate the patient's existing and potential use of the limb. For successful rehabilitation, reconstructive surgery must be individualized.

Rehabilitation in Lower Limb Defects. Children with a lower limb defect should be fitted with a prosthesis at 12 or 15 months of age, the normal age for walking. Very often, a complicated, nonstandard prosthesis must be designed for these patients. Occasionally, if function cannot be achieved with reconstructive surgery, it may be achieved with a properly performed amputation—a good example is the removal of a severely malformed foot to obtain proper fit of a prosthesis. With the prosthesis, the child will look almost normal and be almost normally active.

In the growing child, the amputation should always be through a joint, not across a long bone. Amputation through the diaphysis can result in bone overgrowth. Many times, after an apparently successful amputation, the growing bone perforates distally through the stump, and the

ensuing infection and further overgrowth necessitate multiple surgical procedures. During a joint disarticulation, the growth plate must be preserved to ensure future growth of the stump.

Bone overgrowth can also occur when a severe constriction band syndrome causes a congenital amputation through a long bone. Among the techniques used to control this overgrowth problem are provision of an adequate skin cover and capping the bone end with a silicone implant.

Prostheses. Use of prostheses is successful in children as young as 21 months of age. They can master a voluntary opening hook and eventually become more adept at using a prosthesis than adult amputees. Artificial limbs are used as long

as they are tolerated by the patient, do not cause pain, and are in good working order. Children are readily accepted by playmates once the curiosity about the prosthesis is satisfied.

Children who wear upper limb prostheses are able to dress themselves and put on and take off their artificial limbs without difficulty. The terminal hook device is a very versatile tool, and most patients prefer it to a cosmetic hand. In adolescence, a functioning cosmetic hand may be substituted.

Parents of children with limb defects should keep well informed about rehabilitation programs that include physical therapy, surgery, and prostheses. □

116

Section II

Tumors of Musculoskeletal System

Frank H. Netter, M.D.

in collaboration with

William F. Enneking, M.D. and Ernest U. Conrad, III, M.D.   *Plates 1–34*

Table 1. PRIMARY MUSCULOSKELETAL TUMORS AND USUAL PRESENTING STAGE

Tumors of Bone

Tissue type	Benign	Malignant
Osseous	Osteoid osteoma (2) Osteoblastoma (2-3) Osteoma (1)	Classic osteosarcoma (IIB) Parosteal osteosarcoma (IA) Periosteal osteosarcoma (IIA)
Cartilaginous	Enchondroma (2) Exostosis (2) Periosteal chondroma (2) Chondroblastoma (2-3) Chondromyxoid fibroma (2-3)	Primary chondrosarcoma (IIB) Secondary chondrosarcoma (IA)
Fibrous	Nonossifying fibroma (1-2) Desmoplastic fibroma (2-3) Fibrous dysplasia (NA) Ossifying fibroma (2-3)	Fibrosarcoma of bone (IIB) Malignant fibrous histiocytoma (IIB)
Reticuloendothelial	Eosinophilic granuloma (NA) Hands-Schüller-Christian disease (NA) Letterer-Siwe disease (NA)	Ewing's sarcoma (IIB) Reticulum-cell sarcoma (IIB) Myeloma (III)
Vascular	Aneurysmal bone cyst (2) Hemangioma of bone (2)	Angiosarcoma (IIB) Hemangioendothelioma (IA) Hemangiopericytoma (IA)
Unknown origin	Simple bone cyst (NA) Giant-cell tumor in bone (2-3)	Giant-cell sarcoma (IIB) Chordoma (IB) Adamantinoma (IA)

Tumors of Soft Tissue

Tissue type	Benign	Malignant
Osseous	Myositis ossificans (NA)	Extraosseous osteosarcoma (IIB)
Cartilaginous	Chondroma (2) Synovial chondromatosis (2)	Extraosseous chondrosarcoma (IB)
Fibrous	Fibroma (1-2) Fibromatosis (3)	Fibrosarcoma (I-IIB) Malignant fibrous histiocytoma (IIB)
Synovial	Pigmented villonodular synovitis (2) Ganglion cyst (1)	Synovial sarcoma (IIB)
Vascular	Hemangioma (2-3)	Angiosarcoma (IIB) Hemangioendothelioma (IB Hemangiopericytoma (IB)
Fatty	Lipoma (1) Angiolipoma (3)	Liposarcoma (IA)
Neural	Neurolemmoma (2) Neurofibroma (2-3)	Neurosarcoma (IIB) Neurofibrosarcoma (IIB)
Muscular	Leiomyoma (2) Rhabdomyoma	Leiomyosarcoma (IIB) Rhabdomyosarcoma (IIA)
Unknown origin	Giant-cell tumor of tendon sheath (2)	Epithelioid sarcoma (IB) Clear cell sarcoma (IB) Mesenchymoma (IIB) Undifferentiated sarcoma (IIB)

NA = not applicable (usual presenting stages are shown in Table 2)

Table 2. SURGICAL STAGING SYSTEM FOR MUSCULOSKELETAL TUMORS

		Stage	Grade	Site	Metastasis
Benign	1	Latent	G_0	T_0	M_0
	2	Active	G_0	T_0	M_0
	3	Aggressive	G_0	T_{1-2}	M_{0-1}
Malignant	1A	Low grade, intracompartmental	G_1	T_1	M_0
	1B	Low grade, extracompartmental	G_1	T_2	M_0
	IIA	High grade, intracompartmental	G_2	T_1	M_0
	IIB	High grade, extracompartmental	G_2	T_2	M_0
	IIIA	Low or high grade, intracompartmental, with metastases	G_{1-2}	T_1	M_1
	IIIB	Low or high grade, extracompartmental, with metastases	G_{1-2}	T_2	M_1

Initial Evaluation and Staging of Musculoskeletal Tumors

An understanding of the various tumors of the musculoskeletal system requires a thorough knowledge of clinical presentation, natural history, staging characteristics, histopathology, and response to treatment. A histogenic classification of benign and malignant tumors of bone and soft tissue is presented in Table 1, Page 118.

Further staging studies may be needed to determine the local extent, regional or distant spread, and histogenic diagnosis of the disease.

Radionuclide bone scans are performed to assess multiple sites of involvement, the extent of local intraosseous involvement not apparent on radiographs, and tumor activity.

Tomography is used to detect trabecular or cortical destruction, subtle cortical penetration, and intrinsic density of the tumor.

Computed tomography (CT) is employed for determining the precise location and extent of primary involvement, compartmental involvement, intrinsic density of the lesion, proximity of neurovascular structures, intraarticular or cortical extension, and pulmonary metastasis.

Magnetic resonance imaging (MRI) provides a superior resolution and sensitivity in depicting abnormalities, particularly the extent of soft-tissue lesions and the subtle involvement of the bone marrow in bone lesions.

Angiography is commonly used to assess the tumor's neovascularity (tumor blush) or the details of neurovascular bundle involvement often necessary for planning limb-salvage procedures.

Arthrography is a direct method of determining joint involvement and is especially useful for distinguishing intraarticular (synovial chondromatosis) from extraarticular (chondrosarcoma) cartilaginous tumors.

Staging. The staging system for musculoskeletal tumors shown in Table 2, page 118 represents an assessment of the surgical grade, local extent of disease, and presence or absence of metastases. It is based on the stratification and interrelationship of these three factors and is used to predict the prognosis and response to surgical treatment and the risk of local recurrence or metastasis (see page 149).

The *surgical grade (G)* reflects a tumor's aggressiveness based on its histologic pattern and clinical behavior: benign (G_0); low-grade malignant (G_1); and high-grade malignant (G_2).

The *local extent of disease (T)* defines the primary lesion as intracapsular (T_0, surrounded by an intact capsule of fibrous tissue or reactive bone); extracapsular but intracompartmental (T_1, remaining within an intraosseous, intrafascial-intramuscular, periosteal, or parosseous compartment or potential compartment); and extracapsular and extracompartmental (T_2, extending beyond its compartment of origin or arising within incompletely bounded spaces, such as the popliteal fossa, axilla, or groin).

The designation *M* indicates the presence or absence of *metastases*: no known metastases (M_0); metastases present (M_1). □

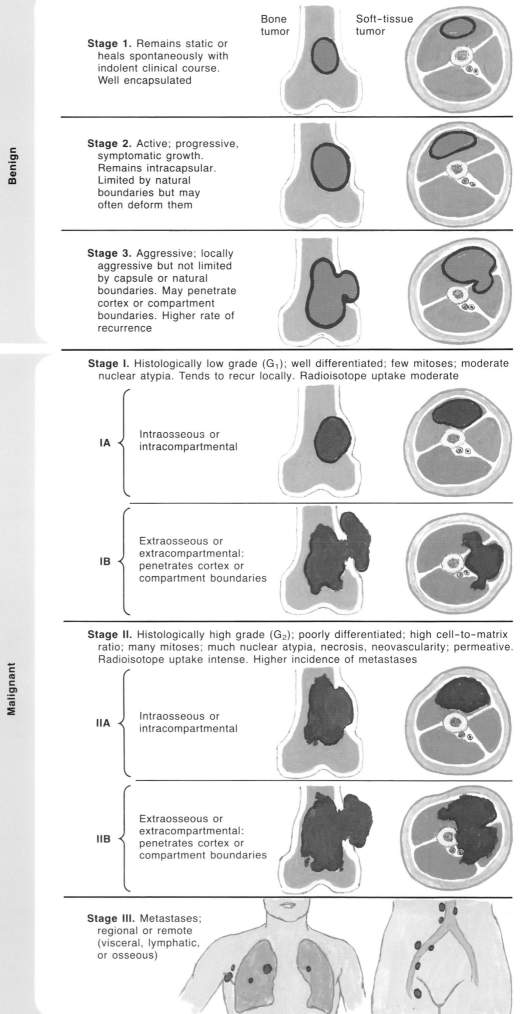

Staging of Musculoskeletal Tumors

Stages 1–3. Histologically benign (G_0); variable clinical course and biologic behavior

Bone tumor   Soft-tissue tumor

Benign

Stage 1. Remains static or heals spontaneously with indolent clinical course. Well encapsulated

Stage 2. Active; progressive, symptomatic growth. Remains intracapsular. Limited by natural boundaries but may often deform them

Stage 3. Aggressive; locally aggressive but not limited by capsule or natural boundaries. May penetrate cortex or compartment boundaries. Higher rate of recurrence

Malignant

Stage I. Histologically low grade (G_1); well differentiated; few mitoses; moderate nuclear atypia. Tends to recur locally. Radioisotope uptake moderate

IA { Intraosseous or intracompartmental

IB { Extraosseous or extracompartmental: penetrates cortex or compartment boundaries

Stage II. Histologically high grade (G_2); poorly differentiated; high cell-to-matrix ratio; many mitoses; much nuclear atypia, necrosis, neovascularity; permeative. Radioisotope uptake intense. Higher incidence of metastases

IIA { Intraosseous or intracompartmental

IIB { Extraosseous or extracompartmental: penetrates cortex or compartment boundaries

Stage III. Metastases; regional or remote (visceral, lymphatic, or osseous)

Benign Tumors of Bone

Osteoid Osteoma

Osteoid Osteoma

Adolescent indicates site of pain on tibia; bony prominence only slight. Pain often dramatically relieved by aspirin

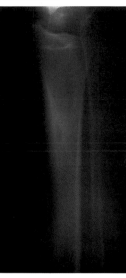

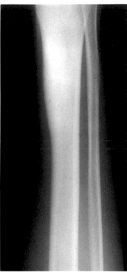

Radiograph of sclerotic lesion of tibial cortex with radiolucent nidus (difficult to see)

Diffuse area of sclerotic cortical thickening apparent during healing phase

Section reveals osteoblastic nidus sharply demarcated from dense, reactive cortical bone (H and E stain)

Sectioned tumor reveals cherry red nidus surrounded by dense, reactive cortical bone

Boy with painful scoliosis. CT scan shows destruction of vertebra by osteoid osteoma

Osteoid osteoma is a benign osseous tumor that occurs primarily in adolescents and less often in children and young adults. The most common site is the proximal femur, and although osteoid osteoma typically involves the diaphysis of long bones, it may also occur in the foot (talus, navicular, or calcaneus) and in the posterior elements of the spine, where it leads to a secondary scoliosis. The typical presenting symptom is well-localized pain that is most severe at night and is relieved by aspirin and other salicylates and prostaglandin inhibitors. In two-thirds of patients, diagnosis is easily made on the basis of a classic history, symptoms, and radiographic and histologic findings. A frequent problem in establishing the diagnosis is the difficulty of locating the nidus on radiographs.

Diagnostic Studies. An intense bony reaction to a small nidus is the radiographic hallmark of osteoid osteoma. Radiographs reveal an oval radiolucent nidus only 3 to 5 mm in diameter and surrounded by a disproportionately large, dense reactive zone. Although usually located in the cortex, a nidus may occur in the subperiosteal and endosteal regions. CT scans at 5-mm intervals are used to confirm a cortical nidus and to help direct the surgical approach. The bone scan usually shows moderate or intense radioisotope uptake.

Radiographic differential diagnosis includes Garré's osteomyelitis (chronic sclerosing osteomyelitis), Brodie's abscess, and stress fracture.

Histologic examination reveals a nidus composed of thick, vascular bars of osteoblastic tissue surrounded by a thin zone of vascular fibrous tissue and then by a dense shell, or margin, of mature reactive cortical bone. The histologic differential diagnosis primarily includes osteoblastoma (Plate 4). Although osteoblastoma is similar to osteoid osteoma in many respects, it is usually larger and has some subtle but distinct histologic differences. Distinguishing osteosarcoma (Plates 15–16) from the small osteoblastic nidus of osteoid osteoma is rarely problematic.

Treatment and Prognosis. Although osteoid osteoma may eventually resolve spontaneously, with spontaneous ossification and the subsequent relief of pain, most patients prefer not to wait 2 to 4 years for resolution. When the nidus is located in a low-stress area such as the metaphysis, en bloc excision with a surrounding small block of reactive bone is the preferred treatment. Alternatively, the overlying margin of reactive bone may be shaved until the nidus is visible as a cherry-red spot that can be removed with curettage. Although intracapsular curettage is associated with a higher recurrence rate than other types of excision, it minimizes the risk of postoperative fracture in high-stress areas such as the femoral neck. Most recurrences result from fragmentation of the lesion, partial excision, or inaccurate localization of the lesion in an inaccessible place.

After complete excision or spontaneous resolution, prognosis is excellent. No cases of malignant transformation have been reported. □

Benign Tumors of Bone
Osteoma

Osteoma

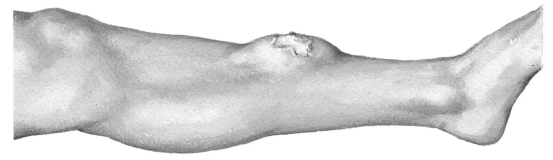

Painless bony mass protrudes from anterior aspect of tibia. Scars due to repeated skin abrasions

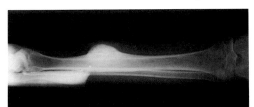

Radiograph reveals globular outgrowth on tibial cortex with sloping extensions (Codman's triangles)

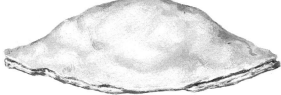

Specimen demonstrates continuity of tumor with overlying periosteum

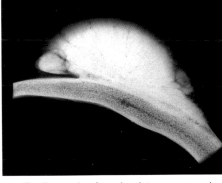

Radiograph of excised tumor reveals densely ossified cortical mass protruding from outer table of skull

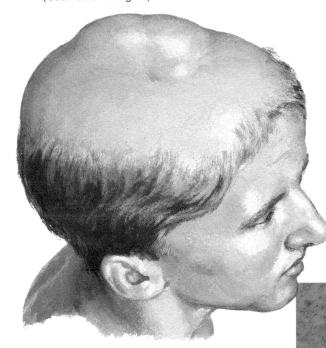

Slowly enlarging, asymptomatic bony mass on dome of head

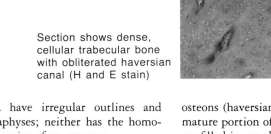

Section shows dense, cellular trabecular bone with obliterated haversian canal (H and E stain)

Osteoma is a rare benign tumor of bone. Like most benign bone tumors, it occurs primarily in adolescents and young adults. The skull, mandible, and middle third of the tibia are the most common sites of involvement. Although osteoma produces no pain or other symptoms, it is visible and palpable as a slowly enlarging bony mass.

Diagnostic Studies. Radiographs reveal a dense, smooth, mature bony mass attached to the surface of the cortex. The hemispheric shape of osteoma has earned it the descriptive term "stuck-on cue ball."

The radiographic differential diagnosis includes osteocartilaginous exostosis (Plate 7) and parosteal osteosarcoma (Plate 17). Exostosis and parosteal osteosarcoma have irregular outlines and occur in the metaphyses; neither has the homogeneous cortical density of an osteoma.

Tomography or computed tomography may be needed to delineate the margins of the tumor and rule out any extension into the medullary canal. Bone scans demonstrate increased radioisotope uptake during active formation of the tumor (stage 2) but little uptake in a mature, usually latent, or inactive, tumor (stage 1).

Histologic examination reveals an outer fibrous layer continuous with the adjacent periosteum, beneath which is a zone of proliferating osteoblasts that produces active intramembranous ossification. The immature bone in turn forms osteons (haversian systems). In the central, more mature portion of the tumor, the haversian canals are filled in, or obliterated, and the bone is strikingly acellular. These necrotic osteons persist, without evidence of remodeling, into the latent stage, surrounded by a shell of living cortical bone.

Treatment and Prognosis. When removal is indicated, an active stage 2 osteoma requires en bloc excision with a marginal margin; a latent stage 1 tumor can be removed in a piecemeal, intracapsular fashion. If the tumor develops in an inaccessible location, it can be monitored until it reaches maturity, then removed with intracapsular excision. The risk of recurrence is minimal. □

Benign Tumors of Bone

Osteoblastoma

Osteoblastoma is an unusual benign osseous tumor. Because of its larger size (>2 cm) and many similarities to osteoid osteoma, it was at one time called giant osteoid osteoma. This tumor is generally seen in a slightly older population than osteoid osteoma, primarily in older adolescents and young adults. There are also important clinical, radiographic, and histologic differences between osteoid osteoma and osteoblastoma. For example, osteoblastoma does not cause well-localized night pain that is relieved by aspirin, and it occurs more often in the posterior elements of the vertebrae (transverse and spinous processes and pedicles) than in the limbs.

Most osteoblastomas are active stage 2 lesions. The more aggressive stage 3 lesion is referred to as pseudomalignant osteoblastoma.

Diagnostic Studies. Plain radiographs show a relatively radiolucent, bone-forming (osteoblastic) lesion that is osteolytic and often has an aneurysmal, or blown-out, appearance. It is surrounded by a thin margin of reactive bone that frequently extends into adjacent soft tissue. The intense bony reaction around osteoid osteoma does not occur with osteoblastoma.

The radiographic differential diagnosis includes osteoid osteoma (Plate 2), aneurysmal bone cyst (Plate 12), eosinophilic granuloma (Plate 11), giant-cell tumor of bone (Plate 14), and osteosarcoma (Plates 15–16).

Bone scans demonstrate an intense radioisotope uptake that helps localize the lesion. Computed tomography confirms the preoperative diagnosis and helps determine the surgical approach; tomography is less useful. Angiography is used for staging aggressive tumors of the spine.

Osteoblastoma

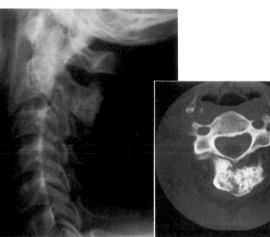

Lateral radiograph of large osteoblastoma of proximal tibia shows bulging, radiolucent zone with thin margin of reactive bone

Radiograph of large osteoblastoma of posterior elements of upper cervical spine. CT scan (right) reveals involvement of spinous process of vertebra with encroachment on lamina

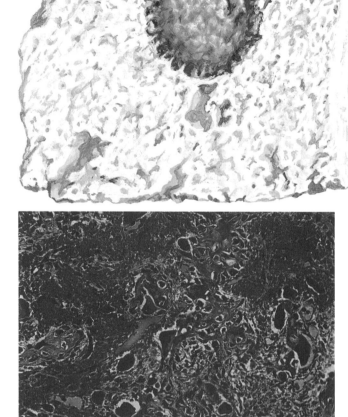

Specimen from neck of scapula, including glenoid margin, shows granular appearance of amorphous ossification in osteoblastoma plus loose, reactive trabecular bone

Section shows many plump, hyperchromatic osteoblasts (chiefly lining spicules of bone and osteoid), numerous giant cells, and vascular background (H and E stain)

Specimen of recurrent pseudomalignant osteoblastoma that filled hollow of sacrum 14 months after intracapsular curettage

The histologic appearance of osteoblastoma is quite similar to that of osteoid osteoma but has a more prominent vascular component. In addition, osteoblastoma has more stromal tissue and giant cells and broader osteoid seams than osteoid osteoma. These characteristics also distinguish osteoblastoma from osteosarcoma. However, the histologic pattern of pseudomalignant osteoblastoma is suggestive of osteosarcoma. Osteoblastoma often contains scattered mitotic figures and a proliferation of immature osteoblasts.

Treatment and Prognosis. En bloc marginal excision of a stage 2 osteoblastoma is usually feasible and is associated with minimal recurrence (≤10% of cases). Active tumors are more likely to recur (10%–30% of cases) after intracapsular procedures, which are usually done to preserve joint function in the spine. The tumor's vascularity may lead to vigorous bleeding during intracapsular procedures. The risk of recurrence after marginal excision of the more aggressive stage 3 tumor is 30% to 50%. Radiation therapy or chemotherapy is not effective.

Although a wide marginal excision is a difficult task in the spinal region, it is nevertheless the treatment of choice for stage 3 osteoblastomas. Pseudomalignant osteoblastoma does not metastasize, but some cases of malignant transformation of aggressive osteoblastoma into osteosarcoma have been reported. □

Benign Tumors of Bone

Enchondroma

Enchondroma

Enchondroma, a benign and asymptomatic cartilaginous tumor of bone, results from a failure of normal endochondral ossification below the growth plate. This intramedullary tumor develops in the adjacent metaphysis and eventually penetrates the diaphysis. Enchondroma represents a dysplasia of the central growth plate. If the dysplastic process occurs in the lateral growth plate, the resulting tumor is called osteocartilaginous exostosis (Plate 7); dysplastic cartilaginous proliferation beneath the perichondrium results in a periosteal chondroma (Plate 6).

Most solitary enchondromas occur in adolescence or young adulthood. Although primarily affecting the small tubular bones of the hands or feet or the proximal humerus, enchondroma may occur anywhere in the skeleton. In rare cases, a benign enchondroma undergoes malignant transformation into secondary chondrosarcoma (Plate 18). The uncommon occurrence of multiple lesions is known as enchondromatosis, or Ollier's disease (see Section I, Plate 83).

Diagnostic Studies. Radiographs show a central radiolucent lesion with a well-defined but minimally thickened bony margin. During the active phase in adolescence, the lesion may slowly enlarge. In the inactive, or latent, phase in adulthood, the cartilaginous tissue may calcify in a diffuse punctate or stippled configuration. These calcifications sometimes appear on the radiograph as subtle "smoke-ring" images. As the lesion matures, it develops a more reactive margin.

Radiographic changes that indicate incipient malignant transformation include radiolucent endosteal destruction ("scalloping"), significant cortical thickening, erosions, penetration and internal "buttressing," and marked endosteal reaction. Additional findings that suggest malignancy are a soft-tissue mass; a large, poorly defined intraosseous lesion; and excessive diffuse calcification.

Bone scans demonstrate radioisotope uptake in the margin, which is related to the activity of the lesion: typically, there is moderate uptake in the active phase and a modest increase during the latent phase after skeletal maturity. A marked increase in the lesion's activity in adulthood suggests malignant transformation; a baseline bone scan should be obtained in patients with multiple lesions or other evidence of increased risk. Computed tomography or magnetic resonance imaging may be used to assess cortical erosion, intralesional density, and exact location. Tomograms may help delineate the bony margin.

Biopsy is often not needed to confirm the diagnosis of enchondroma, since its cartilaginous nature is evident radiographically; in addition, it is often difficult to distinguish between an active benign lesion and a low-grade malignant lesion on the basis of histologic examination alone. Therefore, if there is enough clinical and radiographic evidence for a biopsy, then there is enough evidence for a wide excision. On histo-

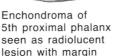

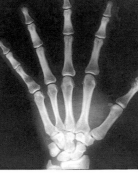

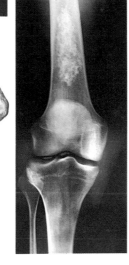

Enchondroma of 5th proximal phalanx seen as radiolucent lesion with margin of reactive bone

Sagittal section of middle phalanx shows digit disarticulation at proximal interphalangeal joint

Involvement of distal femur with calcification. Benign enchondromas usually asymptomatic

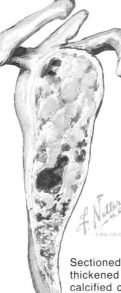

Sectioned scapula shows blade thickened by tumor of pearly gray, calcified cartilage with margin of reactive bone

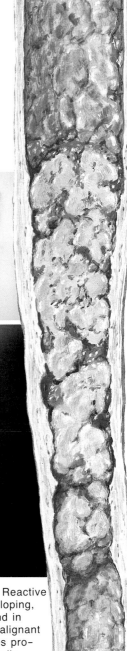

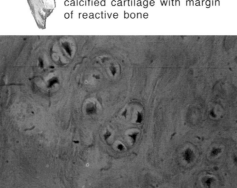

Section shows disorganized cartilaginous tissue with excessive matrix. Nuclear atypia, mitoses, and multiple nuclei not significant in children but suggest malignancy in adults (H and E stain)

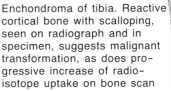

Enchondroma of tibia. Reactive cortical bone with scalloping, seen on radiograph and in specimen, suggests malignant transformation, as does progressive increase of radioisotope uptake on bone scan

logic analysis, stage 2 tumors in children and low-grade, secondary malignant tumors in adults both exhibit marked cellularity, binucleated lacunae, increased cell-to-matrix ratio, and increased mitoses. Since malignant transformation in childhood is very unusual, these findings in a child or adolescent suggest an active benign lesion. In adults, however, these same aggressive features are considered evidence of low-grade chondrosarcoma.

Treatment and Prognosis. Asymptomatic solitary enchondromas are presumed benign and require only periodic clinical follow-ups. If solitary or multiple enchondromas become symptomatic and begin to enlarge, staging studies

(radiographs with or without tomograms, bone scans, and CT scans) are indicated to rule out malignancy. Surgical treatment is needed in any patient with two of the so-called triad of transformation criteria: pain, marked increase of radioisotope uptake on the bone scan, and characteristic radiographic changes. The tumor must be excised with a wide margin of tissue to reduce the risk of recurrence.

The prognosis for benign enchondroma is excellent. The lesion usually becomes latent in adulthood, and only 2% of asymptomatic solitary enchondromas become malignant. In enchondromatosis, however, the risk of malignant transformation is much greater (10% of cases). □

Benign Tumors of Bone
Periosteal Chondroma

Periosteal Chondroma

Painless prominence over lateral aspect of humerus near insertion of deltoid muscle (most common site)

Sectioned humerus shows pearly, translucent, subperiosteal deposits of cartilage over eroded and reactive cortical bone. (Resection of complete bone segment shown here only to depict tumor. En bloc marginal excision usually suffices)

Section reveals cartilaginous component at right overlying reactive bone at left, with partially intervening thin zone of calcified cartilage (H and E stain)

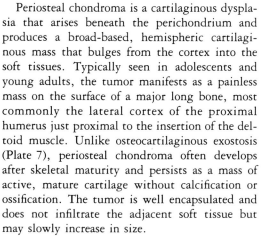

Radiograph demonstrates bulging radiolucent lesion of shaft of humerus

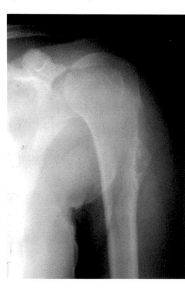

Radiograph shows bone healing well 3 months after marginal cortical excision

Periosteal chondroma is a cartilaginous dysplasia that arises beneath the perichondrium and produces a broad-based, hemispheric cartilaginous mass that bulges from the cortex into the soft tissues. Typically seen in adolescents and young adults, the tumor manifests as a painless mass on the surface of a major long bone, most commonly the lateral cortex of the proximal humerus just proximal to the insertion of the deltoid muscle. Unlike osteocartilaginous exostosis (Plate 7), periosteal chondroma often develops after skeletal maturity and persists as a mass of active, mature cartilage without calcification or ossification. The tumor is well encapsulated and does not infiltrate the adjacent soft tissue but may slowly increase in size.

Diagnostic Studies. Periosteal chondroma appears on radiographs as a radiolucent oval or oblong defect in a shallow, craterlike deformity of the periphery of the cortex. The lesion is underlined by a thin, distinct cortical reaction. The tumor has little or no calcification. Computed tomography is used to demonstrate the extent of cortical involvement and identify the density of the cartilage. The lesion has minimal neovascularity.

The radiographic differential diagnosis includes osteocartilaginous exostosis in younger patients (Plate 7), juxtacortical chondrosarcoma (Plate 18), as well as parosteal and periosteal osteosarcomas (Plate 17).

On gross examination, the lesion has the consistency of mature cartilage without evidence of ossification or calcification. A fine, chalky white line of endochondral ossification is seen at the tumor-bone interface, appearing as a fluorescent band after dynamic tetracycline labeling. Histologic examination reveals an active tumor with lobules of hyaline cartilage. Isolated areas of increased cellularity are occasionally seen, but this finding should be interpreted in light of the clinical, radiographic, and gross findings.

Treatment and Prognosis. Most periosteal chondromas are active stage 2 tumors that require en bloc marginal excision to prevent recurrence. Because of their peripheral location, this can usually be achieved without bone grafting or extensive reconstruction. The main challenge is to remove the entire tumor without rupturing the tumor capsule. Even if the lesion abuts a neurovascular bundle, its smooth surface allows it to be removed easily with blunt dissection.

The risk of recurrence after en bloc marginal excision is less than 10%, and more aggressive excision or adjuvant chemotherapy and radiation therapy are not indicated. Sarcomatous transformation has not been documented, and the rare reports probably reflect the resemblance of periosteal chondroma in the adult to juxtacortical chondrosarcoma. □

Benign Tumors of Bone

Osteocartilaginous Exostosis (Osteochondroma)

Osteocartilaginous exostosis (osteochondroma) is a common developmental dysplasia of the peripheral growth plate that results in a lobulated outgrowth of cartilage and bone from the metaphysis. The classic presentation is an excrescence of trabecular bone capped by a thin zone of proliferating cartilage. An exostosis may develop in any bone that is preformed in cartilage but is usually seen in the long bones. The most common locations are the proximal or distal femur, proximal humerus, proximal tibia, pelvis, and scapula. The tumor develops in adolescence and continues to enlarge during skeletal growth, becoming latent at skeletal maturity.

The initial clinical sign is a hard, painless mass fixed on the bone. Symptoms, when present, are usually due to irritation of the overlying soft tissues that may or may not be associated with a fluid-filled bursa. Variations in the fluid content in the bursa create a fluctuating, palpable mass.

In most patients, the lesion is solitary; however, polyostotic tumors occur in a small subset of patients with a familial form. These multiple hereditary exostoses produce significant deformities such as short stature, clubbing of the radius, and angular deformity of the lower limbs.

Diagnostic Studies. The radiographic appearance of an exostosis is either a flat, sessile lesion or a pedunculated (stalklike) process. It is usually a well-defined metaphyseal projection of bone with mottled density; the cartilaginous cap displays irregular areas of calcification. The radiographic hallmark is the blending of the tumor into the underlying metaphysis. Although a diagnosis is seldom problematic, the presence of a painful and enlarging lesion in an adult may necessitate staging studies to assess the risk of secondary malignant transformation to chondrosarcoma (Plate 18).

Evidence of malignant transformation includes (1) a cartilaginous cap thicker than 1 cm, (2) a sudden or marked increase in radioisotope uptake on the bone scan in an adult patient (inconsistent with the normal latency seen with skeletal maturity), and (3) confirmation by computed tomography or magnetic resonance imaging of a soft-tissue mass or displacement of a major neurovascular bundle.

The radiographic differential diagnosis must consider periosteal chondroma (Plate 6) and

Osteocartilaginous Exostosis (Osteochondroma)

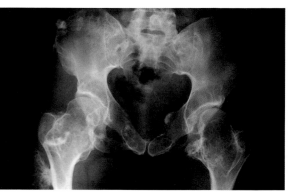

Radiograph shows multiple hereditary exostoses with bilateral involvement of pelvis and proximal femurs

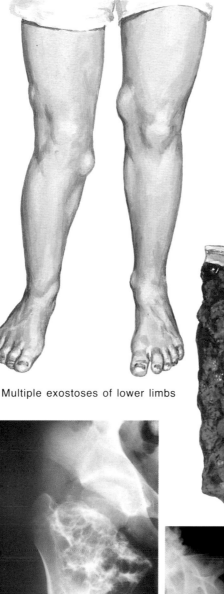

Multiple exostoses of lower limbs

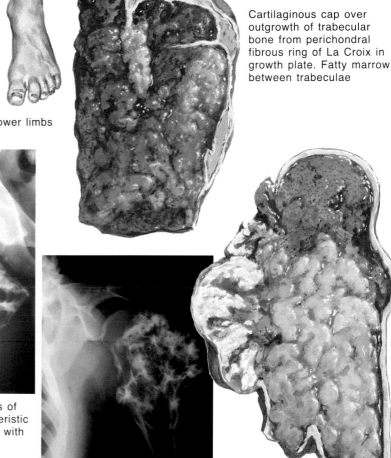

Cartilaginous cap over outgrowth of trabecular bone from perichondral fibrous ring of La Croix in growth plate. Fatty marrow between trabeculae

Solitary benign exostosis of proximal femur. Characteristic mass of trabecular bone with minimal bony reaction

Radiograph and sectioned exostosis of proximal humerus that has undergone malignant transformation to chondrosarcoma

parosteal osteosarcoma (Plate 17). In an adult, a symptomatic "exostosis" that increases in size is more likely to be a parosteal osteosarcoma.

Gross examination reveals an overlying cartilaginous cap separated from the underlying bone by an irregular, chalky white line (zone of calcification). The mass of trabecular bone that makes up the main portion of the exostosis merges into the underlying normal trabecular bone of the metaphysis.

On microscopic examination, the cartilaginous cap is seen to have the same pattern as the normal growth plate: the zones of proliferation, columnization, and calcification exist but in a less organized state. The underlying trabeculae form by endochondral ossification of the cap and contain central cores of calcified cartilage. The trabeculae are not remodeled in response to stress, and the cores of cartilage occur throughout the entire tumor.

Treatment and Prognosis. Marginal excision of an active exostosis, including the cartilaginous cap and the overlying perichondrium, minimizes the risk of recurrence. The deep bony base has minimal activity and may be removed piecemeal. The prognosis for a solitary exostosis is excellent (<5% recurrence following marginal excision). The risk of sarcomatous transformation in solitary exostosis is about 1%, but in multiple hereditary exostoses, the risk approaches 10%. □

Benign Tumors of Bone

Chondroblastoma and Chondromyxoid Fibroma

Chondroblastoma

Chondroblastoma is a painful, benign cartilaginous tumor that arises during adolescence in the secondary ossification center of the proximal humerus, proximal tibia, or distal femur. The majority are active stage 2 lesions, although an aggressive stage 3 form is occasionally seen.

Diagnostic Studies. The radiographic hallmark is an epiphyseal radiolucent lesion with fine punctate calcifications suggestive of a cartilaginous lesion. The tumor is usually bordered by a well-defined margin of reactive bone. Stage 3 chondroblastoma often extends through the growth plate into the metaphysis or through the articular cartilage into the joint.

The radiographic differential diagnosis includes aneurysmal bone cyst (Plate 12), giant-cell tumor of bone (Plate 14), and inflammatory lesions such as pigmented villonodular synovitis (see Section III, Plate 49) and infection. Computed tomography is useful in demonstrating tissue density, extent of epiphyseal involvement, and—often most important—location of the lesion in relation to the articular and epiphyseal cartilages. Bone scans show an increased radioisotope uptake around the margin that is frequently overshadowed by the normal increased activity in the adjacent growth plate.

Gross examination reveals a soft, vascular, reddish purple neoplastic tissue covered by a thin capsule. Histologic examination shows the characteristic "cobblestone" pattern: areas of round, plump chondroblasts (the stones) enmeshed in a sparse chondroid matrix (the mortar between the stones). Clumps of giant cells are seen in areas that contain primarily a spindle-cell stroma. Unique to chondroblastoma is the fine microscopic pattern of calcifications, usually in a "chicken-wire" arrangement, in and around the islands of cartilage.

Treatment and Prognosis. Chondroblastoma often extends through the subchondral bone into the articular cartilage, which makes complete curettage and subsequent reconstruction difficult. A partial injury to the growth plate, resulting from either the tumor or the curettage, often adds to the surgical difficulty. Since most chondroblastomas occur in teenagers who are nearing skeletal maturity, the remaining growth plate can be curetted to promote closure and to prevent late angular deformities. If the tumor occurs in a child with significant growth potential, interposition of fat tissue or a plastic implant may be advisable to prevent premature closure of the growth plate.

The prognosis for chondroblastoma is good; most are active stage 2 tumors with a modest risk of recurrence after curettage. Marginal excision is the treatment of choice, if it does not result in significant disability. Aggressive stage 3 chondroblastoma, most common in the pelvis, recurs in 50% of cases after curettage; cementation of the defect with methylmethacrylate may be

Chondroblastoma

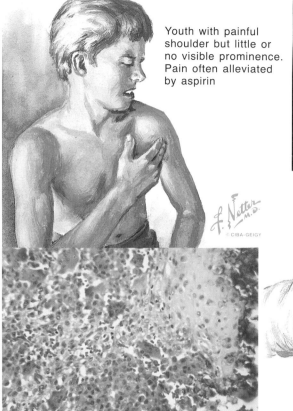

Youth with painful shoulder but little or no visible prominence. Pain often alleviated by aspirin

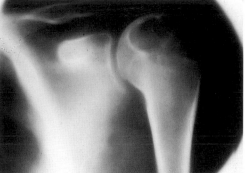

Radiograph reveals ovoid defect in humeral epiphysis extending into metaphysis with fine calcifications

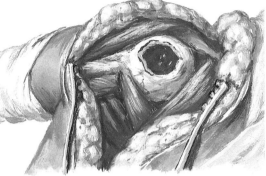

Section shows mixture of chondroblasts and fibrovascular stroma with occasional giant cells (H and E stain)

Curettage of cavity before reconstruction with trabecular bone graft

Chondromyxoid Fibroma

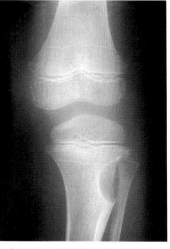

Anteroposterior radiograph shows eccentric radiolucent lesion in proximal tibia with thin margin of reactive bone

Sectioned cartilaginous tumor. Surgical defect repaired with cortical bone graft from iliac crest

Myxomatous cartilage combined with benign fibrous stroma (H and E stain)

added to the curettage. If the aggressive nature of the tumor is recognized before surgery, en bloc excision with a wide margin is usually successful.

Chondromyxoid Fibroma

Chondromyxoid fibroma is a painless, benign cartilaginous lesion of bone. It occurs in adolescents, most often in the metaphyses of major long bones. This lesion most often presents as an active stage 2 lesion and is not known to undergo malignant transformation.

Diagnostic Studies. Radiographs reveal an eccentric radiolucent defect with no evidence of the usual calcification of a cartilaginous tumor. The radiographic differential diagnosis includes nonossifying fibroma (Plate 10) and aneurysmal bone cyst (Plate 12).

Gross examination reveals a soft, gelatinous translucent tissue. Histologic examination shows immature myxoid cartilage with stellate-shaped chondrocytes enmeshed in lightly staining myxomatous chondroid matrix. Intertwined throughout the lesion are strands of benign fibrous tissue and small multinucleated giant cells.

Treatment. Curettage carries a low risk of recurrence in well-encapsulated stage 2 lesions, but the size of the defect often necessitates bone grafting (Plates 30–31). Stage 3 lesions, most often seen in the pelvis, require wide excision to prevent recurrence. □

Benign Tumors of Bone

Fibrous Dysplasia

Fibrous Dysplasia

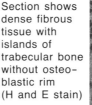

Fibrous dysplasia is a developmental abnormality of bone that results in a haphazard mixture of immature fibrous tissue and small fragments of immature trabecular bone. It occurs slightly more often in females, with onset typically in adolescence. The lesions may occur in one bone (monostotic) or in many (polyostotic), and they are sometimes accompanied by precocious puberty and café au lait pigmentation in females (Albright's syndrome).

Monostotic lesions generally occur in the proximal femur, proximal tibia, mandible, and ribs. Polyostotic disease, which usually presents earlier, may be unilateral or widespread, affecting long bones, hands, feet, and pelvis. Extensive involvement of the proximal femur results in the distinctive "shepherd's-crook" deformity that is characteristic of fibrous dysplasia.

The result of this dysplastic process is a weakened bone that becomes deformed by normal stress or sustains frequent pathologic fractures. Painful stress fractures are especially common in the femoral neck. Although dysplastic bone heals at a normal rate after fracture, the resulting callus is also dysplastic, and the disease persists.

Diagnostic Studies. The classic radiographic feature of fibrous dysplasia is a hazy, radiolucent, or ground-glass, pattern resulting from the defective mineralization of immature dysplastic bone; it is usually strikingly different from the radiographic appearance of normal bone, calcified cartilage, or soft tissue. A small monostotic lesion may be difficult to distinguish from other benign lesions, but extensive polyostotic involvement is likely to produce the characteristic ground-glass density and significant deformity.

The lesions, which develop in the center of the metaphysis or in the diaphysis, are trabeculated and surrounded by a thickened margin of reactive bone. With progression of the disease, the tumor enlarges.

Bone scans demonstrate an intense radioisotope uptake that corresponds exactly to the extent of the tumor visible on radiographs. Tomography depicts the geographic pattern of involvement, and CT scans help evaluate the extent of involvement and provide a better visualization of the ground-glass density of the lesion.

Gross inspection reveals a soft, dysplastic tissue containing small pieces of gritty dysplastic bone. The tumor may exhibit large cystic areas or small nodules of cartilage. The typical histologic pattern is an irregular collection of small pieces of immature bone within a matrix of fibrous tissue. The overall appearance has been likened to that of alphabet soup. The immature trabeculae are not lined with osteoblasts (as in

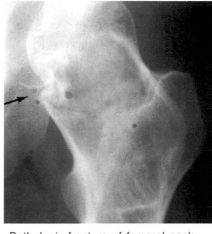

Pathologic fracture of femoral neck and typical ground-glass appearance of bone

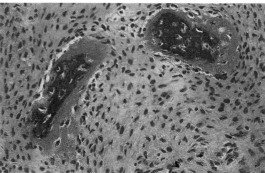

Preoperative (left) and postoperative (right) radiographs of severe monostotic fibrous dysplasia of femur treated for fracture prophylaxis with cortical autograft from fibula

Section shows dense fibrous tissue with islands of trabecular bone without osteoblastic rim (H and E stain)

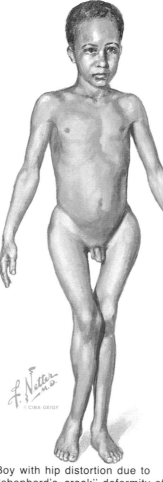

Boy with hip distortion due to "shepherd's-crook" deformity of both femoral necks. Note also deformity of right tibia

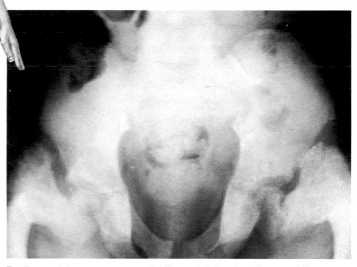

Radiographic appearance of bilateral "shepherd's-crook" deformity; may occur with or without other stigmas of Albright's syndrome (café au lait spots and precocious puberty in females)

ossifying fibroma), do not contain cement lines, and are obviously not aligned according to stress. The fibrous stroma is loosely arranged and immature, replacing the normal marrow. A variable degree of capillary vasculature is seen within the stroma.

The histologic differential diagnosis includes osteoblastoma (Plate 4), osteosarcoma (Plate 15), ossifying fibroma, hyperparathyroidism, and Paget's disease of bone (see CIBA COLLECTION, Volume 8/I, pages 196–199, 236–238).

Treatment and Prognosis. Since more dysplastic bone usually forms after curettage, the goal of management should be prevention of deformity and fracture. This is best accomplished using cortical bone autografts (taken from the fibula), which minimally remodel after incorporation. Alternative treatment methods are reconstruction with cortical bone allografts or fixation with an intramedullary rod. Grafting with cortical bone is particularly appropriate for managing lesions in high-stress areas such as the femoral neck.

The prognosis for monostotic lesions is quite good, but the polyostotic tumors usually remain more active or aggressive and are thus more problematic. Compared with monostotic lesions, polyostotic fibrous dysplasia has a small but significantly higher incidence of malignant transformation to osteosarcoma or fibrosarcoma. □

Benign Tumors of Bone

Nonossifying Fibroma and Desmoplastic Fibroma

Nonossifying Fibroma

Nonossifying fibroma (fibrous cortical defect) is the most common bone lesion. It results from a developmental defect of periosteal cortical bone that leads to a failure of ossification during the normal growth period. This lesion of fibrous origin typically develops in childhood and adolescence, with a slightly higher incidence in males. Although asymptomatic, nonossifying fibroma is an active stage 2 lesion that persists or enlarges throughout childhood. When the tumor occupies more than 50% of the diameter of the bone, the bone is prone to fracture. With skeletal maturation, a nonossifying fibroma becomes latent and ultimately ossifies.

Diagnostic Studies. The lesion commonly develops in the metaphysis of the distal femur or distal tibia and is eccentrically located, usually within or adjacent to the cortex. Radiographs reveal a well-marginated radiolucent zone, with distinct trabeculation producing a multilocular appearance. In addition, nonossifying fibroma usually causes benign cortical thinning, or erosion. The radiographic pattern is usually diagnostic, and further staging studies are seldom indicated.

Gross examination reveals a tumor composed of soft, reddish tan, granulationlike tissue. Histologic features include a combination of dense collagen arranged in a storiform pattern, a scattering of small, multinucleated giant cells, hemosiderin, and lipid-filled histiocytes. The tissue does not contain the degree of hemorrhage and necrosis or the number of giant cells seen in the giant-cell tumor of bone. Although the tissue may resemble the lining tissue of an aneurysmal bone cyst, the lesion does not have a large, central, blood-filled cavity.

Treatment. Intracapsular curettage is usually sufficient, but it may be supplemented with bone grafts or other stabilization techniques for fracture prophylaxis and treatment.

Desmoplastic Fibroma

Desmoplastic fibroma (desmoid tumor) is a rare intraosseous fibroma that typically develops as an aggressive stage 3 tumor. It occurs primarily in young adults but may occur at any age. The long bones—particularly the tibia and the fibula—are the most common sites, although it may occur throughout the skeleton. Its behavior corresponds to that of its soft-tissue counterpart, aggressive fibromatosis (Plate 24).

Diagnostic Studies. Radiographs show a centrally located metaphyseal or diaphyseal lesion, poorly or incompletely contained by a thin margin of reactive bone, which frequently has a trabeculated appearance. It may remain within the bone for some time, surrounded by a thin cortical

Nonossifying Fibroma

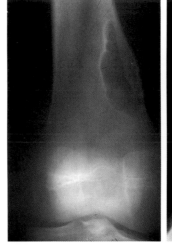

Eccentric radiolucent lesion with margin of reactive bone in metaphysis of distal femur

Both distal tibia and fibula involved; fibula fractured

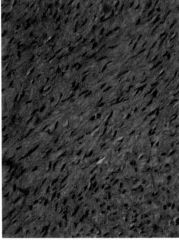

Sectioned proximal tibia with tumor. Reddish tan fibrous core and margin of reactive bone. En bloc excision not usually required as lesions heal eventually, either spontaneously or after curettage

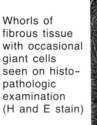

Whorls of fibrous tissue with occasional giant cells seen on histopathologic examination (H and E stain)

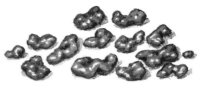

Scrapings from curettage

Desmoplastic Fibroma

Radiograph of distal femur shows bulging, trabeculated, radiolucent lesion with margin of reactive bone

Whitish, rubbery fibrous nodules with rupture into soft tissue

Section shows dense bands of irregularly arranged collagen and mature fibrocytes (H and E stain)

shell, but eventually it extends through the cortex into the soft tissues. The radiographic hallmark is a loculated intraosseous lesion that stimulates very little bony reaction. The radiographic differential diagnosis includes giant-cell tumor of bone (Plate 14) and fibrosarcoma of bone (Plate 19).

Bone scans show increased radioisotope uptake at the margin but very little uptake in the lesion itself. Both bone scans and angiograms demonstrate the relative avascularity of desmoplastic fibroma, and CT scans detect extracompartmental extension and depict the lesion's density. The most characteristic feature is the contrast between the relatively benign findings of the radiographic

and staging studies and the tumor's fairly aggressive clinical behavior.

The lesion is composed of dense, white, fibrous tissue with a rubbery consistency and is easily removed with curettage. The histologic features of dense, irregularly arranged bundles of collagen with an occasional mature fibrocyte closely resemble fibromatosis. Mitoses, vascularity, and necrosis are unusual microscopic findings. The histologic differential diagnosis usually involves low-grade fibrosarcoma of bone.

Treatment. Excision with a wide margin results in local control of the lesion. Recurrence after curettage is frequent, with invasion of the soft tissue. □

Benign Tumors of Bone
Eosinophilic Granuloma

Eosinophilic granuloma belongs to a group of disorders characterized by tumorlike lesions that occur as a result of metabolic defects in the reticuloendothelial system. This group of disorders, called the histiocytoses, or histiocytosis X, also includes Hand-Schüller-Christian disease and Letterer-Siwe disease. The clinical and radiographic manifestations of histiocytoses resemble those of neoplasms, but their clinical course differs from that of malignant reticuloendothelial tumors such as lymphoma, Ewing's sarcoma (Plate 20), leukemia, lymphosarcoma, Hodgkin's disease, and multiple myeloma (Plate 21).

Eosinophilic granuloma usually occurs as a solitary, minimally symptomatic lesion in children under 10 years of age but can occur as multiple tumors at any age and at any site. Low-grade fever, elevated erythrocyte sedimentation rate, and mild peripheral eosinophilia are occasional associated findings. The skull, mandible, spine, ribs, supraacetabular region of the pelvis, and diaphysis of long bones are the usual sites of involvement. Patients with pelvic involvement report a subtle pain in the hip that is exacerbated by movement and ambulation.

Diagnostic Studies. On radiographs, a small lesion may resemble the punched-out radiolucent lesion of multiple myeloma. Involvement of a vertebral body produces the pathognomonic finding of vertebra plana ("coin-on-edge" appearance) subsequent to vertebral collapse. A lesion that occurs in the diaphysis or metaphysis of a limb appears as an oval radiolucent area surrounded by a thick margin of reactive bone. Because of its variable radiographic characteristics, eosinophilic granuloma has been called the great imitator.

Bone scans are used to document the presence of multiple lesions (<10% of cases); an intense radioisotope uptake indicates an active lesion. Computed tomography is helpful in demonstrating the lesion, especially in the spine and hip.

Gross examination of an active lesion reveals a soft, vascular, granulomatous tissue covered with a mature bony capsule. The yellowish, greasy tissue of mature, latent tumors is due to their high lipid content. Histologic characteristics are a mixture of lipid-filled histiocytes, eosinophils, and occasional giant cells with little background stroma. The same histologic pattern is seen in the lesions of the more serious Hand-Schüller-Christian and Letterer-Siwe diseases.

Eosinophilic Granuloma

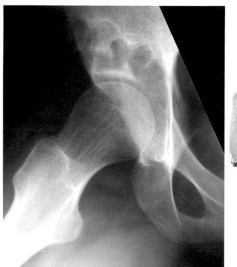

Radiograph shows loculated, bubblelike, radiolucent lesion in supraacetabular region of right ilium

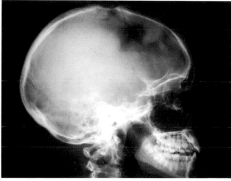

Variegated defects in flat bones of skull

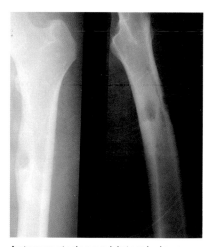

Anteroposterior and lateral views show typical marginated, radiolucent lesions in femoral shaft

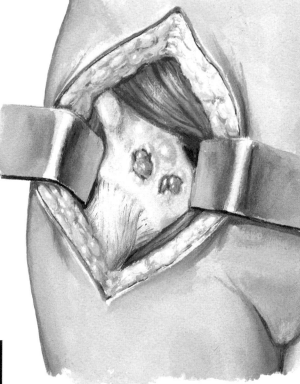

Surgical exploration reveals granuloma eroding through cortex of ilium

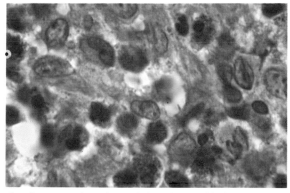

Section reveals pale-staining, foamy histiocytes interspersed with bilobed eosinophils (H and E stain)

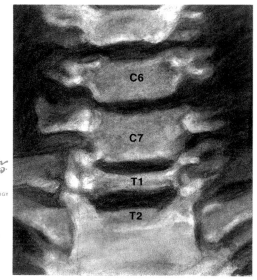

Marked narrowing of 1st thoracic vertebra that led to spinal cord injury in 13-year-old boy. Vertebra plana in young patients strongly suggests eosinophilic granuloma

Treatment and Prognosis. The curettage performed to obtain tissue for diagnosis is also adequate treatment. When the defect is large, bone grafts may be needed to prevent fracture (Plate 31). Chemotherapy or radiation therapy is not indicated for eosinophilic granulomas, since the lesions resolve spontaneously. In a small percentage of patients with a solitary lesion, the visceral manifestations of Hand-Schüller-Christian disease eventually develop, but this transformation is poorly understood and poorly documented. □

Benign Tumors of Bone
Aneurysmal Bone Cyst

Aneurysmal Bone Cyst

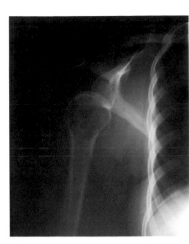

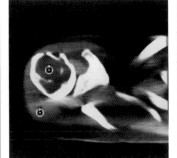

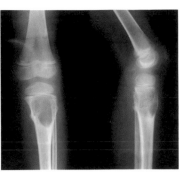

CT scan defines margins and density of lesion

Anteroposterior and lateral views of aneurysmal bone cyst in proximal tibia

Radiograph shows radiolucent lesion in proximal humerus with characteristic ballooned, loculated appearance

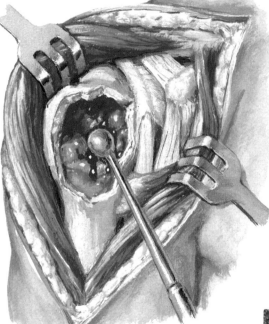

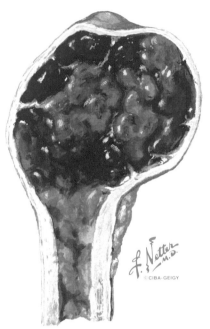

Specimen demonstrates ballooned shape, margin of reactive bone, and characteristic multiloculation. Pockets filled with clotted (cranberry-saucelike) blood

Curettage of cyst before reconstruction of cavity with trabecular bone graft

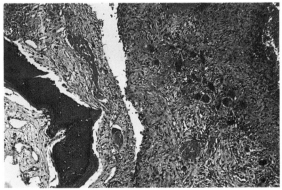

Section shows stroma of benign spindle cells, scattered giant cells, blood, and bone fragments (H and E stain)

The aneurysmal bone cyst is a tumorlike proliferation of vascular tissue that forms a lining around a blood-filled cystic lesion. Occurring most commonly in adolescents and young adults, it develops in the metaphyseal region of long bones, pelvis, or vertebral body, sometimes secondary to another benign or malignant bone lesion.

Diagnostic Studies. A radiolucent lesion with a ballooned expansion of the bone cortices is the radiographic hallmark of an aneurysmal bone cyst. Although some lesions appear to have an aggressive, expansile quality, they remain contained by a thin rim of reactive periosteal bone. In children, these benign lesions seldom penetrate the articular surface of a joint or the growth plate; therefore, evidence of growth plate penetration by an aneurysmal bone cyst indicates the need for careful staging studies to rule out malignancy. The radiographic differential diagnosis includes simple bone cyst (Plate 13), giant-cell tumor of bone (Plate 14), telangiectatic sarcoma, and angiosarcoma (Plate 28).

Bone scans show intense radioisotope uptake in the margin of the lesion, with normal background or diminished uptake in its center (in contrast to osteosarcoma or other high-grade malignant tumors in which the activity is intense throughout the lesion). Computed tomography and magnetic resonance imaging are used to depict the precise anatomic extent and density of the lesion, and especially the thin, limiting margin of reactive bone (which is not well visualized on plain radiographs). A fluid level seen on the CT scan confirms the diagnosis. Angiography, particularly in the late venous phase, reveals a highly neovascular periphery with very little vascularity in the central part. When the tumor occurs secondary to a *benign* lesion, its histologic characteristics are typical of the aneurysmal bone cyst; when it develops secondary to a *malignant* lesion, the histologic features of the underlying malignancy predominate.

Gross examination reveals a thin, distinctly bluish reactive shell overlying the vascular tissue. The proliferative lining tissue of an aneurysmal bone cyst is often difficult to distinguish from that of a giant-cell tumor of bone. It contains a mixture of benign stromal tissue, giant cells, and large amounts of hemosiderin. The tissue usually contains large vascular lacunae lined with giant cells and filled with clotted blood that resembles

cranberry sauce. Because of the preponderance of giant cells, many aneurysmal bone cysts are initially thought to be giant-cell tumors of bone, but a comparison of the distinguishing features of the two lesions usually establishes the diagnosis. When these histologic features also occur in other lesions (eg, chondroblastoma, osteoblastoma, osteosarcoma, eosinophilic granuloma, nonossifying fibroma), they are called secondary aneurysmal bone cysts.

Treatment and Prognosis. The majority of active aneurysmal bone cysts are treated with curettage and bone grafting; the recurrence rate, however, is 20% to 30%. Whenever possible, marginal or wide excision is preferable.

After incision of an active cyst, an alarming amount of bleeding may occur until the lining is completely removed. After complete excision of the cyst, there may be brisk bleeding emanating directly from the bony wall, which can be controlled with coagulation. Curettage may be augmented with cementation with methylmethacrylate, which appears to reduce the risk of recurrence. Aggressive stage 3 lesions have a higher risk of recurrence, particularly in the pelvis and spine where complete surgical exposure and removal are more difficult. Nevertheless, the prognosis for primary aneurysmal bone cyst is excellent, and recurrences can usually be managed with more aggressive curettage or excision. □

Benign Tumors of Bone

Simple Bone Cyst

The simple (unicameral) bone cyst is a membrane-lined cavity containing a clear yellow fluid. Occurring most often in children 4 to 10 years of age, the cysts have a predilection for the metaphysis of long bones, particularly the proximal humerus (50% of cases), proximal femur, and proximal tibia. The lesions remain asymptomatic unless complicated by fracture. They enlarge during skeletal growth and become inactive, or latent, after skeletal maturity.

Active cysts develop in patients under 10 years of age. Typically, the cyst abuts the growth plate and occupies most of the metaphysis; it is expansile with a thin cortical shell, continues to enlarge during observation, and is commonly associated with fracture. The cyst is considered active as it arises and grows adjacent to the growth plate. With growth, it is left behind and becomes increasingly separated from the growth plate and at this point is considered latent.

Latent cysts are seen in patients over 12 years of age. They are separated from the growth plate by 1 to 2 cm and have a thicker bony wall than active lesions. They remain static or diminish in size, show evidence of healing or ossification, and are less likely to result in fracture.

Diagnostic Studies. Radiographs show a central, well-marginated radiolucent defect in the metaphysis, with a symmetric appearance, usually without bony septations or loculations. The metaphysis is expanded, with marked cortical thinning that predisposes to fracture. After fracture, the eggshell-thin fragments are often displaced into the cystic cavity, thus creating the "falling-leaf" sign.

The radiographic differential diagnosis is usually limited to fibrous dysplasia (Plate 9) and aneurysmal bone cyst (Plate 12). In some cases, the even radiolucency of the cyst may be difficult to distinguish from the ground-glass density of fibrous dysplasia. However, monostotic fibrous dysplasia is usually eccentric rather than central and diaphyseal rather than metaphyseal; in addition, the periosteal reaction is greater in fibrous dysplasia than in a simple bone cyst. An aneurysmal bone cyst (and even telangiectatic sarcoma) may also appear as a large radiolucent lesion, making it difficult to distinguish from a simple cyst.

Staging studies are indicated only when radiographs are difficult to interpret. Bone scans show an increased radioisotope uptake around the margin of the cyst, in contrast to the uniform uptake in fibrous dysplasia. Computed tomography may assist in determining the density of the lesion. On angiography, there is no uptake of the contrast material in the cyst cavity itself and very little uptake in the peripheral soft tissue, whereas fibrous dysplasia lesions are vascular. The finding of straw-colored fluid on needle aspiration confirms the diagnosis of a simple cyst.

Manometry may be used to determine the stage of the bone cyst. With an internal pressure of 30 cm H₂O or more, the cyst is considered active. Radiopaque dye injected into an active

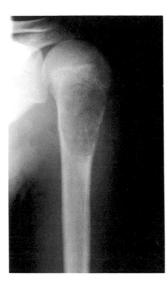

Radiograph shows radiolucent lesion in proximal humerus typical of simple bone cyst abutting growth plate

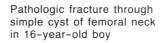

Pathologic fracture through simple cyst of femoral neck in 16-year-old boy

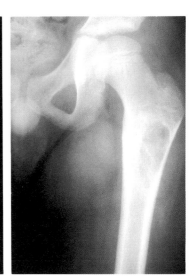

Same patient, 7 months later. Fracture healed, cystic cavity becoming obliterated following limb immobilization

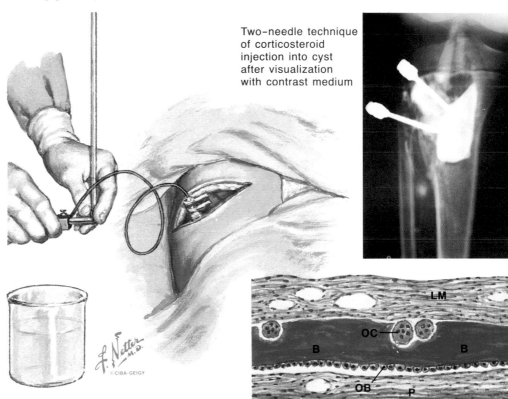

Two-needle technique of corticosteroid injection into cyst after visualization with contrast medium

Manometric measurement of intracystic pressure. In active cysts, pressure averages 30 cm H₂O and pulsates with heartbeat. In latent phase, pressure much lower with no pulsation. Note clear, yellowish fluid aspirated from cyst

High-power section through cyst wall. Beneath lining membrane (LM), osteoclasts (OC) have formed resorption cavities in bony margin (B). Rim of active osteoblasts (OB) has formed on bone subjacent to periosteum (P) (H and E stain)

cyst escapes into the venous system in a few minutes. A latent cyst contains a more viscous fluid and has lower, nonpulsatile pressures resembling venous pressures (6–12 cm H₂O). Communication with the venous system is poor, and the contrast medium clears more slowly.

Histologic examination of an active cyst reveals a mesothelial membrane lining a thin margin of reactive bone. The inner wall of the margin deep to the mesothelial membrane is often covered with a network of osteoclasts. Between the membrane and the osteoclastic activity is a layer of areolar tissue containing fibroblastic and multinucleated giant cells. Latent cysts have a thicker membrane with little

underlying osteoclastic activity, fewer giant cells, and more reactive bone.

Treatment and Prognosis. Simple cysts are treated with curettage and bone grafting; recurrence is high for active cysts (50%) and low for latent cysts (10%). Treatment with injection of corticosteroid is based on the theory that corticosteroids stabilize the mesothelial lining and induce healing of the cyst. Cyst fluid is aspirated with sterile percutaneous needle technique; then 80 to 200 mg of methylprednisolone acetate is infused into the cavity. In more than half of patients studied, the cyst healed following this technique, although multiple injections may have been required. □

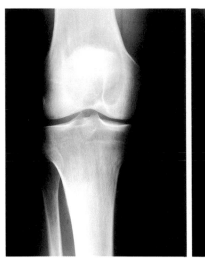

Anteroposterior radiograph shows giant-cell tumor of epiphysis and metaphysis of distal femur extending into but not penetrating subchondral plate

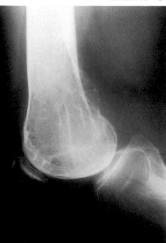

Lateral view reveals radiolucent lesion bulging posteriorly into popliteal fossa

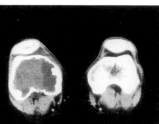

CT scan of right femur reveals marked endosteal erosion by intraosseous lesion

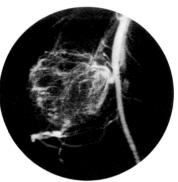

Angiogram demonstrates intense vascularity of tumor area

Pathologic fracture through giant-cell tumor of distal femur

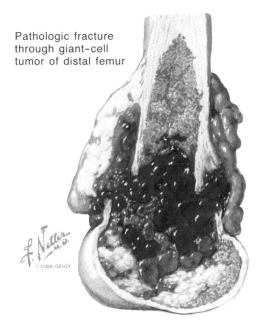

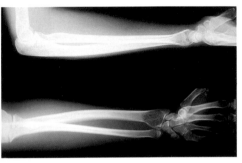

Giant-cell tumor of distal radius

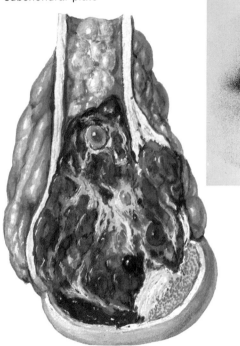

Bone scan demonstrates characteristic "doughnut sign" (also typical of aneurysmal bone cyst)

Sectioned distal femur shows meaty, hemorrhagic tissue with lighter, dense, fibrous areas, small cysts and blood clots, and thin margin of reactive bone with Codman's triangle. Tumor has infiltrated soft tissue

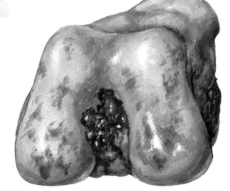

View of femoral condyles. Tumor apparent in spots through thin subchondral plate and articular cartilage; also in intercondylar notch covered by synovial membrane

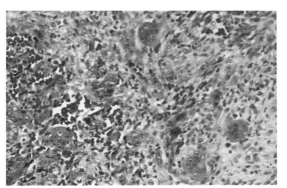

Section shows stroma of spindlelike cells with pale-staining cytoplasm and nuclei, many multinucleated giant cells, vascular channels, and free blood (H and E stain)

SECTION II PLATE 14   Slide 4561

Benign Tumors of Bone
Giant-Cell Tumor of Bone

Giant-cell tumor of bone (osteoclastoma) is a common benign but locally aggressive lesion of unknown histogenesis. It occurs chiefly in men between 20 and 40 years of age. The lesion is typically located in the epiphysis of the distal femur or proximal tibia. Other sites are the distal radius, proximal humerus, distal tibia, and sacrum. The tumor usually enlarges to occupy most of the epiphysis and adjacent metaphysis, penetrating and eroding the subchondral bone and even invading the articular cartilage. (When a tumor in the distal femur extends into the knee joint, however, it usually tracks through the origin of the cruciate ligaments rather than penetrating the cartilage.)

Patients report a deep, persistent intraosseous pain that mimics an internal derangement of the knee. A pathologic fracture or reactive knee effusion is the initial symptom in about one-third of patients; in a small number (<5%), the tumor undergoes benign pulmonary metastases.

Diagnostic Studies. Radiographs reveal a large radiolucent lesion surrounded by a distinct margin of reactive bone. Cortical thinning, endosteal erosion, and trabecularization, or bony septation, of the cavity are associated findings. Bone scans may show decreased radioisotope uptake in the center of the lesion ("doughnut sign"). Tomography distinguishes the irregular bony trabeculation, and CT scans disclose the extent of involvement and bony margination.

Angiography usually demonstrates the tumor's hypervascularity.

Gross examination reveals a soft, friable, reddish brown neoplastic tissue with the consistency of a wet sponge. Some areas are gelatinous or fatty, and some are aneurysmal and cavitated. Histologic features include a generous sprinkling of multinucleated giant cells, a proliferative stroma with vesiculated nuclei, areas of aneurysmal tissue, areas of necrosis, reactive peripheral bone, and occasional mitotic figures and intravascular tumor plugs in venous sinuses.

Treatment. The size and stage of the tumor determine the type of treatment. For stage 1 or 2 lesions, curettage is often combined with bone grafting or cementation. For recurrent or stage 3 lesions, en bloc excision with a wide margin and extensive reconstruction are required. A prior pathologic fracture should be allowed to heal before surgery is attempted. □

Osteosarcoma

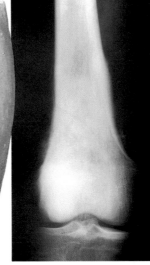

Anteroposterior radiograph (left) shows dense lesion and widened metaphysis of distal femur

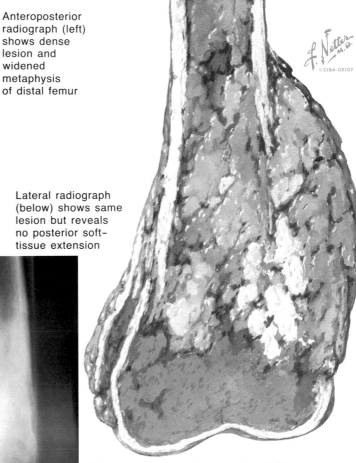

Lateral radiograph (below) shows same lesion but reveals no posterior soft-tissue extension

Mass on left distal femur palpable and tender but only slightly visible

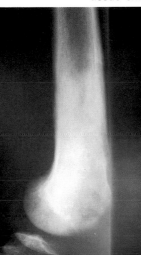

Tumor composed of bone and soft tissue occupies entire metaphysis of distal femur. Actual extension into soft tissue much greater than suggested by staging studies

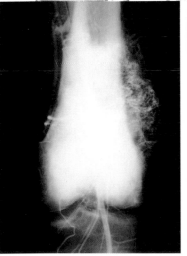

Anteroposterior angiogram demonstrates vascular blush of tumor extending laterally into soft tissue

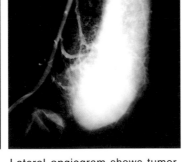

Lateral angiogram shows tumor extending posteriorly but not distorting femoral vessels

Bone scan shows intense radioisotope uptake over tumor area

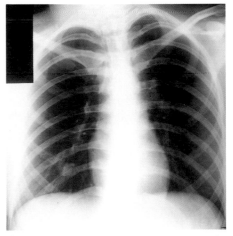

Chest radiograph shows early metastasis in hilus of right lung

SECTION II PLATE 15   Slide 4562

Malignant Tumors of Bone

Osteosarcoma

Classic Osteosarcoma

Classic osteosarcoma (osteogenic sarcoma) is a malignant tumor of bone in which neoplastic osteoid is produced by a proliferating, spindle-cell stroma. It is the most common primary malignant bone tumor of mesenchymal derivation (Plates 15–16). Most osteosarcomas are the classic type; the variant forms, which are distinguished by significant differences in radiographic and microscopic appearance and prognosis, include parosteal and periosteal osteosarcomas (Plate 17) and telangiectatic sarcoma.

Osteosarcoma usually develops in adolescents and affects males slightly more often than females. Although the lesion may occur throughout the skeleton, in 50% of patients, it occurs in the region of the knee (distal femur or proximal tibia). Other common sites are the proximal humerus, proximal femur, and pelvis. Most osteosarcomas originate in long bones in the regions of highest growth velocity, namely, in the metaphyses. The initial symptom is a tender,

bony mass. At the time of diagnosis, most osteosarcomas are stage IIB lesions that have infiltrated the soft tissue. The tumor penetrates the cortex earlier in the metaphyseal region because of the presence of numerous perforating vessels in the cortical wall. In 50% of adolescent patients, the tumor penetrates the growth plate into the epiphysis. "Skip" metastases (small tumor nodules in ostensibly uninvolved areas of the same bone) are found in about 25% of patients. Pulmonary or lymph node metastases are detected at presentation in about 10% of patients.

A significant percentage of osteosarcomas in adults occur in association with Paget's disease of bone (see CIBA COLLECTION, Volume 8/I,

Malignant Tumors of Bone

Osteosarcoma
(Continued)

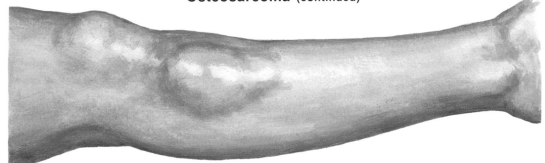

Osteosarcoma of proximal tibia presents as localized, tender prominence

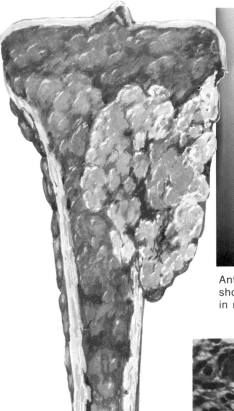

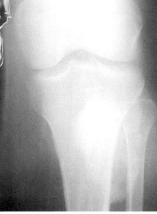

Anteroposterior radiograph shows eccentric, dense lesion in metaphysis of proximal tibia

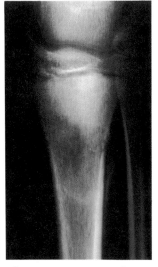

Osteosarcoma sometimes appears as radiolucent lesion

Sectioned proximal tibia. Tumor density fairly uniform with some areas of necrosis and hemorrhage. Neoplasm has penetrated cortex into surrounding soft tissue

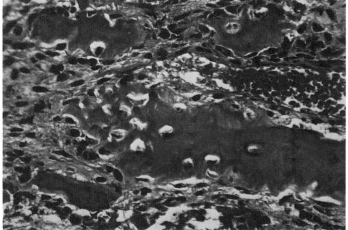

Masses of tumor cells with hyperchromatic nuclei interspersed with foci of malignant osteoid are typical histopathologic findings (H and E stain)

pages 236–238). Severe, unremitting pain and pathologic fracture are the primary clinical manifestations of sarcomatous transformation in Paget's disease. Staging studies are difficult to interpret because manifestations of the pagetic process overshadow the evolving neoplasm.

Diagnostic Studies. Radiographs characteristically demonstrate a permeative destructive lesion in which amorphous neoplastic bone can be detected. Typically, the lesion is predominantly dense, or osteoblastic, but may also have a mixed pattern or appear purely osteolytic. Other major characteristics include early cortical destruction, lack of containment by periosteal new-bone formation, and a poorly defined margin. The incompetent periosteal reaction may take the form of a triangular area of bone at the cortical margins produced by periosteal elevation and reaction (Codman's triangle). On radiographs, the amorphous, neoplastic bone produces a pathognomonic "sunburst" pattern: spicules of neoplastic bone arising perpendicular to the long axis of the limb, unlike the parallel, or "onion-skin," arrangement seen in reactive bone.

Tumors treated with adjuvant chemotherapy often become heavily ossified, and the extent of soft-tissue involvement is clearly visible on radiographs.

In most cases, the radiographic differential diagnosis involves only Ewing's sarcoma (Plate 20); less often, osteosarcoma resembles osteomyelitis or aggressive osteoblastoma (Plate 4).

Results of staging studies reflect the tumor's aggressive nature. Bone scans show intense radioisotope uptake and reveal more widespread involvement than is apparent on radiographs, reflecting the subtle, infiltrative extensions characteristic of high-grade sarcomas. Computed tomography and magnetic resonance imaging provide more detailed information about intraos-

seous involvement and relationship to fascial septa and major muscles; CT scans are also needed to detect radiographically occult pulmonary metastases. Angiography or computed tomography with contrast medium is useful in documenting the tumor's location with respect to the major vessels, its neovascularity, and the extent of soft-tissue involvement.

Staging studies are essential not only to confirm the diagnosis and document the extent of infiltration into the soft tissue, but also to monitor the response to chemotherapy and plan the surgical approach.

Osteosarcomas vary widely in appearance, from hard, white tissue in a heavily mineralized lesion

to a cavitated tumor filled with necrotic and aneurysmal tissue. The microscopic appearance is characterized by a malignant stroma producing amorphous, immature osteoid of trabecular bone. The areas of osteoid may be thin and streamy or they may be large, broad seams. It may be difficult to distinguish nonneoplastic, reactive osteoid from immature neoplastic osteoid, especially if the tissue samples are small.

Treatment and Prognosis. The success of preoperative adjuvant chemotherapy has substantially increased the proportion of lesions that are amenable to wide limb-salvaging excision and significantly improved the prognosis for patients with osteosarcoma.

Malignant Tumors of Bone

Osteosarcoma

(Continued)

Parosteal Osteosarcoma

Parosteal (juxtacortical) osteosarcoma arises between the cortex and muscle as a low-grade stage IA surface tumor, most commonly in adolescents and young adults (Plate 17). It usually presents as a fixed, painless mass on the posterior aspect of the distal femur (50% of cases), the medial aspect of the proximal humerus, or other sites. Parosteal osteosarcoma is distinguished from classic osteosarcoma by its much slower, less aggressive clinical course. The tumor remains separated from the normal bone, especially in the early stage; extension into the underlying bone is associated with a higher incidence of dedifferentiation and pulmonary metastases.

Diagnostic Studies. Radiographs show a dense, heavily ossified, broad-based fusiform mass that appears to encircle the metaphysis. Typically, the tumor is separated from the cortex by a thin, uninvolved, radiolucent zone. Satellite nodules of tumor that are distinctly separate from the main mass are often seen in the peripheral margin. As growth continues, the radiolucent zone between the mass and the underlying bone may be partially or completely obliterated as the cortex becomes involved. Invasion into the overlying displaced soft tissues is rare. Late in the disease, the tumor extends through the underlying cortex to invade the medullary canal as well, converting to a stage IB tumor; about 10% of these tumors exhibit areas of dedifferentiation into high-grade sarcoma and are thus considered stage IIB lesions.

Differential diagnosis includes osteocartilaginous exostosis (Plate 7), myositis ossificans (see Section I, Plate 21), and periosteal chondroma (Plate 6), all of which occur in adolescents.

Histologic features are mature trabeculae with a peculiar pattern of cement lines similar to that seen in Paget's disease of bone. Enmeshed in a low-grade stroma, the trabeculae often contain varying degrees of cartilage that is not obviously malignant. Because of these bland overall features, this tumor is frequently underdiagnosed as benign, leading to inadequate intracapsular or marginal excision and recurrence.

Treatment and Prognosis. Treatment of the parosteal osteosarcoma is wide excision that can usually be accomplished with a limb-salvaging procedure. Unless dedifferentiation (favored by repeated recurrence or prolonged neglect) occurs, the prognosis is good and chemotherapy is not indicated.

Periosteal Osteosarcoma

This uncommon variant of classic osteosarcoma primarily affects young adults, presenting as an enlarging, often painless mass that grows on the external surface of the bone.

Parosteal Osteosarcoma

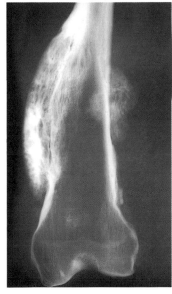

Anteroposterior radiograph shows densely ossified prominence on anterolateral aspect of distal femur. Satellite lesion on opposite side characterizes mass as parosteal osteosarcoma rather than osteoma or osteocartilaginous exostosis

Sectioned femur. Longitudinal tumor has invaded cortex but not medullary canal. Satellite lesion still separated from cortex by cleft; in early stage, primary tumor also separated from cortex by uninvolved zone

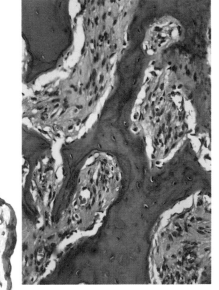

Section shows relatively bland stroma with mature trabecular pattern but without mitoses. Minimal osteoblastic rim on trabeculae helps rule out myositis ossificans or reactive bone (H and E stain)

Periosteal Osteosarcoma

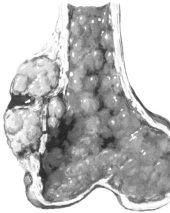

Erosive cartilaginous lesion in periosteum of distal femoral metaphysis. Codman's triangles of reactive bone at margins

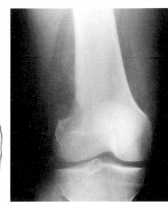

Radiograph reveals craterlike lesion with margin of reactive bone and faint calcification

Highly malignant stroma with cartilaginous and osteoid components (H and E stain)

Diagnostic Studies. Radiographs show a largely external, poorly mineralized mass in a craterlike area of cortical erosion with an irregular margin and periosteal reaction. Extension through the cortex into the bone occurs earlier than in the parosteal variant; when this happens, the incidence of pulmonary metastases is higher and the prognosis worse. The radiographic differential diagnosis includes classic osteosarcoma (Plates 15–16), periosteal chondroma (Plate 6), and juxtacortical chondrosarcoma (Plate 18).

Bone scans show a disproportionate increase in radioisotope uptake throughout the tumor, considering its predominantly radiolucent appearance. Computed tomography depicts a tumor sitting in a shallow cortical defect with only moderate calcification.

On gross examination, the tumor appears to be composed primarily of cartilage; microscopic examination, however, reveals areas of frankly malignant mesenchymal stroma containing neoplastic osteoid scattered in and about the lobules of low-grade mature cartilage.

Treatment and Prognosis. Because of its intermediate aggressiveness and accessible location, the lesion is almost always amenable to excision with a wide margin. Adjuvant systemic chemotherapy is indicated only for higher grade, dedifferentiated tumors. Prognosis for patients with periosteal osteosarcoma is fair. □

Chondrosarcoma

Massive chondrosarcoma of iliac crest

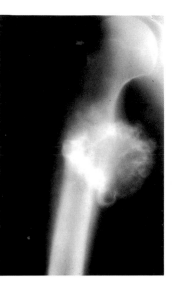

Chondrosarcoma of femur near lesser trochanter. Density characteristic of cartilaginous tumors

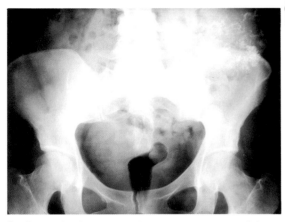

Radiograph of above patient reveals tumor arising in and destroying iliac crest

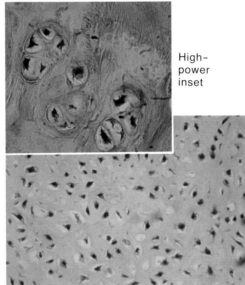

Sectioned tumor shows tough cartilaginous tissue eroding iliac crest

High-power inset

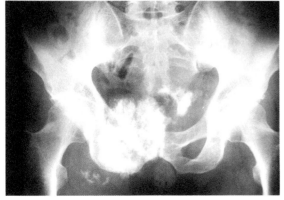

Radiograph of different patient with large chondrosarcoma in region of obturator foramen. Note mottled calcification

Ratio of cells to cartilaginous matrix, amount of cellular atypia and mitoses, and occurrence of multiple nuclei in lacunae vary with degree of malignancy (H and E stain)

Specimen shows tumor has eroded femoral cortex and invaded surrounding cortex

Malignant Tumors of Bone

Chondrosarcoma

Chondrosarcoma is a malignant cartilaginous tumor of bone. Primary chondrosarcoma occurs most often in men between 30 and 50 years of age and tends to affect the pelvis, proximal femur, and shoulder girdle. A persistent, dull, aching pain, like that of arthritis, is the initial manifestation. In about 25% of cases, it is a secondary malignant transformation of a preexisting enchondroma or osteocartilaginous exostosis. Variants of classic chondrosarcoma are dedifferentiated (high grade), clear cell (intermediate grade), or juxtacortical (low grade), based on the histogenic pattern and location.

Diagnostic Studies. Radiographs reveal a subtle, radiolucent, permeative lesion with hazy or speckled calcifications that may be in a diffuse "salt-and-pepper" or more discrete "popcorn" pattern; this appearance is quite different from the "smoke-ring" pattern of benign enchondroma. Primary chondrosarcoma may arise centrally in the medullary canal or peripherally on the external surface of the bone, causing cortical destruction in association with a protruding cartilaginous mass. The pattern of calcification is usually pathognomonic of a cartilaginous process, but the radiographic differential diagnosis must rule out other cartilaginous lesions.

In the diagnosis of classic chondrosarcoma, bone scans are used to evaluate tumor activity, and CT scans are used to assess its exact location and the extent of cortical involvement. Arthrography may be combined with computed tomography if radiographs or tomograms do not clearly show whether the lesion is intraarticular or juxtaarticular.

Histologic examination shows that the degree of cellular activity is reflected by the cell-to-matrix ratio, amount of hyperchromatism of the

Malignant Tumors of Bone

Chondrosarcoma

(Continued)

nuclei, and number of binucleated cells. Wide nuclear variation (pleomorphism), chromatin clumping, and double and triple nuclei are other features of atypia and signs of malignancy. Occasionally, alternating fields of dedifferentiated malignant mesenchymal stroma are present, indicating a more malignant stage II tumor. High-grade cartilaginous lesions frequently have a soft, viscous, jellylike consistency, while low-grade lesions have a firmer consistency with abundant calcification and distinct cauliflowerlike nodules of mature cartilage. While high-grade lesions are poorly differentiated and often difficult to identify as cartilaginous, low-grade lesions are well differentiated but sometimes difficult to distinguish as malignant.

Treatment and Prognosis. Low-grade tumors rarely metastasize or recur locally after wide limb-salvaging excision, in contrast to high-grade tumors, which have a higher rate of recurrence after limb salvage, often require amputation, and are prone to pulmonary metastases. Neither chemotherapy nor radiation therapy is effective. □

Malignant Tumors of Bone

Fibrous Histiocytoma and Fibrosarcoma of Bone

Fibrous Histiocytoma

Malignant fibrous histiocytoma and fibrosarcoma occur less often in bone than in soft tissue and are less common than their benign counterparts, nonossifying fibroma, ossifying fibroma, and desmoplastic fibroma in bone. Before 1970, malignant fibrous histiocytoma and fibrosarcoma of bone were both considered intraosseous fibrosarcomas. At present, they are considered discrete entities, based on histologic appearance and age at onset. Malignant fibrous histiocytoma occurs in older patients than does fibrosarcoma and tends to arise out of Paget's disease of bone or a bone infarct. The tumor has a high rate of metastasis, especially to regional lymph nodes. It usually presents as an aggressive stage IIB sarcoma; quite frequently, a pathologic fracture is the first clinical manifestation.

Malignant Fibrous Histiocytoma of Bone

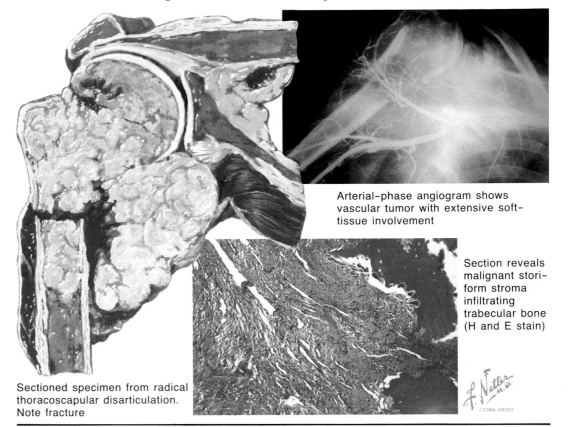

Arterial-phase angiogram shows vascular tumor with extensive soft-tissue involvement

Section reveals malignant storiform stroma infiltrating trabecular bone (H and E stain)

Sectioned specimen from radical thoracoscapular disarticulation. Note fracture

Fibrosarcoma of Bone

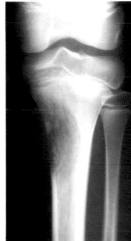

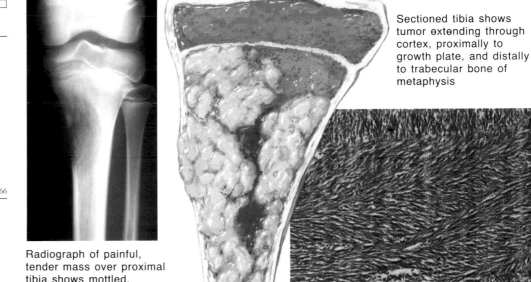

Sectioned tibia shows tumor extending through cortex, proximally to growth plate, and distally to trabecular bone of metaphysis

Radiograph of painful, tender mass over proximal tibia shows mottled, radiolucent, poorly defined lesion with penetration of reactive bone, indicative of malignant sarcoma but not specific for type

Section shows malignant spindle cells and collagen fibers in herringbone pattern with marked nuclear atypia, characteristic of fibrosarcoma (H and E stain)

Diagnostic Studies. Radiographs show a destructive, radiolucent lesion with cortical erosion and a poorly defined, permeative margin. Extensive bony infiltration by the tumor occurs early in the course of the disease. When associated with a radiodense bone infarct, malignant fibrous histiocytoma may be misinterpreted as a sarcomatous transformation of enchondroma. Staging studies are used to define the extent of extraosseous involvement, and special attention should be directed to ruling out metastases to the regional lymph nodes.

The histologic pattern of malignant fibrous histiocytoma of bone resembles that of a poorly differentiated fibrous tumor. The tumor consists of histiocytic cells that secrete collagen lacking the herringbone pattern of fibrosarcoma; these cells are called facultative fibroblasts. The appearance varies from reddish purple, friable neoplastic tissue to yellowish tan histiocytic tissue. The neoplastic areas are composed of large, bizarre, foamy histiocytes; large "supermalignant" giant cells; and a loose storiform stroma of spindle cells. In addition, variable areas of necrosis, mitoses, and grossly abnormal histiocytes are present. Some undifferentiated areas may resemble histiocytic lymphoma; the fibrous areas may suggest fibrosarcoma. A definitive diagnosis may require confirmation with special staining techniques and electron microscopy.

Malignant Tumors of Bone

Fibrous Histiocytoma and Fibrosarcoma of Bone

(Continued)

Treatment and Prognosis. An intraosseous stage IIB malignant fibrous histiocytoma requires excision with a radical margin. If this is not feasible, wide or marginal excision with adjuvant chemotherapy is required, which is often ineffective. The overall prognosis is guarded.

Fibrosarcoma of Bone

Fibrosarcoma of bone occurs most commonly in adolescents or young adults. It usually develops in the major long bones, presenting as a painful, tender mass.

Diagnostic Studies. Radiographs reveal a poorly defined, destructive, radiolucent lesion of the metaphyseal region. Preoperative staging studies are important to differentiate low-grade stage I fibrosarcomas from high-grade stage II lesions. Stage I tumors usually remain within the bone and have a distinct, well-defined margin. High-grade tumors are poorly marginated and produce a permeative, or "moth-eaten," radiographic pattern of bone destruction.

The histologic appearance of fibrosarcoma of bone varies according to the degree of the lesion's aggressiveness. Stage I lesions have less pleomorphism or anaplasia and closely resemble an aggressive, benign desmoplastic fibroma (Plate 10). In stage II tumors, the collagen component is less dominant than in low-grade tumors, and cellularity and atypia are correspondingly greater. Poorly differentiated lesions may require electron microscopic studies to confirm the histogenesis.

Treatment and Prognosis. Limb-salvaging excision with a wide margin suffices for stage IA tumors, whereas stage IIB fibrosarcomas require radical or wide margins with adjuvant chemotherapy or radiation therapy. The prognosis for patients with stage II fibrosarcoma is guarded. □

Malignant Tumors of Bone

Reticuloendothelial Tumors

Ewing's Sarcoma

Ewing's sarcoma is a highly malignant bone tumor derived from the nonmesenchymal elements of the bone marrow. It represents approximately 7% of all primary bone malignancies, is the fourth most common malignancy of bone, and occurs more frequently than osteosarcoma. Onset is primarily between the ages of 10 and 15. Ewing's sarcoma is more common in males than in females and is rare in blacks. It almost always presents as a stage IIB lesion. The primary symptom is an enlarging, tender, bony prominence with an associated large, soft-tissue mass accompanied by constitutional symptoms (fever, malaise, weight loss, lethargy); anemia; leukocytosis; and an elevated erythrocyte sedi-

mentation rate. The most common site, is the femoral diaphysis, followed by the ilium, tibia, humerus, fibula, and ribs. The lesion also has a peculiar predilection for the shaft of the fibula—an area containing little or no hematopoietic marrow. Tumors in the pelvis are typically detected later and are therefore larger, with a poorer prognosis.

Diagnostic Studies. Radiographs show a permeative diaphyseal tumor with a mottled, or patchy, density that indicates the tumor's destructive nature. Cortical involvement frequently produces a reactive, "onionskin" appearance of the periosteum, a pattern of layered ossification that, when associated with an underlying malignant tumor, strongly suggests the diagnosis. The differential diagnosis includes osteomyelitis, osteolytic osteosarcoma (Plate 15), and eosinophilic granuloma (Plate 11).

Bone scans demonstrate intense radioisotope uptake well beyond the limits seen on radiographs and often reveal multiple skeletal lesions. The hypervascularity of the tumor and associated soft-tissue mass are apparent on angiograms, and

computed tomography and magnetic resonance imaging are used to determine its local extent and involvement of the soft tissue.

Histologic features are small, round, neoplastic cells with large, hyperchromatic nuclei and a vague, indistinct cytoplasm and cytoplasmic membrane. These small cells are usually spread out in thick sheets. Mitoses are common, and pseudorosette patterns are typical. The diagnosis is supported by a positive periodic acid Schiff (PAS) stain for glycogen and confirmed by electron microscopy.

Treatment and Prognosis. Management of Ewing's sarcoma has changed significantly since the effectiveness of various combinations of chemotherapy, radiation therapy, and resection has been demonstrated. Pulmonary metastases have been reduced, and patient survival has improved.

Wide surgical excision is preferred over radiation therapy for local control if (1) the involved bone is expendable (eg, fibula, rib, clavicle), (2) radiation treatment would cause significant growth deformity (eg, in young children with growth plate involvement), (3) there is little hope

Ewing's Sarcoma

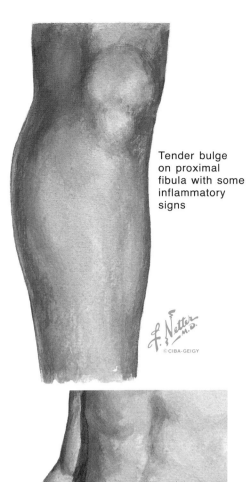

Tender bulge on proximal fibula with some inflammatory signs

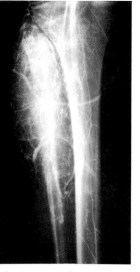

Radiograph reveals mottled, destructive, radiolucent lesion

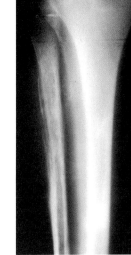

Angiogram shows vascular blush extending into soft tissue

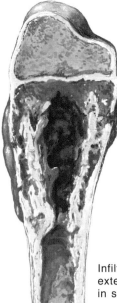

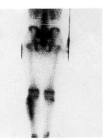

Bone scan shows heavy radioisotope uptake in tumor area. Other hot spots related to normal bone growth

Infiltrative, destructive tumor extending into soft tissue seen in sectioned proximal fibula

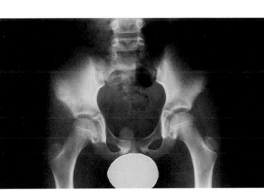

Lesion of mottled density involves anterior superior iliac spine

Sectioned femur shows highly vascular intraosseous and soft-tissue tumor components with much reactive bone

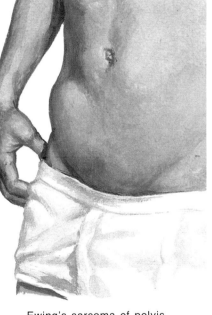

Ewing's sarcoma of pelvis. Scarcely visible but palpable mass in right lower quadrant

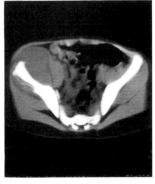

CT scan defines mass filling right iliac fossa

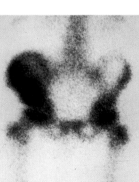

Bone scan shows heavy radioisotope uptake in right iliac wing

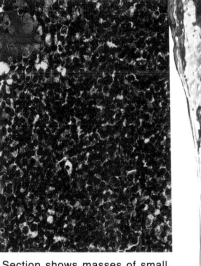

Section shows masses of small, round cells with uniformly sized hyperchromatic nuclei (H and E stain)

SECTION II PLATE 20   Slide 4567

Malignant Tumors of Bone

Reticuloendothelial Tumors
(Continued)

for successful rehabilitation (eg, tumors complicated by ununited pathologic fracture), and (4) previous local irradiation was unsuccessful.

Myeloma

Myeloma is a malignant tumor of plasma cells. It is the most common malignant primary tumor of bone and usually develops in middle age. Myeloma may arise as a single intraosseous tumor (solitary plasmacytoma), but more often it develops as multiple painful lesions throughout the skeleton (multiple myeloma). Associated findings are constitutional symptoms, anemia, thrombocytopenia, and renal failure.

Diagnostic Studies. The results of most staging studies are the same as for other malignant primary tumors. On bone scans, however, myelomas often appear cold. Laboratory findings include anemia, elevated erythrocyte sedimentation rate, hyperuricemia, and hypercalcemia. A homogeneous elevation in gamma-A or gamma-B globulins (paraproteins) on serum immunoelec-

trophoresis and also the presence of Bence Jones proteins in the urine and serum are frequently diagnostic.

Histologic features include aggregates of immature plasma cells with little intervening stroma but with impressive areas of central necrosis. The neoplastic plasma cells are hyperchromatic, and the clumps of chromatin give the cell a "clock-face" or "spoke-wheel" appearance. The round, distinct nucleus is eccentric and has a prominent nucleolus and abundant binucleated plasmacysts.

Treatment and Prognosis. Myeloma is very sensitive to radiation therapy, and reossification of the tumors often occurs within several months.

Myeloma

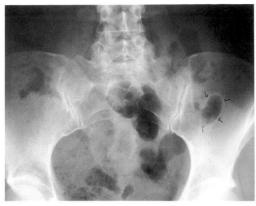

Radiograph of pelvis shows characteristic oval lytic lesion in left ilium

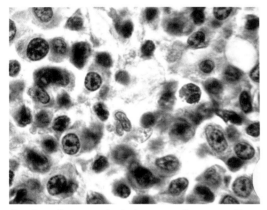

Section shows typical plasma–cell composition of myeloma (H and E stain)

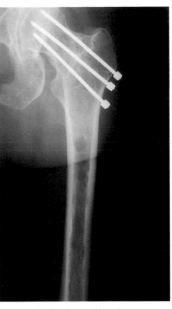

Multiple lesions distal to pathologic fracture of femoral neck (pinned)

Solitary myeloma of tibia with typical reddish gray, crumbling, soft, neoplastic tissue replacing cortices and marrow spaces but, in this case, with no invasion of soft tissue

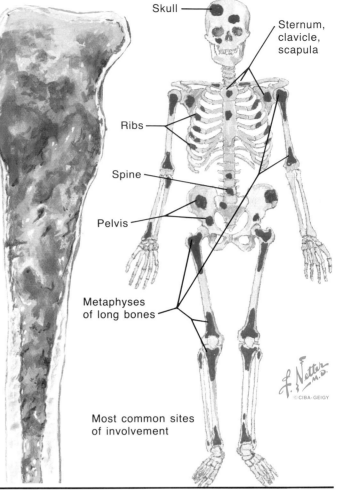

Skull

Sternum, clavicle, scapula

Ribs

Spine

Pelvis

Metaphyses of long bones

Most common sites of involvement

Reticulum-Cell Sarcoma

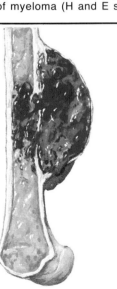

Hypervascular, friable tumor with thin capsule penetrating femoral cortex into soft tissue

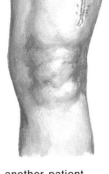

In another patient, mass in thigh disappeared completely after radiation therapy. Note biopsy scar

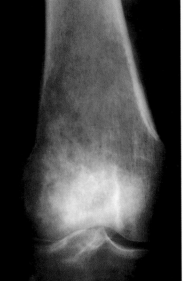

Radiograph reveals diffuse permeation of bone and destruction of distal femur

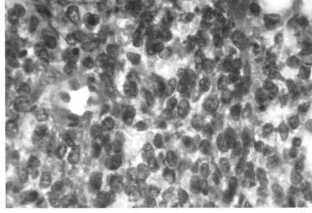

Section shows bizarre tumor cells of various sizes, including many histiocytes (H and E stain)

Malignant Tumors of Bone

Reticuloendothelial Tumors

(Continued)

Large tumors or involvement of high-stress areas necessitate surgical stabilization for fracture prophylaxis (Plate 31). When the disease is disseminated, chemotherapy is indicated but prognosis is guarded, and a 5-year survival remains under 30%.

Reticulum-Cell Sarcoma

Reticulum-cell sarcoma is a primary bone tumor derived from the reticuloendothelial elements of the marrow. It usually develops in middle age, causing localized bone pain with tenderness and effusion in neighboring joints.

Diagnostic Studies. Radiographs show a poorly defined, permeative, osteolytic tumor with minimal periosteal reaction. The lesion begins centrally, permeates rapidly through the cortices, and produces large soft-tissue masses. Differential diagnosis must rule out osteomyelitis, metastatic carcinoma (Plate 23), Ewing's sarcoma (Plate 20), malignant fibrous histiocytoma,

and fibrosarcoma of bone (Plate 19). Reticulum-cell sarcoma is staged differently from sarcomas of mesenchymal origin: stage I, involvement of single lymph node, extralymphatic organ, or bone; stage II, two or more sites, above or below the diaphragm; stage III, involvement on both sides of the diaphragm; and stage IV, diffuse involvement.

Characteristic histologic features are large, foam-filled histiocytes with numerous mitoses and scant stroma. Reticulum stains are positive; periodic acid Schiff (PAS) stains are negative.

Treatment and Prognosis. Stage I tumors are treated with radiation therapy alone; chemotherapy is added for more advanced tumors. □

Malignant Tumors of Bone

Adamantinoma and Giant-Cell Sarcoma

Adamantinoma

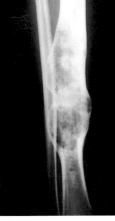

Firm, slowly growing mass. Anterior aspect of tibia most common site

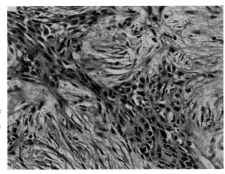

Radiograph shows craterlike radiolucent lesion with "soap-bubble" appearance and margins of reactive bone

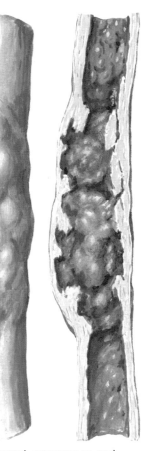

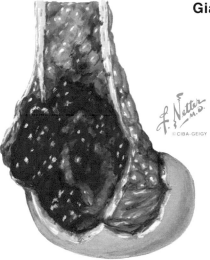

Section shows nests of squamous epitheliallike cells separated by areas of spindle cells (H and E stain)

External appearance and section of excised segment of tibia

Giant-Cell Sarcoma

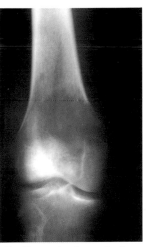

Hemorrhagic metaphyseal–epiphyseal lesion of distal femur penetrating cortex

Radiograph shows lesion with soft-tissue density and permeative margin

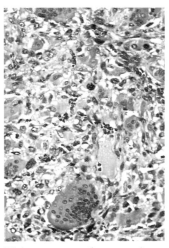

High-power section reveals typical giant cells with multiple mitotic figures (H and E stain)

Adamantinoma

A rare tumor of unknown origin, adamantinoma occurs primarily in young males between 10 and 30 years of age. The mandible or tibia is involved in 90% of patients, but occasionally the tumor develops in the forearm, other long bones, hands, and feet. The clinical manifestation is a firm, slowly enlarging mass that produces minimal disability.

Diagnostic Studies. The radiographic appearance consists of multiple small, oval, radiolucent cortical defects with a distinct margin of reactive bone and a thickened cortex. Adamantinoma typically has a "soap-bubble" appearance with distinct multiloculated lesions that bulge the cortex into the soft tissue. The differential diagnosis includes chondromyxoid fibroma (Plate 8), ossifying fibroma, and monostotic fibrous dysplasia (Plate 9).

Staging studies are indicative of a low-grade stage IA tumor. Tomography may be used to help delineate the cortical radiolucencies, but definitive information about extension along the medullary canal or into adjacent soft tissue is obtained by computed tomography or magnetic resonance imaging.

Histologic examination reveals a classic pseudoglandular appearance that may suggest rounded islands of glandular tissue with a cordlike or "boxcar" arrangement of layers of cells around a slitlike space. These patterns of cuboidal epithelioid cells are intertwined with a dense stroma of fibrous tissue.

Treatment and Prognosis. The treatment of choice is wide excision, usually with a segmental resection of the tibia that can be reconstructed with autograft or allograft bone. More conservative treatment (curettage or marginal excision) is associated with repeated recurrences, which ultimately require amputation, and occasionally with pulmonary metastases. With adequate local control, the prognosis is good.

Giant-Cell Sarcoma

Giant-cell sarcoma is the high-grade malignant counterpart of benign giant-cell tumor of bone. In most cases, the tumor arises as a sarcoma rather than as the transformation of a preexisting benign lesion. Like the benign tumor, giant-cell sarcoma primarily affects young adults.

Diagnostic Studies. The tumor's aggressive nature is apparent on radiographic and histologic examinations. The findings on staging studies are consistent with any high-grade stage IIB tumor, and the diagnosis is suggested only by the epiphyseal location of the tumor. The histologic pattern is dominated by a frankly malignant stroma with many mitotic figures and large, bizarre, multinucleated giant cells with necrosis.

Treatment and Prognosis. Like all stage II lesions, giant-cell sarcoma requires excision with a wide margin. After curettage, recurrence is inevitable, and the incidence of pulmonary metastases, already high, is probably even higher if the tumor has been mistakenly diagnosed as a benign giant-cell tumor of bone and treated with curettage. In this case, the effectiveness of adjuvant radiation therapy or chemotherapy has not been demonstrated, and amputation or radical resection after the curettage is appropriate. □

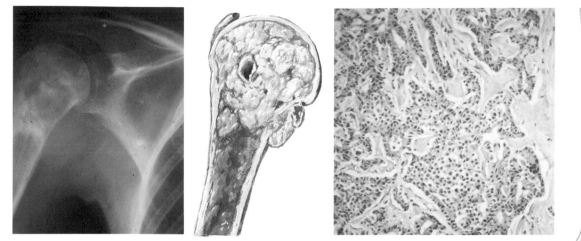

From breast. Tumor of proximal humerus appeared 3 years after mastectomy for carcinoma. Pathology typical of adenocarcinoma of breast (H and E stain)

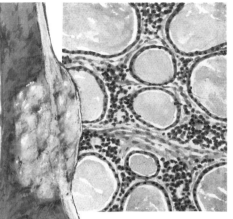

From thyroid gland. Tumor of distal femur was radiolucent on radiograph. Biopsy findings of colloid-containing follicles typical of thyroid carcinoma (H and E stain)

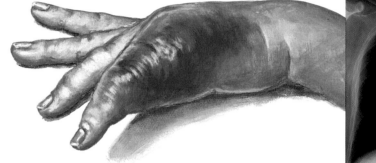

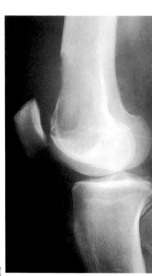

From lung. Initial symptom was painful, erythematous swelling of 5th ray of hand. Chest radiograph showed hilar densities that proved to be source of this unusual metastasis

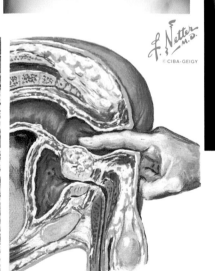

From kidney. Initial symptom was painful mass above knee. Radiograph revealed lytic lesion of femur. Biopsy results indicated adenocarcinoma of kidney, which was confirmed by renal arteriogram and intravenous pyelogram (section below stained with H and E)

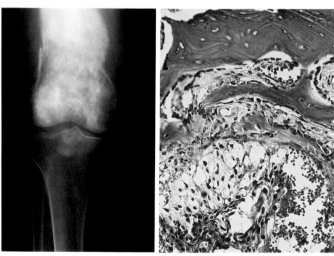

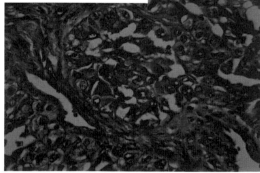

From prostate gland. Fracture of femur was initial manifestation. Radiograph revealed destructive lesion suggestive of osteosarcoma, but histologic findings indicated adenocarcinoma. Elevated acid phosphatase level and results of digital rectal examination confirmed origin (H and E stain)

SECTION II PLATE 23   Slide 4570

Malignant Tumors of Bone

Tumors Metastatic to Bone

Metastatic tumors of the skeleton outnumber primary tumors by 25 to 1. The vast majority occur secondary to carcinoma of the prostate, breast, thyroid, lung, or kidney. The most common sites of involvement are bones containing hematopoietic marrow (eg, the spine, ribs, skull, pelvis, metaphyses of the femur and humerus). The rare metastases to the bones of the hands or feet suggest arterial seeding from a primary lung carcinoma. In children, metastatic skeletal tumors are usually secondary to neuroblastoma, leukemia, or Ewing's sarcoma; in teenagers or young adults, they are generally secondary to lymphoma. Metastasis after age 30 is usually secondary to carcinoma.

Purely osteolytic metastases generally stem from a primary tumor of the lung, kidney, thyroid, or gastrointestinal tract. Metastatic tumors from kidney or thyroid carcinoma are usually hypervascular, and their angiographic appearance may strongly resemble that of an aneurysm. Osteoblastic metastases are most often seen with prostate or breast carcinoma. In many patients, the primary tumor cannot be detected, and staging studies and biopsy are required. In patients with a history of carcinoma, the presence of a solitary tumor necessitates a search for other sites of skeletal involvement. If there is no history of carcinoma, staging studies are warranted before a needle biopsy is done to assess the potential for curative treatment. For multiple metastatic lesions, chemotherapy, hormonal manipulation, and palliative radiation therapy are the therapeutic options. Prognosis for patients with skeletal metastases is poor. □

Benign Tumors of Soft Tissue

Fibroma, Fibromatosis, and Hemangioma

Fibroma

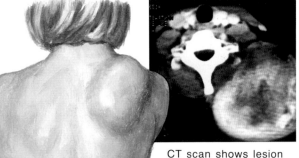

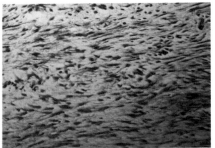

CT scan shows lesion posterolateral to vertebral column

Section shows irregular bands of collagenous fibrous tissue (H and E stain)

Massive fibroma of right suprascapular region

Sectioned fibroma composed of dense, firm, whitish tissue

Plantar fibroma

Fibromatosis

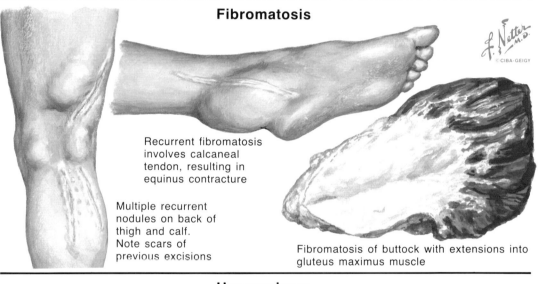

Recurrent fibromatosis involves calcaneal tendon, resulting in equinus contracture

Multiple recurrent nodules on back of thigh and calf. Note scars of previous excisions

Fibromatosis of buttock with extensions into gluteus maximus muscle

Hemangioma

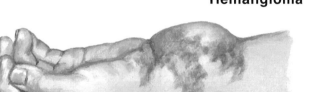

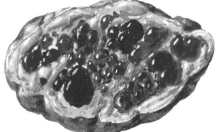

Hemangioma in wrist of young child

Sectioned hemangioma

Fibroma

A fibroma is a solitary, benign fibrous tumor of soft tissue. It may occur at any age, first appearing as an asymptomatic but slowly enlarging soft-tissue mass, usually adjacent to fibrous or fascial structures and frequently in extracompartmental soft tissues. The palmar and plantar aspects of the hands and feet are common sites of involvement. Although originating as an active stage 2 tumor, fibroma is often not detected until it has become inactive, or latent (stage 1).

Diagnostic Studies. On radiographs, tumor margins are sometimes difficult to distinguish from the normal fascial structures. Gross examination reveals a firm, well-encapsulated tumor composed of whitish nodules entangled in masses of fibrous tissue. Vascularity is normal. Older, latent lesions frequently have degenerated necrotic centers. Treatment of fibroma is by marginal excision.

Fibromatosis

The term "fibromatosis" refers to multiple fibrous tumors that, although benign, are significantly more aggressive than solitary fibroma. These lesions often develop in the proximal limbs or the trunk and are also called abdominal and extraabdominal desmoid tumors, depending on whether or not they involve the abdominal wall. Although generally superficial, the tumors are locally invasive, frequently involving adjacent neurovascular structures.

Diagnostic Studies. Staging studies are required for fibromatosis because of the lesions' aggressive behavior and the need to exclude low-grade malignancy. Although the lesions usually develop adjacent to or even adherent to bone, bone scans are often deceptively cold. Angiography shows very little associated neovascularity; on computed tomography, tumor margins are poorly demonstrated because the lesion infiltrates the surrounding fascial or fibrous structures. Histologic examination reveals scattered mature fibrocytes enmeshed in heavy strands of mature collagen.

Treatment and Prognosis. Because the extent of involvement and the aggressiveness of fibromatosis are often underestimated, the surgical margins achieved may be inadequate. Unless the tumors are excised with a wide margin, recurrence is likely. Recurrences are difficult to distinguish from the scarring of previous excisions, thus making subsequent excision even more hazardous. Adjuvant radiation therapy reduces the recurrence rate after marginal or even after intracapsular excision.

Hemangioma

Hemangioma of soft tissue is a benign, vascular tumor that occurs in children, usually in the limbs or the trunk. Sometimes, hemangioma is congenital, appearing as a solitary tumor that infiltrates local tissue and, like fibromatosis, may involve adjacent neurovascular structures. Capillary (small-vessel) hemangiomas are noninvasive and usually smaller and more cellular than cavernous hemangiomas, which are invasive and frequently contain calcifications or phleboliths that are readily seen on radiographs. The most common form is a tumor with infiltrative margins composed of both large and small vessels.

Diagnostic Studies. The most efficient test for demonstrating the cavernous spaces of hemangioma is venography. Magnetic resonance imaging is superior to computed tomography for distinguishing the lesion from surrounding normal tissue. Hemangiomas may infiltrate the adjacent bone and produce areas of osteoporosis, but the bone scans show little or no increase in radioisotope uptake in these areas.

Treatment and Prognosis. Aggressive stage 3 mixed tumors require en bloc wide marginal excision; excision with a smaller margin is associated with a recurrence rate of 30%. Despite their vascular origin, hemangiomas do not metastasize or undergo malignant transformation. □

Benign Tumors of Soft Tissue

Lipoma, Neurofibroma, and Myositis Ossificans

Lipoma

Lipoma, the most common tumor of soft tissue, is a benign tumor usually composed of lobules of mature fat. It occurs in adults, appearing as a soft, slowly enlarging, asymptomatic mass usually located superficially in the subcutaneous tissues or in the fatty planes along the neurovascular bundles. Lipomas that arise in deep tissues may become remarkably large. This tumor often presents as an active stage 2 lesion, later becoming inactive, or latent. Angiolipoma, a variant of lipoma with a vascular component, occurs in children as a deep, intramuscular soft mass. It is distinguished from an ordinary lipoma by a distinct tenderness.

Diagnostic Studies. Lipoma is the one soft-tissue tumor easily recognized by its characteristic radiographic appearance: a crisply marginated radiolucent image. Radiographs may also show calcification in areas of necrosis and metaplastic bone or cartilage.

The usual avascular lipoma appears cold on the bone scan. The pathognomonic density seen on computed tomography is much less than that of liposarcoma or fluid-filled lesions. Angiography is the best method for diagnosing angiolipoma.

Treatment. Marginal excision is successful for lipoma, and recurrences are rare.

Neurofibroma

A neurofibroma is a benign tumor of neural origin. Although it may affect almost any tissue type, it is most commonly found in skin and subcutaneous tissue or associated with nerve fibers. Whether they are solitary or multiple, neurofibromas occur in persons of any age. Multiple neurofibromas are a primary manifestation of neurofibromatosis. Neurofibromas also occur in conjunction with scoliosis, congenital pseudarthrosis of the tibia, and gigantism of a limb. (For a discussion of these conditions, see Section I.)

Most neurofibromas present as active stage 2 tumors, but aggressive stage 3 infiltrative forms may be seen occasionally. Long-standing neurofibromatosis may undergo malignant transformation.

Diagnostic Studies. Staging studies demonstrate an oval, avascular tumor. Neurofibroma is frequently seen as a fusiform mass in continuity with a major nerve best demonstrated by magnetic resonance imaging. Although many neurofibromas are well encapsulated, some actually infiltrate a peripheral nerve, thereby precluding en bloc extracapsular marginal excision and preservation of the nerve. Histologic examination reveals a loose, spindle-cell stroma containing wavy eosinophilic fibrillar material and occasional Verocay bodies, which are composed of amorphous eosinophilic material that is surrounded by spindle-shaped or oval cells.

Lipoma

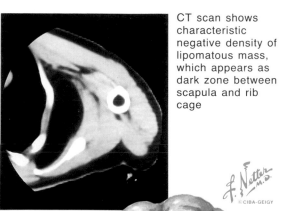

Massive lipoma of axilla

CT scan shows characteristic negative density of lipomatous mass, which appears as dark zone between scapula and rib cage

Sectioned lipoma composed of yellow fat lobules with narrow intervening fibrous septa

Neurofibroma

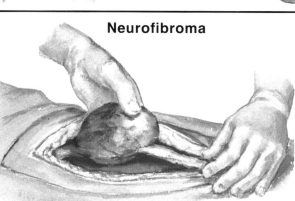

Surgical stripping of large, solitary neurofibroma from sciatic nerve

Section reveals loose, fibrillar, wavy neural strands characteristic of neurofibroma (H and E stain)

Myositis Ossificans

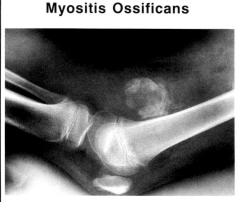

Lateral radiograph shows nodule with peripheral maturation in soft tissue of posterior distal thigh

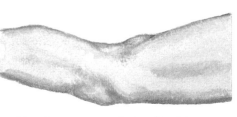

Prominence on posterior distal femur limits flexion

Myositis Ossificans

Myositis ossificans is a nonneoplastic reparative or reactive ossification of soft tissue that usually occurs following blunt trauma. Occasionally, it arises spontaneously in the absence of trauma and is then called pseudomalignant myositis ossificans. It typically occurs in adolescents as a painless, enlarging mass in the upper arm, thigh, or buttocks. This clinical presentation may erroneously suggest an extraosseous osteosarcoma or soft-tissue sarcoma. (For complete discussions of fibrodysplasia [myositis] ossificans progressiva, see Section I, Plate 21, and CIBA COLLECTION, Volume 8/I, page 239.)

Diagnostic Studies. Radiographs reveal a round mass with a distinct margin of mature ossification and a radiolucent center of immature osteoid and primitive mesenchymal tissue. This peripheral maturation—the reverse of that seen in a malignant tumor—is so characteristic of myositis ossificans that documentation with computed tomography clearly offsets the impression of malignancy suggested by the histologic appearance of the central immature area.

Treatment and Prognosis. Mature pseudomalignant myositis ossificans requires only marginal excision. After the 6 to 8 weeks required for maturation, the risk of recurrence is greatly diminished. □

Malignant Tumors of Soft Tissue

Sarcomas of Soft Tissue

The incidence of soft-tissue sarcomas equals that of malignant bone tumors (1 in 100,000 annually), but their diagnosis is often more difficult. Most soft-tissue sarcomas are palpable or symptomatic, yet they are not well visualized on radiographs. As a result, they are frequently managed initially as hematoma, thrombophlebitis, cyst, or abscess. However, the greatest risk to the patient is not the diagnostic delay but rather the inadvertent contamination that may result from inappropriate treatment. About two-thirds of malignant sarcomas recur after initial inadequate local excision.

Limb-salvage procedures (ie, local excision) have replaced amputation as the primary treatment for soft-tissue sarcomas, chiefly as a result of the effectiveness of adjuvant therapy. Despite the efficacy of limb-salvage procedures in obtaining local control, however, pulmonary metastasis remains a significant problem.

Malignant Fibrous Histiocytoma

Malignant fibrous histiocytoma is the most common sarcoma of soft tissue (Plate 26). The cells, of histiocytic derivation, are capable of producing collagen and thus are known as facultative fibroblasts. Malignant fibrous histiocytoma is seen in adults, first appearing either as a large mass involving the deep soft tissues of the proximal limbs and girdles or as a small, superficial, low-grade tumor in the distal limbs. The incidence of early osseous invasion and metastases to regional lymph nodes is high.

Diagnostic Studies. Bone scans of a large stage IIB tumor show increased radioisotope uptake in the adjacent cortex, and marked neovascularity is seen on angiography. Although the extent of soft-tissue involvement and the tumor's relationship to the major neurovascular structures can be estimated by computed tomography, magnetic resonance imaging better demonstrates the differences between normal and neoplastic tissue.

Histologic characteristics include a mixture of fibrous tissue arranged in a typical storiform pattern; areas filled with large, foamy histiocytes; and a scattering of wildly bizarre, atypical cells with obvious mitotic figures. Additional findings include prominent necrosis, vascular invasion, and erythrocyte phagocytosis by bizarre histiocytes.

Treatment and Prognosis. Low-grade stage I tumors usually develop in more peripheral and superficial locations than do high-grade tumors. Treatment with a wide surgical excision is usually adequate, with amputation reserved for multiple recurrences.

Stage II malignant fibrous histiocytoma requires excision with radical margins, whether by resection or amputation. Preoperative radiation therapy or postoperative chemotherapy, or

Malignant Fibrous Histiocytoma of Soft Tissue

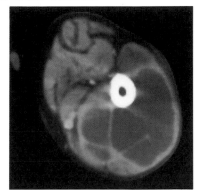

CT scan shows tumor occupying antero-lateral compartment

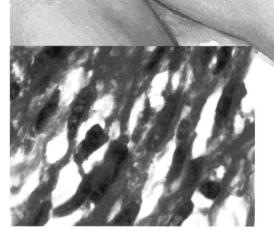

High-power section reveals characteristic pattern of malignant fibrous stroma and histiocytes (H and E stain)

Firm, deeply palpable tumor of anterior proximal thigh

Fibrosarcoma of Soft Tissue

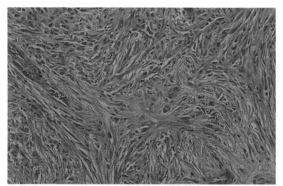

Section shows typical spindle-cell nuclei of malignant fibroblasts arranged in herringbone pattern (H and E stain)

Large, infiltrating tumor encompassing knee typifies high-grade, soft-tissue fibrosarcoma that may occur at many sites

both, may be recommended for these high-grade lesions.

Fibrosarcoma of Soft Tissue

The diagnosis of fibrosarcoma is reserved for the invasive, malignant, spindle-cell tumors with cellular atypia, mitoses, and formation of type I collagen (Plate 26). Fibrosarcoma occurs more often and is also less aggressive in soft tissue than in bone. This tumor can occur at any age and at any stage. It develops more frequently in men and is the most common soft-tissue sarcoma in infants. The lower limb is the typical site, and stage II lesions are usually extracompartmental. Low-grade stage I fibrosarcoma is often difficult

to distinguish from its benign but aggressive counterpart, fibromatosis (Plate 24).

Diagnostic Studies. Radiographs show a lesion with a discrete margin. The bone scan reveals a moderate radioisotope uptake. Angiography demonstrates surprisingly little vascularity within the lesion.

Histologic characteristics are marked cellular atypia, abundant collagen in a herringbone pattern, and a distinct pseudocapsule. A stage I tumor has less cellularity and atypia and more mature collagen than a stage II tumor; in children, a stage I lesion can be confused with aggressive juvenile fibromatosis, a diagnostic difficulty that affects treatment choices.

Malignant Tumors of Soft Tissue

Sarcomas of Soft Tissue

(Continued)

Synovial Sarcoma

Synovial sarcoma is derived from the synovial tissues found along fascial planes, in periarticular structures, and rarely, in joints (Plate 27). An enlarging, painful, juxtaarticular mass is the primary clinical manifestation. Occurring most frequently as a stage IIB lesion in the lower limbs, it also may appear as a stage I tumor in the hands or feet where it may be confused with a ganglion (see Section III, Plate 47).

Diagnostic Studies. Radiographs show a hazy, soft-tissue density and, the majority of cases, discrete intrinsic calcifications. Evidence of regional lymph node involvement strongly supports the diagnosis.

Bone scans show marked radioisotope uptake, and significant neovascularity is noted on angiography. The lesion is often adjacent to major neurovascular structures, and accurate localization is best provided by computed tomography or magnetic resonance imaging.

Histologic examination reveals a biphasic pattern, with intermixed areas of "glandular," synoviallike cells and spindle-shaped fibrous cells. The synovial cells often have an acinar, or ductal, arrangement around acellular "slits" containing mucin, while the fibrous component may be arranged in the herringbone pattern of fibrosarcoma. Some lesions have a predominant spindle-cell component and are thus called monophasic synovioma.

Treatment and Prognosis. Low-grade lesions can be controlled with a wide excision, but the treatment of high-grade tumors requires either radical resection or wide surgical excision plus radiation therapy. Despite adequate local control, the incidence of both regional and pulmonary metastases is high, and prognosis for patients with synovial sarcoma is poor.

Liposarcoma

Liposarcoma, a tumor derived from fat tissue, occurs in two forms: the usually low-grade myxoid liposarcoma and the high-grade pleomorphic liposarcoma (Plate 27). Myxoid liposarcoma occurs in young adults; pleomorphic liposarcoma is more common in older patients. An enlarging but painless mass in the buttocks (the most common site), proximal thigh, or upper arm is the characteristic presentation.

Diagnostic Studies. Liposarcoma is markedly vascular, which is best demonstrated by angiography and is reflected by the marked increase in radioisotope uptake in the early phase of the bone scan. The radiolucency noted on computed tomography may suggest the histogenesis in low-grade, well-differentiated lesions with a high fat content.

Synovial Sarcoma

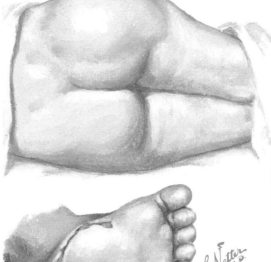

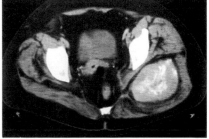

CT scan shows tumor with calcification posterolateral to right ilium

Tumor of medial plantar aspect of foot. Note scar of biopsy incision

Section shows typical biphasic pattern with accumulation of eosinophilic mucinous material (H and E stain)

Liposarcoma

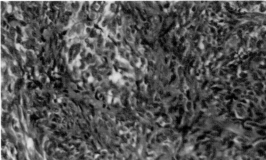

CT scan reveals mixture of benign (low-density) and sarcomatous (high-density) areas of tumor

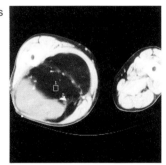

Large liposarcoma of posterior thigh

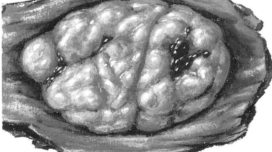

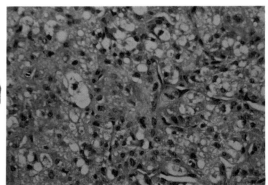

Excised tumor with muscle at margin; tumor darker and firmer than benign lipoma

Section shows characteristic malignant lipoblasts (H and E stain)

Histologic examination of myxoid liposarcoma reveals a fine reticular vascular pattern, whereas pleomorphic lesions have amorphously arranged, large vascular lakes. In myxoid liposarcoma, lipoblasts are dispersed in the anastomosing capillary framework; in the pleomorphic tumor, the vasculature is less structured. In both types, however, the vascularity results in a characteristic, almost cherry red color of the tumor. The more aggressive pleomorphic liposarcoma, which tends to invade bone, contains large, pyknotic, bizarre, mononucleated cells in combination with immature lipoblasts.

Treatment. Stage I myxoid lesions are treated with wide surgical excision, whereas stage II pleomorphic lesions require wide excision supplemented with radiation therapy or radical resection or amputation.

Neurosarcoma

Neurosarcoma (malignant schwannoma or fibrosarcoma of nerve sheath) is an extracompartmental tumor that develops from the sheaths (Schwann cells) of peripheral nerves (Plate 28). Although typically a primary lesion occurring along proximal major nerve trunks, neurosarcoma occasionally develops as a secondary transformation of neurofibromatosis. This large tumor is high-grade but is usually asymptomatic until it causes neurapraxia.

Malignant Tumors of Soft Tissue

Sarcomas of Soft Tissue
(Continued)

Diagnostic Studies. Gross inspection reveals a large fusiform mass. Rather than being displaced by the tumor, the associated nerve enters the proximal pole of the tumor and exits the distal pole. The fibrillar pattern is loose and undulating with increased cellularity, multiple mitoses, and the typical wavy eosinophilic pattern of neural tissue with comma-shaped nuclei. In an undifferentiated lesion, electron microscopic examination is needed to distinguish it from fibrosarcoma.

Treatment and Prognosis. Wide excision with a wide margin, when practical, or radical amputation is the treatment of choice. In patients with concomitant neurofibromatosis, determining adequate surgical margins may be complicated by the difficulty in distinguishing benign neurofibroma from neurosarcoma. Prognosis for patients with primary neurosarcoma is more favorable than for those with malignant transformation of neurofibromatosis.

Myosarcoma

Myosarcoma describes sarcomas of smooth muscle (leiomyosarcoma) and those of skeletal muscle (rhabdomyosarcoma) (Plate 28). Leiomyosarcoma arises extracompartmentally from the intestinal walls in the abdomen; in the limbs, it develops from the smooth muscle of arterial walls. It is not a transformation of benign leiomyoma. Rhabdomyosarcoma takes two forms: embryonal rhabdomyosarcoma, which occurs in the head and neck, and adult rhabdomyosarcoma, which develops in the limbs.

Diagnostic Studies. Angiography or computed tomography with contrast medium shows the marked vascularity of leiomyosarcomas. Early invasion of adjacent bone may result in multiple osteolytic lesions. The histologic picture is not dominated by vessels but by smooth muscle spindle cells with blunt-ended nuclei that resemble cigars.

The adult form of rhabdomyosarcoma is a high-grade lesion with histologic findings characterized by a background of undifferentiated malignant cells admixed with malignant myoblasts that appear as large, racquet-shaped "tadpole" or "strap" cells. The embryonal form has a glandular pattern and lacks the large, racquet-shaped myoblasts. In both types of rhabdomyosarcoma, because of its close histologic resemblance to malignant fibrous histiocytoma, the presence of cross-striations in the malignant cells must be established by electron microscopy to validate the diagnosis.

Treatment and Prognosis. Chemotherapy has improved survival tof patients with both forms of rhabdomyosarcoma, and tumors in the limbs, often intracompartmental, are amenable to wide excision. Patients with stage IIB leiomyosarcoma

Neurosarcoma

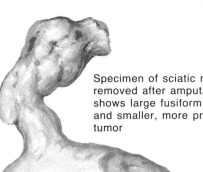

Specimen of sciatic nerve removed after amputation shows large fusiform tumor and smaller, more proximal tumor

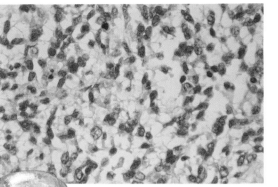

Section reveals round, hyperchromatic nuclei mixed with myxomatous, undulating spindle-cell stroma indicative of neural origin (H and E stain)

Myosarcoma

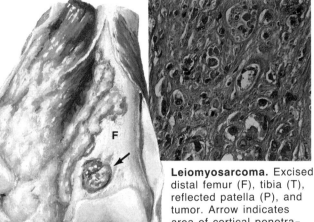

Leiomyosarcoma. Excised distal femur (F), tibia (T), reflected patella (P), and tumor. Arrow indicates area of cortical penetration. Section (above) shows transversely and longitudinally sectioned malignant smooth muscle cells (H and E stain)

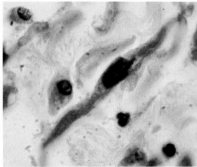

Rhabdomyosarcoma. High-power section demonstrates typical "strap" cells. Cross-striations seen under oil immersion (H and E stain)

Angiosarcoma

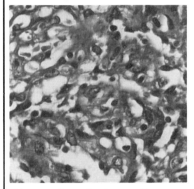

Hemangiopericytoma. Eccentric hyperchromatic nuclei of pericytic cells surrounding vascular spaces (H and E stain)

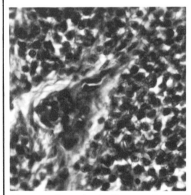

Hemangioendothelioma. Central hyperplastic capillary surrounded by malignant endothelial cells (H and E stain)

who have major neurovascular involvement often require amputation.

Angiosarcoma

Angiosarcoma describes high-grade sarcomas of vascular origin, both hemangioendothelioma, more common in bone than in soft tissue, and hemangiopericytoma, more common in soft tissue than in bone (Plate 28). Soft-tissue angiosarcomas occur in middle-aged persons, in the abdominal viscera or limbs. When the tumor arises in bone, it frequently extends up and down the bone or even adjacent bones, with a distinctive pattern of multiple, discrete "soap-bubble" lesions.

Diagnostic Studies. The permeative, invasive nature of the lesion is evident on computed tomography and magnetic resonance imaging, and its intense vascularity is demonstrated by angiography. Bone scans show marked radioisotope uptake. The histologic features include multiple, fine neoplastic capillaries coursing through a background of endothelial cells with infrequent mitoses. In hemangioendothelioma, the histologic pattern is dominated by neoplastic endothelial cells; in hemangiopericytoma, by neoplastic pericytes.

Treatment. Both types of angiosarcomas require either wide surgical margins with adjuvant radiation therapy or radical amputation. ☐

Tumor Biopsy

Successful management of a tumor is based on an accurate histologic diagnosis. If a malignant neoplasm is suspected, incisional biopsy is the standard technique for obtaining an adequate amount of tissue for histologic study. Open incisional biopsy, which involves cutting into the lesion, is superior to closed trocar or needle techniques because a larger tissue sample can be obtained for histologic study and thus a more reliable diagnosis. En bloc excisional biopsy, actually an intracapsular or marginal excision of the tumor, carries a higher risk of wound contamination than incisional biopsy, as it involves more tissue exposure and dissection.

The risk of wound contamination with incisional biopsy can be minimized by a strict adherence to the following surgical principles.

Correct Placement of Incision. In a limb, a longitudinal incision is used. The biopsy incision is placed in the line of the planned subsequent excision so that the biopsy tract can be excised en bloc with the lesion at the time of the definitive procedure.

Minimal Dissection of Soft Tissue. The surgical approach for biopsy should be direct, with minimal dissection of soft tissue. Muscle, fascia, and capsule or pseudocapsule are preserved for later closure.

Avoidance of Neurovascular Structures and Adjacent Joint. The biopsy site should be selected carefully to avoid exposure of major vessels, nerves, and joint capsules, thus preventing their contamination and necessitating subsequent sacrifice.

Adequate Specimen. During the biopsy procedure, frozen sections should be evaluated to ensure the adequacy of the tissue specimen. Cultures are performed routinely, and additional tissue can be obtained for histochemical stains, electron microscopy, flow cytometry, and other special studies as needed.

Strict Hemostasis. If practical, a tourniquet should be used to prevent bleeding. Before the tourniquet is released, the tumor capsule is closed meticulously. Strict hemostasis should be achieved with coagulants before wound closure. Holes in bone that may leak tumor cells are plugged with methylmethacrylate cement.

Tight Wound Closure. The pseudocapsule and fascial layers should be closed meticulously. Neat skin closure is best accomplished with short skin or subcuticular sutures.

Complications. A poorly conceived and executed incisional biopsy may lead to a dissecting hematoma, which may contaminate previously uninvolved tissues. Thus, a subsequent excision of the tumor often requires a wider surgical margin. Widespread contamination may preclude a limb-salvage procedure or greatly increase the risk of local recurrence after limb-salvaging excision.

Alternative Biopsy Procedures. Excisional and closed biopsies are both alternatives to open incisional biopsy. En bloc excisional biopsy is done for accessible, presumptively benign tumors. Closed biopsy may be done by aspiration for cytologic studies or by trocar technique, which obtains thin cores of tissue. Aspiration with a fine-gauge needle obtains a thin film of cells that often yields useful information on cytologic examination. Accuracy of the results, however, requires both homogeneous tissue samples and the pathologist with unusual expertise. The aspiration technique is most useful for the diagnosis of soft-tissue sarcomas, metastatic carcinomas, and marrow-cell tumors. A closed biopsy is faster than an incisional biopsy and can be performed on an outpatient basis with minimal risk of hematoma and contamination. □

Tumor Biopsy

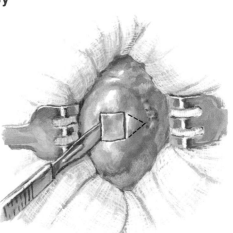

Proposed incision site for tumor removal

Biopsy incision longitudinal (not transverse); placed to permit inclusion of biopsy tract in definitive tumor excision. Neurovascular bundle must be avoided and shortest route to tumor used, with least removal of soft tissue

Wedge-shaped specimen must be adequate size and include both intraosseous and extraosseous tissue. Contamination of soft tissue with tumor cells must be avoided. Strict hemostasis must be achieved before closure. Bone defect plugged with cement

Specimen may be used for
frozen section, fixation for histopathologic study, electron microscopy, study with special stains

Multiple cultures

Wound closed neatly with short sutures

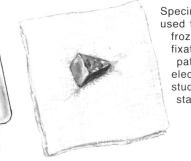

Needle biopsy (for aspiration or tissue sample)

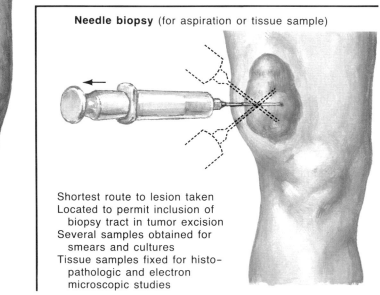

Shortest route to lesion taken
Located to permit inclusion of biopsy tract in tumor excision
Several samples obtained for smears and cultures
Tissue samples fixed for histopathologic and electron microscopic studies

Surgical Margins for Musculoskeletal Tumors

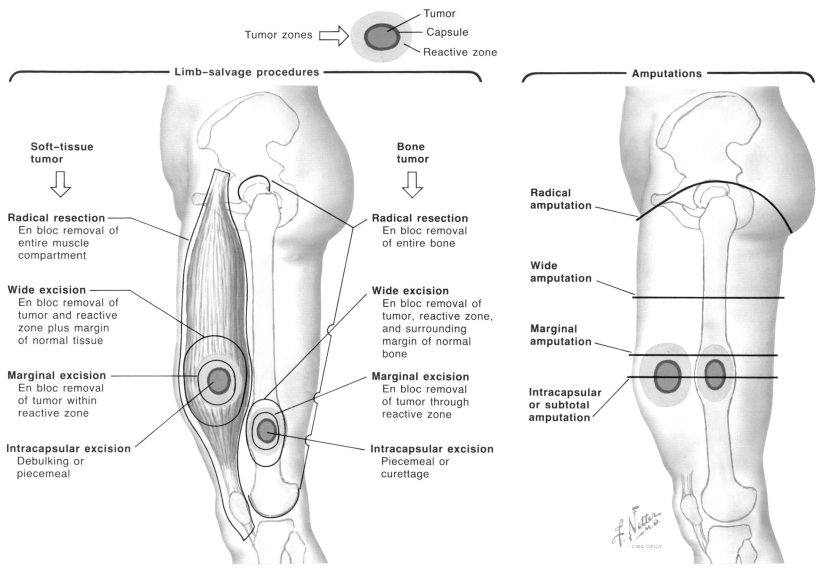

Tumor zones → Tumor / Capsule / Reactive zone

Limb-salvage procedures

Soft-tissue tumor ⇩

Radical resection
En bloc removal of entire muscle compartment

Wide excision
En bloc removal of tumor and reactive zone plus margin of normal tissue

Marginal excision
En bloc removal of tumor within reactive zone

Intracapsular excision
Debulking or piecemeal

Bone tumor ⇩

Radical resection
En bloc removal of entire bone

Wide excision
En bloc removal of tumor, reactive zone, and surrounding margin of normal bone

Marginal excision
En bloc removal of tumor through reactive zone

Intracapsular excision
Piecemeal or curettage

Amputations

Radical amputation

Wide amputation

Marginal amputation

Intracapsular or subtotal amputation

Surgical Margins

The surgical removal of a tumor is most accurately described by stating the procedure and the surgical margin achieved—the amount and type of the nonneoplastic surrounding tissue. The four basic surgical margins are intracapsular, marginal, wide, and radical. Each margin may be achieved with local excision or by amputation. The procedure can be expressed, for example, as excision with a wide margin or simply as wide excision. Although described in surgical terms by the level of the dissection, the surgical margins also reflect the progressive natural barriers to tumor extension by the (1) capsule or pseudocapsule, (2) reactive zone, and (3) surrounding normal tissue and fascial planes. The reactive zone, or margin, represents the reaction of the normal host tissue to the tumor and consists of a proliferation of mesenchymal, neovascular, and inflammatory tissue.

An *intracapsular margin* is obtained when the surgical dissection extends through the reactive zone and the capsule or pseudocapsule into the tumor itself. A *marginal margin* describes a plane

of dissection through the reactive zone just outside the capsule or pseudocapsule. A *wide margin* is achieved when the dissection plane is through normal tissue outside the reactive zone; thus, the tumor and its pseudocapsule are excised along with an intact "cuff" of normal tissue. A *radical margin* describes removal of the tumor and the entire natural compartment (bone, muscle compartment) that contains it. The recurrence rate for both benign and malignant musculoskeletal tumors in relation to the surgical margin is tabulated below.

Although marginal, wide, or radical margins may all be free of tumor cells, the marginal margin, because of the closer proximity of the surgical margin to the tumor, is more likely to leave behind microscopic fragments of tumor and thus lead to local recurrence. Similarly, a wide margin, despite removal of a cuff of normal tissue,

still has a higher risk for leaving residual tumor cells than does a radical procedure.

The term "contaminated margin" refers to a recognized intraoperative violation of the lesion, followed by closure and subsequent adjustment of the plane of dissection. For example, a contaminated wide excision indicates that the tumor was inadvertently entered during the excision, the exposed tissues were contaminated by leakage from the tumor, the opening was closed, and the contaminated tissues were excised to obtain a wide margin.

The adequacy of the surgical margin is estimated by gross and microscopic examination of the excised specimen. Gross inspection is particularly important in distinguishing whether a wide margin or a radical margin has been obtained, because the microscopic appearance of each is free of tumor cells. □

Recurrence (%): Surgical Margin Versus Stage (after surgery only)

Surgical margin	Stage						
	Benign			Malignant			
	1	2	3	IA	IB	IIA	IIB
Intracapsular	0	30	70	90	90	100	100
Marginal	0	0	50	70	70	90	90
Wide	0	0	10	10	30	30	50
Radical	0	0	0	0	0	10	20

Reconstruction Following Partial Excision or Curettage (Fracture Prophylaxis)

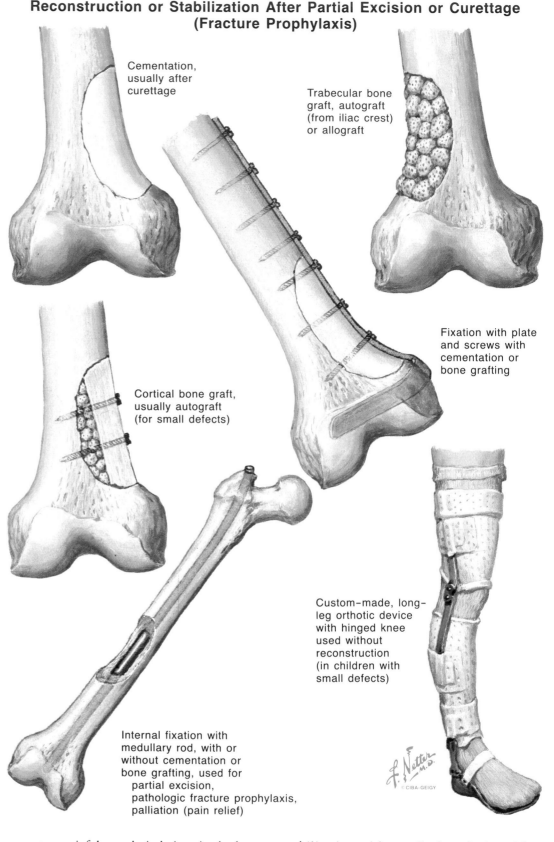

Reconstruction or Stabilization After Partial Excision or Curettage (Fracture Prophylaxis)

Cementation, usually after curettage

Trabecular bone graft, autograft (from iliac crest) or allograft

Cortical bone graft, usually autograft (for small defects)

Fixation with plate and screws with cementation or bone grafting

Internal fixation with medullary rod, with or without cementation or bone grafting, used for partial excision, pathologic fracture prophylaxis, palliation (pain relief)

Custom-made, long-leg orthotic device with hinged knee used without reconstruction (in children with small defects)

The excision of a tumor with removal of one cortex (wide fenestration) and curettage of the metaphysis is a common treatment for active or aggressive benign tumors or metastatic bone lesions. Reconstruction of the resulting surgical defect depends on its size and location and the age of the patient. In a child or young adult with a small cortical defect, for example, the weakened bone can be managed with a protective plaster cast or an orthotic device while the defect heals; these devices are also used to protect against postoperative injury following a complicated reconstruction procedure.

Excision of active or aggressive benign tumors often requires a wide surgical margin, which leaves a large defect that increases the risk of pathologic fracture. In these instances, the defect can be reconstructed with cortical bone autografts or allografts, or with cementation. For example, cementation following curettage of an active stage 2 giant-cell tumor of bone lowers the risk of tumor recurrence and postoperative fracture. An additional advantage of this technique is the resulting immediate stabilization of the affected joint, which contributes to faster and more effective rehabilitation. When necessary, curettage plus cementation may be combined with internal fixation to preserve the integrity of a fragile remnant of cortex.

Reconstruction of large metaphyseal defects with bone grafting involves the selection of appropriate cortical and trabecular bone autografts or allografts. Small, stable defects are successfully reconstructed with grafts or strips of trabecular bone; larger, less stable defects require use of cortical bone to provide good support. Autografts are easily obtained from the iliac crest (trabecular bone) or from the fibula (cortical bone), with minimal morbidity and no risk of immunologic (allogenic) rejection.

The potential for pathologic fracture is a common problem associated with metastatic carcinoma or marrow-cell tumors. These tumors often present as painful osteolytic lesions in the lower limb, with pain on ambulation reflecting significant intrinsic bone weakness. The risk of pathologic fracture in a tubular bone is significant when the tumor occupies 50% or more of the bone diameter or produces a cortical defect longer than 2.5 cm. Prophylactic surgical stabilization should be considered in patients who are at significant risk for pathologic fracture or who have fractures or painful tumors that prevent ambulation. Stabilization of tubular bones is best accomplished with intramedullary rod fixation with or without cementation.

When the tumor is located in the proximal femur, the femoral neck may require prophylactic stabilization with a nail-plate device. After removal of a tumor in the distal femur, the stabilizing device may be inserted retrogradely through the knee, with additional curettage and cementation as needed; this allows early knee motion despite the arthrotomy. Destructive tumors in the acetabulum may be treated with curettage and cementation or with total hip replacement, but the remaining proximal, uninvolved ilium requires careful stabilization. Treatment of symptomatic tumors of the humerus also includes surgical stabilization after tumor removal, preferably with an intramedullary rod, because coaptation splinting does not alleviate painful rotational instability. □

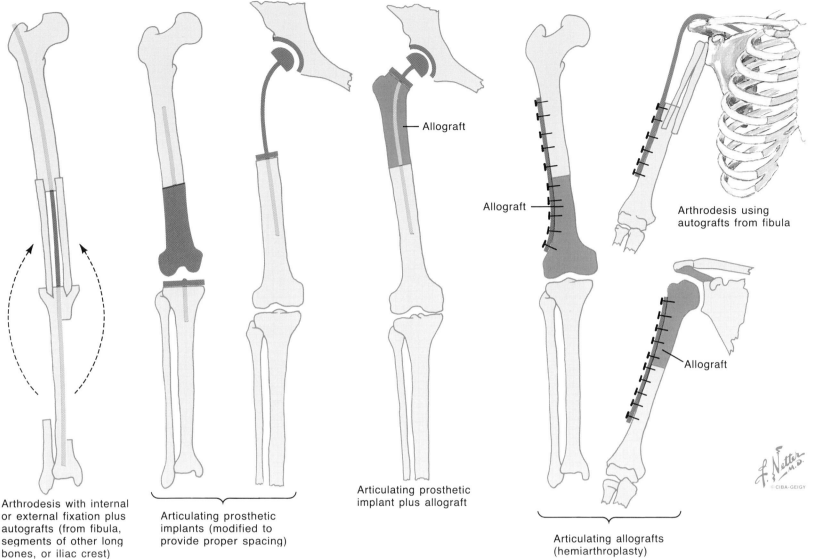

Arthrodesis with internal or external fixation plus autografts (from fibula, segments of other long bones, or iliac crest)

Articulating prosthetic implants (modified to provide proper spacing)

Allograft

Allograft

Articulating prosthetic implant plus allograft

Arthrodesis using autografts from fibula

Allograft

Articulating allografts (hemiarthroplasty)

SECTION II PLATE 32   Slide 4579

Limb-Salvage Procedures

A major development in the management of musculoskeletal tumors in the limbs is the increasing effectiveness of limb-salvage procedures with adjuvant chemotherapy, especially in patients with osteosarcoma. For many lesions, patient survival rates once attainable only with amputation are now being achieved with a combination of preoperative chemotherapy and limb-salvage surgery.

Two principles are recognized in limb-salvage surgery: careful, adequate excision of the tumor followed by optimal functional reconstruction of the limb. These dual objectives are frequently contradictory, and the desire to preserve tissue and optimize the reconstruction may subtly seduce the surgeon to compromise the surgical margins.

Obtaining adequate margins often requires sacrifice of bone, cartilage, joint, and soft tissue. Limb-salvage procedures are practical when major neurovascular bundles can be safely spared and tissue removal does not preclude functional reconstruction.

Patients should be informed of the increased risks of local recurrence, distant metastases, and death associated with limb-salvage procedures. Their life-style and expectations should be carefully considered when selecting the reconstructive procedure. Most patients with stage IA, IB, and IIA tumors can be successfully treated with limb-salvage procedures, but in many patients with stage IIB tumors, only amputation can minimize the likelihood of recurrence. In addition, amputation may still be needed if the limb-salvage procedure is followed by recurrence, deep infection, vascular insufficiency, or neurologic deficit. Since the initial emotional shock of the diagnosis often prevents the patient from comprehending all the aspects to be considered in treatment, many detailed discussions between physician and patient are essential before a rational decision can be reached.

Reconstruction of Joint

Following excision of a soft-tissue sarcoma, the defect is usually reconstructed with a local tissue transfer to obliterate dead space or avoid wound complications. Large soft-tissue excisions, most commonly in the thigh, may involve the transfer or rotation of a muscle or skin flap, split-thickness skin grafts, or neurovascular grafts.

The soft-tissue reconstructions described above are frequently combined with a bone or joint resection following en bloc excision of a tumor.

Less extensive resections of, for example, one condyle require "unicondylar" reconstructions, while more extensive procedures, usually for high-grade stage IIB lesions, involve en bloc resection of the entire joint (extraarticulation), including the intact joint capsule and contiguous ligaments. When half of the joint or the whole joint is resected, the reconstructive procedures used are arthroplasty, arthrodesis, and pseudarthrosis (Plates 32–34).

Arthroplasty. Successful arthroplasty depends on a surrounding musculature that has good power, vasculature, and innervation. The optimal result of arthroplasty is a painless, stable joint with good range of motion. Unstable motion is neither functional nor painless and leads to early deterioration of the reconstructed joint. Restricted motion, usually associated with pain, results in limited function and thus a poor result.

Arthroplasty may be achieved with (1) implantation of a prosthetic joint or partial joint (see Section IV), (2) transplantation of an articulating bone allograft, or (3) a composite technique—a combination of prosthesis plus bone allograft (Plate 32). Use of bone allograft offers the advantage of a biologic implant that has the potential for gradual incorporation and remodeling. However, it is associated with a high rate of complications such as rejection of the graft, infection, fracture, and nonunion at the graft-host junction. The risk of a serious complication necessitating

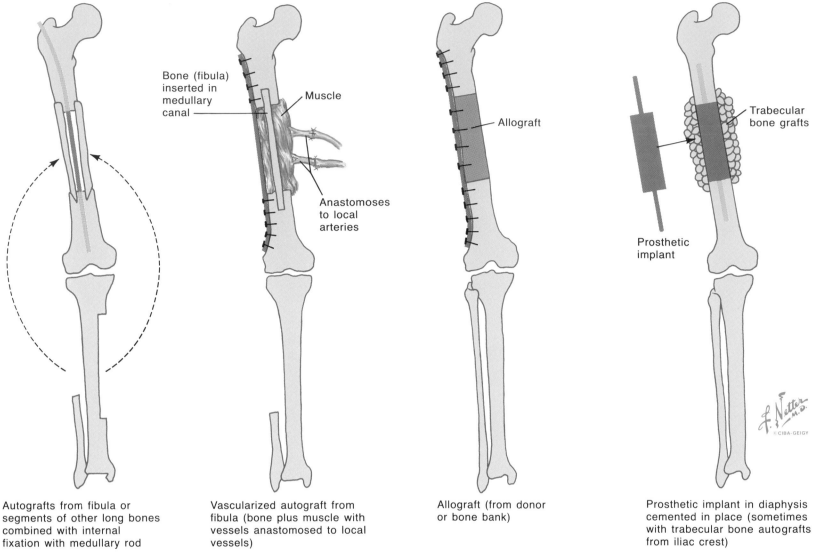

Autografts from fibula or segments of other long bones combined with internal fixation with medullary rod

Vascularized autograft from fibula (bone plus muscle with vessels anastomosed to local vessels)

Allograft (from donor or bone bank)

Prosthetic implant in diaphysis cemented in place (sometimes with trabecular bone autografts from iliac crest)

SECTION II PLATE 33   Slide 4580

Limb-Salvage Procedures
(*Continued*)

removal of the graft or another operative procedure—including amputation—is as high as 30%. Reconstruction with an allograft joint is most appropriate in young patients who, because of their age, are poor candidates for prosthetic joint replacement.

Arthrodesis. In this technique, the resected bone is replaced with bone grafts that achieve fusion of the joint. Arthrodesis is most successful in the knee, shoulder, hip, and wrist; it is a more complicated procedure following tumor removal than when it is used to treat the arthritic joint, and the incidence of delayed union or nonunion is 20%. Since a well-innervated musculature is not a prerequisite for arthrodesis, resection with a greater margin is thus possible. A successful arthrodesis results in a durable limb that will last a lifetime. Its chief disadvantage is permanent joint stiffness and loss of motion.

Arthrodesis of the shoulder may be accomplished with intercalary grafting with bone allograft, vascularized fibular autograft, or dual conventional

fibular autografts, all of which require rigid internal fixation with a plate (Plate 32). It is the best alternative when the tumor excision requires sacrifice of the axillary nerve, a major portion of the deltoid muscle, or the rotator cuff. In patients without deltoid power for abduction, shoulder arthroplasty provides only a spacer with limited functional results. Patients with shoulder arthrodesis have limited but powerful abduction provided by the scapulothoracic musculature. When the arm is fused in a position that allows proper positioning of the hand, upper limb function is excellent; the significant functional loss results from the loss of rotation of the upper limb at the shoulder.

Arthrodesis of the hip is usually successful in young patients who have had minimal resection of the proximal femur. However, after en bloc resection of the whole hip, including the acetabulum, fixation of the femur to the remaining iliac wing is so difficult that the incidence of nonunion and functional failure is very high. When the acetabulum and abductor mechanism can be preserved, the preferred method of reconstruction is hemiarthroplasty with a custom-made prosthesis or arthroplasty with a combination of prosthesis and bone allograft (Plate 32).

Arthrodesis of the knee is best suited to young patients whose life-style or occupation imposes heavy functional demands on the joint. It can be used to reconstruct a bone resection of as much

as 20 cm in length and is accomplished with conventional bone autografts. (Resection of a greater amount of bone necessitates reconstruction with bone allograft.) Usually, a segment is removed from the fibula and the anterior hemicortex of the tibia or femur of the same limb and placed anterior and posterior to a full-length intramedullary rod that spans the defect and stabilizes the limb. However, in 10% of cases, significant complications occur that prevent good function. An *articulating allograft* (hemiarthroplasty) is an alternative to knee fusion in a young patient.

Reconstruction of Diaphysis

Reconstruction of the diaphysis (intercalary procedure) after tumor removal is achieved with bone grafts or prosthetic implants, or both (Plate 33). Grafting alternatives include use of conventional dual fibular autografts, bone allografts, and vascularized fibular autografts.

Fibular Bone Grafts. Fibular autografts, combined with intramedullary rod or plate fixation, offer excellent stabilization. Bone allograft is even more readily available and can also be combined with intramedullary rod or plate fixation.

Transplantation with a vascularized fibular graft with microscopic arterial and venous anastomoses is a complex procedure requiring significantly longer operating time than other bone-grafting techniques. It offers the potential of a

Limb-Salvage Procedures
(Continued)

Tikhoff-Linberg Procedure for Tumors of Scapula and Proximal Humerus

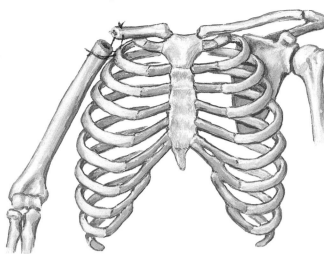

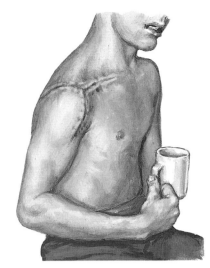

Scapula and proximal humerus removed. Remaining humerus stabilized by suturing to clavicle and 2nd rib

Patient now has flail shoulder but acceptable elbow flexion and good hand and finger function

Rotationplasty for Sarcoma of Distal Femur

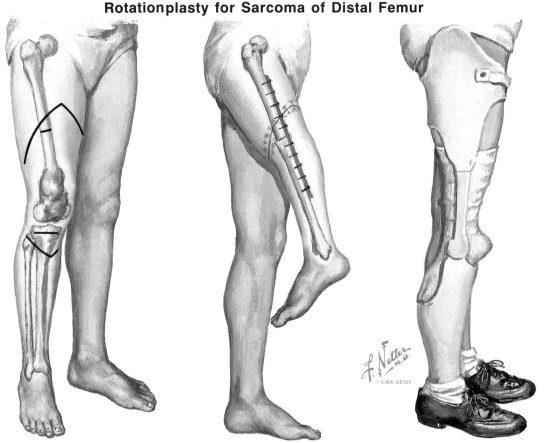

Osteosarcoma of distal femur. Skin incisions and lines of bone resection indicated

Midportion of limb removed. Distal segment rotated 180°, and tibia united to femur

Patient wearing prosthesis. Ankle joint now serves as knee joint

viable graft that has the ability to remodel and hypertrophy much more rapidly than a conventional fibular graft. Usually placed within the medullary canal, this type of graft is fixed with one or two long plates.

Prosthetic Implant. A segmental diaphyseal defect may be reconstructed using a porous prosthetic implant inserted into the medullary canal (Plate 33). Trabecular bone autograft may be added around the implant to produce an enveloping sleeve of bone.

Pseudarthrosis

Reconstruction with a pseudarthrosis (flail joint) is performed after a radical resection of the shoulder or hip or as revision of a failed reconstruction. Although functionally inferior to a painless arthroplasty or arthrodesis, it is superior to an arthroplasty or arthrodesis complicated by instability, pain, and infection. A pseudarthrosis requires only soft-tissue reconstruction. The resultant joint is excessively mobile but has little or no stability.

Tikhoff-Linberg Shoulder Girdle Resection. This procedure is a classic example of reconstruction by a pseudarthrosis after en bloc interscapulothoracic resection of the upper humerus and scapula (Plate 34). It has traditionally been used as an alternative to amputation for sarcomas that involve the shoulder girdle but not the brachial plexus and vessels. While the original procedure involved complete resection of the scapula and the lateral half of the clavicle, later modifications preserved a greater portion of the clavicle, when appropriate, to support the remaining limb and give it a moderate amount of stability. In the procedure used at present, the proximal humerus is suspended from the remaining clavicle with a

heavy suture or the biceps brachii tendon(s), or with an intramedullary rod cemented in the humerus and attached proximally to the clavicle or the first or second rib. This reconstruction allows normal hand-and-finger function with consistent relief of pain.

Rotationplasty

This reconstructive procedure is used in a skeletally immature patient after en bloc extraarticular resection of osteosarcoma about the knee (Plate 34). The technique was devised by Van Nes in 1950 for the reconstruction of severe congenital defects of the femur and has been widely used in Europe to treat sarcoma in young

children; treatment with bone allograft or prostheses is not suitable because they cannot grow with the child.

After resection of the diseased bone, the remaining tibia is rotated 180° to the proximal femur and fixed to it with plates. The redundant vessels are carefully looped in the soft tissues. The length of the newly created limb is adjusted so that the ankle is positioned at the level that will match the level of the contralateral knee at completion of growth. The rotated ankle functions as a knee joint, and the foot serves as the stump of a below-knee amputation. Rotationplasty provides a much better functional result than above-knee amputation. □

Section III

Rheumatic Diseases

Frank H. Netter, M.D.

in collaboration with

Mack L. Clayton, M.D., George Hammond, M.D., Morris H. Susman, M.D., Alfred B. Swanson, M.D., and Genevieve de Groot Swanson, M.D.   *Plate 59*

Mack L. Clayton, M.D. and Morris H. Susman, M.D.   *Plates 50–58*

Chester W. Fink, M.D.   *Plates 17–20*

Richard H. Freyberg, M.D.   *Plates 1–13, 21–37*

George Hammond, M.D.   *Plates 38–39, 42–49, 60–61*

George Hammond, M.D. and Stuart C. Kozinn, M.D.   *Plates 40–41*

H. Ralph Schumacher, Jr., M.D.   *Plates 14–16*

Alfred B. Swanson, M.D. and Genevieve de Groot Swanson, M.D.   *Plates 62–73*

Rheumatic Diseases

Joint Pathology in Rheumatoid Arthritis

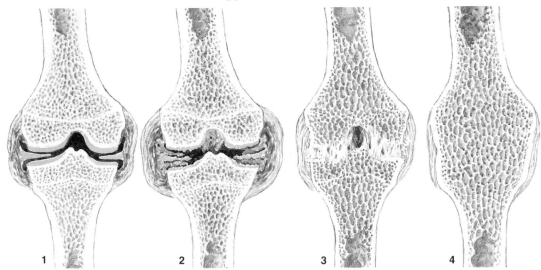

Progressive stages in joint pathology. 1. Acute inflammation of synovial membrane (synovitis) and beginning proliferative changes. 2. Progression of inflammation with pannus formation; beginning destruction of cartilage and mild osteoporosis. 3. Subsidence of inflammation; fibrous ankylosis. 4. Bony ankylosis; advanced osteoporosis

The term "rheumatic disease" refers to any illness characterized by pain and stiffness in or around the joints. These diseases are divided into two main groups: disorders that involve the joints primarily (the different forms of arthritis) and disorders that—while not directly affecting the joints—involve connective tissue structures around the joints (the periarticular disorders, or nonarticular rheumatism). The many types of arthritis and nonarticular disorders differ from one another in etiology, pathogenesis, pathology, and clinical features. This section focuses on the more commonly encountered rheumatic conditions.

Rheumatoid arthritis and osteoarthritis (also called degenerative joint disease) are the most common forms of arthritis. Both of these chronic conditions are characterized by pain, stiffness, restricted joint motion, joint deformities, and disability, but their differences in pathogenesis, pathology, and clinical features must be distinguished because the prognosis and treatment of the two diseases differ.

Rheumatoid Arthritis

Rheumatoid arthritis is a chronic, systemic illness with widespread involvement of connective tissue. Although rheumatoid arthritis may begin at any age, onset is usually in the fourth or fifth decade. Occurring in all parts of the world, it affects females two to three times more often than males.

The major characteristic of rheumatoid arthritis is inflammation of many joints (polyarthritis), usually the joints of the limbs. Although partial remissions are common, they are often followed by relapses and progression of active disease. If unchecked, the joint inflammation causes irreversible damage to the articular cartilage and bone, resulting in joint deformity, disability, and crippling.

Joint Pathology

The evolution of the pathologic changes in the joint provides the key to understanding the clinical nature of the disease (Plate 1). Rheumatoid

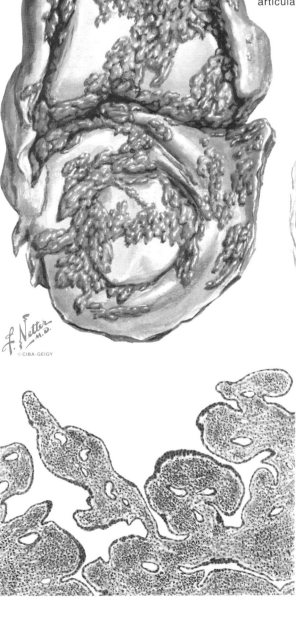

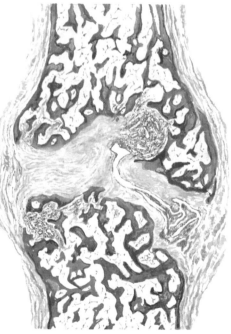

Knee joint opened anteriorly, patella reflected downward. Thickened synovial membrane inflamed; polypoid outgrowths and numerous villi (pannus) extend over rough articular cartilages of femur and patella

Section of proximal interphalangeal joint shows marked destruction of both articular cartilages and subchondral bone; replacement by fibrous and granulation tissue, which has obliterated most of joint space and invaded bone

Section of synovial membrane shows villous proliferation with extensive lymphocytic and plasma cell infiltration and numerous blood vessels. Synovial lining cells are elongated and arranged in palisade formation

Early and Moderate Hand Involvement in Rheumatoid Arthritis

Rheumatic Diseases
(Continued)

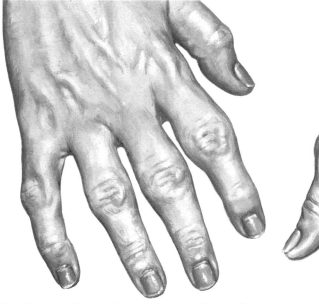

Fusiform swelling of fingers due to inflammation of proximal interphalangeal joints is typical of early involvement

Moderate involvement of proximal interphalangeal, metacarpophalangeal, and wrist joints

Advanced changes include subcutaneous nodules and beginning ulnar deviation of fingers

arthritis is basically an inflammatory disease of connective tissue. In the joint, the inflammation begins in the synovial membrane (synovitis). The synovial membrane becomes edematous and infiltrated with mononuclear cells, primarily lymphocytes and plasma cells. This produces diffuse proliferation of the synovial membrane, and synovial fluid accumulates. In this early stage, the articular cartilage and subchondral bone are not involved.

As the disease progresses, the inflamed synovial membrane continues to proliferate, and villous projections grow into the joint cavity (villous synovitis). The villi become infiltrated with lymphoid cells, which may form follicular collections. The proliferations spread along the cartilage surface (pannus formation), eroding and thinning the cartilage. The proliferative inflammation often invades the subchondral bone. Osteoporosis develops in the metaphyseal bone, weakening it, sometimes enough to cause erosion of the supporting cortical bone and disrupt the joint.

As the disease becomes more chronic, fibroblasts infiltrate the inflamed joint capsule, which becomes thickened and boggy. The pannus progresses, causing more destruction and joint deformity. The progressive inflammation causes irreversible destructive changes in cartilage and bone. After months or years of periods of active disease and partial remissions, the inflammation subsides, but the fibrous tissue increases and further restricts motion, leading to *fibrous ankylosis*. The stiffened, deformed joint may become solidly fused by bony bridges across the joint space; this final stage is thus called *bony ankylosis*. Pain lessens as the inflammation subsides, but the joint damage persists, accounting for the stiffened and deformed joints, crippling, and incapacitation.

Clinical Manifestations

Early in the course of the illness, joint involvement is characterized by signs and symptoms of polyarthritis in the limbs, usually in a symmetric distribution. In pauciarticular (oligoarticular) onset rheumatoid arthritis, only one or a few joints are involved. The affected joints become diffusely swollen, warm, and tender. Joint movement is painful, and the swelling of the joint capsules creates a feeling of stiffness. Generalized stiffness is also noted after long periods of inactivity, especially on arising in the morning. Depending on the severity of the illness, morning stiffness may last 1 or 2 hours, making routine daily activities difficult. Even early in the illness, the patient may be partially incapacitated.

Although the progression of joint inflammation follows no fixed pattern, usually several pairs of joints in the limbs are affected first. After months or even years, other joints may become involved, including the acromioclavicular, sternoclavicular, and temporomandibular joints, and even tiny joints such as the cricoarytenoid articulations. It is common, however, for some joints to be spared even if the disease remains active for many years and the joints involved early undergo severe crippling changes. The factors that determine the distribution of the disease and the severity of the inflammatory process in any joint remain unexplained.

Early and Moderate Hand Involvement

The joints of the hands and wrists are among the most frequent sites of involvement (Plate 2).

Rheumatic Diseases

(Continued)

Advanced Hand Involvement in Rheumatoid Arthritis

Marked ulnar deviation of meta-carpophalangeal joints, boutonniere deformity of thumb, synovitis of wrist

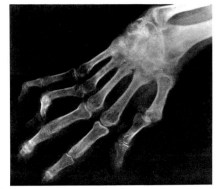

Radiograph shows cartilage thinning at proximal interphalangeal joints, erosion of carpus and wrist joint, osteoporosis, and finger deformities

Crippling involvement of metacarpophalangeal and interphalangeal joints of both hands. Swan–neck deformity of many fingers, boutonniere deformity of thumbs, and numerous subcutaneous nodules

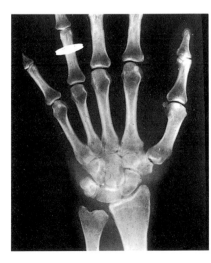

Radiograph (left) shows early loss of articular cartilage and osteopenia

Same patient after 14 years (right). Carpus, wrist joint, and ulnar head com–pletely eroded

In the fingers, some or all of the proximal interphalangeal joints are often bilaterally affected, whereas the distal interphalangeal joints are seldom involved. Because the inflammatory swelling occurs only at the middle joints, the affected fingers become fusiform in the early stages of disease. The metacarpophalangeal and wrist joints may also become inflamed. At first, there is little restriction of motion in the involved joints, but stiffness, swelling, and pain prevent the patient from making a tight fist, thus weakening grip strength. Except for soft-tissue swelling, radiographs reveal no abnormalities.

Advanced Hand Involvement

As the disease progresses and the inflammation invades the joints, destroying articular cartilage and bone, joint motion becomes severely limited and joint deformities develop (Plate 3). Flexion deformities frequently occur at the proximal interphalangeal and metacarpophalangeal joints. The patient cannot fully extend or flex the fingers, and the grip becomes progressively weaker. Radiographs reveal cartilage thinning, bone erosions at the joint margins, and metaphyseal osteoporosis. After years of chronic inflammation, joint damage becomes severe; the joint capsule stretches; muscles atrophy and weaken; and tendons stretch, fray, and even rupture. All of these changes result in severe, incapacitating deformities.

A number of hand deformities are seen in the late stages of rheumatoid arthritis. For example, the muscles on the ulnar side of the fingers and wrist may overpower those of the radial group, causing ulnar deviation of the fingers at the metacarpophalangeal joints; the wrists may also be affected. The swan-neck deformity of the finger is common, as is the boutonniere deformity of the thumb, which is caused by hyperextension of the proximal interphalangeal joint and flexion at the metacarpophalangeal joint. The long extensor tendon may rupture near the distal interphalangeal joint, leaving the distal phalanx permanently flexed. Prolonged disease may lead to permanent subluxation or dislocation of the finger joints,

and severe cartilage and bone erosion at the wrist may literally destroy the carpus. In this late stage of the disease, radiographs help to define the severity of the structural damage and deformities.

Foot Involvement

Joint involvement in the foot resembles that in the hand, except for deformities that are determined chiefly by the foot's weight-bearing function (Plate 4). The toes usually become hyperextended, or cocked up, at the metatarsophalangeal joints and flexed at the proximal interphalangeal articulations (hammertoes). The joint capsules, fasciae, and tendons become stretched and weakened, and the metatarsal and longitudinal arches

flatten. Standing and walking exert great pressure on the osteoporotic metatarsal heads, causing severe erosion of the metatarsals. Frequently, plantar callosities develop under the metatarsal heads. Hallux valgus with bunion formation is also common. Cartilage thinning of the intertarsal joints is usually so severe that the tarsus becomes quite rigid, adding strain to the inflamed ankle joint. These structural changes make walking both difficult and painful.

Knee, Shoulder, and Hip Involvement

Inflammation of the large joints of the limbs causes a boggy and diffuse swelling of the soft tissues of the joints. In the elbows and knees, this

Foot Involvement in Rheumatoid Arthritis

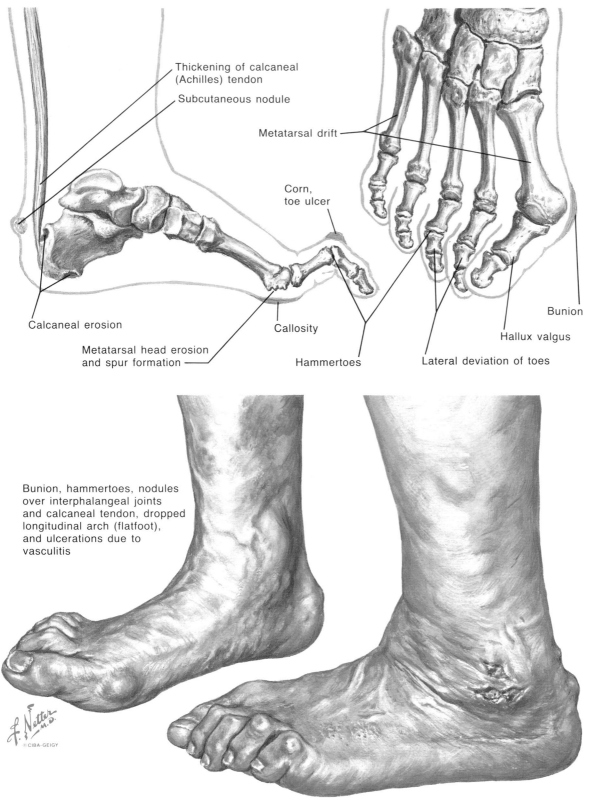

Thickening of calcaneal (Achilles) tendon

Subcutaneous nodule

Metatarsal drift

Corn, toe ulcer

Calcaneal erosion

Metatarsal head erosion and spur formation

Callosity

Hammertoes

Lateral deviation of toes

Hallux valgus

Bunion

Bunion, hammertoes, nodules over interphalangeal joints and calcaneal tendon, dropped longitudinal arch (flatfoot), and ulcerations due to vasculitis

Crippled foot with multiple nodules and callosities under metatarsal heads, hallux valgus with metatarsus varus, bunion, splayfoot, and hammertoes

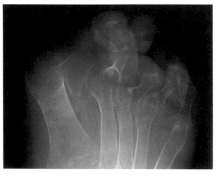

Radiograph shows severe erosion of metatarsal heads and bases of proximal phalanges, subluxation of metatarsophalangeal joints, marked osteoporosis, and severe hallux valgus

SECTION III PLATE 4   Slide 4585

Rheumatic Diseases

(Continued)

swelling is easily observed on physical examination (Plate 5). Involvement of the hip and shoulder joints, on the other hand, cannot be detected by inspection and palpation because the hips and, to a lesser degree, the shoulders lie deep beneath the skin and are well covered by fleshy muscles. Examination for range of motion elicits pain and

restricted movement if the joints are inflamed. In these large, well-covered joints, radiographs are required to evaluate the damage to the articular cartilage.

Flexion deformities can develop quickly at the knees and hips, making walking and arising from a sitting position difficult and painful. Extensive damage to the large joints in the limbs may cripple the patient, necessitating use of a cane, crutch, or walker, or confinement to a wheelchair or a bed.

Extraarticular Manifestations

Rheumatoid arthritis is a systemic illness—not just a disease of the joints—and thus has a variety

of nonarticular, or extraarticular, manifestations (Plates 6–7). Some of these features are occult, with little clinical importance, but others are clinically significant. In some cases, extraarticular features are the dominant clinical signs. Many rheumatologists prefer the term "rheumatic disease" to "rheumatoid arthritis," because of the extraordinarily broad range of nonarticular manifestations that, while integral to the illness, are not directly related to joint inflammation and its consequences.

Rheumatoid inflammation may be nodular or diffuse and may occur in parenchyma and connective tissues throughout the body. It therefore produces a variety of pathologic lesions in many

Knee, Shoulder, and Hip Joint Involvement in Rheumatoid Arthritis

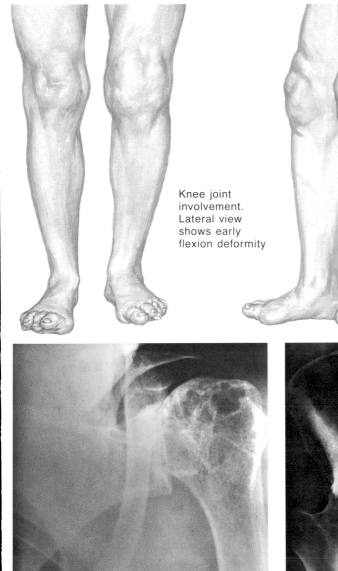

Knee joint involvement. Lateral view shows early flexion deformity

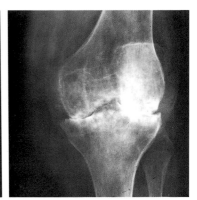

Radiograph shows thinning of cartilage in both compartments of knee joint

Same patient 4 years later. Progression of bone erosion and marked osteoporosis

Severe crippling deformities of multiple joints

Shoulder joint involvement. Severe osteoporosis in head of humerus and thinning of cartilage at glenohumeral joint

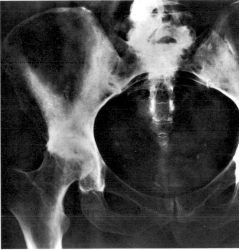

Hip joint involvement. Thinning of articular cartilages and flattening and medial migration of femoral head

Flexion contracture of hip joint

SECTION III PLATE 5 Slide 4586

Rheumatic Diseases
(Continued)

locations. The inflammation of the nonarticular connective tissue has the same characteristics as the synovitis: it is a proliferative inflammatory reaction containing lymphocytes, macrophages, and plasma cells. The lymphocytes often cluster in a follicular pattern.

Rheumatoid Nodules. In about 15% of cases, nodules develop in connective tissue along tendons, at tendon sheaths, in bursa and joint capsules, and in the subcutaneous connective tissue around bony prominences (Plate 6). A common place for nodules to occur is a few centimeters distal to the olecranon process of the ulna. The nodules in subcutaneous tissue are freely movable; those that originate in the periosteum are firmly attached to the underlying bone. Rheumatoid nodules occur singly or in aggregate in clusters, and they vary in size from 1 mm to more than 2 cm in diameter.

When surrounded by soft tissue, rheumatoid nodules are painless, but nodules located over

bony prominences are often painful when pressure is exerted on them. For example, nodules around the ischial tuberosity cause pain when the patient sits on a firm seat, and nodules over spinous processes or the occipital protuberance make lying supine on a firm surface painful. Similarly, those occurring on the plantar surface of the foot cause discomfort when standing or walking. Nodules located over the knuckles, toes, or knees may restrict motion in the underlying joint.

The presence of rheumatoid nodules greatly aids diagnosis of rheumatoid arthritis because they occur with no other form of chronic arthritis. However, nodular swellings near joints and along the border of the ulna are associated with

Crippled hand with subcutaneous nodules over knuckles, swan-neck deformity of middle finger, ulnar deviation of fingers, and muscle atrophy

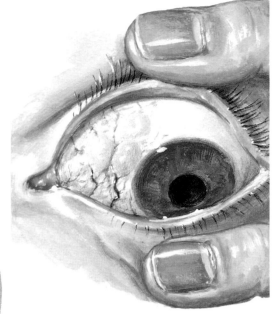

Nodular episcleritis with scleromalacia

Subcutaneous nodule just distal to olecranon process, and another in olecranon bursa

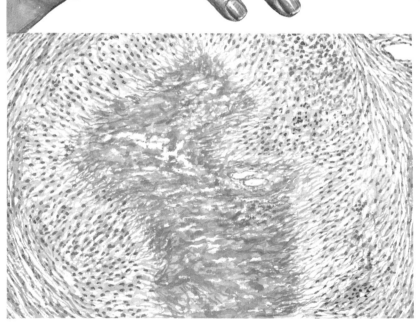

Section of rheumatoid nodule. Central area of fibrinoid necrosis surrounded by zone of palisading mesenchymal cells and peripheral fibrous tissue capsule containing chronic inflammatory cells

Radiograph shows rheumatoid nodule in right lung. Lesion may be misdiagnosed as carcinoma until identified by biopsy or postsurgical pathologic analysis

SECTION III   PLATE 6   Slide 4587

Rheumatic Diseases
(Continued)

other illnesses (eg, urate deposits, or tophi, in gout). If the nature of the nodular swelling is not clear, excision and microscopic study of the tissue are advised. Characteristic histopathologic features of rheumatoid nodules are (1) a central zone of fibrinoid degeneration surrounded by (2) an intermediate zone of palisading epithelioid cells

and (3) an outer coat of granulation tissue infiltrated with lymphocytes and plasma cells.

Pulmonary Involvement. Rheumatoid nodules may develop in the parenchyma of the lung (Plate 6). On radiographs, a solitary nodule often cannot be differentiated from a neoplasm, but histologic study of the lesion reveals the pathologic features of a rheumatoid nodule. Caplan's syndrome is a unique form of pneumoconiosis that may be a granulomatous response to chronic exposure to silica dust. It is especially prevalent in coal miners. Widely distributed and particularly prevalent in the periphery, the nodules usually appear abruptly, with little or no evidence of prior pneumoconiosis. They may occur before,

during, or after the onset of arthritis. Patients with Caplan's syndrome usually have a high serum titer of rheumatoid factor. Progressive interstitial fibrosis and pleurisy with or without effusion are other pulmonary manifestations of rheumatic disease.

Cardiac Involvement. In the myocardium, rheumatoid nodules may cause cardiac conduction defects. Pericarditis may occur but is rarely symptomatic; if effusion develops, the fluid, like rheumatoid pleural effusion, has a very low sugar content. This characteristic effusion is a helpful diagnostic finding. Constrictive pericarditis and valvular granulomatous lesions (usually aortic) are rare.

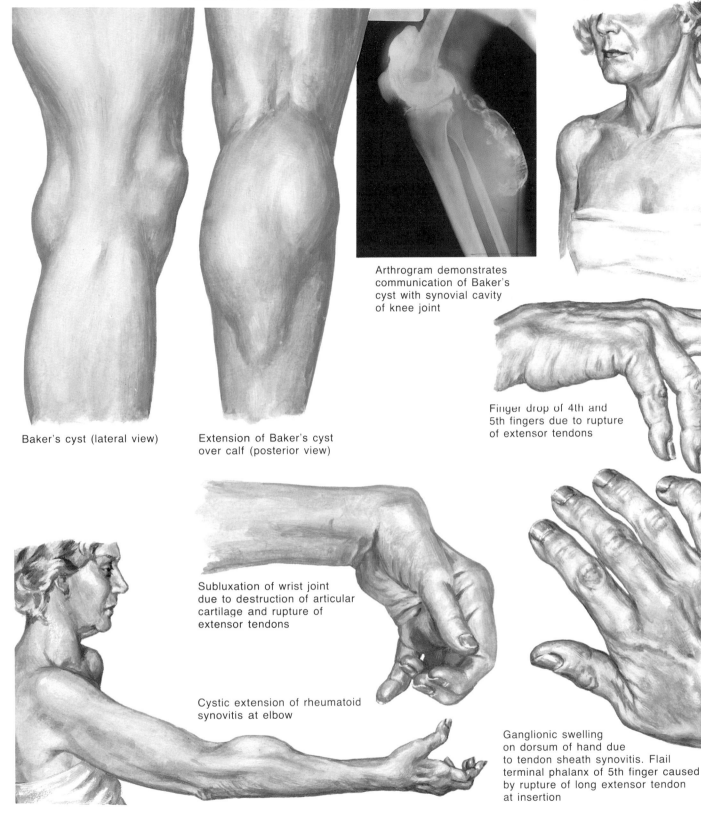

Baker's cyst (lateral view)

Extension of Baker's cyst over calf (posterior view)

Arthrogram demonstrates communication of Baker's cyst with synovial cavity of knee joint

Soft-tissue cystic swelling of capsules of both shoulders

Finger drop of 4th and 5th fingers due to rupture of extensor tendons

Subluxation of wrist joint due to destruction of articular cartilage and rupture of extensor tendons

Cystic extension of rheumatoid synovitis at elbow

Ganglionic swelling on dorsum of hand due to tendon sheath synovitis. Flail terminal phalanx of 5th finger caused by rupture of long extensor tendon at insertion

SECTION III PLATE 7   Slide 4588

Rheumatic Diseases

(Continued)

Ocular Changes. Keratoconjunctivitis is commonly associated with rheumatoid arthritis. Granulomatous scleritis occurs less often but may lead to scleromalacia perforans (Plate 6).

Nervous System Involvement. The dura mater is another site of rheumatoid nodules. A more frequent clinical manifestation, however, is peripheral neuropathy due to inflammation in the arterioles supplying the nerve. Peripheral nerve compression from localized articular or nonarticular inflammation surrounding the nerve (eg, compression of the median nerve in carpal tunnel syndrome) is also common. Ulnar neuropathy and radial nerve palsy are seen less often.

Periarticular Fibrous-Tissue Manifestations. In many cases, the inflammation affects specialized periarticular fibrous-tissue structures, most commonly tendons, tendon sheaths, and bursae (Plate 7). The periarticular inflammation has the same proliferative and invasive characteristics as synovitis. Tendonitis and tenosynovitis may cause the tendon to rupture, and in some patients, the periarticular inflammation causes as much pain, stiffness, and disability as the arthritis. Muscle weakness and atrophy occur in late stages of rheumatoid arthritis.

Rheumatoid Vasculitis. Now recognized as a major manifestation of rheumatoid arthritis, vasculitis is classified by pathologic changes into three main categories: (1) intimal proliferation of digital arteries causing ischemic areas in the nail fold, nail edge, or digital pulp; (2) subacute lesions in small vessels of muscles, nerves, heart, and other tissues; and (3) widespread fulminant necrotizing arteritis of medium and large vessels. Leukocytosis, scleritis, neuropathy, mesenteric

Rheumatic Diseases

(Continued)

Immunologic Features in Rheumatoid Arthritis

Immunofluorescence studies of synovium

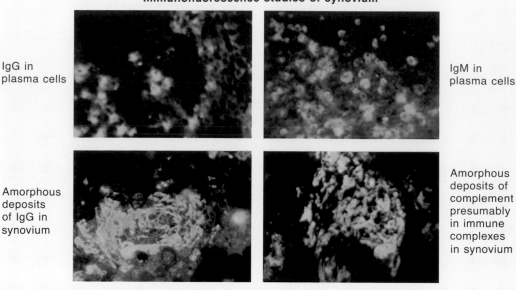

IgG in
plasma cells

IgM in
plasma cells

Amorphous
deposits
of IgG in
synovium

Amorphous
deposits of
complement
presumably
in immune
complexes
in synovium

Latex fixation test for rheumatoid factor

Serum containing rheumatoid factor causes agglutination of latex
particles coated with human IgG (commercially available)

Negative
result

Positive
result

infarction, and ischemic skin ulceration or gangrene are commonly associated with occlusive or necrotizing arteritis.

Rheumatoid arthritis complicated by vasculitis is associated with severe and long-standing joint inflammation, elevated serum titers of rheumatoid factor, diminished serum complement levels, rheumatoid nodules and other extraarticular manifestations, and a poor prognosis. The detection of IgG, IgM, and complement components in the inflamed arterial wall supports the hypothesis that rheumatoid vasculitis is due to the deposition of soluble immune complexes in the vessel wall (Plate 8).

Other Manifestations. Mild-to-moderate anemia is typical of active disease, with the exception of mild cases, and is largely due to a relative failure of bone marrow production because of increased uptake and abnormal storage of iron by the reticuloendothelial system and the phagocytic cells of the inflamed, hyperplastic synovial membrane. Unless an iron deficiency supervenes, the erythrocytes are normocytic and only slightly hypochromic. Impaired absorption of iron from the gastrointestinal tract and, in some cases, bleeding into the gastrointestinal tract caused by salicylates or other therapeutic drugs also contribute to the development of anemia.

Osteoporosis in the metaphyses of bones adjacent to inflamed joints begins early. In advanced disease, especially when weight-bearing activity is curtailed, the osteoporosis becomes generalized and often severe.

Although generalized lymphadenopathy is a frequent finding, splenomegaly occurs in only about 5% of patients. When accompanied by leukopenia, the disorder is known as Felty's syndrome. Leukopenia, if severe, may lead to serious infection. Other manifestations of Felty's syndrome include rheumatoid nodules, chronic leg ulcers, peripheral neuropathy, thrombocytopenia, anemia (often severe), keratoconjunctivitis sicca, as well as increased myeloid activity, and very high titers of rheumatoid factor.

In the late stage of rheumatoid disease, secondary amyloidosis may occur, but this is relatively uncommon.

Immunologic Features

The serum of most patients with rheumatoid arthritis contains immunoglobulins, or antibodies, against gamma globulin (IgG), which are called *rheumatoid factors*. The latex fixation tests commonly used in the diagnosis of rheumatoid arthritis detect only the IgM class of rheumatoid factor, which is most prevalent; however, IgG and, to a lesser extent, IgA rheumatoid factors are also found. All classes of rheumatoid factor act as antibodies to IgG (which acts as antigen) to form immune complexes. In rheumatoid arthritis, some rheumatoid factor is produced in the synovium. Some of the IgG and IgM shown in plasma cells (Plate 8) consists of rheumatoid factor. Immune complexes containing rheumatoid factor, IgG, and complement are prominent in vacuoles of synovial fluid cells as well as in synovial macrophages and interstitium.

Rheumatoid factor–containing immune complexes can activate complement, thus releasing chemotactic factors, and can then be phagocytized by polymorphonuclear neutrophils, leading to release of leukotrienes, proteolytic enzymes, and generation of destructive oxygen-free radicals. Complement activation also generates proinflammatory anaphylatoxins. Complexes are often sequestered in cartilage, where they may provide a reservoir of immune response–stimulating antigen and may attract pannus cells toward this tissue. The immune complexes also appear to be

important in extraarticular disease because they deposit in vessel walls and cause vasculitis.

The *latex fixation test* detects the presence of rheumatoid factors in serum. The patient's serum is combined with a suspension of latex particles coated with IgG. Rheumatoid factors, if present, become fixed to the IgG-coated particles, forming a precipitate. The titer of rheumatoid factor in the serum determined by tube dilutions approximately parallels the severity of the disease. Rheumatoid factor is thought to play an important role in *perpetuating* disease activity by way of its immunologic reactions with IgG, but most likely it does not initiate the disease. The initiating factor (or factors) is still unknown; a variety of infectious agents have been considered, but none has been confirmed.

A genetic predisposition is an important factor in determining the immune response to the still-unknown initiating factors. The class II antigen HLA-DR4 is associated with an increased incidence of rheumatoid arthritis in many populations, but it is not present in all patients with rheumatoid arthritis. Early disease is associated with synovial microvascular lesions, proliferation of lining cells, and infiltration by small numbers of mononuclear cells. The antigen-processing cells (macrophages and dendritic cells) release interleukin-1, which stimulates the proliferation of lining cells and release of a variety of prostaglandins and collagenase. Interleukin-1 can also act on chondrocytes and T lymphocytes (T cells). In patients with rheumatoid arthritis, the synovium becomes heavily infiltrated with lymphocytes, including a higher percentage of helper

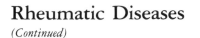

Rheumatic Diseases

(*Continued*)

Variable Clinical Course of Adult Rheumatoid Arthritis: Prognosis Difficult in Early Stage

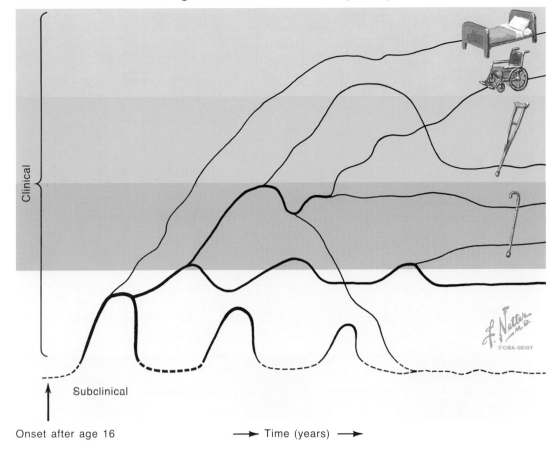

Subclinical

Onset after age 16   ⟶ Time (years) ⟶

T cells. The latter activate B cells, leading to plasma-cell formation, and also release a number of lymphokines that can have various modulating effects on inflammation. Other factors released from monocytes and mast cells interact as the disease evolves into the proliferative and erosive process typical of rheumatoid arthritis.

Analysis of synovial fluid shows pathologic changes characteristic of rheumatoid arthritis: increased volume; increased leukocyte count (>10,000/mm³), with a preponderance of mononuclear or polymorphonuclear cells at different stages of disease and in different patients. Activated T lymphocytes are commonly present. There is poor viscosity due to diluted and denatured hyaluronate and low complement levels. Synovial fluid leukocytes often contain inclusion particles that are made up of IgG, rheumatoid factor, and complement. Many of the modulators of inflammation discussed above can be identified in joint fluid in rheumatoid arthritis but are not routinely measured.

The increase in the erythrocyte sedimentation rate (ESR) usually correlates with the severity of the disease activity. This laboratory test is therefore of some value in the diagnosis of patients with the less classic form of the disease and in monitoring the course of the illness.

Etiology and Pathogenesis

Although the etiology of rheumatoid arthritis is not yet understood, many causative factors have been proposed, including infectious microorganisms such as *Streptococcus*, *Mycoplasma*, and *Erysipelothrix*; metabolic and biochemical derangements; abnormal physiologic change (eg, altered blood flow); neurogenic factors; and genetic aberrations. Many investigators propose that a viral infection is the initial event, although viral particles have not been demonstrated by electron microscopy or recovered from joint tissues, nor has the persistence of virus (slow virus) been established. Another hypothesis is that the disease results from a spontaneous autoimmune reaction in genetically susceptible persons.

It is widely believed that rheumatoid arthritis develops in a person with a genetic predisposition

following exposure to an infectious agent (possibly viral). It is also possible that the illness results from an inappropriate immune response to a ubiquitous pathogenic agent. In the absence of an established cause, physicians can only evaluate each clinical and laboratory abnormality in relation to the disease and speculate on its etiologic significance.

Results of numerous laboratory studies have clarified the major role of immunologic reactions in the pathogenesis and perpetuation of rheumatoid inflammation as follows: infiltration of the synovial membrane with lymphoid cells and macrophages, often with follicular formation; detection of IgG and synthesis of rheumatoid factor by plasma cells in the synovial membrane and nearby lymph nodes; diminished complement components in synovial effusion; presence of IgG, IgM, and complement components in inclusion bodies in synovial cells; presence of antigen-antibody complexes (especially IgG-IgG rheumatoid factor) in synovial fluid; and existence of IgG-IgM rheumatoid factor complexes and complement components in rheumatoid arthritis cells in synovial fluid. These observations have led to the following proposed sequence of events in the course of rheumatic disease: (1) An unknown causative factor (antigen), carried to the joint by the circulation, initiates synovitis. (2) The antigen establishes itself in the joint cavity and stimulates the local production of antibody (and secondarily, rheumatoid factor). (3) The antigen and antibody interact, forming immune complexes, and the interaction of the resulting immune complex with rheumatoid factor in the synovial membrane and fluid stimulates a sequence of events that generates chemotactic factors. (4) These chemotactic factors attract cellular elements of the blood into the perivascular space.

(5) Polymorphonuclear leukocytes and macrophages in the vessel wall and perivascular space phagocytize immune complexes, using receptors for IgG and complement component C3 on their surface. (6) Engulfment follows, with release of lysosomal hydrolytic enzymes that destroy cartilage and mediate proliferation of granulation tissue, which invades bone, adding to the joint damage. Cartilage is also injured by the mediator interleukin-1 released by macrophages in the lining and sublining layers of the synovial membrane. Interleukin-1 stimulates the chondrocytes to release lysosomal enzymes in the interior of the cartilage.

In a small group of patients with rheumatoid factor, soluble immune complexes are present in the serum. These immune complexes contain IgM and IgG rheumatoid factors and IgG and deposit in the walls of blood vessels, causing vasculitis.

Clinical Course and Prognosis

The clinical course of rheumatoid arthritis is characterized by remissions and relapses. In the first few months after onset, the course of the disease cannot be predicted because it is so variable (Plate 9). Only repeated observation of the patient with active disease allows the physician to determine the prognosis. Factors associated with a poor prognosis include persistence of active illness for longer than a year, presence of rheumatoid nodules, high serum titers of rheumatoid factor, and extraarticular manifestations.

Early and prolonged remission is more likely if the disease is mild at onset. Although partial or even complete remission may occur at any time and continue for a long time, complete remission is seldom seen after 3 or 4 years of continuously active disease.

Rheumatic Diseases

(Continued)

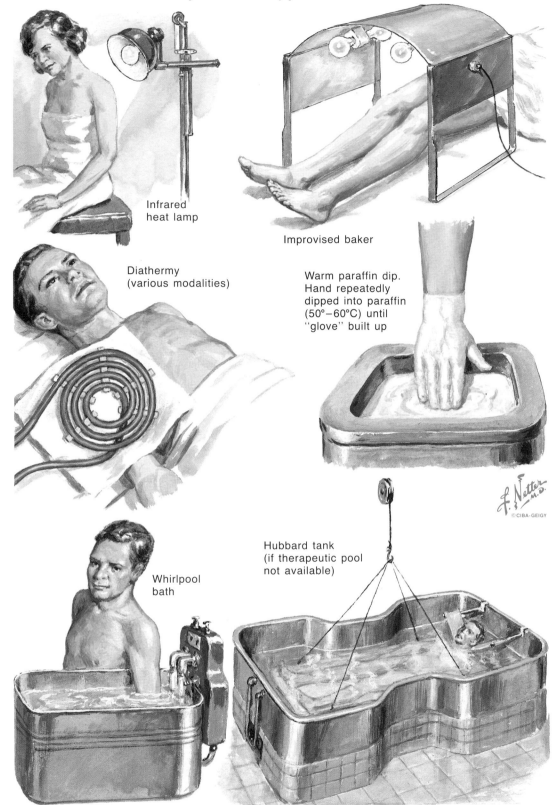

Infrared heat lamp

Improvised baker

Diathermy (various modalities)

Warm paraffin dip. Hand repeatedly dipped into paraffin (50°–60°C) until "glove" built up

Whirlpool bath

Hubbard tank (if therapeutic pool not available)

Although appropriate therapy cannot completely arrest the disease process, it does relieve joint pain, allows patients to be more active, and helps to avoid disability and incapacitation. However, studies of large groups of patients in arthritis study centers indicate that the effectiveness of treatment—regardless of the type—diminishes as the disease becomes more chronic. The amount of joint damage and disability is greater after 10 years of continuously active disease than after 5 years and is greater still after 15 years.

Diagnosis

Early in the course of the disease, when synovitis and mild systemic illness are the only clinical manifestations, it is often very difficult to distinguish rheumatoid arthritis from other rheumatic diseases. As there is no reliable laboratory test for rheumatoid arthritis, diagnosis depends on the judgment of a well-informed physician, usually based on frequent physical examinations and laboratory studies performed over many months. The most significant diagnostic findings are synovitis in many joints (especially paired joints in the limbs); systemic signs and symptoms; elevated ESR; circulating rheumatoid factor in serum; and rheumatoid nodules. However, circulating rheumatoid factor may not be detected for many months after the onset of illness, and many patients remain seronegative. Likewise, radiographic changes become visible only after months of persistent joint inflammation.

Diagnosis is not difficult after the illness has become chronic or when any of the following manifestations are present: rheumatoid nodules; rheumatoid factor in serum; characteristic joint deformities; and radiographic evidence of articular cartilage thinning, subchondral bone destruction, joint deformity, or ankylosis.

Criteria. The following criteria, formulated by the American Rheumatism Association, are a reliable basis for accurate diagnosis:

- Morning stiffness
- Pain and tenderness in at least one joint
- Joint swelling due to thickening of soft tissue and/or increased joint fluid (not bony overgrowth) in at least one joint

- Swelling of at least one other joint within 3 months of onset of the second and third criteria
- Bilateral, symmetric joint swelling. (Finger and toe joint involvement need not be absolutely symmetric; terminal interphalangeal involvement does not satisfy this criterion)
- Rheumatoid nodules
- Radiographic changes typical of rheumatoid arthritis (including decalcification of bone adjacent to inflamed joints)
- Positive latex fixation test for rheumatoid factor
- Poor precipitation of mucin clots in synovial fluid

- Characteristic findings in the synovial membrane with three or more of the following signs: marked villous hypertrophy; proliferation, often with palisading, of synovial lining cells; abundant infiltration of inflammatory cells (chiefly lymphocytes and plasma cells) that tend to form lymphoid follicles; deposition of compact fibrin on synovial surface or in interstitium; foci of necrotic cells
- Characteristic histopathologic findings in nodules: granulomatous foci with central zones of cell necrosis surrounded by proliferative fixed cells and peripheral fibrosis infiltrated with chronic inflammatory cells, predominantly in perivascular sites

Rheumatic Diseases
(Continued)

Exercises for Upper Limbs

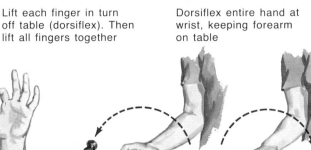

Place hand and forearm flat on table, palm down. Spread fingers apart and bring together

Lift each finger in turn off table (dorsiflex). Then lift all fingers together

Dorsiflex entire hand at wrist, keeping forearm on table

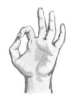

Open and clench hand successively, spreading fingers widely on opening

Touch each finger in turn to thumb, pinching firmly

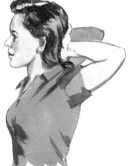

Grasp hammer firmly by handle, holding arm snugly to side. Rotate forearm so that hammerhead swings from side to side. Degree of resistance can be varied by gripping closer to or farther from hammerhead

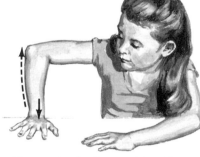

Place palm firmly on table with forearm horizontal. Raise elbow as high as possible while pressing down on table

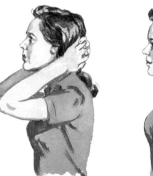

Place hands behind head. Draw elbows back as far as possible, simultaneously pulling chin in and pushing head back

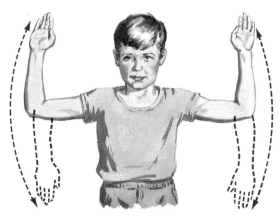

Extend arms sideways with elbows flexed 90°. Swing hands and forearms down and up, thus rotating shoulders

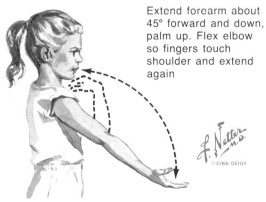

Extend forearm about 45° forward and down, palm up. Flex elbow so fingers touch shoulder and extend again

A diagnosis of *classic* rheumatoid arthritis requires seven of these criteria to be met; the clinical features listed in the first five criteria must persist for at least 6 weeks. A diagnosis of *definite* rheumatoid arthritis is made on the basis of five criteria, including at least one of the first five, which must be present for 6 weeks or longer. If only three criteria exist, including at least one of the first five for 6 weeks, the diagnosis of rheumatoid arthritis is considered only *probable*. *Possible* rheumatoid arthritis is suggested by the presence of two of the six following features for at least 3 weeks: (1) morning stiffness, (2) tenderness or pain on motion, (3) history (or observation by physician) of joint swelling, (4) subcutaneous rheumatoid nodules, (5) elevated ESR, and (6) iridocyclitis.

Exclusions. Even if the required criteria are met, the diagnosis of rheumatoid arthritis is not tenable if any of the following 17 findings exist:

- High serum concentration of lupus erythematosus (LE) cells
- Typical erythematous dermatitis of systemic lupus erythematosus
- Histologic evidence of polyarteritis nodosa, dermatomyositis, tuberculous arthritis, or sarcoidosis
- Definite diagnosis of scleroderma not limited to fingers
- Clinical picture of rheumatic fever
- Typical attacks of gouty arthritis, especially if relieved by colchicine therapy
- Tophi
- Clinical picture of acute infectious arthritis, especially if there is evidence of bacteria in inflamed joints, acute focus of infection, or arthritis closely associated with a systemic disease of known infectious etiology
- Tubercle bacilli in inflamed joints
- Clinical picture of Reiter's syndrome
- Unilateral shoulder-hand syndrome
- Clinical picture of hypertrophic pulmonary osteoarthropathy
- Neuroarthropathy
- Alkaptonuria and ochronosis

- Erythema nodosum
- Multiple myeloma
- Leukemia or lymphoma

Careful application of these criteria and exclusions can minimize errors in diagnosis. The many exclusions underscore the importance of differentiating rheumatoid arthritis from the many illnesses that have similar features. Thus, differential diagnosis requires a complete and detailed medical history, a complete physical examination, and supplemental laboratory and radiographic studies. The clinical examination and appropriate laboratory studies may have to be repeated every 2 or 3 months in order to refine the diagnosis. Examination of the joints alone is not sufficient

because accurate diagnosis also depends on the recognition of *extraarticular* pathology.

Although no one laboratory test is diagnostic for rheumatoid arthritis, results of serologic studies and immunofluorescent microscopy—considered along with all the other criteria—help to establish the diagnosis; examination of synovial fluid also contributes valuable information (Plates 14–16). The latex fixation test for rheumatoid factor, although useful, cannot differentiate rheumatoid arthritis from other illnesses characterized by chronic joint inflammation, such as systemic lupus erythematosus. Moreover, rheumatoid factor is not detected in approximately 20% of patients with rheumatoid arthritis

Rheumatic Diseases
(Continued)

Standing with arms at side, raise arms sideways in wide arc as high as possible over head and return to side

Swing arms forward and up instead of sideways. Exercises may also be done in lying or sitting position

and may be found in patients with other rheumatic diseases as well as in some apparently healthy persons, usually over 60 years of age. Also, antinuclear antibodies may be present in the serum of some patients with rheumatoid arthritis.

In most patients, it is easy to distinguish rheumatoid arthritis from osteoarthritis, the other common form of chronic arthritis, because of the basic difference in joint pathology (Plates 21–24). Also, rheumatoid arthritis is a chronic systemic inflammatory disease that usually affects young and middle-aged persons, whereas osteoarthritis is a localized degenerative disease that involves weight-bearing joints (and often the distal interphalangeal joints) in elderly persons. However, rheumatoid arthritis and osteoarthritis may coexist in older persons.

Polyarthritis is a prominent component of systemic lupus erythematosus, a multisystem disease. The joint inflammation in systemic lupus erythematosus is clinically indistinguishable from that of rheumatoid arthritis; therefore, differentiation of these two diseases is difficult or impossible, especially in the early stages. The immune system plays an important role in the pathogenesis and course of each of these diseases. However, the abnormal immunologic features of each illness differ sharply and, consequently, proper laboratory studies of the immune response play an important diagnostic role in differentiating them. Because the involvement of the central nervous system and visceral organs is more serious than the polyarthritis of systemic lupus erythematosus, discussion and illustration of this illness are not included in this section but can be found in CIBA COLLECTION volumes on the heart, kidneys, and respiratory system (see Volume 5, page 180; Volume 6, pages 141–143; and Volume 7, page 261).

Treatment

Patient education is a key factor in the success of the treatment program. Understanding the nature of the disease helps the patient to maintain a proper outlook and to function within the limitations imposed by its changing course. Pessimism should be avoided. Many persons fear permanent crippling and incapacitation. These

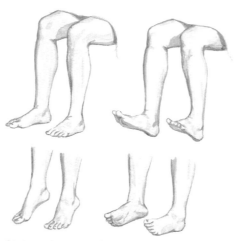

Lying on back, alternately draw each knee up as close as possible to chest, lower, and extend

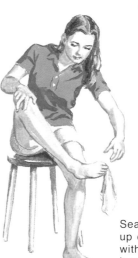

Sitting with legs hanging over table edge, extend knee against resistance (supplied by another person)

Sitting with soles flat on floor, first raise toes as high as possible, return to starting position, raise heels, and finally turn soles inward to face each other

Seated on stool, pick up cloth or other object with toes and deliver it to opposite hand

patients need to be reassured that the degree of severity varies, that the disease is often mild, that complete remissions occur, and that although there is no cure, proper treatment can control or even slow disease progression, in most cases preventing serious deformity and incapacitation. The physician should emphasize the remitting nature of the disease and the benefits of cooperation with a proper treatment program.

No single treatment is adequate for rheumatoid arthritis. Rather, management of the disease is a balanced, integrated program of many treatment modalities designed specifically for each patient. Treatment must also be altered periodically as the disease progresses. The program

should be aimed at relief of discomfort; maintenance of good muscle strength and maximal joint motion; prevention of deformity; suppression of the inflammatory process; maintenance of proper nutrition; maintenance of general health by eliminating or controlling complications and/or unrelated concurrent disease; correction of joint deformities, if present; and rehabilitation of crippled patients.

The chief complaint of most patients with rheumatoid arthritis is pain—joint pain, myalgia, and stiffness. Consequently, analgesia is the primary goal of every therapeutic program. Medication, physical therapy, and nonweight-bearing rest are the standard methods of pain relief.

Devices Used to Rest Inflamed Joints and Prevent Deformities

Rheumatic Diseases

(Continued)

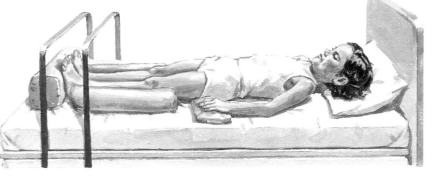

Sandbags keep joints in alignment. Cushioned foot board may be used in place of sandbag to support feet at right angle. Cradle keeps weight of blankets off feet; bed board under mattress

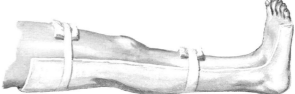

Rest splint for wrist and hand. If only wrist treated, cast may be shortened distally to permit finger function

Rest splint for knee, ankle, and foot. Foot at right angle and in slight varus rotation, cast molded to arch. If only foot and ankle treated, cast may be shortened to below knee

Analgesic and Antiinflammatory Medication. Over the years, acetylsalicylic acid (aspirin) and other salicylic acid derivatives have been the most commonly used analgesic medications for rheumatic pain. Used in adequate amounts and in properly divided doses, aspirin is a reliable, usually well-tolerated, and inexpensive analgesic. For many rheumatologists, aspirin is still the drug of choice in the initial treatment of rheumatoid arthritis. If aspirin is not tolerated in the amounts needed for pain relief and antiinflammatory effects, aspirin substitutes, known as nonsteroidal antiinflammatory drugs (NSAIDs), can be used. As NSAIDs may be toxic in older patients, their use must be supervised by an experienced physician alert to the signs of toxicity.

The antiinflammatory effect of NSAIDs is comparable to, or greater than, that of aspirin, and the incidence of gastrointestinal side effects is considerably lower. For these reasons, and because NSAIDs are administered only once or twice daily, some physicians prefer them to aspirin.

Physical Therapy

Heat when applied to painful joints, muscles, and connective tissue via warm baths, warm compresses, poultices, heating pads, infrared lamps, diathermy, ultrasonography, paraffin dips, and whirlpool or therapeutic baths is most effective in relieving the discomforts of rheumatoid arthritis, especially aching and stiffness (Plate 10). Specific techniques, such as appropriate exercises, also help maintain muscle strength and joint motion and prevent deformity.

Rest and Splints

Abundant rest is essential, especially early in the illness, and complete bed rest may be necessary for short periods (Plate 13). However, a balanced and moderate program of rest and therapeutic exercises must be maintained. Although excessive use of an inflamed joint aggravates the synovitis and increases pain, especially in weight-bearing joints, prolonged and complete immobility quickly leads to marked stiffness, even irreversible ankylosis. Slings, braces, splints, and rest molds can be used to rest and support affected limbs but must be removable for daily exercising. Sandbags, footboard, and bed board are used to maintain the joints in proper alignment and prevent deformities.

Exercises

Therapeutic exercises help to maintain good muscle strength and joint motion (Plates 11–12). The exercises should be nonweight bearing, extend through the full range of motion, and be performed only within the limits of pain. When joints are severely inflamed, assisted exercises or isometric exercises may be required. Underwater exercise (in a therapeutic pool or Hubbard tank) simultaneously relieves the force of gravity and provides heat to enhance the value of the exercise (Plate 10).

Treatment of Progressive Disease

The basic conservative measures described above are appropriate in the initial treatment of all patients with rheumatoid arthritis. In fact, many patients require no additional treatment, although those with more severe, prolonged, and worsening disease may need more potent means of suppressing the inflammatory process. These measures primarily include administration of antiinflammatory agents such as gold preparations, penicillamine, hydroxychloroquine, methotrexate, corticosteroids, and immunosuppressive or cytotoxic agents. Because these antiinflammatory agents may cause serious toxic reactions, their use involves a calculated risk and must be supervised by an experienced rheumatologist and monitored with all appropriate clinical and laboratory studies to detect early toxicity. The drugs should be administered only when the risk of crippling from unrelenting progressive disease clearly outweighs the risk of toxicity. Many physicians first try gold salts, penicillamine, or hydroxychloroquine. Only if these agents are inadequate or poorly tolerated should corticosteroids or a cytotoxic agent be substituted.

Local treatment of inflamed joints may supplement the prolonged systemic treatment. These measures include medication (chiefly intraarticular steroid injection), correction of flexion contractures by splinting, and surgery. Recently, arthroscopy has been used to excise proliferative synovial tissue from chronically swollen large joints.

Flexion contractures and other mild deformities that develop early in the illness may respond to nonsurgical procedures such as physical therapy. However, damaged articular cartilage, bone, ligaments, and tendons resulting in deformity usually require surgery. Many surgical advances have contributed to the treatment of rheumatoid arthritis, including repair of ruptured tendons, realignment of angulated joints, stabilization of unstable joints, and release of ankylosed joints. Surgery, if needed, should be done as an adjunct to active chemotherapy. Badly damaged joints seen in late disease require replacement with a total joint prosthesis (see Section IV).

Management of the patient is usually the responsibility of the primary physician, and treatment most often takes place in the home. However, the team approach has advantages in the planning of treatment, evaluation of response, and adjustment of therapy in response to changes in the course of the disease. This can best be provided in a rheumatism center equipped with appropriate facilities and a staff of medical, surgical, and allied health professionals.

Although rheumatoid arthritis cannot be cured, it can usually be controlled to enable the patient to live a reasonably comfortable, active, and useful life without severe crippling and incapacitation. □

Synovial Fluid Examination

Techniques for Arthrocentesis

After the careful history and physical examination, aspiration of joint fluid (arthrocentesis) with laboratory analysis is probably the most valuable procedure in the evaluation of joint disease. Analysis of joint fluid is the only way to begin determining exactly what pathologic process is occurring in a joint, and it is the only method to confirm the presence of infectious arthritis or crystal-induced arthritis such as gout or pseudogout. In a study of 180 consecutive patients with knee effusions, about 20% of the initial diagnoses suggested by clinical signs and history were changed after analysis of joint fluid.

While this procedure is too important to be limited to rheumatologists and orthopedists, these specialists should be consulted for joints that are difficult to aspirate, such as the hips and temporomandibular joints. Other joints are aspirated as shown on Plate 14. The knee is probably easiest to aspirate because simply positioning the needle beneath the patella ensures that it has penetrated the joint. Sites for arthrocentesis are frequently on the extensor surface and should be distant from larger vessels and nerves.

The joint aspirated should be one that is symptomatic and swollen. The area is cleaned and the site for needle puncture marked on the skin. The skin is infiltrated with a solution of 1% xylocaine for superficial anesthesia, or some analgesia is obtained with a quick application of ethyl chloride spray. The aspiration needle should be at least a 20 gauge (22-gauge needles may be needed for finger joints).

Gloves should be worn for any procedures involving the handling of body fluids. One hand is used to identify the anatomic landmarks, with care not to touch the needle. The initial thrust should be decisive; if fluid is not readily obtained, the position of the needle can be readjusted a little without withdrawing it. A 10-ml syringe is usually easiest to use unless the effusion is massive. A little fluid can be obtained from almost any joint, even knees and digits that appear clinically normal. An assistant may be needed to help "milk" fluid into the area of the needle. Only 1 ml of fluid is required for a thorough synovial fluid analysis, but more fluid may be removed, if needed, to relieve symptoms in a distended joint. Even drops of fluid can allow identification of crystals or infectious agents.

The same procedure is used for intraarticular injections of depot corticosteroids. This treatment provides temporary relief for some patients with severe osteoarthritis, rheumatoid arthritis, or other types of inflammatory arthritis. Triamcinolone hexacetonide and prednisolone tebutate are examples of steroids appropriate for injection. Synovial fluid should always be examined as part of the injection procedure and injection avoided if there are any signs of joint infection.

Based on the clinical signs and the symptoms reported by the patient, the specific tests and stains needed are determined before aspiration

Techniques for Aspiration of Joint Fluid

Knee. Needle inserted horizontally at medial or lateral margin of patella to pass beneath patella. 20-gauge needle used for most joints

Ankle. Needle inserted just above and lateral to medial malleolus and medial to extensor hallucis longus tendon

Shoulder. Needle inserted at or just below coracoid process and medial to head of humerus

Elbow. With joint flexed 90°, needle inserted below lateral epicondyle and above olecranon

Finger joints. With joint partially flexed, 20- to 22-gauge needle inserted obliquely from dorsomedial or dorsolateral aspect

Wrist. With joint slightly flexed, needle inserted just distal to radius at ulnar margin of extensor pollicis longus tendon (demarcation of anatomic snuffbox)

(Plates 15–16). If infection is suspected, some fluid must be kept in the sterile syringe for prompt delivery to the laboratory.

Complications from joint aspiration are very rare. Iatrogenic infection occurs in less than 1 of 7,000 patients. To avoid this problem, the route of aspiration should not be through areas of cutaneous inflammation. Hemarthrosis resulting from a traumatic arthrocentesis ("bloody tap") is a very rare complication, and cautious aspiration can be done even in patients being treated with anticoagulants. No special care is needed after the procedure, but rest for 1 to 2 days may increase the effect of injected corticosteroids.

Gross Inspection

Analysis of joint fluid must begin with gross inspection. The fluid's appearance—clarity, presence of blood, and viscosity—often gives clues to the diagnosis and thus influences the physician's selection of laboratory tests.

The *clarity* of the fluid is assessed by expressing a small amount of fluid out of the plastic syringe into a glass tube. (Plastic tubes have a slight

Synovial Fluid Examination

(Continued)

opacity that may confuse the results.) Printed words viewed through normal and noninflammatory joint fluid can be read easily (Plate 15). Cloudy fluid is not typical of uncomplicated osteoarthritis and therefore suggests an inflammatory disease such as rheumatoid arthritis. An opaque, pasty fluid is most often due to pus, thus indicating the presence of infection, but a thick, purulent-appearing fluid occasionally results from massive numbers of crystals, amyloid, or in rheumatoid arthritis, degenerated synovial villi (rice bodies). Not all infections cause pus, so some cloudy, nonopaque fluids can also be due to infections.

Bloody fluid in the joint (hemarthrosis) suggests numerous diagnostic possibilities, including trauma (with or without fracture), pigmented villonodular synovitis, synovioma, tumors in or near the joint, hemangioma, neuropathic joint disease (Charcot's joint), severe joint destruction, hemophilia and other bleeding disorders, von Willebrand's disease, anticoagulant therapy, myeloproliferative disease with thrombocytosis, thrombocytopenia, scurvy, ruptured aneurysm, and arteriovenous fistula. Hemarthrosis may, however, be idiopathic.

Viscosity can be crudely estimated by the ability of fluid to string out after being expressed from the syringe. In most noninflammatory diseases, the synovial fluid retains its normal viscosity, stringing out 1 inch or more. Joint fluid from patients with hypothyroidism or ganglion cysts may be very viscous and produce strings of many inches. In contrast, reduced levels of hyaluronate, which decreases viscosity and makes the fluid drop from the syringe more like water, characterize the synovial fluid in inflammatory diseases such as rheumatoid arthritis and gout.

Bacteriologic Cultures

If joint infection is suspected, the aspirated fluid should be left in the syringe, capped under sterile conditions, and promptly transported to the microbiology laboratory. The diseases under consideration must be noted so that the fluid can be appropriately cultured for gonococci, anaerobic organisms, mycobacteria, or fungi.

Microscopic Examination

Crystal-induced arthritis is definitively diagnosed only from examination of wet preparations of joint fluid for the presence of intracellular or extracellular crystals (2–20μm). Occasionally, crystals are also found in tissue or tophi. Two drops of fluid are expressed onto a clean glass slide, which is promptly covered with a clean glass slip. Fluid on a slide can be preserved for a few hours, or a fresh drop preparation can be taken for each examination from fluid kept in a tube. The fluid should be examined on the day it is obtained because small numbers of calcium pyrophosphate dihydrate (CPPD) crystals can dissolve overnight, and with time, artifactual urate-like crystals can form from degenerating cells.

Gross appearance
A. Normal. Clear to pale yellow, transparent
B. Noninflammatory. Slightly deeper yellow, transparent
C. Inflammatory. Darker yellow, cloudy, translucent (type blurred or obscured)
D. Septic. Purulent, dense, opaque
E. Hemarthrosis. Red, opaque. Must be differentiated from traumatic tap

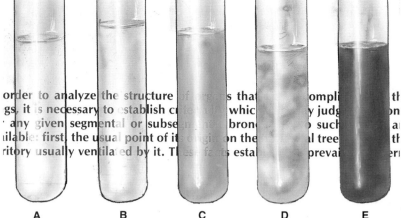

A   B   C   D   E

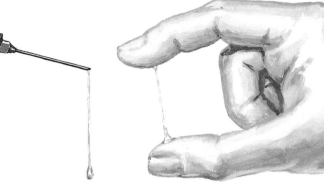

Viscosity. Drop of normal or noninflammatory fluid expressed from needle will string out 1 in. or more, indicative of high viscosity. Inflammatory fluid evidences little or no stringing. Viscosity may also be tested between *gloved* thumb and forefinger

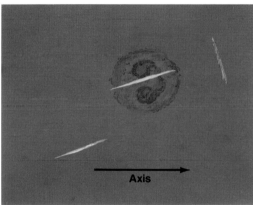

Intracellular and extracellular monosodium urate crystals, indicative of gout, seen on compensated polarized light microscopy. Crystals appear as needles or rods, bright yellow when parallel to axis of slow vibration of a red plate compensator, blue when perpendicular to axis (negative elongation)

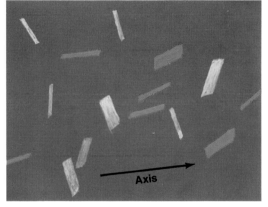

Calcium pyrophosphate dihydrate (CPPD) crystals, indicative of pseudogout, appear as rhomboids or rods, blue when parallel to axis, yellow when perpendicular to it (positive elongation)

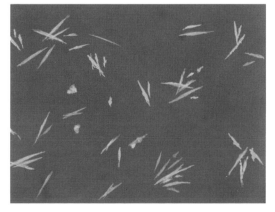

Adrenocorticosteroid crystals resulting from prior joint injection may appear as positively or negatively elongated rods or granules. May be mistaken for urate or CPPD crystals

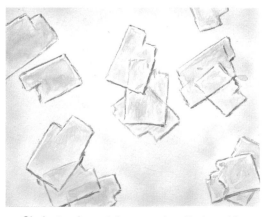

Cholesterol crystals, occasionally found in synovial or bursal fluids of patients with rheumatoid arthritis. Crystals are plate-like, with characteristic notched corners

Synovial Fluid Examination
(Continued)

In the clinic or office, the fluid can be examined with a light microscope; a more definitive identification can be made with a compensated polarized light microscope (Plate 15). Urate crystals are usually rods or needles; CPPD crystals are rods or rhomboids. The presence of depot corticosteroid crystals and cholesterol may confuse the diagnosis. Cholesterol crystal plates are seen most frequently in chronic rheumatoid arthritis; they are larger than other crystals and, since they are rarely phagocytized, probably do not have a significant role in joint inflammation.

The leukocyte count helps determine if the joint effusion reflects an inflammatory, noninflammatory, or infectious (septic) disease. Leukocyte counts in synovial fluid require heparinized fluid and 0.3% saline as diluent because the usual leukocyte-counting fluid causes clumping of the synovial fluid, leading to inaccurate counts.

Leukocyte counts greater than 2,000/mm³ usually cause some gross loss of transparency in the fluid, but confirmation that this is due to leukocytosis is important. A classification of joint effusions based in large part on leukocyte counts has been developed. Counts over 75,000/mm³ strongly suggest the presence of infection, but in some infectious conditions, such as gonococcal arthritis, leukocyte counts are much lower. Also, very high counts in the septic range are occasionally seen in rheumatoid, psoriatic, and crystal-induced arthritis.

Noninflammatory effusions usually contain three or fewer leukocytes per high-power field. Not all noninflammatory effusions are due to osteoarthritis. Other causes are traumatic arthritis, acromegaly, Gaucher's disease, hemochromatosis, hyperparathyroidism, ochronosis, Paget's disease of bone, mechanical derangement, erythema nodosum, villonodular synovitis, tumors, aseptic necrosis, Ehlers-Danlos syndrome, sickle-cell disease, amyloidosis, hypertrophic pulmonary osteoarthropathy, pancreatitis, osteochondritis dissecans, neuropathic joint disease, Wilson's disease, and epiphyseal dysplasias.

The wet preparations that had been examined for crystals can be used to provide a rough estimate of the leukocyte count. Other findings may also be noted (Plate 16). For example, fibrils may be due to cartilage collagen, suggesting cartilage damage. Fat droplets, which usually indicate trauma, can also occur in pancreatic disease with synovial fat necrosis. Examination may reveal large organisms such as fungi or amyloid clumps, entire synovial villi, or foreign bodies, which may need further histologic examination. Crystals of apatite deposition disease, seen in calcific tendonitis or in patients undergoing dialysis, create irregular, shiny, negatively birefringent intracellular or extracellular chunks (2–20µm) visible on wet preparations; individual crystals can be seen only on electron microscopy.

Single drops of joint fluid can be placed on a glass slide and smeared out into a thin preparation as for a blood smear. Air-drying preserves

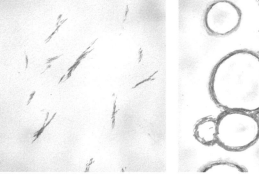

Cartilage fragments, may appear in synovial fluid taken from osteoarthritic joint (unstained, wet preparation)

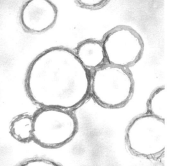

Fat droplets, frequently noted in traumatic arthritis, some inflammatory disorders, and pancreatic disease with synovial fat necrosis (unstained, wet preparation)

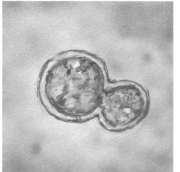

Budding blastomycete, a fungus that rarely appears in synovial fluid of fungal infections. Diagnostic of blastomycosis (unstained, wet preparation)

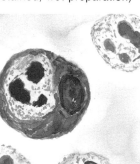
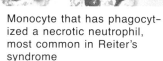

LE cell, seen virtually only in systemic lupus erythematosus (Wright's stain)

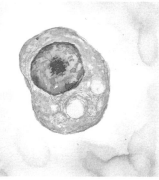

Monocyte that has phagocytized a necrotic neutrophil, most common in Reiter's syndrome

Synovial lining cell (large cell with nucleus usually filling less than 50% of cytoplasm), often seen in noninflammatory aspirates

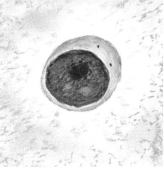

Activated T lymphocyte (large cell with prominent nucleus and nucleolus), most common in rheumatoid arthritis

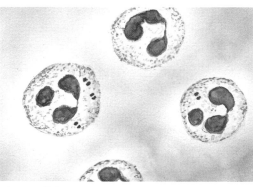

Intracellular gram-negative cocci, seen in only about 25% of cases of gonococcal arthritis (Gram's stain). Gram-positive organisms such as staphylococci seen more often. Diagnosis of tuberculous, gonococcal, or anaerobic infections may require culture on special media

the cells for staining later in the day. If infection is being considered, smears should be stained with Gram's stain. Identification of pathologic organisms can guide the choice of initial antibiotic therapy, but failure to find bacteria on a Gram's-stained preparation does not exclude infectious arthritis.

Wright's stain to identify joint fluid cells is also valuable in synovial fluid analysis. A differential count with more than 95% polymorphonuclear neutrophils suggests bacterial infection or crystal-induced disease (Plates 33–34) even if the leukocyte count is not very high. An inflamed joint space produces an ideal medium for the development of LE cells, which are seen almost exclusively in systemic lupus erythematosus. Mononuclear cells that have phagocytized necrotic neutrophils are seen commonly in Reiter's syndrome (Plate 28), other seronegative spondyloarthropathies, or (occasionally) gout or pseudogout (Plates 33–35). Large cells seen in blood smears include synovial lining cells, most common in noninflammatory disorders, and activated lymphocytes, which are common in rheumatoid arthritis and should not be confused with the rare tumor cell found in joints. Tumor cells from metastases usually occur in clusters or glandular arrays. Large vacuolated cells are usually macrophages and are often seen in fluids from chronically inflamed joints. □

Systemic Juvenile Arthritis

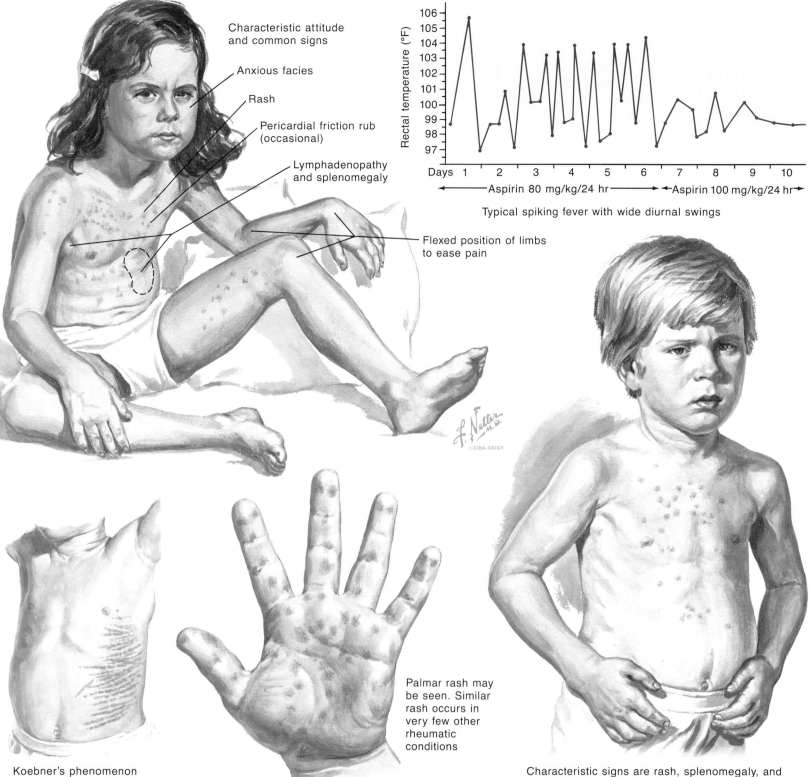

Characteristic attitude and common signs

Anxious facies

Rash

Pericardial friction rub (occasional)

Lymphadenopathy and splenomegaly

Flexed position of limbs to ease pain

Aspirin 80 mg/kg/24 hr ← → Aspirin 100 mg/kg/24 hr

Typical spiking fever with wide diurnal swings

Koebner's phenomenon after scratching skin

Palmar rash may be seen. Similar rash occurs in very few other rheumatic conditions

Characteristic signs are rash, splenomegaly, and axillary adenopathy causing bulging of pectoral folds

SECTION III PLATE 17   Slide 4598

Juvenile Arthritis

Since the clinical, laboratory, and genetic features of rheumatoid arthritis in children differ significantly from those of classic adult rheumatoid arthritis, many rheumatologists have discarded the term "juvenile rheumatoid arthritis" in favor of "juvenile arthritis." The disease has a variable onset and course, making it impossible to develop diagnostic criteria that fit every case. The primary diagnostic criterion is swelling in one or more joints that persists for at least 6 weeks; joint pain or tenderness on palpation plus limitation of movement is acceptable evidence of joint disease activity in a previously diagnosed case. Other manifestations (eg, uveitis) occurring at any time must also be considered in refining the diagnosis.

Based on the manifestations seen in the first 6 months of the disease (the onset period), juvenile arthritis takes three forms: systemic onset, polyarticular onset, and pauciarticular onset.

Systemic Onset Arthritis

About 20% of children with juvenile arthritis have the systemic onset form. The disease may begin at any time during childhood, and both sexes are affected about equally. The major signs of systemic onset juvenile arthritis are a high, spiking fever; characteristic rash; arthritis in one or multiple joints; hepatosplenomegaly; and lymphadenopathy (Plate 17).

The fever in systemic onset arthritis rises above 102°F and falls to normal or below once (quotidian pattern) or twice (double quotidian) during every 24 hours. While the rise and fall are usually rapid, the pattern of fever may otherwise be quite variable. In some children, the temperature is significantly elevated much of the time, with only short afebrile periods; in others, the duration of the fever spikes is shorter. Single spikes

Juvenile Arthritis
(Continued)

tend to occur in the late afternoon or evening. In patients with a more hectic fever, administration of aspirin or another nonsteroidal antiinflammatory drug (NSAID) may change the fever pattern to a once-a-day spike or return the temperature to normal.

The rheumatoid rash tends to occur simultaneously with the fever, often disappearing completely during afebrile periods (Plate 17). It may be generalized or develop only in warmer areas such as the axillae and medial thighs or on the palms and soles. The typical rash is macular; individual lesions are pale pink with relatively indistinct margins and somewhat paler centers. When the rash is extensive, the macules tend to coalesce. About 20% of children with a typical fever pattern have a maculopapular or pruritic rash, and 10% have no rash. In a few children, macules appear along scratch marks made in the skin (Koebner's phenomenon). This manifestation, which may not appear immediately, should not be confused with the rapid appearance of the wheal-and-flare response normally seen after scratching.

Severe arthralgia and myalgia are common, particularly during febrile periods. The 30% of children who have no initial evidence of joint involvement may seem to be completely normal during the afebrile periods. During the first 6 months of disease, however, arthritis develops in at least five joints in over 80% of children with systemic onset arthritis.

Localized or generalized adenopathy is common; occasionally, the swelling of a single node or groups of nodes is massive, resembling that of cancer. Biopsy findings usually indicate a reactive hyperplasia. Hepatosplenomegaly is also common.

About 25% of patients with systemic onset arthritis have symptoms or signs of pericarditis or pleuritis, or both. In asymptomatic children, echocardiography may reveal a small amount of pericardial fluid, but this is usually of little clinical significance; rarely, the amount of pericardial fluid is sufficient to cause cardiac tamponade and require aspiration. Pericardial effusions are usually associated with pleural effusions, and myocarditis frequently accompanies pericarditis. Since affected children are very sensitive to digitalis, the usual dose should be decreased by at least one half. A pericardial friction rub may be localized to a small area, usually the lower sternum. Patients with pericardial irritation show a reluctance to lie down because of increased chest pain.

Ocular involvement of any type is uncommon in patients with the systemic onset form. Central nervous system involvement, including seizures, has been reported but appears to be rare.

The majority of deaths due to juvenile arthritis have occurred in children with the systemic onset form. In many countries, the leading cause of

death in patients with juvenile arthritis is renal failure secondary to amyloidosis. Amyloidosis appears to be significantly less common in the United States. These regional differences suggest a genetic factor in the etiology of secondary amyloidosis.

Laboratory Findings. Laboratory tests may help in the diagnosis of systemic onset arthritis, but antinuclear antibody (ANA) and rheumatoid factor tests are negative. Most patients have a modest-to-marked leukocytosis (15,000–25,000/mm³); occasionally, the count may be as high as 50,000/mm³. Polymorphonuclear leukocytes predominate, and there is a significant percentage of young cells. In most children, the platelet count is also elevated. Thrombocytopenia is rare. Normochromic, normocytic anemia with a normal mean corpuscular volume (MCV) develops initially, but with continuing disease activity, the hemoglobin level decreases, followed by a fall in MCV and development of a microcytic, hypochromic anemia. Serum levels of iron are usually low with a normal-to-high iron-binding capacity. Serum ferritin levels may be normal to significantly elevated and probably reflect the generalized inflammatory disease. Although the anemia is unresponsive to administration of iron, reticulocytosis and a rapid rise in hemoglobin value occur with disease remission. During the febrile phase, urinalysis may reveal intermittent or persistent proteinuria or increased red or white cell counts. Liver function may be abnormal, even before treatment with salicylates or other NSAIDs.

Polyarticular Onset Arthritis

About 20% to 25% of children with juvenile arthritis exhibit the polyarticular onset form, which is characterized by involvement of five or more joints and the absence of significant systemic manifestations. In many children, the disease is chronic and progressive, leading to significant deformities. About 25% of patients with polyarticular onset arthritis have high serum levels of IgM rheumatoid factor. This finding led to the classification of polyarticular onset arthritis into two distinct types: rheumatoid factor positive (late onset) and rheumatoid factor negative (onset throughout childhood).

Polyarticular onset arthritis affects both large and small joints, including the cervical spine, temporomandibular joints, and growth centers of the mandible. The distribution is generally symmetric.

Radiographs of the involved cervical spine initially reveal a loss of the normal curve; with time, the apophyseal joints (most often of C2–3) may narrow and eventually fuse (Plate 20). The fusion may affect the whole cervical spine or only segments. Since limitation of motion is most significant in extension and lateral motion, some children hold the head in a position of fixed flexion (Plate 20). Anterior subluxation of C1 on C2 is a potentially serious complication seen with extensive fusion below C2.

Arthritis of the cervical spine is often associated with involvement of the temporomandibular joints, frequently accompanied by poor growth of the mandible and crowding of the teeth (Plate 20). Growth of the maxilla is rarely affected. If temporomandibular joint involvement is unilateral, the lower jaw shifts significantly when the mouth is opened.

In the hands and feet, the arthritis affects multiple joints in a symmetric pattern. Attenuation

of supporting structures and damage to tendons, tendon sheaths, and attachments lead to joint laxity and subluxation. The metacarpophalangeal and proximal interphalangeal joints of the hands are affected first, followed by the distal interphalangeal joints (Plate 18).

Rheumatoid Factor–Positive Polyarthritis. This juvenile version of adult rheumatoid arthritis usually develops in girls over 10 years of age. The arthritis, which involves multiple large and small joints, is erosive and chronic. Erosions in the small joints may be evident radiographically as early as 6 months after onset of disease, and the destructive synovitis may continue for 10 years or longer.

Subcutaneous rheumatoid nodules are common, usually developing at or distal to the elbow on the extensor surface. Constitutional manifestations of rheumatoid factor–positive polyarthritis include low-grade fever, easy fatigability, mild-to-moderate anemia, and poor weight gain. Uveitis (iridocyclitis) does not occur, and episcleritis is rare.

This progressive form of the disease may lead to significant deformities in the limbs and spine. However, because patients are in late childhood or adolescence at onset, growth of the vertebral bodies is not significantly disturbed even when the spinous processes are fused.

Rheumatoid Factor–Negative Polyarthritis. Approximately 75% of patients with polyarticular onset arthritis do not have IgM rheumatoid factor in the serum, and the rheumatoid factor test rarely becomes positive after the first year of disease onset. In contrast to rheumatoid factor–positive disease, which primarily affects girls, about 25% of patients in this subgroup are boys.

The arthritis may start at any age, but in about one half of patients, onset occurs before age 6. In younger children, parents generally notice only one or two swollen joints, only to have the rheumatologist identify many more.

The inflammatory process is usually less severe than in rheumatoid factor–positive polyarthritis. Large and small joints are affected, but erosions usually develop later. Early radiographs reveal only osteoporotic changes.

Tenosynovitis on the dorsum of the wrist and tarsus is common, but flexor tenosynovitis is also seen, usually in the hand. Involvement of the finger joints is often symmetric. In young children, swelling of the joints may be partially masked by diffuse swelling of the entire finger (fusiform swelling, Plate 18). Periostitis and widening of the digits are occasionally seen on radiographs.

Subcutaneous nodules are uncommon. Chronic, asymptomatic uveitis develops in a small number of patients and is usually associated with a positive ANA test.

The long-term prognosis for patients with rheumatoid factor–negative polyarthritis varies. In some patients, the disease is controlled by NSAIDs alone or it goes into long-term remission, leaving minimal deformities. In others, the course of the disease resembles rheumatoid factor–positive arthritis, only less severe.

Pauciarticular Onset Arthritis

Pauciarticular onset arthritis occurs in 55% to 60% of children with juvenile arthritis. The arthritis is limited to fewer than five joints during the onset period, although more joints may

Juvenile Arthritis
(Continued)

become involved after the initial 6-month period. In patients whose involvement ultimately extends beyond a few joints, the disease resembles rheumatoid factor–negative polyarthritis and produces more dysfunction than was predicted from the original, limited involvement. Disease activity may be intermittent and even recur in previously uninvolved joints, even after years of remission, making an early prognosis difficult. Systemic signs are rare, but a number of patients eventually exhibit features of other diseases, primarily psoriasis. Two small subgroups have been identified. Uveitis develops in one group, made up primarily of females with early onset arthritis. Males with late onset arthritis (after age 9) make up the other group. However, the majority of patients with pauciarticular onset arthritis do not fit in these subgroups.

The knee is the joint most often affected in pauciarticular onset disease, and monarticular involvement is common. The ankles are the next most common site of involvement, followed by the wrists, elbows, and hips. The small joints of the hands and feet, the cervical spine, and the jaw are affected less often than in polyarticular onset arthritis.

In some children, the joint contains only a small amount of fluid, which is difficult to demonstrate, particularly in the early stages. The bulge sign is used to confirm the presence of small amounts of fluid in the knee (Plate 18). The bulge is elicited by compressing or stroking proximally the medial side of the knee, moving fluid into the suprapatellar bursa and the lateral compartment. Rapid compression of the lateral compartment moves fluid back to the medial side, resulting in a bulging of the medial compartment. The effusion may also be demonstrated by compressing the suprapatellar bursa or by distally stroking the lateral compartment.

In monarticular involvement, overgrowth of the involved limb may occur because of increased blood supply; this is seen most frequently with arthritis of one knee. With remission or treatment, the growth may decrease, allowing growth in the uninvolved limb to catch up. However, the overgrowth occasionally continues even after clinical signs of inflammation have disappeared. If the limb-length discrepancy is predicted to be greater than 2.5 cm, early epiphyseal stapling or epiphysiodesis of the affected side may be indicated (see Section I, Plate 85).

Pauciarticular Arthritis With Uveitis. A potentially blinding uveitis may develop in some children with pauciarticular onset arthritis. The ocular

Joint Involvement in Juvenile Arthritis

Swelling of proximal interphalangeal, metacarpophalangeal, and wrist joints in polyarticular onset disease. Involvement usually symmetric

Fusiform swelling of fingers. Most common in young patients in early stage of disease

Involvement of left knee with valgus deformity of lower leg and flexion contracture of knee

Bulge sign
Medial side of knee compressed or stroked proximally to move fluid away from medial compartment (upper picture). Lateral side is quickly compressed or stroked distally; bulge appears medial to patella (lower picture)

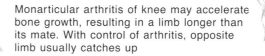

Monarticular arthritis of knee may accelerate bone growth, resulting in a limb longer than its mate. With control of arthritis, opposite limb usually catches up

Juvenile Arthritis
(Continued)

Ocular Manifestations in Juvenile Arthritis

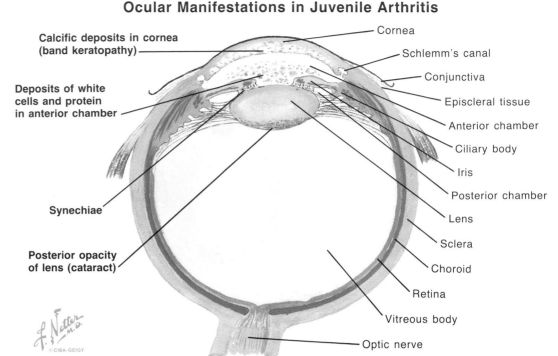

inflammation usually begins within a year of the onset of arthritis, and nearly always within the first 5 years. Rarely, the uveitis becomes evident before the joint manifestations, and the inflammation in joints and eyes may not be present at the same time. The patients most at risk are girls who are under 5 years of age at the onset of arthritis and who have knee or ankle involvement and a positive ANA test.

Since the uveitis is asymptomatic, periodic slit lamp examination to detect inflammation in the early stage is mandatory in all children with juvenile arthritis. The early changes are not seen with the ophthalmoscope.

The inflammation primarily affects the iris and ciliary body, and slit lamp examination reveals white cells and protein in the anterior chamber (Plate 19). Fibrin strands may develop between the iris and the anterior surface of the lens (synechiae), resulting in a fixed or irregular pupil. White cells and protein deposited on the surface of the cornea may calcify, resulting in band keratopathy, which can totally obstruct vision. Cataracts may be caused by a combination of factors, including inflammation, blocked Schlemm's canal, increased pressure, and corticosteroid therapy. Although careful follow-up and aggressive treatment have improved the prognosis for patients with uveitis, a small but significant proportion of patients do not respond satisfactorily and suffer significant loss of vision.

Pauciarticular Onset Arthritis in Older Boys. A second distinct subgroup is made up primarily of boys age 9 or older at the onset of peripheral arthritis.

The arthritis usually involves the knees, ankles, and hips, and exclusive involvement of the hip is not uncommon. Inflammation at the insertions of tendons or fascia into bone causes pain in the heel and tenderness in the heel and arches. Uveitis with pain and redness in the eyes is seen in about 20% of patients, but the duration of inflammation is usually short.

In some patients, radiographic changes in sacroiliac joints or mild back pain or limitation of motion of the lower spine develops with time. Some patients eventually manifest other features consistent with a diagnosis of juvenile ankylosing spondylitis or psoriatic arthritis. Most patients, even those with sacroiliac joint or back involvement, are essentially asymptomatic by 30 years of age, which suggests that this disease probably represents yet another form of juvenile arthritis rather than the ankylosing spondylitis or psoriatic arthritis seen in adults.

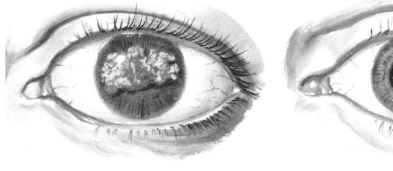

Deposits in anterior chamber seen on slit lamp examination

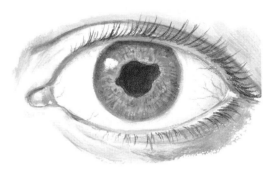

Irregular pupil due to synechiae

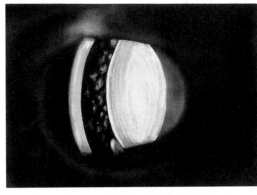

Band keratopathy

Cataract

The histocompatibility of the human leukocyte antigen 27 (HLA-B27) is detected in a large percentage of patients in this subgroup (80% in our series). Children should not be included in this subgroup solely because of the presence of HLA-B27, which is also found in children with other types of juvenile arthritis at the same frequency as in the general population. The same disease may develop in younger boys, in girls with HLA-B27, and in children with involvement of more than four joints.

Differential Diagnosis

Systemic onset arthritis may resemble a number of other diseases. When joint inflammation

is absent, it may be confused with infectious or inflammatory diseases. When joint inflammation is present, infectious arthritis, osteomyelitis, and cancer, especially leukemia, must be ruled out. Other diagnostic possibilities include a variety of connective tissue diseases, inflammatory bowel disease, various types of systemic vasculitis, and occasionally, reactions to infections or drugs.

Polyarticular onset arthritis must be differentiated from other joint diseases such as systemic lupus erythematosus and acute rheumatic fever. Unlike these conditions, however, polyarticular onset arthritis rarely has significant systemic manifestations.

Juvenile Arthritis
(Continued)

Sequelae of Juvenile Arthritis

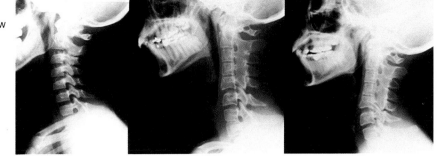

Radiographs show progression of arthritis of cervical apophyseal joints from only upper vertebrae to almost entire cervical spine

Pauciarticular onset arthritis, especially monarticular involvement, can be confused with trauma, joint conditions such as osteochondritis, viral-induced synovitis, and Lyme disease.

Laboratory studies are usually not very helpful in making the diagnosis. While a positive ANA test in a young girl with pauciarticular onset arthritis is a helpful clue, uveitis detected on slit lamp examination is a more valuable diagnostic finding. In other patients with juvenile arthritis, a positive ANA test may only lead to confusion with other connective tissue diseases. A high serum titer of rheumatoid factor helps to establish the diagnosis of polyarticular onset arthritis. However, a common error is to diagnose juvenile arthritis in a child without arthritis on the basis of a low, and therefore nondiagnostic, titer of rheumatoid factor.

Although useful in research studies, genetic typing is of little clinical value at present. There is a significantly increased frequency of HLA-B27 in older males with pauciarticular onset disease and an increased frequency of HLA-DR4 in children with rheumatoid factor–positive polyarthritis, similar to that seen in adult rheumatoid arthritis. Similarly, HLA-DR5 and HLA-DRw8 are often found in patients with pauciarticular onset arthritis (with the exception of the older male sub-group) and in those with rheumatoid factor–negative polyarthritis. However, as the same markers are present in many normal people, their demonstration is of value only in population studies, not in individual patients.

Treatment

The treatment of juvenile arthritis is multifaceted, requiring a coordinated team approach. Ideally, the family physician, rheumatologist, orthopedist, pedodontist, ophthalmologist, and physical therapist should all be involved in the treatment program.

The drugs, physical therapy programs, and surgical procedures used in adults with rheumatoid arthritis are also appropriate for children with juvenile arthritis (see pages 168–169). Drug doses, timing of additions of second-line (remittive) drugs such as gold or immunosuppressive agents, and some other aspects of therapy differ.

Most children with mild arthritis require only treatment with NSAIDs. Since these drugs may take over 30 days to effect any improvement, a trial of any drug should last at least a month before another medication is tried. If the response is not satisfactory, several NSAIDs may have to

Receding chin results from early closure of ossification centers of mandible

Fixed forward position of head due to involvement of joints in cervical spine

Extensive multiple deformities. Amyloid hepatosplenomegaly occurs primarily in systemic onset form; rare in United States

be tried sequentially before resorting to a second-line drug. Because juvenile arthritis undergoes spontaneous remission more often than adult rheumatoid arthritis, remittive agents, which are usually administered for years, are added later in children than in adults. However, patients with rheumatoid factor–positive polyarthritis and those with rapidly progressive arthritis require earlier therapy with second-line drugs.

Corticosteroids should be used sparingly in children. Oral corticosteroids may be indicated in some patients with systemic onset arthritis, and short-term, low-dose treatment is helpful for patients unable to function because of severe disease. Topical (and, occasionally, oral) corticosteroids are needed for uveitis, and intraarticular injection of a slow-release form is used when involvement of a single joint is the major problem.

Children with juvenile arthritis should attend school like normal children, but they require frequent rest periods and daily physical therapy. Swimming and bicycle riding are excellent exercises and should be encouraged. Engaging in activities usual for their age is not sufficient, since most children will avoid using the stiff, painful joints, and disuse quickly leads to joint contractures and muscle atrophy. In general, other than avoiding activities likely to injure the joints, children with juvenile arthritis should lead as normal a life as possible. □

Osteoarthritis

The most common joint disease, osteoarthritis, is a noninflammatory, progressive disorder characterized by the deterioration of articular cartilage and formation of new bone in the subchondral region and at joint margins. The best descriptive term is "degenerative joint disease," which correctly indicates the fundamental pathologic change; however, the designation "osteoarthritis," which incorrectly implies an inflammatory mechanism, continues to be the most popular label.

Although many factors influence its onset and the speed of joint deterioration, osteoarthritis is an inherent part of aging and is therefore common in elderly persons. Secondary osteoarthritis, the term used to designate degenerative joint disease appearing as a sequel to other forms of arthritis, injury, internal derangement, or dysplasia of the joint, usually develops in younger persons.

Evidence of osteoarthritis has been found in the skeletal remains of prehistoric animals and humans. Today, the true prevalence is difficult to determine because mild or early degenerative joint disease may be asymptomatic. In asymptomatic persons, osteoarthritis is often discovered accidentally on radiographs taken in connection with nonrheumatic diseases.

Pathology

Unlike rheumatoid arthritis, osteoarthritis is not a *systemic* disease; instead it is a degenerative process that is *localized* in joint structures, primarily articular cartilage and subchondral and marginal bone.

Changes in Articular Cartilage. The earliest recognized degenerative change is a diminished content of proteoglycans, which consist principally of chondroitin sulfate and smaller amounts of keratan sulfate bound to a core protein. (For a discussion of the composition of cartilage see CIBA COLLECTION, Volume 8/I, page 174.) This leads to a softening of the cartilage that develops in a focal distribution near the articular surface, chiefly in the central portion of the joint where the weight bearing and the stress of joint movement are concentrated. The cartilage surface over these softened areas begins to fray and fibrillate; cracks develop and extend more deeply into the cartilage. Clusters of chondrocytes proliferate around cracks in the deeper portion of the cartilage. As degeneration progresses, the entire cartilage becomes thin, and the surface becomes rough from the focal ulcerations (Plate 21). Eventually, the articular surface is denuded of cartilage. Since adult cartilage has no blood supply, regeneration is virtually impossible; these changes are therefore irreversible.

Changes in Bone. New bone forms at two sites—in subchondral bone and at joint margins. In subchondral tissue, the new bone grows chiefly beneath the eroded cartilage surface, thus

becoming the articular surface. The new bone becomes smooth, glistening, and sclerotic, or eburnated. Beneath the joint surface, the bone marrow undergoes mucoid and fibrous degeneration, which leaves cystic areas of rarefaction surrounded by new bone and fibrous tissue. The apex of the "cyst" is usually located beneath eburnated bone; sometimes the cyst develops at the site of ligament attachments. Because much of the trabecular bone disintegrates, the bone structure weakens and may even crumble.

The most characteristic pathologic feature is the growth of osteophytes at the margins of affected joints (nodule or spur formation). The osteophyte, which consists of bone growing from the

joint margin, usually follows the contour of the articular surface within the capsule and ligamentous attachments; it may even grow into the joint space and be covered by cartilage that merges into the synovial lining.

Changes in Soft Tissue. The synovial and capsular tissues may show mild-to-moderate inflammation and fibrous thickening in joints severely deranged by extensive damage to cartilage and bone. These soft-tissue changes are thought to be caused by stress, strain, and mechanical irritation that are secondary to the degenerative changes. Fibrosis and even cartilaginous metaplasia may develop along ligaments and tendons around the affected joints.

Joint Pathology in Osteoarthritis

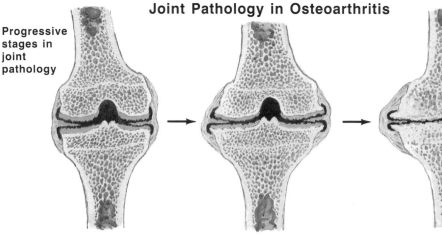

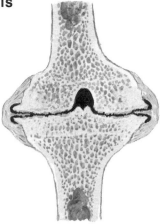

Progressive stages in joint pathology

Early degenerative changes with surface fraying of articular cartilages

Further erosion of cartilages, pitting, and cleft formation. Hypertrophic changes of bone at joint margins

Cartilages almost completely destroyed and joint space narrowed. Subchondral bone irregular and eburnated; spur formation at margins. Fibrosis of joint capsule

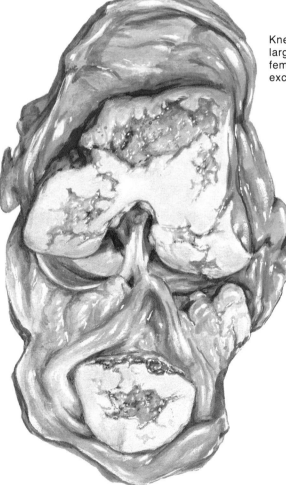

Knee joint opened anteriorly reveals large erosion of articular cartilages of femur and patella with cartilaginous excrescences at intercondylar notch

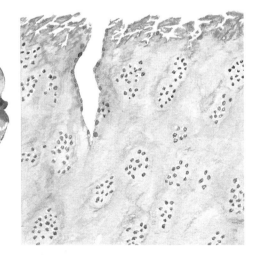

Section of articular cartilage shows fraying of surface and deep cleft. Hyaline cartilage abnormal with clumping of chondrocytes

Osteoarthritis

(Continued)

Pathogenesis

The pathogenesis of osteoarthritis is poorly understood. It is clear that degeneration of cartilage is an inherent part of the aging process, but several features of the disease suggest that other factors contribute to the degenerative process—for example, the wide variation in age at onset and the fact that some persons exhibit little or no symptomatic arthritis.

Several chemical, metabolic, genetic, and mechanical factors are believed to contribute to joint disintegration. For example, the articular cartilage in arthritic joints differs significantly in chemical composition and metabolism from cartilage in healthy joints. The role of chondrolytic enzymes in producing these chemical changes is not clear.

Genetic factors appear to influence the development of Heberden's nodes, the nodular swellings at the terminal joints of the fingers (Plate 22). A single gene, dominant in females and recessive in males, is believed to be involved in the inheritance. Microtraumas caused by daily "wear and tear" on articular cartilage in weight-bearing joints contribute significantly to the degenerative process, as do friction in the joint and pressure in an immobilized joint. Mechanical factors that predispose to osteoarthritis are excessive body weight, postural abnormalities, and joint instability.

Clinical Manifestations

The signs and symptoms of osteoarthritis depend on the joint or joints affected. Most commonly involved are the weight-bearing joints and some joints of the hand.

Pain and restricted movement are the major clinical manifestations. The patient is usually comfortable at rest but finds weight bearing and moving the affected joints painful. Aching during rainy weather, stiffness after inactivity, and crepitation are other frequent complaints.

Physical examination reveals irregular hard swellings at the joint margins, tenderness, pain and crepitation with joint movement, and usually, a limited range of motion. Although signs of synovitis—warmth and erythema over the joint—are usually absent, a diffuse swelling exists if there is joint effusion.

Knee Joint Involvement

Of the large joints, the knee is most often affected. Because the knee is so crucial in the lever action of the leg and in ambulation, osteoarthritis in this joint can be both very painful and disabling, especially when it is bilateral. The medial compartment of the knee is usually more severely damaged than the lateral compartment. Often, the tibial plateau breaks down, cystic changes form in the weight-bearing portion of

Hand Involvement in Osteoarthritis

Early Heberden's nodes with inflammatory changes

Chronic Heberden's nodes. 4th and 5th proximal interphalangeal joints also involved in degenerative process

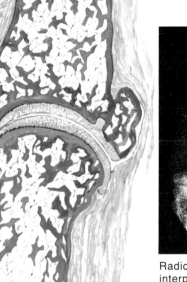

Section through distal interphalangeal joint shows irregular, hyperplastic bony nodules (Heberden's nodes) at articular margins of distal phalanx. Cartilage eroded and joint space narrowed

Radiograph of distal interphalangeal joint reveals late-stage degenerative changes. Cartilage destruction and marginal osteophytes (Heberden's nodes)

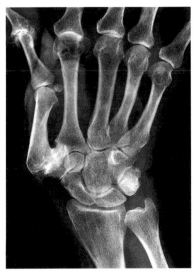

Late-stage degenerative changes in carpometacarpal articulation of thumb

the femoral condyles, and chondromalacia often develops in the patella. The structural damage in the joint causes much pain, restriction of motion, and crepitation. Subluxation and angular deformities are late sequelae.

Hand Involvement

Some clinical manifestations are unique to particular joints. Heberden's nodes, hallmarks of osteoarthritis, develop only at the terminal joints of the fingers (Plate 22). While the cartilage of the distal interphalangeal joint is degenerating, osteophytes grow from the dorsomedial and lateral aspects of the base of the distal phalanx to produce these nodular protuberances. Flexion deformity usually results when the pathologic changes are severe. Early in their development, the nodes are tender and painful; when mature, they are asymptomatic and have only cosmetic significance. Heberden's nodes are more common in women and are often familial. Bouchard's nodes, similar to but less common than Heberden's nodes, develop at the proximal interphalangeal finger joints.

In the wrist, the first carpometacarpal articulation is the most common joint to undergo the degenerative changes of osteoarthritis. This joint is affected much more often in women. Local tenderness and pain, usually severe, are exacerbated by firm grasping and by moving the wrist.

Hip Joint Involvement in Osteoarthritis

Osteoarthritis

(Continued)

Hip Joint Involvement

Osteoarthritis of the hip (malum coxae senilis) is the most crippling and painful form of degenerative joint disease. Standing and walking often cause severe localized hip pain that may radiate to the medial aspect of the thigh and knee. The articular cartilage becomes thin, cysts form in the femoral head and acetabulum, the bone softens and crumbles, and the femoral head flattens. Osteophytes grow around the rim of the acetabulum (Plate 23). As a result, joint motion becomes markedly restricted, leading to a fixed deformity of the hip in flexion, adduction, and external rotation. Unilateral hip joint involvement is usually secondary to other hip joint disease or injury. Bilateral hip involvement may cause complete disability.

Spine Involvement

Degenerative disease of the spine occurs to some degree in almost every person past middle age, but the severity and speed of progression vary greatly. Two types of spinal degeneration are seen in osteoarthritis: one affects the intervertebral discs and their adjacent vertebrae and the other affects the diarthrodial, or apophyseal, joints.

Degeneration of the cartilaginous discs with secondary pathologic changes is much more common than facet disease. With aging, the intervertebral discs lose water, the proteoglycan content decreases, the amount of collagen increases, and the gelatinous central core (nucleus pulposus) becomes hard and brittle. Defects develop in the surrounding fibrous material (annulus fibrosus), which becomes fibrillated. Fissures develop in the annulus fibrosus, through which the nucleus pulposus may herniate. The disc deteriorates and becomes thin, and disc fragments—sometimes the entire degenerated disc—may become displaced and press on the spinal nerve roots. The vertebrae on either side of the thin disc become closer, putting a strain on the facets (Plate 24). Bony spurs grow and protrude from the vertebral margins, sometimes uniting to form a bony bridge between the vertebrae. Intervertebral disc degeneration occurs chiefly where movement is greatest—in the cervical, lower thoracic, and lumbar regions. Movement of the spine causes localized pain, which is intensified by strenuous activity, especially lifting heavy objects.

Degeneration of spinal facets usually occurs in the cervical and lumbar regions in older persons. The degenerating articular cartilage becomes thin, the surface and margins become rough, and spurs grow from the bony edges. Joint motion is restricted and painful, and crepitation is common, especially in the cervical spine.

Neuropathies augment the clinical problems of degenerative disease of the spine. Spurs growing from vertebral margins adjacent to degenerated discs and from facet borders may narrow the

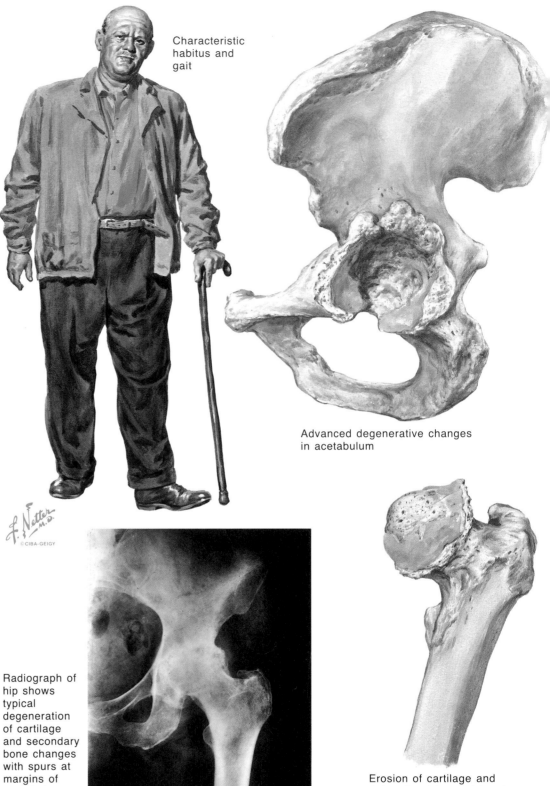

Characteristic habitus and gait

Advanced degenerative changes in acetabulum

Radiograph of hip shows typical degeneration of cartilage and secondary bone changes with spurs at margins of acetabulum

Erosion of cartilage and deformity of femoral head

foramina through which the spinal nerves exit. Pressure on and irritation of the nerve roots cause neuralgia, paresthesia, or paresis. Neuralgic pain in the occipital region and about the shoulders and arms is due to spurs in the cervical region; sciatic pain is caused by nerve root pressure from a protruding degenerated disc or spurs in the lumbar region. In the cervical spine, compression of the spinal cord from large osteophytes or from displaced degenerated discs may lead to an uncommon but serious neurologic complication manifested by upper motor neuron or long tract signs. The same type of spinal cord compression, spinal stenosis, may also occur in the lumbar spine, leading to claudication and lower limb weakness.

Laboratory Studies

Hematocrit reading, blood cell counts, erythrocyte sedimentation rate (ESR), and results of serum protein electrophoresis, blood chemistry studies, urinalysis, and other laboratory tests are usually normal unless other diseases exist. If severe degenerative changes cause a secondary (traumatic) synovitis, the ESR may be slightly elevated. Rheumatoid factor is occasionally detected in the serum of elderly persons, with or without clinical osteoarthritis. However, the titer is always low, and this finding has no diagnostic significance. Synovial fluid analysis reveals no abnormalities except a slight increase in cells.

Spine Involvement in Osteoarthritis

Osteoarthritis
(Continued)

Radiographs reveal the only diagnostic findings: cartilage thinning, osteophytes (nodes, spurs, and bony bridging), and deterioration of bone.

Diagnosis

Diagnosing osteoarthritis and differentiating it from rheumatoid arthritis are usually not difficult. The localization of pathology to one or a few weight-bearing joints of the lower limbs, the spine, the distal interphalangeal finger joints, and/or wrist joints in otherwise healthy older persons, together with normal results of laboratory studies and characteristic radiographs, confirms the diagnosis. However, the abnormalities seen in radiographs of the spine often do not parallel the clinical findings: extensive and severe pathologic changes may be seen in radiographs when the patient has only mild pain and disability. On the other hand, only minor osteophytic or degenerative changes seen in conventional radiographs of the spine may be accompanied by severe arthritic symptoms if the abnormalities are in a critical area. Myelography is helpful in confirming and localizing disc protrusion. Spinal cord impingement may be detected with myelography and computed tomography.

Treatment

Since pain and disability result from severe degeneration of the weight-bearing joints, rehabilitative surgery, including total joint replacement, effectively relieves discomfort and restores good joint function.

Treatment should accomplish the following objectives: (1) relieve pain; (2) avoid trauma to or excessive use of affected joints; (3) correct factors that produce strain on involved joints (eg, overweight, vigorous weight-bearing exercise); (4) prevent or retard progression of degenerative changes; and (5) maintain or restore joint function.

Medications. Analgesics such as aspirin are the drugs of choice in the treatment of osteoarthritis. The considerations discussed in drug therapy for rheumatoid arthritis (see pages 168–169) apply equally to osteoarthritis. However, administration of gold salts and corticosteroids has no place in the treatment of this degenerative, essentially noninflammatory, localized joint disorder. The benefits of NSAIDs may be largely due to their inherent analgesic effect. Intraarticular administration of corticosteroids may provide short-term relief in early developing Heberden's nodes and severely degenerated joints complicated by secondary traumatic synovitis. More investigation is required to determine whether any medication can retard the progress of degenerative joint disease.

Rest. Weight-bearing activity should be minimized, and all strenuous activity should be avoided. Weight bearing can be redistributed from

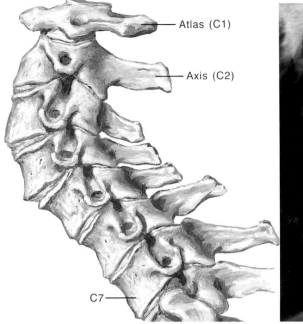

Atlas (C1)

Axis (C2)

C7

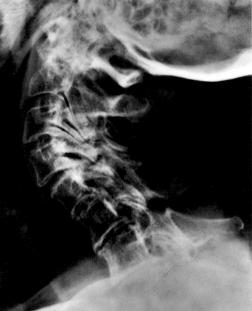

Extensive thinning of cervical discs and hyperextension deformity with narrowing of intervertebral foramina. Lateral radiograph reveals similar changes

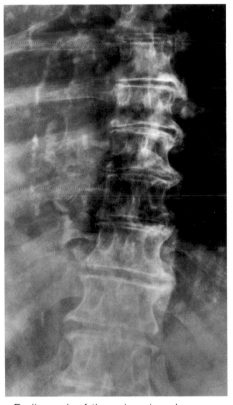

Radiograph of thoracic spine shows narrowing of intervertebral spaces and spur formation

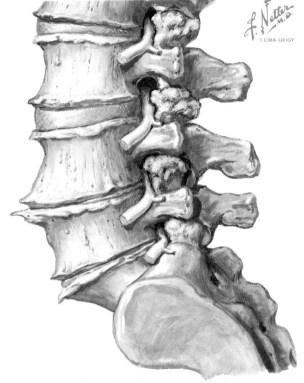

Degeneration of lumbar intervertebral discs and hypertrophic changes at vertebral margins with spur formation. Osteophytic encroachment on intervertebral foramina compresses spinal nerves

the lower to the upper limbs by the proper use of canes, elbow-length or axillary crutches, or a walker. It is most important to reduce excessive body weight and to correct poor posture. A firm bed with a bed board helps to relieve strain on the spine, and use of a firm armchair with a straight back and a high seat avoids straining a degenerated spine and the joints in the lower limbs.

Physical Therapy. The general principles of physical therapy outlined for rheumatoid arthritis (see page 169) should be followed for osteoarthritis. In particular, local heat and appliances to restrict joint motion help to relieve the pain and stiffness. Use of traction and a support collar can

significantly reduce pain in the cervical region, and a firm corset or brace can be used to support the low back region.

Surgery. If the patient is otherwise healthy, joint replacement, when performed before significant degenerative changes have occurred, can help to correct abnormal weight bearing. Total joint replacement of the hip and knee is now a common procedure, allowing thousands of persons to regain painless joint movement (see Section IV). Surgery may also be required to relieve unrelenting pain, eliminate pressure and irritation of spinal nerve roots and spinal cord, correct spinal deformity, stabilize the spine, and rehabilitate severely affected patients. □

Ankylosing Spondylitis

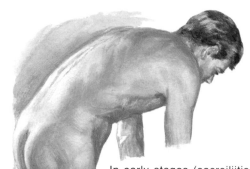

In early stages (sacroiliitis only), back contour may appear normal but flexion may be limited

In more advanced sacroiliac plus lower spine involvement, back is straightened with "ironed-out" appearance

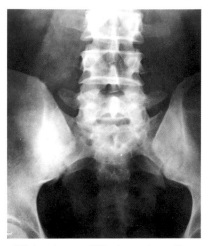

Bilateral sacroiliitis is early radiographic sign. Thinning of cartilage and bone condensation on both sides of sacroiliac joints

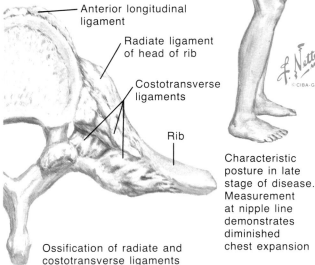

Anterior longitudinal ligament

Radiate ligament of head of rib

Costotransverse ligaments

Rib

Ossification of radiate and costotransverse ligaments limits chest expansion

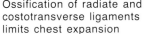

Characteristic posture in late stage of disease. Measurement at nipple line demonstrates diminished chest expansion

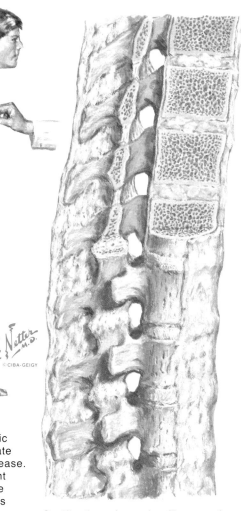

Ossification of annulus fibrosus of intervertebral discs, apophyseal joints, and anterior longitudinal and interspinal ligaments

Ankylosing spondylitis is a form of spinal arthritis characterized by the calcific bridging of the intervertebral spaces that eventually stiffens the spine. It primarily affects young men (only 10%–15% of cases occur in women). Onset of clinical manifestations usually occurs in the late teens or early twenties.

Initially, the sacroiliac joints become inflamed bilaterally, and the disease then spreads up the spine. The speed of progression varies considerably from patient to patient, and advancement may stop at any spinal level. In some patients, there is only pelvic and lumbar spine involvement, while in others, the entire spine is affected.

Pathology

The primary pathologic change is an inflammatory process in the pelvic joints and apophyseal and costovertebral articulations; the hips are affected in about 50% of patients and the shoulders in about 33%. The synovitis is indistinguishable from that of rheumatoid arthritis, and the inflammation can destroy the articular cartilage, which leads to ankylosis of the joint. Perispinous (subligamentous) calcification greatly exacerbates stiffening of the spine.

Because the joint pathology of ankylosing spondylitis and rheumatoid arthritis is so similar, this form of spondylitis was thought to be rheumatoid arthritis of the spine. However, there are more differences than similarities between these two disorders. The following features characterize ankylosing spondylitis but not rheumatoid arthritis: (1) predominance in young men, (2) absence of rheumatoid nodules and other nonarticular manifestations of connective tissue inflammation, (3) absence of rheumatoid factor, and (4) occurrence of perispinous calcification. In addition, the diseases respond differently to some forms of treatment. Ankylosing spondylitis is now considered to be a disease that is distinctly different from rheumatoid arthritis. This conclusion is further supported by the presence of HLA-B27, which is usually not found in patients with classic rheumatoid arthritis. This histocompatibility antigen is considered an important genetic factor in the pathogenesis of the disease.

Clinical Manifestations. In the early stage of the disease, patients complain of low back pain that extends into the buttocks. Frequently, the pain is severe early in the morning and may awaken the patient from sleep. Other early signs and symptoms include difficulty in arising from bed because of pain and muscle spasm in the low back; tenderness on pressure and percussion of the sacroiliac joints and lumbar spine; painful,

Ankylosing Spondylitis
(Continued)

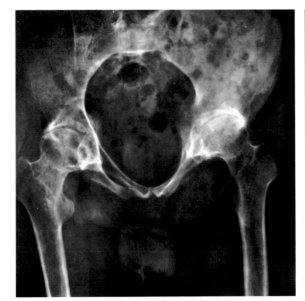

Radiograph shows complete bony ankylosis of both sacroiliac joints in late stage of disease

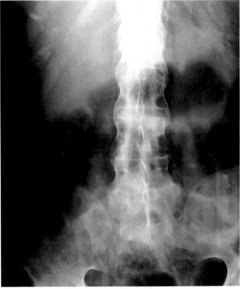

"Bamboo spine." Bony ankylosis of joints of lumbar spine. Ossification exaggerates bulges of intervertebral discs

Complications

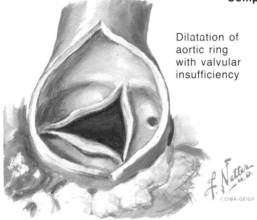

Dilatation of aortic ring with valvular insufficiency

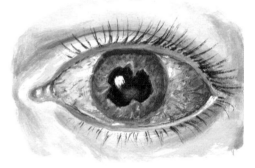

Iridocyclitis with irregular pupil due to synechiae

restricted motion of the low spine; and flattening of the normal lumbar lordosis (Plate 25). As the disease progresses up the spine, the thoracic spine becomes painful, and movement is limited; chest expansion is restricted as the costovertebral joints become involved. If the cervical spine becomes affected, movement of the head and neck also becomes painful and restricted.

After years of disease activity, the inflammation subsides and pain abates, but since the ankylosis is irreversible, the spine remains rigid with some degree of deformity and variable incapacitation. In advanced disease, the thoracic spine becomes considerably kyphotic, and the neck and head assume a fixed forward position. Affected hips are also painful, and movement is restricted; a complete, incapacitating ankylosis may result.

Constitutional manifestations of ankylosing spondylitis are usually mild and limited to fatigue, anorexia, and weight loss. In the active stage of the disease, the erythrocyte sedimentation rate is elevated, and mild anemia may occur.

Radiographic Findings. Radiographs of the pelvis and spine help to confirm the diagnosis. In the early stage of the disease, radiographic changes are seen only in the sacroiliac joints. First, the bone on both sides of the sacroiliac joint and the bony borders are indistinct (Plate 25). Later, the cartilage space narrows, and erosions appear in the bordering bone. In the late stages, radiographs show complete ankylosis of the sacroiliac joints (Plate 26). After the disease has progressed to involve the lumbar and thoracic spine, the facet borders become indistinct; then the cartilage space appears narrowed, and later, bony ankylosis is apparent. Ossification of the annulus fibrosus is usually first seen at the

L1–2 and T11–12 levels; later, the perispinous calcification spreads upward and downward. In severe, advanced disease, the calcification is continuous throughout the spine, producing a "bamboo-spine" appearance on the radiograph (Plate 25). Late in the disease, there is radiographic evidence of bony ankylosis in many facets together with the perispinous calcification. In affected hips and shoulders, radiographic changes are similar to those seen in rheumatoid arthritis.

Two infrequent but serious complications may develop late in patients with severe disease. Disturbances in cardiac conduction, usually first-degree atrioventricular (AV) block, are detected in about 10% of patients; dilatation of the aortic ring and insufficiency of the aortic valve may develop in some of these patients (Plate 26). Iridocyclitis in one or both eyes may result in synechiae and impaired vision if it is severe and untreated.

Treatment and Prognosis. The prognosis for ankylosing spondylitis is better than for rheumatoid arthritis. The evolution of the disease may cease at any time, occasionally before it progresses to the upper spine. In all patients, disease activity and pain subside completely after a number of years. Reduced chest expansion, especially when associated with kyphosis of the thoracic spine and aortic insufficiency, embarrasses pulmonary function and predisposes to respiratory

infection. Apart from these problems, the patient usually lives a comfortable, normal life span, handicapped only by rigidity of the spine and restricted motion of hips and shoulders due to the ankylosis.

The principles and objectives of treatment are the same as those for rheumatoid arthritis. Although aspirin successfully relieves pain in some patients, other NSAIDs are generally superior and less toxic. Administration of corticosteroids should be reserved for severe disease not adequately suppressed by NSAIDs or aspirin. Other essential therapeutic elements include abundant rest, especially early in the disease; use of a firm mattress on a bed board and a firm armchair with a high seat; application of heat; a program of active, nonweight-bearing exercises for the spine, hips, and shoulders; as well as deep-breathing exercises. As the disease activity lessens, medications may be decreased and eventually discontinued, but exercises should be continued to maintain range of motion. If hip involvement causes severe pain and incapacitation, total hip replacement should be considered (see Section IV). Marked rigid kyphosis may be corrected with spinal osteotomy; however, this severe deformity can often be avoided with a program of physical therapy and exercises, use of proper bed and chair, and avoidance of occupations that predispose to kyphosis, such as driving a taxi or truck, gardening, and farming. □

Psoriatic Arthritis

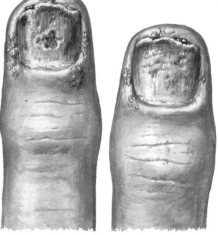

Pitting, discoloration, and erosion
of fingernails with fusiform swelling
of distal interphalangeal joints

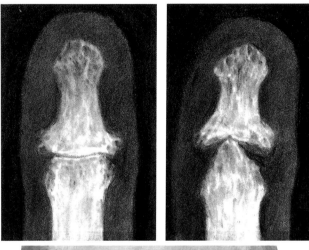

Psoriatic patches on dorsum of
hand with swelling and distortion
of many interphalangeal joints
and shortening of fingers due
to loss of bone mass

Radiographic changes in distal
interphalangeal joint.
Left: in early stages, bone
erosions seen at joint margins.
Right: in late stages, further loss
of bone mass produces "pencil
point in cup" appearance

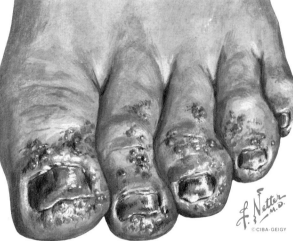

Toes with sausagelike swelling,
skin lesions, and nail changes

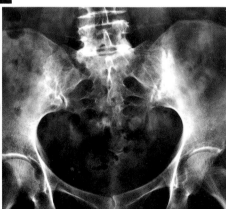

Radiograph of sacroiliac joints shows
thin cartilage with irregular surface
and condensation of adjacent bone in
sacrum and ilia

About 10% of persons with psoriasis have some form of inflammatory joint disease. Although this association has been recognized for more than a century, the features that characterize psoriatic arthritis as a separate clinical entity have been identified only recently.

Clinical Manifestations. Onset of the skin disease may long precede the arthropathy, but occasionally, the reverse is true. The distinguishing features of psoriatic arthritis are (1) a predilection for the distal joints of the fingers and toes, frequently accompanied by psoriatic involvement of only a few other joints of the limbs; (2) destructive and mutilating changes of the phalanges adjacent to the inflamed joints, which produce the radiographic appearance of a "whittling" or "pencil point in cup" of the proximal phalanx and a "cupping" of the central portion of the base of the apposing distal phalanx, with bony proliferation of the borders; (3) shortening, angulation, and telescoping of the fingers due to extensive bone resorption in the phalanges; and (4) frequent involvement of the sacroiliac joints and spine, which simulates ankylosing spondylitis.

Other features that differentiate this disorder from rheumatoid arthritis include (1) absence of both rheumatoid factor and rheumatoid nodules; (2) presence of HLA-B27 in the serum of 90% of patients with sacroiliitis and spondylitis; (3) more frequent remissions of the arthropathy (usually simultaneous with the remission of psoriasis); (4) characteristic radiographic evidence of gross destruction of isolated small joints, with marked osteolysis and bone erosion; (5) "fluffy" periostitis of the shafts of long bones; and (6) nonmarginal as well as marginal syndesmophytes as features of spondylitis.

Laboratory Studies. Although there are no specific laboratory tests for the diagnosis of arthritis associated with psoriasis, the erythrocyte sedimentation rate is elevated in proportion to the extent and activity of the synovitis. Mild anemia may occur. The serum uric acid level may be elevated, especially when psoriasis is extensive and active; the increase may be due to the rapid turnover of cells in the cutaneous lesions. The pathology of the synovitis is indistinguishable from that of rheumatoid arthritis, and synovial fluid analysis reveals only an exudative, polymorphonuclear cell response.

Treatment. Therapeutic measures are the same as those indicated for rheumatoid arthritis, with specific therapy for the skin lesions. Patients with mild involvement often respond well to aspirin or other nonsteroidal antiinflammatory drugs. As in rheumatoid arthritis, administration of gold salts is beneficial in refractory cases. Corticosteroids should be reserved for treatment of severe and rapidly progressive disease; if used, triamcinolone is the drug of choice. Antimalarial drugs, however, are contraindicated. Methotrexate and other immunosuppressive drugs may be very effective, but because of the potential hazards associated with their use, they should be used only in very severe disease. Surgical procedures are performed to correct deformities and replace joints (see Section IV). □

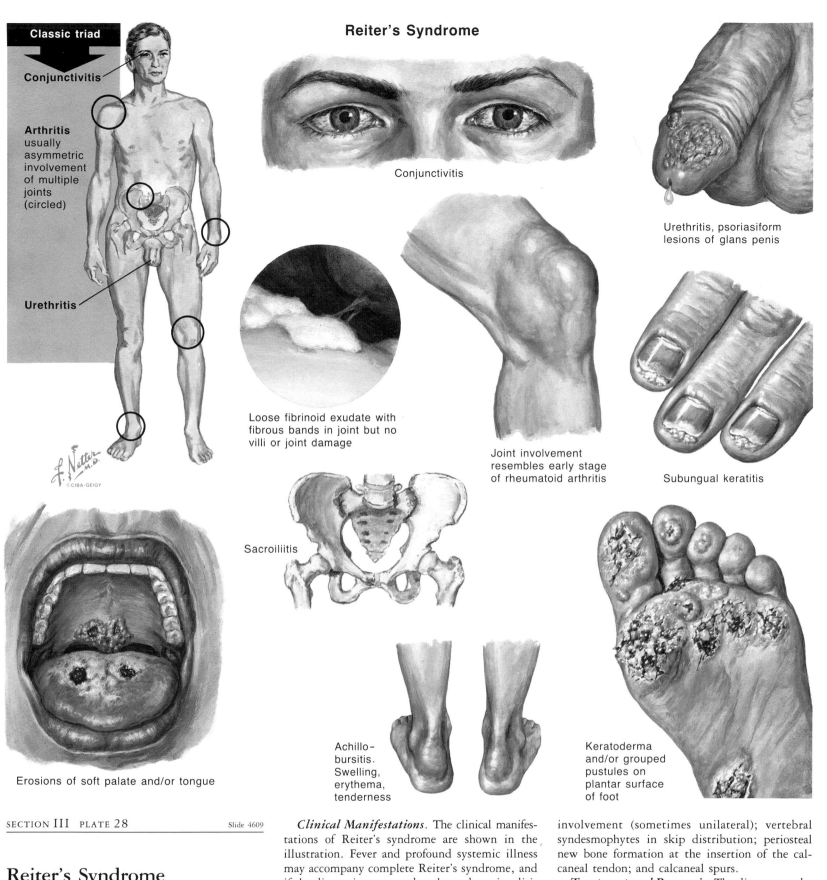

Reiter's Syndrome

Classic triad

Conjunctivitis

Arthritis usually asymmetric involvement of multiple joints (circled)

Urethritis

Conjunctivitis

Urethritis, psoriasiform lesions of glans penis

Loose fibrinoid exudate with fibrous bands in joint but no villi or joint damage

Joint involvement resembles early stage of rheumatoid arthritis

Subungual keratitis

Sacroiliitis

Erosions of soft palate and/or tongue

Achillo-bursitis. Swelling, erythema, tenderness

Keratoderma and/or grouped pustules on plantar surface of foot

SECTION III PLATE 28   Slide 4609

Reiter's Syndrome

Reiter's syndrome has been considered a clinical triad of urethritis, conjunctivitis, and arthritis. It is now accepted that a specific type of dermatitis is another characteristic of the disease, and diagnosis of complete Reiter's syndrome requires the presence of at least three of these four signs.

Of unknown cause, the disease usually occurs in males (90% of cases). It is no longer considered a venereal disease that is caused by a single etiologic agent but is believed to be triggered by prostatitis or bowel inflammation caused by different infectious agents.

Clinical Manifestations. The clinical manifestations of Reiter's syndrome are shown in the illustration. Fever and profound systemic illness may accompany complete Reiter's syndrome, and if the disease is severe and prolonged, pericarditis and myocarditis may occur, sometimes leading to heart block, dilatation of the aortic ring, and aortic valve insufficiency. Several clinical features are similar to those of psoriatic arthritis, and in several instances, Reiter's syndrome has gradually evolved into typical psoriatic arthritis.

The clinical and histologic characteristics of synovitis are nonspecific. In about 90% of cases, HLA-B27 is found on lymphocytes.

Radiographic Findings. Rarefaction of bone near the inflamed joints is visible on radiographs (in chronic disease, articular cartilage destruction and joint deformities are also apparent); sacroiliac involvement (sometimes unilateral); vertebral syndesmophytes in skip distribution; periosteal new bone formation at the insertion of the calcaneal tendon; and calcaneal spurs.

Treatment and Prognosis. The disease may be self-limiting, lasting only a few weeks or months, although attacks may last as long as a year and most patients have persistent joint activity for years. The lesions of the mucous membrane and skin heal without scar. About 50% of patients suffer recurrences, and residual joint deformities may occur.

Therapy for the arthritis component consists of NSAIDs, analgesics, and physical therapy. Tetracycline may be beneficial in patients in the early febrile stage, especially if urethritis is also present, and may shorten the active disease and prevent recurrences. The value of antibiotics, however, is controversial. □

Infectious Arthritis

Joint inflammation caused by specific pathogenic microorganisms invading joint tissues and the joint cavity is known as infectious arthritis. Although almost every known bacteria and some viruses, yeasts, and fungi have been implicated, the microorganisms most commonly responsible for acute infectious arthritis in adults are gonococci, staphylococci, pneumococci, meningococci, colon bacilli, and salmonellae. The incidence of pyogenic arthritis is higher in children than in adults, and the most common causative organisms are *Staphylococcus aureus*, β-hemolytic streptococci, pneumococci, *Haemophilus influenzae*, and various gram-negative bacilli. Factors that predispose to the development of infectious arthritis are bacteremia and susceptibility in the host and the tendency of some organisms, such as gonococci, to invade joints (infectious arthritis develops in approximately 80% of persons with gonococcal bacteremia). In addition to being blood borne, microorganisms may invade the joint tissues from juxtaarticular infection, or they may be introduced by intraarticular injection, penetrating wound, or surgery.

Pathogenesis. Microorganisms first invade the synovial membrane and subsynovial tissues, where they propagate. This incites an acute inflammatory process characterized histologically by infiltration with polymorphonuclear cells and later with lymphocytes and mononuclear cells, tissue proliferation, and neovascularization. If the inflammatory process spreads into the joint cavity, a purulent exudate develops in the joint space, producing what is called a septic joint. Enzymes released from the bacteria and leukocytes rapidly destroy articular cartilages and bone, causing severe structural damage and joint dysfunction; ankylosis may result.

Clinical Manifestations. Gonococcal arthritis typifies infectious arthritis caused by bacteremia. A few days after the onset of genitourinary gonorrhea, when gonococci invade the bloodstream, a mild-to-moderate fever and polyarthralgia or polyarthritis are the presenting signs and symptoms. After a few days, the fever abates, the generalized arthralgia subsides, and severe acute inflammation localizes in a few joints (occasionally only one), usually the large joints in the limbs. Joint pain and tenderness are severe, and signs of inflammation are intense. The patient may be incapacitated. Sparse cutaneous lesions, which at first have hemorrhagic centers that later develop into small pustules, frequently appear on the limbs and trunk.

Leukocytosis, an elevated erythrocyte sedimentation rate, and sometimes mild anemia are present during the invasive stage of pyogenic arthritis. Radiographs of untreated septic joints first show

Infectious Arthritis

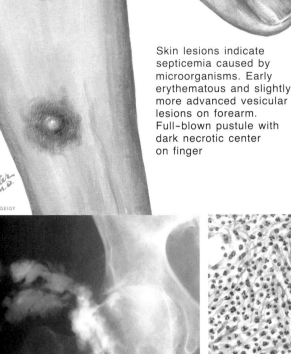

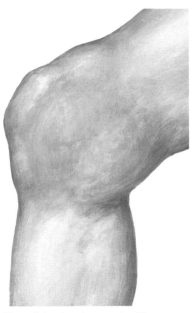

Skin lesions indicate septicemia caused by microorganisms. Early erythematous and slightly more advanced vesicular lesions on forearm. Full-blown pustule with dark necrotic center on finger

Knee joint involvement with swelling and erythema

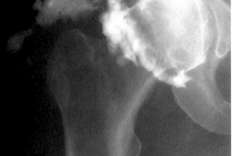

Arthrogram shows destruction of cartilage and bone (aspiration yielded purulent fluid)

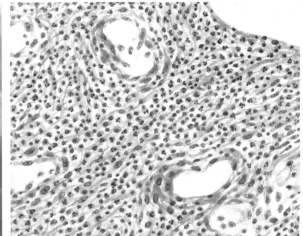

Biopsy specimen of synovial membrane shows infiltration with polymorphonuclear cells, lymphocytes, and mononuclear cells, and tissue proliferation with neovascularization

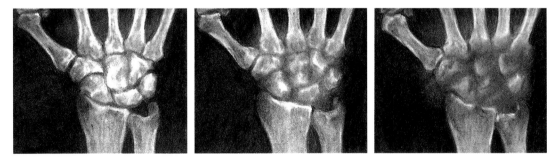

Rapid progression of wrist involvement within 4 weeks, from almost normal (left) to advanced destruction of articular cartilages and severe osteoporosis (right)

a blurring of the joint margins, soon followed by thinning of the cartilage space, roughened subchondral bone, and severe osteoporosis.

Diagnosis. Prompt identification and treatment of infectious arthritis are essential to prevent irreversible joint damage. Infectious arthritis should be suspected in all cases of acute articular inflammation in one or two large joints of the limbs and in all cases of monarticular arthritis in young adults and children whose illness begins with chills and fever. The causative organism should be determined immediately by examination of all bodily discharges, repeated blood cultures, and especially analysis of smears and culture of fluid from the inflamed joint. As soon as the causative

agent is isolated and the antibiotic susceptibilities identified, appropriate parenteral antimicrobial therapy should be instituted and continued until the infection is cured. If septic joint is suspected and the causative infectious agent has not yet been identified, initial therapy should be instituted as for a staphylococcal infection. Infected joint fluid, especially if purulent, should be aspirated daily until the infection is controlled. Septic joints that respond slowly to systemic treatment may require surgical drainage. Response to treatment must be monitored assiduously and changes of antibiotic, dosage, or type of drainage made when indicated. Patients with joint damage and residual dysfunction require rehabilitation. □

Tuberculous Arthritis

Tuberculous Arthritis

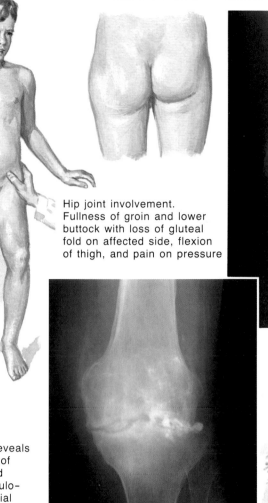

Hip joint involvement. Fullness of groin and lower buttock with loss of gluteal fold on affected side, flexion of thigh, and pain on pressure

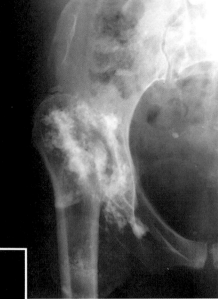

Advanced hip joint involvement shows extensive destruction

Radiograph reveals degeneration of knee joint and calcified granulomatous material

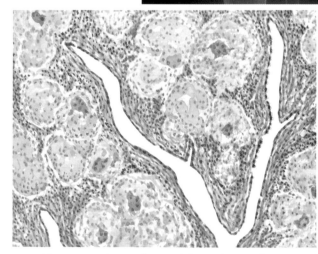

Biopsy specimen of synovial membrane shows conglomerate caseating tubercles

Tuberculous osteomyelitis of spine (Pott's disease) with angulation and compression of spinal cord

Since the advent of effective antibiotic therapy and the eradication of bovine tuberculosis in milk cattle, the incidence of tuberculous arthritis has declined sharply. However, because of its seriousness, the possibility of tuberculosis must always be considered, especially in cases of monarticular arthritis in children and young adults.

Clinical Manifestations. Tuberculous arthritis usually involves only one joint. In order of frequency, the joints affected are the spine, hip, knee, elbow, ankle, sacroiliac, shoulder, and wrist. The onset of symptoms is insidious. In children, the first symptom is often a limp or severe muscle spasm that occurs at night. Clinical examination reveals a "doughy" swelling (without erythema) of joints in the limbs, with fluid accumulation and early, severe, localized muscle atrophy. When the spine is involved (Pott's disease), walking and negotiating steps are painful. Pott's disease often causes anterior wedging of the vertebrae, resulting in an angular kyphosis that is evident on physical examination. Signs of spinal cord compression varying from reflex changes to paraplegia may occur. In late-stage infection, draining sinuses may develop around the affected area.

Radiographic Findings. Radiographs help to establish the diagnosis. The earliest observable change is the decalcification of bone near the diseased joint. Later, marked irregularity and narrowing of the cartilage space indicate subchondral bone invasion. Decreased density of cortical bone

is evidence of regional atrophy of bone. In advanced disease, bone necrosis may be extensive, resulting in complete destruction of the joint architecture. Soft-tissue shadows of abscesses may be evident.

Laboratory Studies. The tuberculin skin test is usually strongly positive. In about 50% of patients, chest radiographs show pulmonary tuberculosis. Laboratory tests are usually needed to confirm the diagnosis. Peripheral blood count may show a relative increase in mononuclear cells.

Synovial fluid analysis reveals a marked decrease in sugar content and a white blood cell count of more than 10,000/mm³ with a high content of mononuclear cells. Examination of stained smears

of synovial fluid seldom shows acid-fast bacilli, but results of culture or guinea pig inoculation are usually positive. The most specific diagnostic procedure is the demonstration of typical caseating tubercles in the inflamed synovial membrane or in regional lymph nodes; acid-fast bacilli can usually be found in cultures of biopsy tissue. If simpler tests are not definitive, a biopsy of synovial or lymph node tissue, or both, should be carried out.

Treatment. Prolonged chemotherapy with isoniazid and rifampin, which may be supplemented with ethambutol, is usually curative, even in advanced cases. Surgical drainage, synovectomy, or fusion is required in rare cases. □

Hemophilic Arthritis

Hemophilic Arthritis

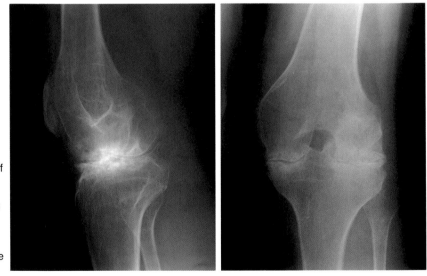

Swelling of right knee joint and atrophy of thigh muscles in young boy are signs of hemophilic arthritis resulting from repeated hemarthroses. Purpuric patches on left leg and knee are from recent hemorrhages

Morbidity in the hemophilic patient is caused by hemorrhage and its consequences. Bleeding into the joint (hemarthrosis) occurs in at least 80% of patients, and the resulting inflammation is one of the more serious forms of arthritis. Hemarthrosis usually begins in childhood and recurs until adulthood, when it becomes infrequent. Trauma to the joint is the immediate cause of bleeding, although the injury may be mild and go unnoticed until the hemorrhage is recognized. The most commonly involved joints are those most vulnerable to injury: knees, elbows, and ankles; less often, shoulders, hips, and small joints of the hands and feet.

Hemarthrosis initiates an acute inflammatory reaction in the joint, which becomes swollen, warm, very tender, and painful to move. Fever and leukocytosis are common associated findings. When joint hemorrhage and synovitis are mild, the arthritis may resolve completely in a few days; if they are severe, the joint inflammation may persist for several months. Repeated hemarthroses cause a chronic joint inflammation that is characterized by villous proliferation of the synovial membrane and infiltration of plasma cells and lymphocytes. Hemosiderin is deposited in the hypertrophied synovial membrane, and progressive fibrosis develops, leading to flexion contracture of the joint. Intraosseous bleeding causes cysts to form in the subchondral bone. In approximately 50% of affected joints, the articular cartilage is eroded, creating permanent joint damage and disability. Extensive bleeding into the muscles around the affected joint may cause hematomas that compress adjacent nerves or blood vessels, or both, further restricting joint motion.

Radiographic Findings. Soft-tissue shadows indicate acute hemorrhage into the joint. After repeated hemarthroses, joint radiographs reveal cartilage thinning, narrowing of joint space, rough subchondral bone, marginal spurs, bone cysts, and thick joint capsule. These same findings are seen in the older patient with osteoarthritis. Radiographic findings unique to hemophilic arthritis are soft-tissue densities of hemosiderin deposits, hypertrophy of epiphyses adjacent to the affected joint, enlargement of the radial head, flattening of the articular surface ("squaring") of the patella, slipped capital femoral epiphysis, and sometimes, deformity or even destruction of the femoral head.

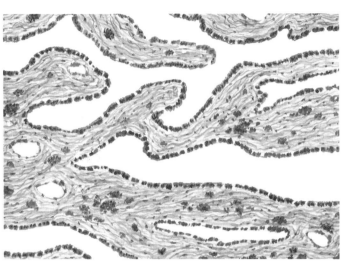

Synovial membrane in chronic disease shows extensive deposits of hemosiderin in lining cells and synovial stroma; reactive fibrosis

Radiographs of left knee joint show narrowing of joint space (due to loss of articular cartilage), irregular articular surfaces, osteophyte formation, and cyst formation in subchondral bone secondary to multiple hemarthroses

Treatment. Because prophylaxis is an important part of the management, the patient should make every effort to prevent joint trauma and, in particular, avoid contact sports. Prompt treatment for acute hemarthrosis helps to minimize structural damage that can cause chronic joint disability. The affected joint should be immobilized immediately, and ice packs and antiinflammatory drugs used to reduce pain. (A nonsalicylate analgesic is recommended because the anticoagulating effect of salicylic acid derivatives prolongs bleeding.) Severe hemorrhage requires the administration of a factor VIII concentrate. Intraarticular administration of corticosteroid helps to inhibit both inflammation and bleeding. Also, orally administered prednisone in large doses has been effective in decreasing the amount of factor VIII needed to stop bleeding.

After administration of a coagulation factor, blood from the distended joint can be aspirated to relieve pain and reduce articular damage. After the bleeding and synovitis have subsided, an active exercise program is started to restore full joint motion. Use of traction, wedging casts, or progressive-extension casts can reduce flexion contractures. Surgery to correct joint deformities, once extremely dangerous, is now safe if sufficient coagulation factor is used to control hemorrhage; this modality has greatly enhanced the rehabilitation of the disabled patient. □

Neuropathic Joint Disease

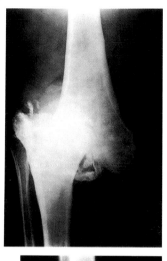

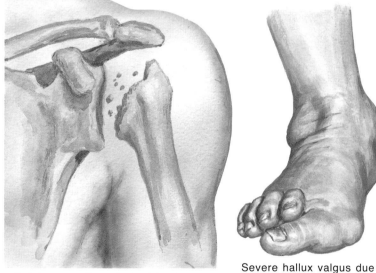

Neuropathic (Charcot's) knee joints in tabes dorsalis

Complete destruction of knee joint due to syphilitic neuropathic joint disease. Bone fragmentation with loose bodies, tissue calcification, and fistula formation

Radiograph shows severe degeneration of knee joint in diabetic neuropathic joint disease

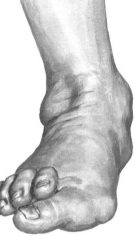

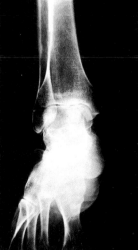

Painless swelling of shoulder joint in syringomyelia with extensive loss of bone mass, effusion, and detritus

Severe hallux valgus due to diabetic neuropathic joint disease. Ankle also involved

Degeneration of ankle joint in diabetic neuropathic joint disease

Neuropathic joint disease (Charcot's joint) is a chronic degenerative disorder caused by a disturbance of the nerve supply to the affected joint. It is most common in males over 40 years of age. Diagnosis is based on typical clinical and radiographic findings and requires identification of the underlying neurologic disorder.

Many different diseases can cause the arthropathy. Even though tertiary syphilis has declined markedly since the advent of effective antibiotic treatment, tabes dorsalis still is the most common underlying cause of neuropathic joint disease, followed by (in order of frequency) diabetic neuropathy, syringomyelia, myelomeningocele, and a group of miscellaneous neurologic disorders. The loss of proprioception and pain sensation leads to the relaxation of the ligaments and other structures that support the joint. Joint instability results, and later, injuries related to either daily activities or the neurologic dysfunction initiate the destruction of bone and cartilage.

The joints affected depend on the primary neurologic disorder. Tabes dorsalis most frequently involves the knee, hip, ankle, and lower thoracic and lumbar vertebrae. In diabetic neuropathy, the tarsal, metatarsal, and ankle joints are most often affected; in syringomyelia, the elbow or shoulder is the site of involvement.

Clinical Manifestations. Insidious swelling or instability (or both) of the involved joint is usually the first abnormality noted, followed by effusion and joint destruction. Pain, however, is mild. Physical examination reveals an enlarged, hyper-

mobile, and slightly tender joint with a large effusion. The effusion and enlargement gradually increase. Late in the disease process, the prominent sign is crepitation caused by the extensive destruction of cartilage and bone and the accumulation of intraarticular loose bodies. In diabetic neuropathy, the foot widens and the ankle becomes irregularly swollen.

Radiographic Findings. At first, radiographs may appear basically normal, revealing only joint effusion. Later, loss of cartilage and resorption and fragmentation of bone create a radiographic appearance of numerous loose bodies and unusually shaped osteophytes at the joint margins. The joint looks like a "bag of bones."

Treatment. Because the neuropathy causing the joint disorder is usually either advanced (as in syphilis) or not amenable to therapy, treatment does not often alter the progression of the joint destruction. Supportive measures such as the use of braces and splints to stabilize the joint and crutches or a walker may help to decrease the disability.

Arthrodesis (joint fusion), although the preferred surgical procedure for unstable joints, is often unsuccessful because of nonunion or infection. If infection occurs in a foot, ankle, or knee that has been destroyed by advanced neuropathic joint disease and if antibiotic therapy is unsuccessful, amputation should be considered. □

Gout and Gouty Arthritis

Gout is a disturbance of purine metabolism in which the concentration of uric acid in the blood and body tissues is elevated. Gouty arthritis is a direct result of the deposition of urate crystals in the joint. Primary gout, also described as classic or idiopathic gout, is an inherited inborn error of metabolism. Secondary gout is a consequence of elevated uric acid levels precipitated by another illness or induced by a drug.

For a discussion of uric acid metabolism and the origin of hyperuricemia in primary gout, see CIBA COLLECTION, Volume 4, pages 239–241.

Primary Gout

Primary gout occurs chiefly in males (90% of patients). Although the genetic factors underlying the hyperuricemia are presumably present at birth, the disorder produces no clinical signs or symptoms until the hyperuricemia develops at puberty in males or at a later age in females. Clinical manifestations of gout usually do not appear until middle age in males (30–50 years) and later in females (Plate 33).

Pathogenesis. Although it is known that the excessive concentration of uric acid in the blood is responsible for gouty arthritis, the physiologic and chemical changes that lead to the attack are not completely understood. Many factors can induce an acute attack of gouty arthritis, among them excessive ingestion of alcoholic (especially fermented) beverages, overeating, prolonged exposure to cold, surgery, use of diuretics, and dehydration. The immediate cause of the acute synovitis is the precipitation of monosodium urate crystals in the synovial membrane and joint cavity; thus, the attack is crystal induced. Polymorphonuclear leukocytes vigorously phagocytize the urate crystals, and a complex chain of events, which is not fully understood, results in an acute inflammation. Enzymes released from the phagocytizing leukocytes are the presumed cause of erosion of the articular cartilage, which occurs after prolonged, severe inflammation, but other factors such as interleukin-1 (IL-1), which can activate chondrocytes, may also be involved.

Clinical Manifestations. Almost always, the first clinical evidence of gout is acute arthritis in one or a few peripheral joints. A fulminant synovitis begins abruptly, typically during the night, frequently involving the first metatarsophalangeal joint. This acute involvement of the great toe is known as *podagra*. The affected joint becomes very swollen, red, hot, tender, and excruciatingly painful (Plate 33). Fever and leukocytosis may accompany the attack, and the erythrocyte sedimentation rate is usually increased. If untreated,

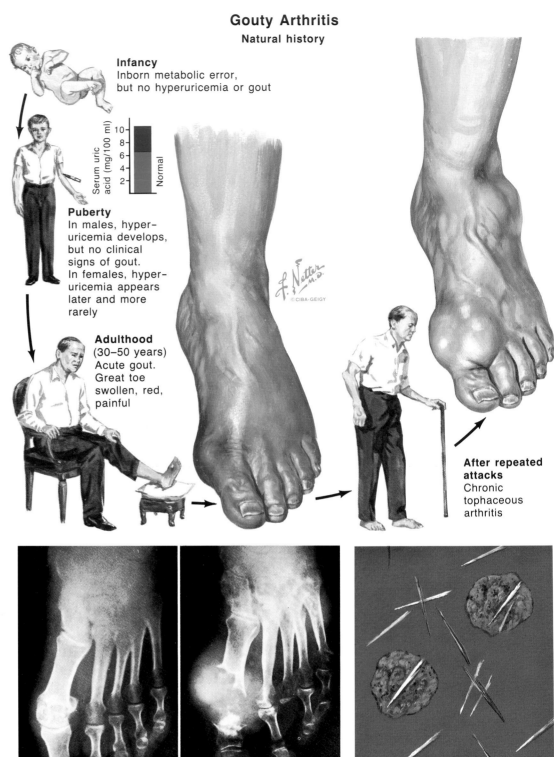

Gouty Arthritis
Natural history

Infancy
Inborn metabolic error, but no hyperuricemia or gout

Puberty
In males, hyperuricemia develops, but no clinical signs of gout. In females, hyperuricemia appears later and more rarely

Serum uric acid (mg/100 ml) 10 8 6 4 2 Normal

Adulthood
(30–50 years) Acute gout. Great toe swollen, red, painful

After repeated attacks
Chronic tophaceous arthritis

Early tophaceous gouty arthritis → Same patient 12 years later, untreated

Free and phagocytized monosodium urate crystals in aspirated joint fluid seen on compensated polarized light microscopy

acute monarticular gouty arthritis lasts 3 or 4 days; if several joints are severely inflamed, the attack may persist 2 or 3 weeks. As the inflammation subsides, there is desquamation of the overlying skin after which the joint returns to normal, and the patient remains asymptomatic until the next attack. After several attacks at 1- or 2-year intervals, the intercritical period is shorter, and the gouty episodes tend to be more severe, last longer, and involve several joints.

After several years of recurrent acute arthritis and persistent hyperuricemia, deposits of monosodium urate, called *tophi*, form in joint structures (and other tissues). Tophi are the hallmark of chronic gout, occurring in 50% of patients.

They cause structural damage to articular cartilage and adjacent bone, resulting in chronic arthritis. In this late stage of the disease, known as *chronic tophaceous gout*, the affected joints show irregular knobby swelling and signs of chronic inflammation. Joint motion is limited and painful, deformities develop, and sinuses tend to form at the swollen joint, from which a calcific exudate drains from the underlying urate deposits.

Radiographs show marked destruction of bone and cartilage and "punched-out" areas in the bone caused by the urate deposits (Plate 33).

Tophi often form in extraarticular structures as well, especially in the extensor tendons of the fingers and toes, the olecranon and infrapatellar

Gout and Gouty Arthritis
(Continued)

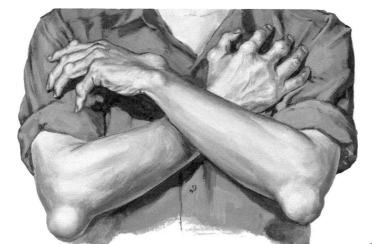

Tophaceous deposits in olecranon bursae, wrists, and hands

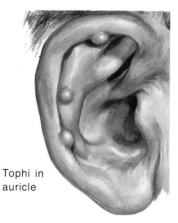

Tophi in auricle

bursae, the calcaneal tendon, the cartilage of the external ear, and the parenchyma of the kidney (Plate 34). Urate deposits in the kidney usually cause chronic gouty nephritis and urate renal stones.

Diagnosis. Diagnosis is problematic only in the first or early attacks of acute arthritis. Gout should always be suspected when acute synovitis develops in a few small joints, especially in the great toe of an older person, particularly a male. A history of gout in close relatives and the finding of hyperuricemia strongly support the diagnosis. Additional evidence is a quick and complete resolution of the synovitis after oral or intravenous administration of high (nearly toxic) doses of colchicine early in the attack. Nonsteroidal antiinflammatory drugs (NSAIDs) produce similar results. The presence of urate crystals in synovial fluid taken from the inflamed joint confirms the diagnosis.

Late in the disease, the presence of tophi, characteristic radiographic findings, or urate kidney stones make the diagnosis obvious.

Secondary Gout

Gout may also be a consequence of the overproduction of uric acid caused by an increased turnover of nucleic acid in such myeloproliferative disorders as polycythemia, myeloid metaplasia, acute and chronic granulocytic leukemia, multiple myeloma, sickle cell anemia, and other hemoglobinopathies. Decreased excretion of uric acid is another cause of secondary gout. This occurs with prolonged use of diuretics and in nephritis due to lead poisoning (saturnine gout).

Clinical and radiographic manifestations of secondary gout are similar to those of primary gout, except for some minor differences: there is a higher prevalence in females; usually, the hyperuricemia is extremely significant; the episodes of synovitis last longer; and tophi develop less frequently. In any patient with no family history of gout, an underlying causative disorder should be suspected.

Treatment

For *acute gouty arthritis*, administration of colchicine is the traditional treatment. Used properly, colchicine can effectively abort or hasten the resolution of the inflammation; however, there is little margin of safety between the adequate therapeutic dose and overdose, which causes severe gastrointestinal disturbances. Indomethacin is equally effective and usually better tolerated than

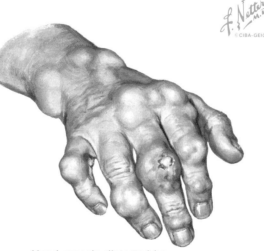

Hand grossly distorted by multiple tophi (some ulcerated)

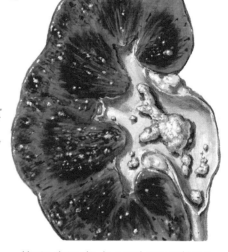

Urate deposits in renal parenchyma, urate stones in renal pelvis

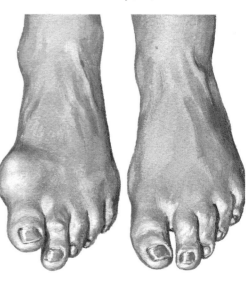

Resolution of tophus after 27 months of treatment with uricosuric agents

colchicine and has therefore become the treatment of choice for acute gout. Other NSAIDs may also be effective.

In the intercritical period, if the hyperuricemia is not excessive and the attacks are mild and infrequent, small daily doses of colchicine may suffice as prophylactic treatment. When the serum uric acid concentration is persistently high or attacks are frequent, and in all cases of chronic tophaceous gout, the serum uric acid level should be reduced to the normal range and maintained there for the rest of the patient's life. In most cases, this can be accomplished with administration of adequate daily dosages of a well-tolerated uricosuric agent, commonly probenecid or the

xanthine oxidase inhibitor allopurinol. Severe gout may require concurrent therapy with both agents. Frequent determinations of the serum uric acid concentration are required to monitor the effective dosage. Management also includes dietary changes to avoid excessive intake of food (particularly purine-rich foods) and alcoholic beverages and to reduce body weight to normal. This treatment program, which must be continued for the rest of the patient's life, can virtually eliminate acute attacks of gouty arthritis, prevent the deposition of new urate crystals, and reduce existing tophaceous deposits. With proper treatment and patient compliance, gout can nearly always be controlled. □

Articular Chondrocalcinosis (Pseudogout)

Articular Chondrocalcinosis (Pseudogout)

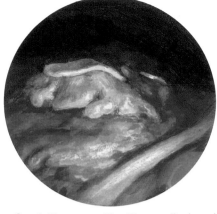

Crystalline synovitis. Biopsy disclosed calcium pyrophosphate crystals seen under polarized light microscopy

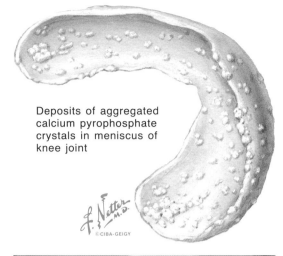

Deposits of aggregated calcium pyrophosphate crystals in meniscus of knee joint

Articular chondrocalcinosis refers to the deposition of calcium-containing salts in the hyaline cartilage and fibrocartilage of joints. In particular, the deposition of calcium pyrophosphate dihydrate (CPPD) crystals in the joint causes a symptomatic disorder known as calcium pyrophosphate dihydrate deposition disease, which is typically manifested as acute arthritis. Because the attacks of arthritis resemble classic gout due to hyperuricemia, this type of arthritis is called pseudogout. Other calcium phosphate salts have been identified in the menisci, but nearly all synovial fluid aspirated from joints affected with pseudogout contains CPPD.

The mechanism of CPPD deposition in articular cartilage is not yet understood. Serum calcium, phosphate, and alkaline phosphatase levels are normal, as is urinary calcium excretion. The synovitis of pseudogout is induced by crystals of CPPD in synovial fluid, and trauma to the joint and surgery are two factors that can provoke an attack. A popular but unproven hypothesis for the pathogenesis of the acute attack is the discharge of CPPD crystals from deposits in hyaline cartilage into the joint space. The crystals then induce inflammation by the same mechanism as the urate crystal–induced synovitis of gout (Plates 33–34). The speed of onset of the attack may be related to the rate of CPPD crystal release into the joint space, and the severity of the synovitis can be determined by the quantity of crystals released.

Clinical and Radiographic Manifestations. Pseudogout affects men somewhat more often than women, and patients are generally middle-aged or elderly. It involves one or a few joints of the limbs, most often the knee. The onset of acute synovitis is abrupt, and the inflammation reaches peak intensity more slowly than in true (urate) gout. The attack is also somewhat less painful. A self-limiting disorder, an episode of pseudogout lasts from 1 or 2 days to a few weeks. Between attacks, the patient remains asymptomatic.

In about 5% of patients with chondrocalcinosis, a subacute polyarthritis occurs that resembles rheumatoid arthritis and lasts many months. This manifestation occurs along with the attacks of acute synovitis typical of pseudogout.

About half of older patients with chondrocalcinosis (mostly women) also exhibit progressive degenerative changes in many joints (osteoarthritis). The knee joint is the most common site of involvement, followed by the wrist, metacarpo-

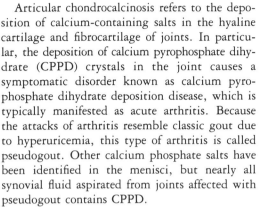

Anteroposterior radiograph of knee reveals densities due to calcific deposits in menisci

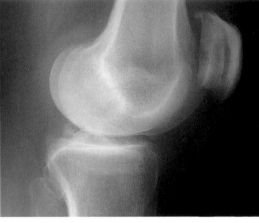

In lateral radiograph, calcific deposits in articular cartilage of femur and patella appear as fluffy white opacities

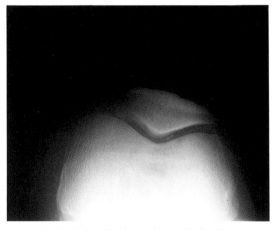

Axial ("skyline") view of knee joint in flexion demonstrates calcinosis of articular cartilages of patella and femur

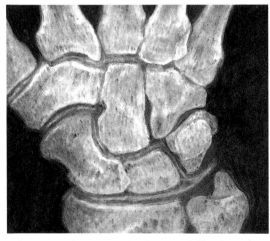

Drawing of radiograph shows calcific deposits in articular cartilages of carpus as fine lines between carpal bones and in radiocarpal joint

phalangeal, hip, shoulder, elbow, and ankle joints. Most joints with radiographic signs of chondrocalcinosis are asymptomatic, even in patients with synovitis in other joints. Thus, articular chondrocalcinosis does not necessarily imply the existence of pseudogout.

On radiographs of the joint, chondrocalcinosis appears as a fine line of CPPD crystals arranged parallel to the cartilage surface. Diagnosis of pseudogout should be suspected in all cases of acute synovitis in a large joint of an older person whose serum uric acid level is normal. Diagnosis requires the radiographic demonstration of chondrocalcinosis and the finding of CPPD crystals on microscopic examination of aspirated joint fluid.

Treatment. Aspiration of fluid from the inflamed joint, coupled with intraarticular injection of a corticosteroid, is often sufficient to relieve symptoms of acute pseudogout arthritis. Oral administration of a nonsteroidal antiinflammatory drug (NSAID) is a helpful adjunct. The response to treatment with colchicine is unpredictable but occasionally dramatic. Some patients may benefit from a short-term course of oral corticosteroid therapy. Treatment of chronic arthritis associated with chondrocalcinosis is the same as that for osteoarthritis. It is not possible to halt the progressive deposition of CPPD crystals in articular cartilage or to remove CPPD crystals that have already been deposited. □

Nonarticular Rheumatism

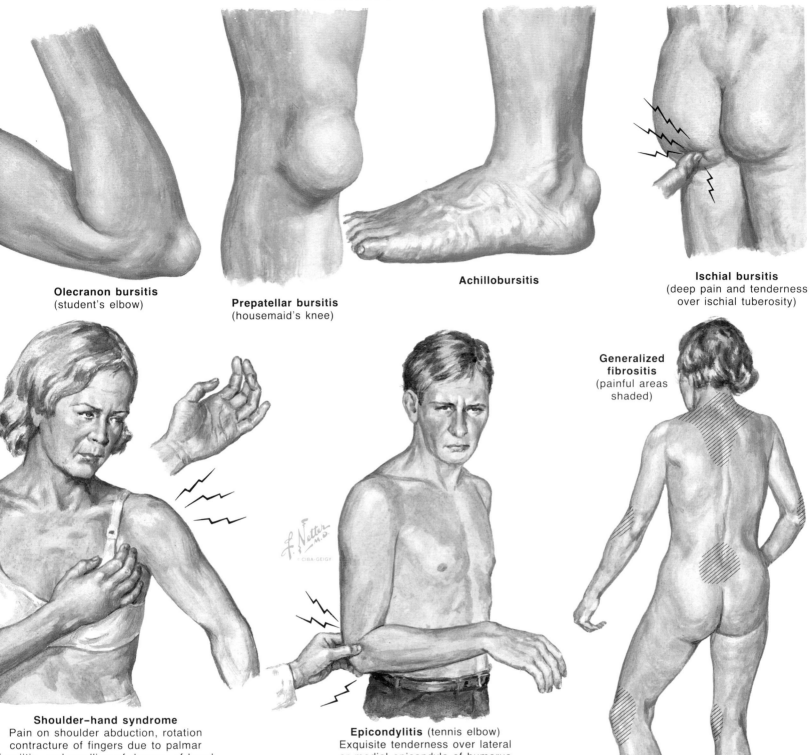

Olecranon bursitis
(student's elbow)

Prepatellar bursitis
(housemaid's knee)

Achillobursitis

Ischial bursitis
(deep pain and tenderness
over ischial tuberosity)

**Generalized
fibrositis**
(painful areas
shaded)

Shoulder–hand syndrome
Pain on shoulder abduction, rotation
contracture of fingers due to palmar
fasciitis, and swelling of dorsum of hand

Epicondylitis (tennis elbow)
Exquisite tenderness over lateral
or medial epicondyle of humerus

Nonarticular Rheumatism

Nonarticular rheumatism refers to a diverse group of inflammatory disorders that affect only the nonarticular connective-tissue structures. The nonarticular inflammation is often localized to a specialized fibrous-tissue structure adjacent to a joint, frequently the shoulder, elbow, wrist, or ankle. Tendonitis, tendon attachment syndrome, tenosynovitis, and bursitis are common examples. The major symptoms—pain, stiffness, and restricted motion—are the same as those of joint disease.

Sometimes the problem may affect structures around several joints, as in palmar and plantar fasciitis, or it may be a combination of disorders, as in the shoulder-hand syndrome, which comprises tendonitis and periarticular fasciitis at the shoulder plus fasciitis, tendonitis, and tenosynovitis of the hand. Presumed involvement of the fibrous tissue of large muscles around the shoulders, back, and hips is called generalized fibrositis, or muscular rheumatism.

Nonarticular rheumatic disorders can be differentiated from arthritis (this is important because treatment and prognosis differ) by accurate localization of tenderness and pain and by the absence of clinical and radiographic signs of joint pathology and systemic disease.

Localized nonarticular rheumatism may result from a direct blow or from repeated, prolonged, or strenuous use of the joint in activities to which the patient is unaccustomed. However, the conditions are usually self-limiting and resolve without residual pathology. An exception is generalized fibrositis, which is a chronic condition; its etiology and pathogenesis are still not known.

Treatment includes rest of the inflamed part, application of heat, and use of salicylates or nonsteroidal antiinflammatory drugs (NSAIDs). Injection of corticosteroid into the inflamed bursa or tendon sheath and around the inflamed tendinous attachment usually results in prompt symptomatic relief and arrest of the inflammation. In rare cases, severe acute inflammation requires a short-term course of systemic corticosteroid treatment. □

Polymyalgia Rheumatica and Giant-Cell Arteritis

Polymyalgia Rheumatica

Polymyalgia rheumatica is a form of nonarticular rheumatism characterized by severe pain and stiffness in the proximal musculature and a very high erythrocyte sedimentation rate (ESR). Although it occurs in both sexes, it is more common in women. Almost all patients are over 50 years of age (average age at onset is 65–70 years).

The etiology of polymyalgia rheumatica is not understood. Follow-up studies have failed to reveal a neoplasm or another rheumatic disease as the causative factor. The relationship between polymyalgia rheumatica and giant-cell arteritis, however, has generated great interest.

Clinical Manifestations. Pain and stiffness, which rapidly become severe, develop in the neck and shoulders, interscapular region, low back, and about the hips. Morning stiffness is marked but muscle weakness and atrophy are absent. Fever, which is often high, is a systemic characteristic, and anorexia, weight loss, apathy, and malaise may be pronounced. Although the muscles appear normal on physical examination, the affected muscles, sternum, and rib cage are tender. Early in the disease, synovitis may be noted in one or two large joints, most often in the knee. Radiographs, electromyograms, and muscle biopsy reveal no abnormality.

Laboratory Studies. The ESR is often more than 100 mm/hr Westergren. Anemia is a common finding, with a hematocrit reading often as low as 0.30. Rheumatoid factor and antinuclear antibodies are absent, and muscle enzyme levels are normal.

Diagnosis is based on characteristic clinical findings and the absence of physical signs and radiographic and laboratory findings to support other, more common rheumatic diseases. A dramatic response to the administration of corticosteroids provides reliable supporting evidence.

Treatment. Prednisone in an initial daily dosage of 20 to 30 mg eliminates symptoms and restores normal physical activity within 24 to 48 hours. The daily dose of prednisone can be reduced rapidly to 7.5 to 10 mg, with a further reduction after several weeks. In many cases, treatment with prednisone can be discontinued after several months, although it may be required for 1 or 2 years in patients with severe disease. The dosage and duration of treatment needed to keep the patient asymptomatic and the ESR normal are monitored by periodic trial reductions.

The prognosis for polymyalgia rheumatica is very good. Complete resolution, without residual effects, can be expected within a few months to 2 years, although there may be a recurrence of the disease.

Polymyalgia Rheumatica; Giant-Cell Arteritis

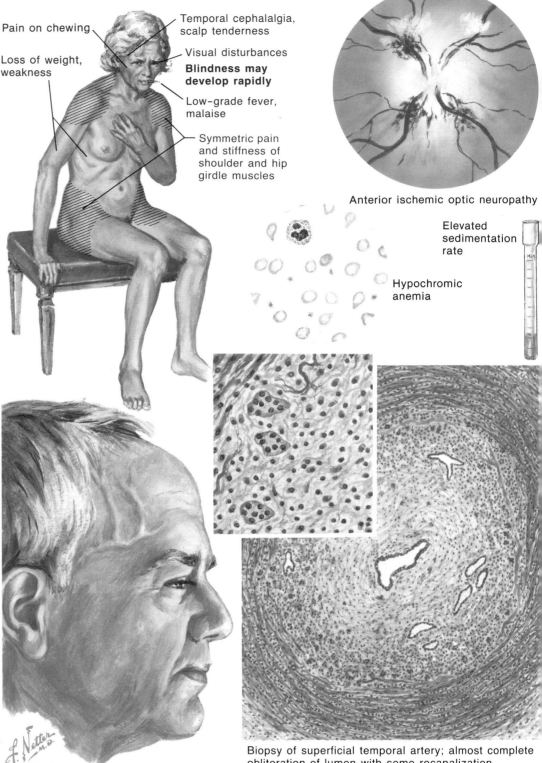

Pain on chewing

Temporal cephalalgia, scalp tenderness

Loss of weight, weakness

Visual disturbances

Blindness may develop rapidly

Low-grade fever, malaise

Symmetric pain and stiffness of shoulder and hip girdle muscles

Anterior ischemic optic neuropathy

Elevated sedimentation rate

Hypochromic anemia

Rigid, tender, nonpulsating temporal arteries may be visible or palpable

Biopsy of superficial temporal artery; almost complete obliteration of lumen with some recanalization. High-power insert shows infiltration with lymphocytes, plasma cells and giant cells; fragmentation of elastica

Giant-Cell Arteritis

Severe temporal headache and visual loss—even blindness—occur in some elderly patients, either independently or in conjunction with polymyalgia rheumatica. The temporal arteries are prominent and tortuous, and biopsy of a branch reveals giant-cell arteritis, characterized by inflammation of the tunica media and tunica intima, fibroblastic proliferation, giant-cell infiltration, and partial occlusion of the lumen by thrombus. These pathologic findings are also observed in 10% to 15% of patients with polymyalgia rheumatica who have no signs and symptoms of arteritis. In addition, at autopsy giant-cell arteritis

has been found in medium and large arteries without involvement of the temporal arteries or association with polymyalgia rheumatica. Giant-cell arteritis is now recognized as a systemic disease that has a segmental distribution and involves only some medium and large arteries.

Much clinical and pathologic evidence exists to link polymyalgia rheumatica and giant-cell arteritis, but whether all patients with polymyalgia rheumatica have occult giant-cell arteritis and whether there is causal relationship are questions that require further investigation. Treatment of temporal arteritis with prednisone produces dramatic results. It may prevent blindness and may even be lifesaving. □

Tendonitis and Bursitis of Shoulder

Tendonitis and Bursitis of Shoulder

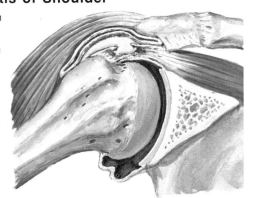

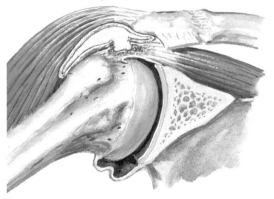

Abduction of arm causes repeated impingement of greater tubercle of humerus on acromion, leading to degeneration and inflammation of supraspinatus tendon, secondary inflammation of bursa, and pain on abduction of arm. Calcific deposit in degenerated tendon produces elevation that further aggravates inflammation and pain

Calcific deposit may rupture spontaneously beneath floor of bursa, with relief of pain and inflammation

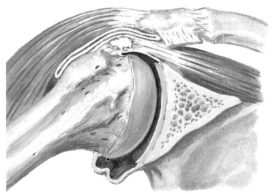

Deposit may rupture spontaneously into bursa and be resorbed, relieving pain and acute inflammation

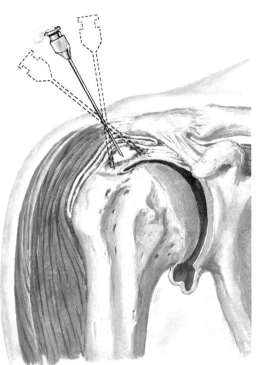

Chronic tendonitis and bursitis with calcific deposit in tendon and minimal inflammation. Chronic deposits do not rupture spontaneously but may be resorbed

Needle rupture of deposit in acute tendonitis promptly relieves acute symptoms. After administration of local anesthetic, needle introduced at point of greatest tenderness. Several probings may be necessary to reach deposit. Toothpastelike deposit may ooze from needle. Irrigation of bursa with saline solution using two needles often done to remove more calcific material. Corticosteroid may be injected for additional relief

Tendonitis and secondary bursitis of the shoulder—also referred to as painful arc syndrome, subdeltoid (subacromial) bursitis, calcific tendonitis, and impingement syndrome—usually causes shoulder pain in middle-aged persons of both sexes.

The anatomic configuration of the shoulder contributes to the physiologic degeneration that gradually develops in the rotator (musculotendinous) cuff in persons more than 40 years of age. In young persons, impingement syndrome most often results from overuse or acute trauma. The incidence of impingement syndrome leading to disability is higher in persons with occupations in which the arms are constantly elevated. When the arm is abducted, the poorly vascularized supraspinatus tendon of the rotator cuff is pinched between the greater tubercle of the humerus, the acromion, and the coracoacromial ligament. This repeated trauma accelerates and intensifies normal degenerative changes. The fibers of the tendon become frayed, fibrillated, avascular, and even necrotic, occasionally leading to a tear of the rotator cuff. For unknown reasons, a calcific deposit may also develop in the degenerating area.

As a result, an acute or chronic inflammatory process develops in the surrounding viable tendon and in the overlying floor of the subdeltoid bursa. The swelling, which is increased by a deposition of calcium salts, encroaches on the space between the greater tubercle of the humerus and the acromion, and the increased impingement

causes pain with certain movements of the shoulder (Plate 38).

Acute Calcific Tendonitis and Bursitis

Clinical and Radiographic Manifestations. Acute calcific tendonitis and bursitis of the shoulder is extremely painful but self-limiting, usually lasting 6 to 14 days. Acute inflammation and swelling occur around a degenerated area in a tendon, usually the supraspinatus, and in the bursa. A sudden onset of disabling shoulder pain causes the patient to guard and splint the arm against the body. Some patients report previous attacks. The primary signs are exquisite tenderness directly over the inflamed rotator cuff and

calcific deposit and severe pain that greatly restricts active motion. Radiographs usually reveal a fluffy deposit of calcium in the region of the supraspinatus tendon.

Treatment. The patient's preference and the stage of the disease determine the type of treatment. If the acute pain is subsiding, indicating spontaneous rupture of the calcium deposit, symptomatic treatment is sufficient. Oral analgesic medication, rest with the arm in a sling for a few days, and progressive exercises as symptoms permit often result in a prompt recovery.

If severe pain persists, some patients still elect symptomatic care and wait for spontaneous rupture or resorption of the calcific deposit, which

Tendonitis and Bursitis of Shoulder

(Continued)

Surgery for Acute and Chronic Calcific Tendonitis and Bursitis of Shoulder

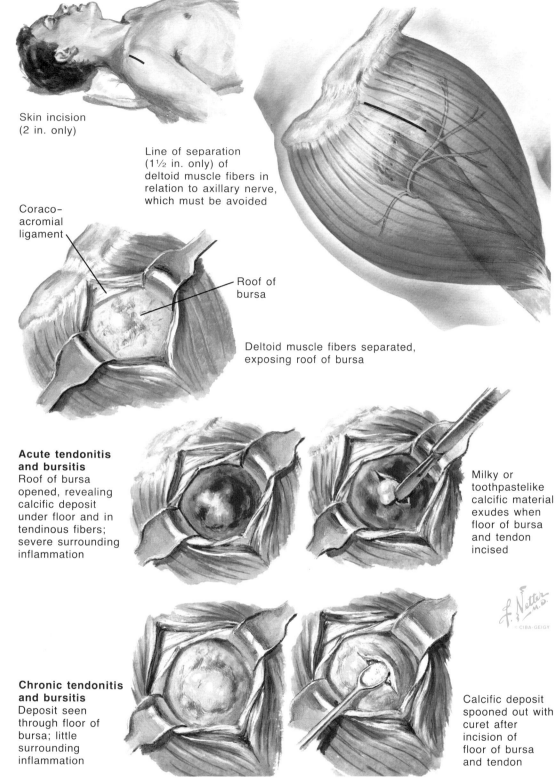

Skin incision (2 in. only)

Line of separation (1½ in. only) of deltoid muscle fibers in relation to axillary nerve, which must be avoided

Coraco-acromial ligament

Roof of bursa

Deltoid muscle fibers separated, exposing roof of bursa

Acute tendonitis and bursitis
Roof of bursa opened, revealing calcific deposit under floor and in tendinous fibers; severe surrounding inflammation

Milky or toothpastelike calcific material exudes when floor of bursa and tendon incised

Chronic tendonitis and bursitis
Deposit seen through floor of bursa; little surrounding inflammation

Calcific deposit spooned out with curet after incision of floor of bursa and tendon

usually occurs 4 to 10 days after onset of symptoms (Plate 38). A course of nonsteroidal antiin-flammatory drugs (NSAIDs) helps relieve pain and inflammation.

To shorten the duration of severe pain, some patients choose a more aggressive treatment such as rupture of the deposit with needle puncture. Under aseptic conditions and local anesthesia, one or two needles are inserted into the zone of maximum tenderness and into the calcific deposit. Aspiration of the milky or toothpastelike material confirms the rupture. Before the needle is withdrawn, the bursa is often irrigated with saline solution and injected with a corticosteroid. The essential part of this procedure is rupture of the deposit. If the severe pain has not been relieved, the needle puncture has failed to rupture the calcific deposit and may need to be repeated. After the puncture, conservative symptomatic treatment is prescribed, and progressive exercises and use of the arm are begun as soon as possible.

Refractory cases occasionally require evacuation of the calcific material with a surgical procedure. A short anterolateral incision is used to split the deltoid muscle; the bursa is opened and the deposit located and incised. The calcific material is evacuated and the wound closed (Plate 39).

Chronic Tendonitis

More common than acute calcific tendonitis, chronic tendonitis of the rotator cuff refers to the inflammation of the tendinous tissues surrounding a degenerated zone in the rotator cuff and associated mild subdeltoid bursitis. A calcific deposit may also be present. The mild swelling of this lesion, often enlarged by a calcific deposit, increases the painful impingement of the cuff on the acromion (Plate 38).

Clinical Manifestations. The primary complaint is a dull, aching pain of varying intensity in the deltoid area. Symptoms, which are chronic and intermittent, are precipitated and intensified by abduction and rotation or forward flexion of the shoulder. The discomfort, however, is often mild and usually not disabling; night pain is common.

Physical examination reveals normal active and passive shoulder motion, with pain occurring when the shoulder is abducted and flexed beyond 60°. A normal range of passive motion distinguishes this condition from adhesive capsulitis (Plate 42). Mild, local tenderness of the rotator cuff is another common manifestation. Because tears of the rotator cuff (Plate 44) sometimes accompany chronic tendonitis and bursitis, the examination should include a test to determine the strength of the initiation of abduction and the patient's ability to maintain the arm in an abducted position against gravity and resistance. A subacromial injection of lidocaine and corticosteroid aids in the diagnosis of chronic tendonitis by relieving

Tendonitis and Bursitis of Shoulder

(Continued)

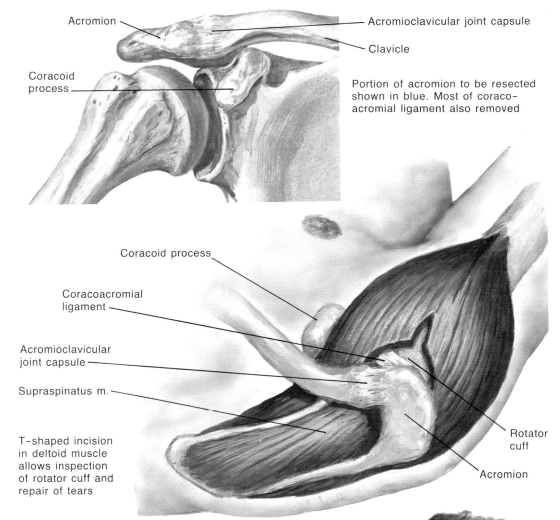

Acromion

Acromioclavicular joint capsule

Clavicle

Coracoid process

Portion of acromion to be resected shown in blue. Most of coraco-acromial ligament also removed

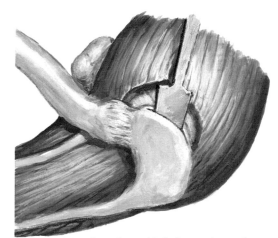

Coracoid process

Coracoacromial ligament

Acromioclavicular joint capsule

Supraspinatus m.

T-shaped incision in deltoid muscle allows inspection of rotator cuff and repair of tears

Rotator cuff

Acromion

pain and restoring active range of motion. The patient with a large tear of the rotator cuff does not regain strength after the subacromial space is anesthetized. Radiographs may or may not demonstrate a calcific deposit. An arthrogram to establish the diagnosis of a torn rotator cuff may be indicated in certain cases.

Treatment. More than 90% of cases of chronic tendonitis resolve spontaneously, but the recovery time varies. Conservative measures to relieve symptoms and prevent complications include avoiding activities that move the shoulder in the painful arc of motion, in addition to pendulum and range-of-motion exercises, normal use of the arm, and use of salicylates. Needling procedures with corticosteroid injections are ineffective. The physician should reassure the patient of the benign nature of the problem.

In a few patients, disabling shoulder pain persists despite conservative treatment. Simple removal of the dry calcific material, which is often not well localized in a cavity but is infiltrated among tendon fibers, is usually unsuccessful in relieving symptoms. In these cases, an anterior acromioplasty, or partial acromionectomy, frequently yields good results. Although good results have been reported following complete acromionectomy, the more conservative partial acromionectomy is favored at present.

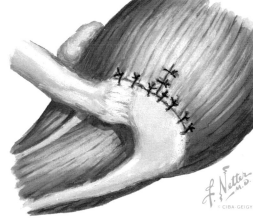

Anterolateral portion of inferior surface of acromion removed with osteotome and coracoacromial ligament released

Deltoid muscle securely repaired with sutures through acromioclavicular joint capsule and fibrous stump of coracoacromial ligament or with wires through small drill holes in acromion

The following conditions must be met before partial acromionectomy is performed: (1) the pain must be sufficiently severe to cause considerable disability; (2) the pain must have been present long enough to make it reasonably certain that spontaneous improvement and cure will not take place in the foreseeable future; and (3) there must be a complete active or passive range of motion in the shoulder joint. Any calcific deposit discovered at the time of surgery need not be touched, as it is absorbed spontaneously after the surgery.

Surgical management is performed with an open acromioplasty or an arthroscopic procedure (Plates 40–41). If a rotator cuff tear is suspected,

repair can be combined with the open acromioplasty. Surgery is recommended in patients with severe symptoms of impingement that do not resolve after a minimum of 6 months of conservative treatment.

Open Acromioplasty (Partial Acromionectomy)

The patient is placed supine in a semi-sitting position (Plate 40). The arm is draped free to allow distraction and rotation of the humerus during the procedure. A superior incision from the clavicle to the tip of the acromion is marked on the skin. The incision can be extended to gain access to tears of the rotator cuff.

Tendonitis and Bursitis of Shoulder

(Continued)

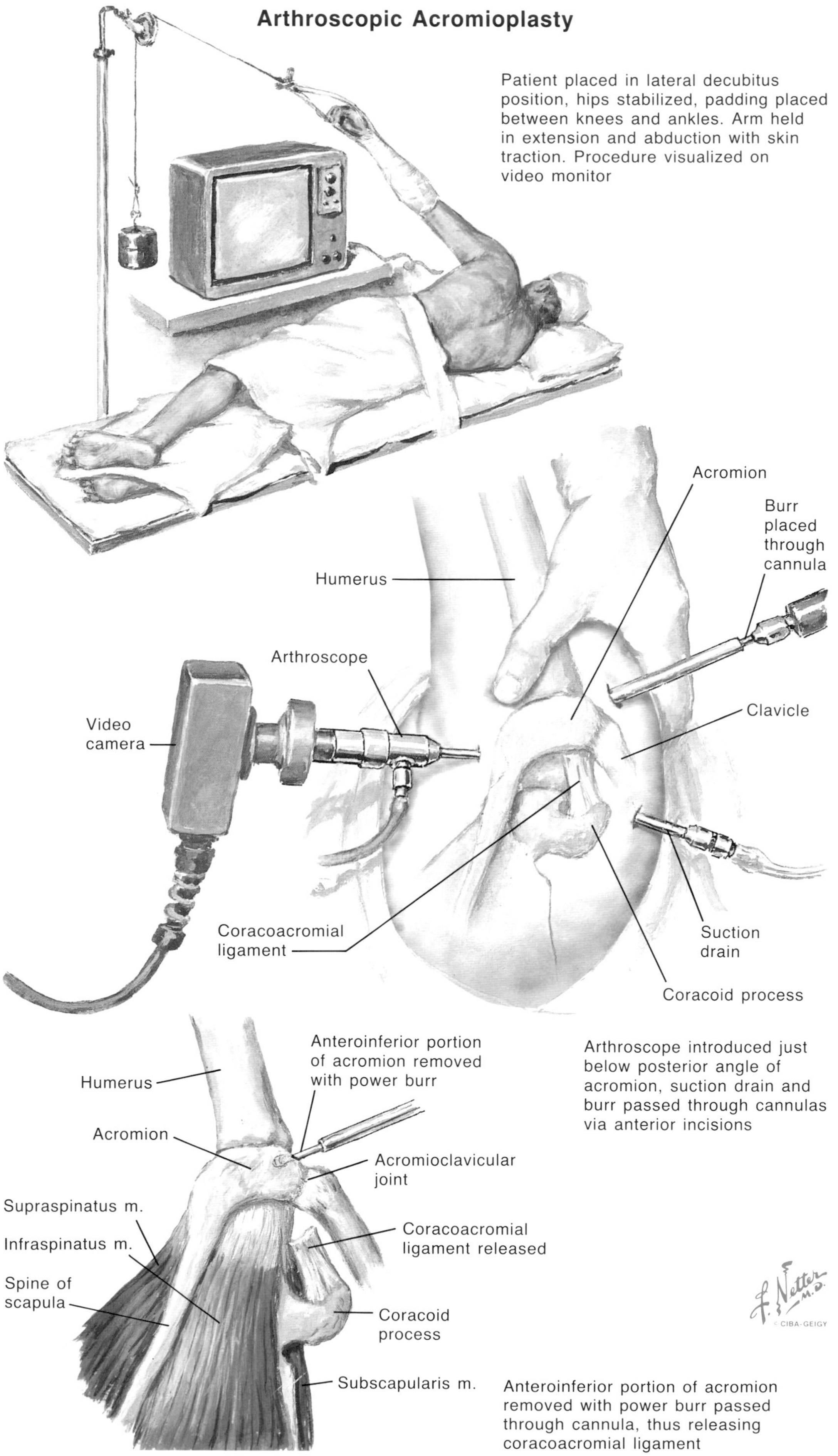

Arthroscopic Acromioplasty

Patient placed in lateral decubitus position, hips stabilized, padding placed between knees and ankles. Arm held in extension and abduction with skin traction. Procedure visualized on video monitor

Humerus

Arthroscope

Acromion

Burr placed through cannula

Video camera

Clavicle

Coracoacromial ligament

Suction drain

Coracoid process

Arthroscope introduced just below posterior angle of acromion, suction drain and burr passed through cannulas via anterior incisions

Humerus

Anteroinferior portion of acromion removed with power burr

Acromion

Acromioclavicular joint

Supraspinatus m.

Infraspinatus m.

Spine of scapula

Coracoacromial ligament released

Subscapularis m.

Coracoid process

Anteroinferior portion of acromion removed with power burr passed through cannula, thus releasing coracoacromial ligament

The deltoid muscle is released from its insertion on the anterior acromion. Small drill holes are made in the acromion for later repair of the deltoid muscle. When the arm is distracted, allowing visualization of the subacromial space, fibrous adhesions and a hypertrophic bursa beneath the acromion are usually seen. A bald spot on the humeral head indicates the presence of a rotator cuff tear, which may also need repair (Plate 44). The anteroinferior bony surface of the acromion is removed with an osteotome or power burr, and the coracoacromial ligament is released. A smooth range of motion, including full elevation, should be documented under direct vision before the wound is closed. The arm is placed in a sling, and passive motion exercises are begun on the fourth day after surgery. At 8 weeks, strengthening exercises for the deltoid muscle are added. Full recovery after an open acromioplasty may take 4 to 6 months.

Arthroscopic Acromioplasty

In recent years, subacromial decompression using standard arthroscopic equipment and a power burr has gained popularity (Plate 41). The patient is placed in the lateral decubitus position, and the involved arm is elevated 30° to 45° with 10 lb of traction. Incisions for the insertion of the arthroscopic tools are marked on the skin. Both the joint and bursal sides of the rotator cuff can be visualized, as can the coracoacromial ligament and the tip of the power burr. The same amount of bone is removed from the anteroinferior area of the acromion as in the procedure for open acromioplasty.

The arm is placed in a sling for 3 to 8 days, followed by physical therapy to increase range of motion and then by cuff-strengthening exercises. The rehabilitation period after arthroscopic acromioplasty usually takes up to 3 months. □

Adhesive Capsulitis of Shoulder

Adhesive Capsulitis of Shoulder (Frozen Shoulder)

Markedly limited range of motion on right side compared with left side. Slight abduction capability largely due to elevation and rotation of scapula. All joint motions restricted and painful at extremes. Atrophy of shoulder muscles

Posterior view reveals atrophy of scapular and deltoid muscles. Broken lines, indicating position of spine of scapula and axis of humerus on each side, show little or no motion in right shoulder

Adhesions of peripheral capsule to distal articular cartilage

Adhesions obliterating axillary fold of capsule

Coronal section of shoulder shows adhesions between capsule and periphery of humeral head

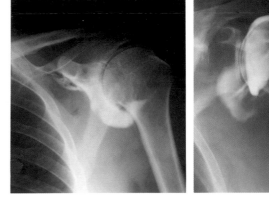

Anteroposterior arthrogram of normal shoulder (left). Axillary fold and biceps brachii sheath visualized. Volume of capsule normal. Anteroposterior arthrogram of frozen shoulder (right). Joint capacity reduced. Axillary fold and biceps brachii sheath not evident

Adhesive capsulitis, also called frozen shoulder, adhesive bursitis, and checkrein shoulder, is a distinct clinical entity associated with pain and a limited range of active and passive motion. Occurring twice as often in women, it is rarely seen in patients under 40 or over 70 years of age. Although the cause is unclear, immobility of the arm is a factor in 50% of cases. For example, minor injuries and bursitis may often cause the patient to avoid moving the arm; immobilization for arm fracture in a cast and sling is another frequent precipitating event.

A low-grade inflammatory process develops involving the capsule, synovial membrane, and rotator (musculotendinous) cuff. As a result, adhesions form between the folds of the capsule and between the capsule and the head of the humerus (Plate 42). The mobility of the biceps brachii tendon may be reduced by the inflammation of its synovial sheath. There are no adhesions in the subdeltoid bursa.

Clinical and Radiographic Manifestations

The onset of pain and stiffness in the shoulder is usually gradual, but the symptoms increase and the pain radiates down the arm, causing considerable disability. Specific motions and positions of the arm aggravate the discomfort. Patients often appear apprehensive and depressed and may have a low pain threshold.

A definite limitation of both active and passive shoulder motion is found on physical examination. The restricted motion, which is partially masked by scapulothoracic motion, can vary from mild to complete loss of glenohumeral movement (frozen shoulder). Persistent capsulitis results in atrophy of the deltoid and scapular muscles (Plate 42).

No abnormality is usually detected on radiographs except bone demineralization due to disuse. The presence of a calcific deposit is considered an incidental finding, not the primary cause of the symptoms. Occasionally, if the diagnosis is in doubt, an arthrogram may be performed.

Treatment

Adhesive capsulitis may be self-limiting, running a protracted course of as long as 1 to 2 years. Some cases are marked by a gradual but complete recovery of the normal range of motion.

Prevention is most important because no treatment promotes an early cure of the established disease. In many patients, simple exercises that move the shoulder through a full range of motion in all conditions that promote inactivity of the arm effectively prevent the condition from developing.

Adhesive Capsulitis of Shoulder

(Continued)

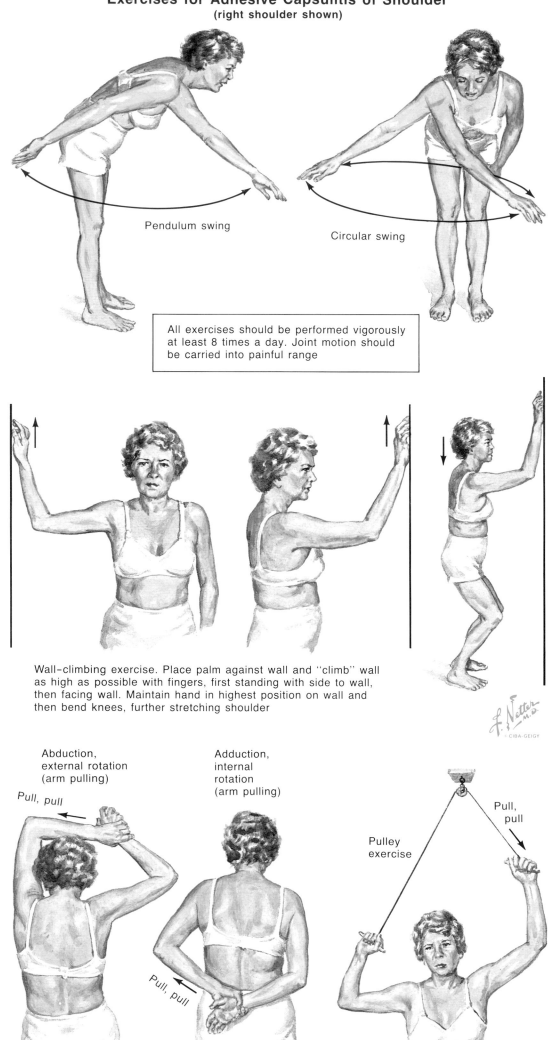

Exercises for Adhesive Capsulitis of Shoulder
(right shoulder shown)

Pendulum swing

Circular swing

All exercises should be performed vigorously at least 8 times a day. Joint motion should be carried into painful range

Wall-climbing exercise. Place palm against wall and "climb" wall as high as possible with fingers, first standing with side to wall, then facing wall. Maintain hand in highest position on wall and then bend knees, further stretching shoulder

Abduction, external rotation (arm pulling)

Pull, pull

Adduction, internal rotation (arm pulling)

Pull, pull

Pulley exercise

Pull, pull

Conservative treatment of established adhesive capsulitis includes analgesia, sedation for sleep, encouragement to use the shoulder as normally as possible, and, most important, a program of active and passive stretching exercises. Successful treatment requires the cooperation of the patient. Both the physician and the physical therapist should instruct the patient in pendulum and stretching exercises that move the shoulder into the painful zone of flexion, abduction, and rotation (Plate 43). Adequate analgesia is most important because it allows the patient to use the arm and perform the stretching exercises vigorously; an oral corticosteroid may also be helpful during the early phase of treatment. The physician must see the patient at regular intervals to offer encouragement, monitor the response to treatment, and add more strenuous exercises as motion increases. These duties should not be relegated to the physical therapist. With this program, most patients gradually recover in 4 to 6 months. If the patient does not cooperate in the exercise program or normal use of the shoulder, there is little hope of improvement with any form of therapy.

In a few refractory cases, manipulation of the shoulder with the patient under general anesthesia may be considered, but it should never be done unless the patient has demonstrated full cooperation in an intensive exercise program that has failed to bring improvement. Otherwise the manipulation will fail, since the exercises must be carried out just as strenuously after the procedure. It should be stressed that manipulation must be gentle inasmuch as forceful manipulation may be associated with serious complications (muscle tears, dislocation of shoulder). □

Tears and Ruptures of Rotator Cuff

Tears and Ruptures of Rotator Cuff

Extensive rupture of left cuff. To bring about abduction, deltoid muscle contracts strongly but only pulls humerus upward toward acromion while scapula rotates and shoulder girdle is elevated. 45° abduction thus possible

Test for partial tear of cuff is inability to maintain 90° abduction against mild resistance

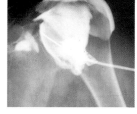

Communication between shoulder joint and subdeltoid bursa is pathognomonic of cuff tear

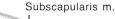

Subscapularis m.

Thickened, edematous biceps brachii tendon

Humerus

Biceps brachii tendon

Infraspinatus m.

Supraspinatus m.

Acute rupture (superior view). Often associated with splitting tear parallel to tendon fibers. Further retraction results in crescentic defect as shown at right

Retracted tear, commonly found at surgery. Broken line indicates extent of debridement of degenerated tendon for repair

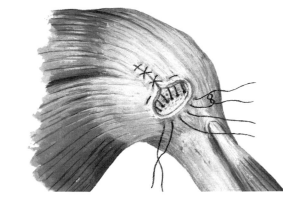

Repair. If freshened edges of tear cannot be brought together, notch is created in humerus just beneath articular surface to allow attachment of tendon through drill holes in bone, using strong sutures

The tendons of the subscapularis, supraspinatus, infraspinatus, and teres minor muscles join together and insert into the tubercles of the humerus and into the shoulder capsule. These conjoined tendons and capsule form the rotator (musculotendinous) cuff, which surrounds the shoulder joint on the anterior, superior, and posterior aspects. Repeated abduction and forward flexion of the shoulder may cause friction and impingement of the cuff tendons between the tubercles of the humerus, the acromion, and the coracoacromial ligament. This repeated rubbing causes degenerative changes in the tendons, which become worn and weakened. Consequently, minor injuries may cause tears or ruptures of the cuff.

Ruptures of the cuff vary from small transverse rents to massive ruptures of all the tendons. The most common is a transverse rupture of the supraspinatus tendon at its insertion, combined with a longitudinal rent through the cuff. The divergent muscular forces of the cuff enlarge the tear, which gradually becomes a crescentic or triangular defect, exposing the head of the humerus and the biceps brachii tendon.

Clinical Manifestations. These ruptures are common and occur most often in middle-aged persons, usually from a minor accident such as a fall on the outstretched arm and hand; however, in some cases, there is no recognized injury. A sharp pain is felt in the shoulder, which gradually subsides to chronic discomfort associated with varying degrees of disability in the shoulder.

Diagnosis is problematic in the early, acutely painful phase. However, as the pain subsides, physical examination is possible and reveals tenderness over the tear just proximal to the greater tubercle of the humerus. Pain and weakness usually limit active abduction of the shoulder, but the range of passive motion is characteristically normal if the manipulation is performed carefully. The range of active abduction of the shoulder varies with the amount of pain and the severity of the tear. The patient may be able to abduct the arm fully against gravity but can neither initiate this movement nor maintain the shoulder at 90° of abduction against mild resistance. Severe ruptures prevent true abduction of the shoulder against gravity, but scapular rotation may account for a small degree of weak abduction (45°–60°). Atrophy of the supraspinatus and infraspinatus muscles is visible 2 to 3 weeks after injury, but atrophy of the deltoid muscle, a characteristic of most painful shoulder conditions, is absent.

Radiographic Findings. Usually, no abnormality is found on radiographs of the shoulder, and a calcific deposit in the cuff is rare. Diagnosis

can be established by arthrography. In this procedure, a radiopaque dye is injected into the joint, and its appearance in the subdeltoid bursa indicates a complete tear of the cuff; normally, there is no communication between the shoulder joint and the bursa.

Treatment. Since many ruptures of the rotator cuff resolve spontaneously, early surgical repair is not indicated unless the tears are massive. Moderate or mild tears require about 2 to 3 weeks of close observation and conservative measures such as analgesic medication, sling support for the arm during the acute period, gentle but progressive exercises, and increasing use of the arm as the pain decreases and function returns. About 50%

of patients regain good shoulder function with this regimen.

If function continues to improve, conservative treatment should be continued, but insufficient improvement and significant loss of function necessitate surgical intervention. The torn cuff is adequately exposed and a partial acromionectomy performed. The margins of the defect are excised to healthy tendinous tissue, and the tear is sutured without excessive tension, gradually reducing the size of the defect. The edge of any remaining defect in the cuff is sutured to the denuded area of the lateral aspect of the humeral head and tubercle. A postoperative program of rehabilitation is essential for optimal results. □

Rupture of Biceps Brachii Muscle

Rupture of Biceps Brachii Muscle

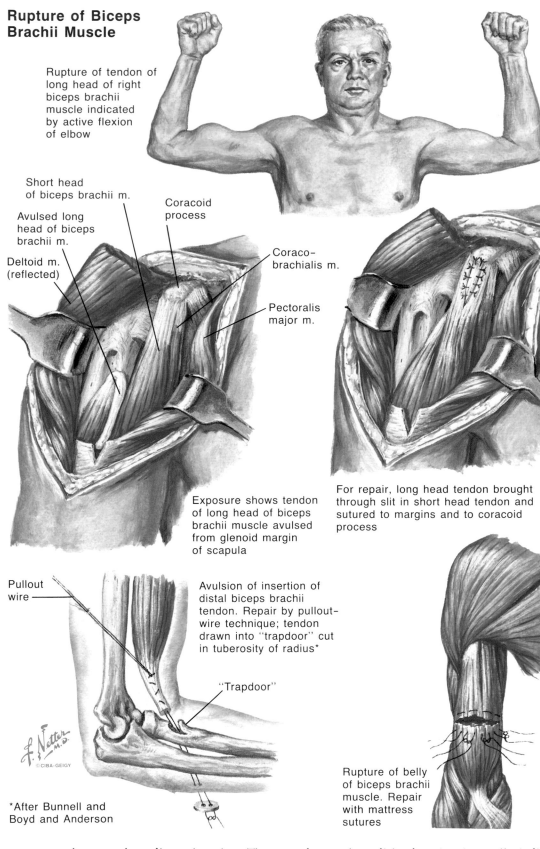

Rupture of tendon of long head of right biceps brachii muscle indicated by active flexion of elbow

Short head of biceps brachii m.

Avulsed long head of biceps brachii m.

Deltoid m. (reflected)

Coracoid process

Coraco-brachialis m.

Pectoralis major m.

Exposure shows tendon of long head of biceps brachii muscle avulsed from glenoid margin of scapula

For repair, long head tendon brought through slit in short head tendon and sutured to margins and to coracoid process

Pullout wire

Avulsion of insertion of distal biceps brachii tendon. Repair by pullout-wire technique; tendon drawn into "trapdoor" cut in tuberosity of radius*

"Trapdoor"

*After Bunnell and Boyd and Anderson

Rupture of belly of biceps brachii muscle. Repair with mattress sutures

Rupture of Tendon of Long Head. The most common site of rupture of the biceps brachii muscle is the tendon of the long head. The rupture may occur in the shoulder joint, in the intertubercular (bicipital) groove, or at the musculotendinous junction. Avulsion of the tendon from the supraglenoid tubercle also occurs.

Middle-aged persons are most prone to this type of rupture, probably as a result of attritional and degenerative changes in the tendon, similar to those in the rotator cuff of the shoulder. The rupture may be spontaneous or the result of a muscular strain such as lifting a heavy object.

The patient often experiences a sharp pain at the time of rupture. Mild swelling and ecchymosis of the upper anterior arm and weakness of flexion of the elbow and supination of the forearm then develop. Although the early pain and weakness largely dissipate, the arm deformity persists. The muscle belly of the long head retracts into the lower third of the arm and is both visible and palpable as a soft lump when the elbow is flexed or the forearm supinated, particularly against resistance. There is little loss of power because the short head of the biceps brachii muscle and the brachialis and flexor muscles of the forearm remain intact.

Since the disability is mild, surgical repair is not necessary. However, because surgery produces optimal functional and cosmetic results, it is indicated in young, athletic patients and in those who perform heavy physical labor. The usual repair procedure consists of excision of the intraarticular proximal segment of the tendon and fixation of the distal segment either in or near the intertubercular groove or into the coracoid process and conjoined tendon of the short head of the biceps brachii and coracobrachialis muscles. End-to-end suture is applicable only if the rupture occurs at or near the musculotendinous junction. The results of repair are usually excellent.

Avulsion or Rupture of Distal Tendon. This uncommon injury, which is associated with degenerative changes in the tendon at or near its insertion in the radial tuberosity, is usually caused by a sudden, forceful flexion of the elbow against resistance. Since the bicipital aponeurosis usually remains intact, the upward retraction of the entire muscle belly is minimal, and the power of flexion remains good. However, supination of the forearm is considerably weakened. The symptoms—moderate aching and weakness—are permanent and lead to a moderate disability of the arm. Surgical repair, which consists of reattaching the tendon to the radial tuberosity, is usually indicated but is not mandatory unless the bicipital aponeurosis is also ruptured. Results are good.

Rupture of Belly of Biceps Brachii Muscle. This injury occurs rarely, usually as a result of violent strain. Prominent symptoms are swelling and ecchymosis. If the tear is incomplete, treatment consists of immobilizing the elbow in a position of flexion greater than 90° until healing occurs. Surgical treatment is indicated when the tear is complete, usually associated with a palpable sulcus. The laceration is repaired with mattress sutures. In extensive or neglected tears, reinforcement of the repair with fascia lata may be necessary. □

De Quervain's Disease, Trigger Finger, and Ganglion of Wrist

De Quervain's Disease

De Quervain's disease is a stenosing tenosynovitis of the abductor pollicis longus and the extensor pollicis brevis tendons at the styloid process of the radius (Plate 46). It is most common in women between 30 and 50 years of age. The etiology remains uncertain but may be related to friction between the tendons, their fibrous sheath, and the underlying bony groove caused by movement of the thumb and wrist. The resulting inflammation causes thickening and stenosis of the synovial sheath of the first compartment of the extensor retinaculum (dorsal carpal ligament).

Clinical Manifestations. Pain develops over the styloid process of the radius, radiating up the forearm and down the thumb. Occasionally, the pain occurs suddenly following a strain of the wrist. The aching pain, aggravated by use of the hand, gradually intensifies and may sometimes cause considerable weakness and disability.

Examination shows a sharp tenderness over the styloid process of the radius, and a visible swelling and palpable thickening of the fibrous sheath may be detected. Sharp pain at this site is often produced by active extension and abduction of the thumb against resistance. Finkelstein's test usually causes severe pain (Plate 46).

Treatment. Often, symptoms are relieved by injecting corticosteroid into the sheath or placing the forearm, wrist, and thumb in a cast for about 1 month, or both. If the pain recurs and persists after this treatment, surgery is indicated. Under local anesthesia, a short transverse incision is made over the sheath on the lateral aspect of the wrist; care must be taken to avoid the sensory branches of the superficial branch of the radial nerve. The thickened sheath is opened with a longitudinal incision through the first compartment, freeing the involved tendons. Great care must be exercised to locate and free all the tendons in the compartment because aberrant tendons and anatomic variations in the tendons and sheaths are common in this area. The incision is then closed. Prognosis is excellent.

Trigger Finger

Trigger finger is the result of localized tenosynovitis of the superficial and deep flexor tendons in the region of the fibrous sheath (annular ligament, or pulley) at a metacarpal head (Plate 47). It occurs most often in the middle or ring fingers (occasionally in the thumb) of middle-aged women, but its exact cause has not been determined. Trigger finger may also be associated with rheumatoid arthritis involving several fingers.

The localized inflammation causes a thickening and narrowing of the sheath, and a nodular or fusiform enlargement develops in the tendons distal to the pulley. These changes interfere with—and may actually prevent—the smooth gliding of the tendons through the fibrous sheath.

Clinical Manifestations. In the early stage, the nodule produces a slightly painful clicking or

Finkelstein's test. Physician grasps patient's thumb and fingers, holding forearm with other hand, then quickly deviates wrist to ulnar side. This causes severe pain over styloid process of radius

Point of exquisite tenderness over styloid process of radius and sheath of involved tendons

Superficial branch of radial n.

Extensor retinaculum   Skin incision

Extensor pollicis longus, extensor pollicis brevis, abductor pollicis longus tendons

Course of abductor pollicis longus and extensor pollicis brevis tendons through 1st compartment of extensor retinaculum, transverse incision, and relation of sensory branches of radial nerve and synovial sheaths

1st compartment of extensor retinaculum opened along ulnar margin, releasing tendons. Note mild inflammation of epitendineum of tendons and slight inflammatory thickening of retinaculum

grating as it passes through the constricted sheath when the finger is flexed and extended. As the pathologic changes in tendon and sheath advance, flexion of the finger is arrested in the middle range; as more force is required to pull the nodule through the constricted pulley, the finger snaps painfully into full flexion or extension. Later, the tendon nodule may not pass through the stricture, and the finger is partially fixed in extension or flexion, usually the latter. Passive manipulation of the flexed finger may force the nodule through the sheath, producing a painful snap into extension.

On examination, the patient can usually demonstrate the trigger finger and may be able to

demonstrate the finger locking in flexion; flexion and extension produce crepitation. Palpation over the metacarpal head reveals a tender nodule that moves with the tendon.

Treatment. Although trigger finger often subsides spontaneously, a cortisone injection into the tendon sheath may alleviate the triggering. If painful triggering continues, a minor operation can provide permanent relief. A ¾-inch transverse incision is made just distal to the distal flexion crease over the metacarpal head, exposing the flexor tendons and sheath. The constriction is relieved by completely incising the thickened pulley longitudinally along its radial or ulnar aspect, taking care to avoid the digital nerves.

Stenosing Tenosynovitis of Flexor Tendons of Finger (Trigger Finger)

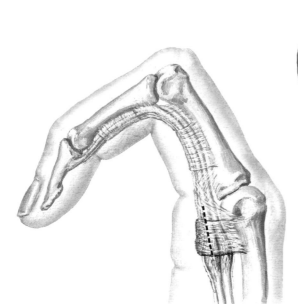

Inflammatory thickening of fibrous sheath (pulley) of flexor tendons with fusiform nodular enlargement of both tendons. Broken line indicates line for incision of lateral aspect of pulley

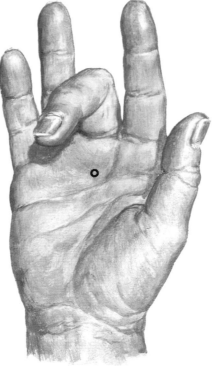

Patient unable to extend affected finger. It can be extended passively, and extension occurs with distinct and painful snapping action. Circle indicates point of tenderness where nodular enlargement of tendons and sheath is usually palpable

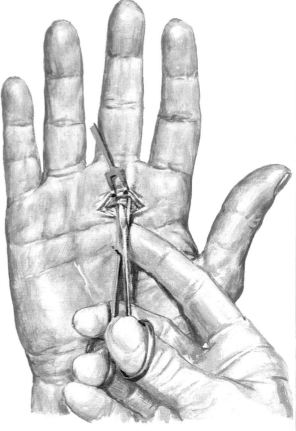

Incision of thickened pulley via small transverse skin incision just distal to distal flexion crease releases constriction, permitting flexor tendons to glide freely and inflammation to subside

Ganglion of Wrist

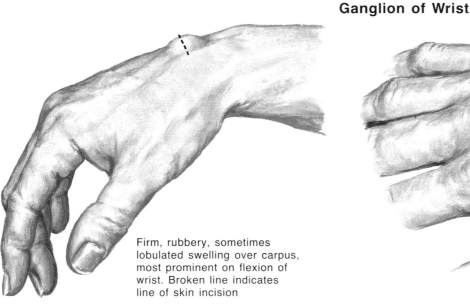

Firm, rubbery, sometimes lobulated swelling over carpus, most prominent on flexion of wrist. Broken line indicates line of skin incision

Extensor tendon retracted

Carpal ligaments and capsule

Excision of ganglion via transverse incision

De Quervain's Disease, Trigger Finger, and Ganglion of Wrist
(Continued)

The patient can now actively flex and extend the finger freely and comfortably.

Ganglion of Wrist

A ganglion is a cystic lesion that is found closely associated with a joint capsule or tendon sheath

(Plate 47). It is often seen in young adults but rarely in children; most frequently, it forms in the hand and wrist and less often in the ankle, foot, and knee. The most common site is the dorsum of the wrist just lateral to the common extensor tendons of the fingers. A ganglion usually occurs singly and may be multilocular; it consists of an outer fibrous coat and an inner synovial lining and contains a clear, colorless, gelatinous fluid.

Although the etiology is uncertain, perhaps the most accepted theory is that a ganglion results from cystic degeneration of connective tissue near joints or tendon sheaths. Repeated trauma appears to be a causative factor in about 50% of cases.

Clinical Manifestations. The only finding may be a slowly growing, localized swelling, but most patients report intermittent aching and mild weakness.

On examination, the cyst is firm, smooth, rubbery, rounded, slightly fluctuant, and at times tender. It is usually fixed but may be slightly movable if it involves a tendon sheath.

Treatment. Some ganglia disappear spontaneously. Treatments such as traumatic rupture, aspiration, and injections are associated with a high recurrence rate. Complete surgical excision of the ganglion and the ligamentous tissue at its base is the treatment of choice and usually prevents recurrence. □

Dupuytren's Contracture

Dupuytren's Contracture

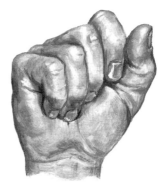

Only extension of involved fingers is limited. Flexion is not impaired because tendons are not involved

Flexion contracture of 4th and 5th fingers (most common). Dimpling and puckering of skin. Palpable fascial nodules near flexion crease of palm at base of involved fingers with cordlike formations extending to proximal palm

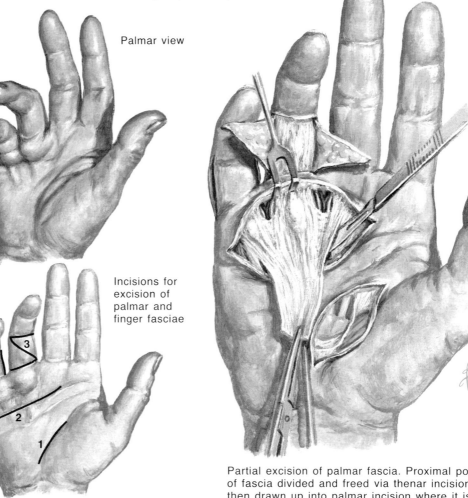

Palmar view

Incisions for excision of palmar and finger fasciae

1 and 2 = incisions just distal to thenar and distal palmar creases; 3 and 4 = alternative Z and midlateral finger incisions

Partial excision of palmar fascia. Proximal portion of fascia divided and freed via thenar incision, then drawn up into palmar incision where it is further dissected with care to avoid neurovascular bundles. Dissection then continued into fingers. Buttonholing of skin must be avoided. Nodules and cordlike fascial thickening apparent

Dupuytren's contracture is a progressive thickening and contracture of the palmar aponeurosis (fascia) that results in flexion deformities of the finger joints. Although its cause is unknown, trauma is not a factor, and an increased familial incidence suggests a genetic component. Dupuytren's contracture chiefly affects middle-aged white men, particularly those of northern European descent. It most commonly affects the ring and little fingers, followed infrequently by middle finger involvement. It rarely affects the index finger or the thumb.

Clinical Manifestations. The first sign of the condition is a slowly enlarging, firm, and slightly painful nodule that appears under the skin near the distal palmar crease opposite the ring finger; other nodules may form at the bases of the ring and little fingers. Subcutaneous contracting cords develop later; they extend proximally from the nodule toward the base of the palm and distally into the proximal segment of a finger.

Flexion contractures gradually develop in the metacarpophalangeal joint and later in the proximal interphalangeal joint of the involved finger. The degree of the flexion deformities and their development rate vary, depending on the extent of thickening and contracture in the palmar fascia. Some contractures develop quickly over a few weeks or months; others take several years. Long remissions may occur, only to be followed by exacerbations and increasing deformity. As the flexion deformity progresses, secondary contractures occur in the skin, nerves, blood vessels, and joint capsules. Because there is no tendon involvement, active flexion of the fingers remains complete. Involvement is usually bilateral, and in 5% of patients, similar contractures occur in the feet.

Serious changes occur in the skin overlying the involved fascia. The short fascial fibers that extend from the palmar aponeurosis to the skin contract and draw folds of skin inward, producing dimpling, pitting, fissuring, and puckering. The subcutaneous fat atrophies, and the skin becomes thickened, less mobile, and attached firmly to the underlying involved fascia. These changes occur particularly in the region of the distal palmar crease on the ulnar side of the palm. Except for the nodules, cords, and finger contractures, the patient has few complaints. Developing nodules may be slightly painful and tender. Finger deformities interfere with use of the hand, leading to disability in patients with certain occupations. The stages are not distinct and description of them is not essential.

Treatment. Surgery is the only effective treatment and should be done before the skin has deteriorated and the skin, nerves, and joint capsules have become too contracted. Surgical repair should not be performed before contractures develop.

Partial fasciectomy, the most common treatment, removes all of the thickened and contracted aponeurosis without excision of the uninvolved portion. After surgery, the fingers are splinted in the corrected extended position.

Complete fasciectomy, a more radical procedure, involves excision of all palmar fascia in the palm and fingers. Occasionally, a preliminary fasciotomy and 2 to 3 weeks of exercises are used to lengthen skin, nerves, and joint capsules before complete fasciectomy.

In both partial and complete fasciectomy, tourniquet hemostasis is essential. Skin flaps must be reflected very carefully to avoid buttonholing of the skin and necrosis and the subsequent need for skin grafts. In addition, great care must be taken to avoid any damage to the nerves and blood vessels that may be surrounded and distorted by the hypertrophic fibrous tissue. Careful hemostasis is very important. Prolonged postoperative care, which may require several months, is necessary to obtain optimal results.

Fasciotomy is reserved for poor-risk, elderly persons and as a preliminary procedure to fasciectomy in patients who have marked contractures; tight, adherent skin; and shortening of nerves and joint capsules. The results are better when this procedure is done in the residual stage of the contracture rather than during active progression of the disease. ☐

Pigmented Villonodular Synovitis and Meniscal Cysts

Pigmented Villonodular Synovitis

This diffuse or circumscribed xanthomatous lesion develops in synovial tissue and involves the joints, bursae, and tendon sheaths. Its etiology is unclear, but an inflammation of unknown origin is the most commonly accepted cause.

Diffuse Villonodular Synovitis. This condition typically occurs in adults between 20 and 40 years of age. A single joint of the lower limb, most frequently the knee, is the most common site of involvement. The synovial membrane becomes thickened and diffusely covered with long, tangled, reddish and yellow-brown villi, which may mat together to form plaques. Later, both sessile and pedunculated rubbery nodules appear. Hemosiderin-bearing stromal cells, lipid-bearing foam cells, and multinucleated giant cells are seen on microscopic examination.

Late in the disease, the pathologic changes may cause pressure indentation of bone and sometimes actual invasion of bone at the articular margins with subsequent bone destruction.

The predominant symptom is a chronic, slowly increasing swelling of the joint that is associated with mild aching. Acute episodes of pain with increased joint swelling may occur intermittently and are attributed to pinching of villi between the joint surfaces, with subsequent hemorrhage. Because the course of the disease is usually benign, diagnosis and treatment are often delayed. Examination of a palpable joint shows a diffuse, slightly warm and tender, boggy swelling. A valuable diagnostic finding is the aspiration of bloody, brown, or serosanguineous fluid from a chronically swollen, *uninjured* joint.

Radiographic examination reveals an increase in joint fluid and a thickened synovial membrane. Late in the disease, superficial erosions of cortical bone near the joint margin and irregular areas of bone destruction may be present.

The best treatment is complete synovectomy, performed through an open incision. If the entire synovial membrane cannot be excised, localized disease recurs, and radiation therapy may be indicated. If bone destruction is present, the abnormal tissue is excised and a significant bone defect filled with bone grafts.

Circumscribed Villonodular Synovitis. This more common form occurs in joints, bursae, and tendon sheaths. The characteristic lesion is a sessile or pedunculated, yellow to reddish brown nodule with localized villous proliferation around its base. Symptoms are mild, consisting of intermittent swelling and aching. Slight swelling and a localized nodule may be noted on examination. The tenosynovitis, also called xanthomatous giant-cell tumor of the tendon sheath, is the most common manifestation of circumscribed villonodular synovitis, occurring primarily in the hand or

Pigmented Villonodular Synovitis

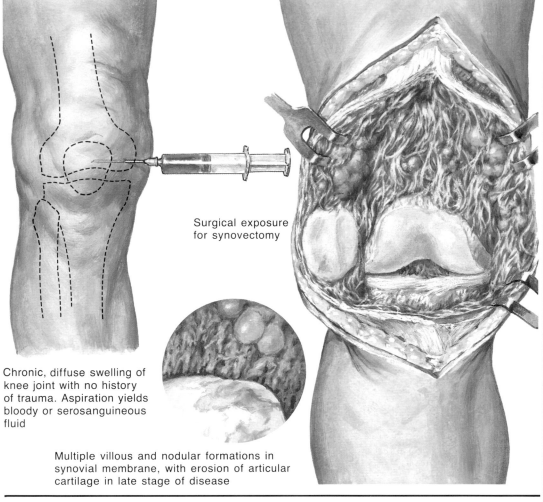

Surgical exposure for synovectomy

Chronic, diffuse swelling of knee joint with no history of trauma. Aspiration yields bloody or serosanguineous fluid

Multiple villous and nodular formations in synovial membrane, with erosion of articular cartilage in late stage of disease

Meniscal Cysts

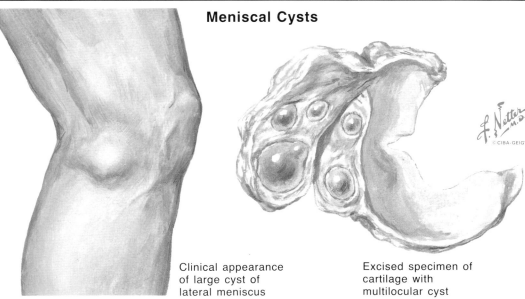

Clinical appearance of large cyst of lateral meniscus

Excised specimen of cartilage with multilocular cyst

foot where it presents as a discrete, firm, slowly enlarging nodule.

Treatment is complete excision of the nodular lesions in joints, tendon sheaths, and bursae.

Meniscal Cysts

Cysts of the meniscus (semilunar cartilage) of the knee are the most frequent cause of swelling at the lateral or medial joint line. The lateral cartilage is involved much more frequently than the medial. Although the etiology of these cysts is unknown, they may be due to trauma that causes cystic or mucoid degeneration in fibrocartilage and fibrous tissue. Patients vary in age from adolescence to middle age.

The cysts develop in the periphery of the middle third of the meniscus and in the adjacent soft tissues within the joint capsule. Usually multilocular and lined with endothelium, they contain a clear, gelatinous material.

Persistent aching in the cyst area is the main symptom. Examination reveals a tense, palpable, and often visible swelling at the joint line over the middle third of the meniscus, usually just anterior to the lateral collateral ligament. The tumor, which moves with the tibia, is most prominent on extension of the knee and tends to disappear on flexion. Excision of the entire meniscus and cyst is indicated if pain and disability are significant. □

Forefoot Deformities in Rheumatoid Arthritis

Forefoot Deformities in Rheumatoid Arthritis

Forefoot deformities are some of the most painful and debilitating manifestations of rheumatoid arthritis. Forefoot involvement often occurs early in the disease, and pain in this area may precede the appearance of overt synovitis. The initial symptoms are pain on weight bearing and swelling and warmth in the forefoot, with deformities developing months or years later.

Typical forefoot deformities include hallux valgus and bunion, hammertoes with contracted dorsal soft tissues, widened forefoot (splayfoot), and depressed metatarsal heads. Excessive pressure from weight bearing on the depressed metatarsal heads causes the formation of large, tender, and at times, ulcerated callosities on the plantar aspect. Pressure from ill-fitting shoes also causes corns and smaller callosities on the dorsal surfaces of the deformed lesser toes, as well as over the medial prominence of the first metatarsal. Associated pronation of the great toe increases pressure on the first metatarsal head and, as on the plantar side, leads to a painful callosity or an enlarged bursa.

The deformities of the lesser toes are due to synovitis of the metatarsophalangeal joints. As the synovitis progresses, the intrinsic muscles of the foot are overpowered by the long extensor and flexor tendons, leading to flexion, or cock up, deformities, similar to those associated with paralysis of the intrinsic muscles of the foot. The flexor tendons sublux laterally and migrate dorsally until they no longer flex the proximal phalanges. As the abnormal biomechanics of the foot persist, the depression and associated prominence of the metatarsal heads increase.

Rheumatoid synovitis and tendon imbalance also cause deformity of the great toe; in particular, involvement of the abductor hallucis tendon increases the valgus orientation. The important sesamoids in the flexor hallucis brevis tendon are displaced away from their normal position under the first metatarsal head, and thus their weight-bearing function is diminished. Rigid hyperextension or valgus deformities may also develop in the interphalangeal joint, further contributing to the painful symptoms.

It is important to note that associated rheumatoid deformities of the hindfoot and midfoot further disturb the biomechanics of the foot, exacerbating the pain and disability of forefoot problems. Talonavicular involvement is the usual precursor of hindfoot valgus deformity, and early recognition allows preventive stabilization with talonavicular arthrodesis (Plate 58). Advanced hindfoot valgus is usually associated with frank rupture of the tibialis posterior tendon. Synovitis in the midfoot and soft-tissue changes, including tenosynovitis of the tibialis posterior tendon, combine to increase midfoot pronation. Both hindfoot valgus deformity and midfoot hyperpronation are features of the hypermobile pronated foot (flatfoot).

Weight-bearing radiographs of the foot are essential in the analysis of deformities. Erosion of

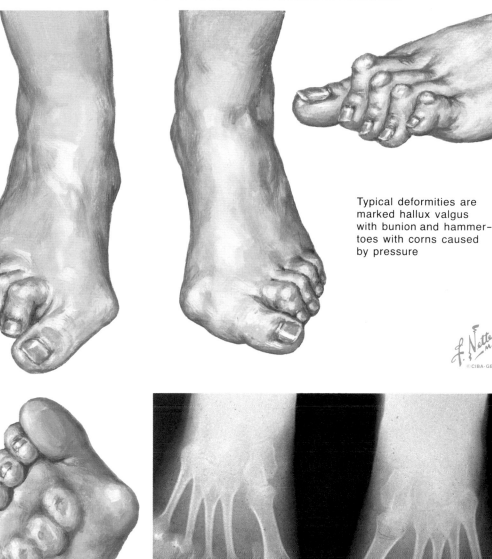

Typical deformities are marked hallux valgus with bunion and hammertoes with corns caused by pressure

Painful plantar callosities over metatarsal heads greatly impair walking

Radiograph reveals severe deformities of forefoot. Hallux valgus, dislocations of metatarsophalangeal joint with lateral deviation of toes. Note also displacement of sesamoids, which results in increased pressure on head of 1st metatarsal

the metatarsal heads and bases of the proximal phalanges is usually greater than first suspected from the clinical evaluation. Joint spaces are narrowed, and anteroposterior views usually reveal subluxation or complete dislocation of the metatarsophalangeal joints, in which the proximal phalanges actually overlap the metatarsal heads (the so-called gun-barrel sign). This is evident when the proximal phalanges are dislocated and flexed 90°.

The hallux valgus varies in severity, but in some cases, the proximal phalanx is dislocated almost completely from the articular surface of the first metatarsal. The widened forefoot is apparent on radiographic examination as well,

along with an associated increase in the angle of the first and second metatarsals, which may have preceded the onset of rheumatoid arthritis.

Many patients obtain relief with good medical management and proper conservative treatment with shoes and supports. Surgery is needed in chronic deformities of the forefoot with pressure problems and continued pain. Forefoot reconstruction by metatarsophalangeal arthroplasty has produced good results for 35 years and has a longer track record than any other arthroplasty in the lower limb. Continued pain and deformity in the hindfoot are generally treated with arthrodesis to correct the deformity and provide a stable hindfoot. □

Conservative Management of Rheumatoid Foot Deformities

Conservative Management of Rheumatoid Foot Deformities

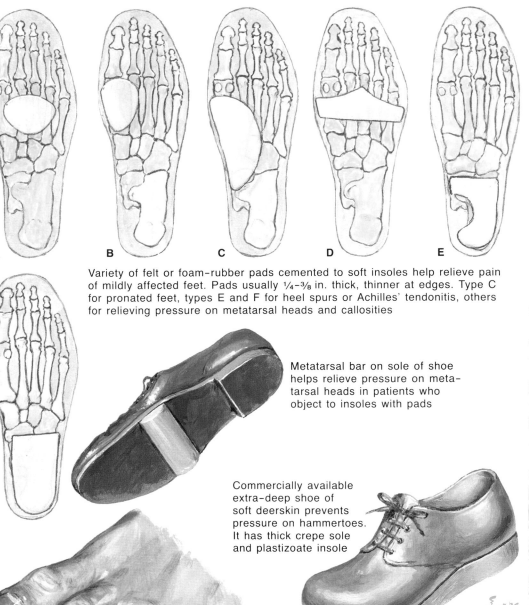

Variety of felt or foam-rubber pads cemented to soft insoles help relieve pain of mildly affected feet. Pads usually 1/4-3/8 in. thick, thinner at edges. Type C for pronated feet, types E and F for heel spurs or Achilles' tendonitis, others for relieving pressure on metatarsal heads and callosities

Metatarsal bar on sole of shoe helps relieve pressure on metatarsal heads in patients who object to insoles with pads

Commercially available extra-deep shoe of soft deerskin prevents pressure on hammertoes. It has thick crepe sole and plastizoate insole

Repetitive stretching exercises for hammertoes may help avoid surgery in nonrigid feet

Ready-made or custom-made orthotic devices for pronated feet; pads may be added as needed

The goal of conservative management of rheumatoid foot deformities is relief of abnormal areas of pressure. In long-standing deformities, pressure is the chief cause of pain after the active synovitis has subsided. (For a discussion of general conservative measures in rheumatoid arthritis, see pages 168–169.)

Patients with early foot involvement should use proper shoes with simple orthopedic supports (orthotics) and perform exercises to maintain the flexibility and mobility of all the toes and the tarsal and hindfoot joints. Passive stretching of the tightened dorsal soft tissues and extensor tendons is particularly important.

Basic oxford shoes with closed toes and low or medium heels are recommended, with metatarsal pads, long arch supports, or heel wedges added as necessary. Arch supports should be made of firm rubber and covered with leather; steel and hard plastic are usually too rigid for the rheumatoid foot. The supports, which are custom-made for each patient, often require secondary adjustments. Shoes with a very large toe box are also available and, with special plastizoate inserts, help relieve pressure on the deformed foot. Some

patients can comfortably wear running shoes, which are also useful in postoperative management (Plates 55–56).

In some patients, even advanced rheumatoid foot disorders can be treated satisfactorily without surgery. Although the extra-deep shoe with a plastizoate liner can be worn by most patients, those with severe deformities require a sandal or a custom-made shoe with special inserts.

Success of treatment depends on supervision of the shoe correction and close cooperation with a knowledgeable pedorthist (shoe expert). However, even after they have worn proper, comfortable shoes, many patients choose surgery so that they can wear fashionable ones. Nevertheless,

wearing comfortable, spacious shoes is essential after surgery, and simple metatarsal pads with or without long arch supports are sometimes needed.

A brace is occasionally helpful for severe valgus deformity of the hindfoot, although it usually provides only temporary relief before surgical stabilization is required. A simple, external short leg brace with an inner 'T' strap is prescribed for minor pain in the ankle joint. For severe pain, a double upright brace that limits ankle motion may be used. Braces made of newer materials such as polypropylene are currently being used to provide rigid support for deformities of the foot and ankle. □

Surgical Reconstruction of Severe Rheumatoid Forefoot Deformity

Surgical Reconstruction of Severe Rheumatoid Forefoot Deformities

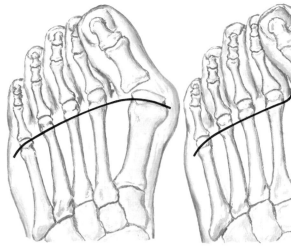

Previously, single transverse dorsal incision over metatarsal heads, curved proximally at each end, usually used for all toes

Now, transverse dorsal incision for all lesser toes plus longitudinal dorsomedial incision for great toe more common

If circulation is marginal or previous scars are present, three longitudinal dorsal incisions may be preferable for access to all metatarsophalangeal joints

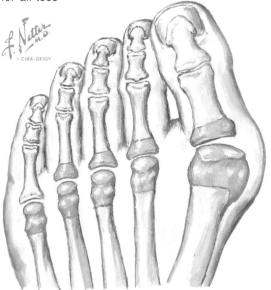

Portions of metatarsals and proximal phalanges removed (blue-shaded areas). Fifth proximal phalanx usually not removed

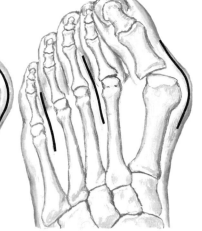

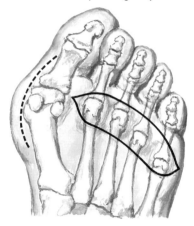

In some cases with marked depression of metatarsal heads, plantar approach with elliptic skin excision may be preferable for lesser toes. Metatarsal heads of lesser toes removed but not phalangeal bases. Separate dorsomedial incision used for great toe, and both phalangeal base and metatarsal head removed

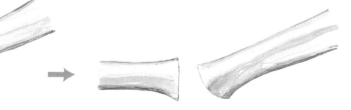

All cut bone ends beveled to provide better, relatively flat weight-bearing surface (or double-hinged silicone implant may be inserted)

Reconstruction of the forefoot in rheumatoid arthritis involves careful joint resection, maintenance of soft-tissue balance, realignment of the digits, and in some techniques, interposition of tissue or prosthetic implants into the joints. The surgical approach to the lateral forefoot is usually via a transverse dorsal incision at the base of the second through the fifth toes, with great care to preserve the longitudinal dorsal veins. Extensor tenotomies are performed to improve exposure, but the severed tendon will not heal if dorsal soft-tissue contractures and metatarsophalangeal dislocations occur.

The dorsal surgical approach to the lesser toes has been criticized because the lesser toes tend to remain "off the ground" and "floppy" even years after surgery. Current methods employ Kirschner wire fixation to reduce postoperative instability. Wire fixation improves realignment of the digits and promotes healing of the soft tissues and formation of a fibrous joint.

Before resecting the metatarsal heads, it is essential to expose all the metatarsal heads and necks of the lesser toes (or the bases of the proximal phalanges of the second through fourth toes when dislocation of the dorsal phalanges prevents direct access to the metatarsal necks). The metatarsal is cut at the junction of the head and neck, and careful attention must be given to the gradual reduction of the length of the metatarsals from the second through the fifth toes. The metatarsal neck is cut in a plantar direction to produce a smooth, beveled plantar surface for weight bearing. The cut surfaces of the metatarsal necks are meticulously smoothed with a rasp or file to eliminate any sharp edges that would cause pain during weight bearing. The only surgical procedures performed on the fifth toe are extensor tenotomy and resection of the fifth metatarsal head, with plantar and lateral beveling to avoid lateral pressure on the distal end of the metatarsal.

In flexion, or cock-up, deformities of the lesser toes (hammertoes), the toes are passively manipulated (but not hyperextended) before phalangeal resection. This manual osteoclasis is an important part of the surgical procedure and may possibly reduce the recurrence rate of digital deformities. The bases of the second, third, and fourth proximal phalanges are then resected.

In the foot with greatly impaired circulation or scars from previous incisions, three longitudinal dorsal incisions are made to expose the great toe and the metatarsophalangeal joints of the lesser toes. The rheumatoid forefoot with severe depression of the metatarsal head, hammertoes, and hypertrophy of plantar skin and subcutaneous and synovial tissue may require a plantar surgical approach. Resection of the proximal phalanges is more difficult with the plantar approach, and resection of the metatarsal heads is usually adequate. Most important in this procedure is the

excision of skin and soft tissue, in which a 1.5- to 2-cm wide elliptic strip of skin is removed. Closure of the surgical skin defect pulls the dorsally displaced toes into a more normal position in relation to the resected ends of the metatarsal shafts.

A procedure for cavus deformities in paralytic feet described by Hoffman is now used for the rare case of cavus foot in rheumatoid arthritis (usually in a child with juvenile arthritis). Resection of the phalangeal bases is eliminated, and a relatively larger portion of the distal metatarsal is resected. This decreases the longitudinal arch, reduces pain in the metatarsals, and improves the overall appearance of the cavus foot. □

Interpositional Arthroplasty for Toes

Plantar Ligament (Plate) Interpositional Arthroplasty for Lesser Toes

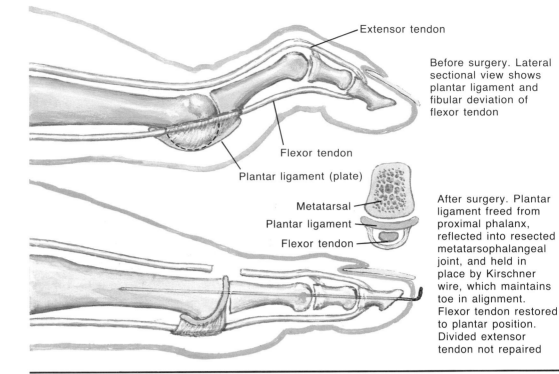

Before surgery. Lateral sectional view shows plantar ligament and fibular deviation of flexor tendon

After surgery. Plantar ligament freed from proximal phalanx, reflected into resected metatarsophalangeal joint, and held in place by Kirschner wire, which maintains toe in alignment. Flexor tendon restored to plantar position. Divided extensor tendon not repaired

Capsular Interpositional Arthroplasty for Great Toe

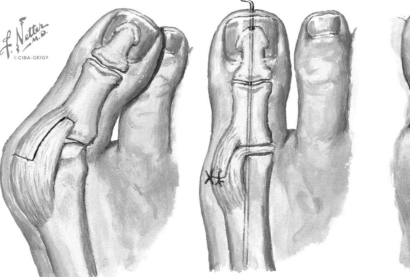

Capsule incised and one portion freed from its attachment to base of proximal phalanx

After joint resection, one portion of capsule turned into joint between cut bone ends, fixed with Kirschner wire. Remaining capsule used to close joint and help secure good alignment

Flexor hallucis brevis tendons freed from insertion into proximal phalanx, allowing sesamoids to move proximally and thus continue their weight-bearing function under newly formed metatarsophalangeal joint

Plantar Ligament (Plate) Interpositional Arthroplasty for Lesser Toes

Interpositional arthroplasty is a recent refinement in the reconstruction of the forefoot. The plantar ligament, or plate, is a thick, somewhat fibrocartilaginous structure that is functionally and anatomically like the palmar ligament in the metacarpophalangeal joint region of the hand. Easily identified on the plantar aspect of the proximal phalanx of the lesser toes, the plantar ligament can be reflected proximally and used as an interpositional graft after resection of the metatarsophalangeal joint. This procedure is not done if the base of the proximal phalanx is not resected or if the plantar ligament is extremely attenuated.

Rheumatoid arthritis often results in fibular deviation of the flexor tendons in the forefoot. Plantar plate interpositional arthroplasty, supplemented with Kirschner wire fixation through the interposed plantar ligament into the metatarsal shaft, realigns the flexor tendon while improving the function and appearance of the toe. The procedure is also thought to enhance the quality of the resultant fibrous joint. Kirschner wire fixation is not used when circulation is impaired, as in patients with rheumatoid vasculitis or diabetic vascular disease. In these patients, there is concern about possible impairment of the circulation if wire fixation is used. The alternative technique is to interpose the plantar ligament and suture it to the distal end of the metatarsal through a small drill hole in the cut end of the metatarsal. This technique allows rapid mobilization after surgery, which is important in older patients.

Capsular Interpositional Arthroplasty for Great Toe

The standard medial capsular interpositional arthroplasty of the metatarsophalangeal joint of the great toe produces a durable, pain-free joint with some motion. A longitudinal dorsomedial incision is made to expose the first metatarsal head and associated medial prominence and the proximal one-third to one-half of the proximal phalanx of the great toe. The metatarsal head is resected and the cut end shaped, leaving the length of the

first metatarsal equal to that of the second metatarsal. The base of the proximal phalanx is also resected; the amount of bone to be removed is determined by the selected procedure, ie, simple resection arthroplasty (Plate 52), reconstruction with a prosthetic implant (Plate 54), or interpositional graft (Plate 53).

The sesamoids are released from the plantar surface of the first metatarsal head, which allows them to move proximally and continue their weight-bearing function under the newly shaped distal metatarsal. Failure to do this leads to uneven, painful weight bearing at the resected metatarsophalangeal joint even if an implant is used. The sesamoids are excised only if bone degeneration,

hypertrophic osteophytic proliferation, or ankylosis is present.

A part of the usually excessive medial capsule is interposed into the new metatarsophalangeal joint. The remaining part of the medial capsule is used for capsulorrhaphy, which accomplishes both closure and realignment of the great toe. Although fixation of the capsular interpositional graft with Kirschner wires is now commonly used, it is possible to suture the medial capsule directly over the distal end of the first metatarsal to avoid using wire fixation. As in the case of the lesser toes, however, wire fixation improves alignment of the great toe and promotes better soft-tissue healing and fibrous joint formation. □

Silicone Implant Resection Arthroplasty

Silicone Implant Resection Arthroplasty for Rheumatoid Forefoot Deformity (after Swanson)

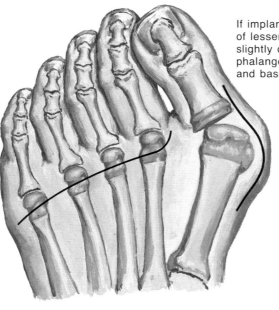

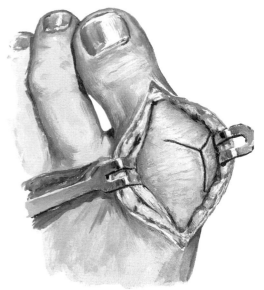

If implant is for great toe, metatarsal heads of lesser toes removed via transverse incision, slightly curved as pictured, but bases of proximal phalanges of those toes left intact. Metatarsal head and base of proximal phalanx of great toe removed

Curved longitudinal dorsolateral incision used for great toe. Extensor tendon retracted, and Y-shaped incision made in dorsolateral aspect of joint capsule down to bone

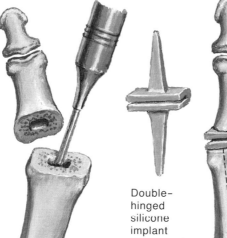

After removal of 1st metatarsal head and base of proximal phalanx, both bones drilled to receive implant stems

Double-hinged silicone implant (Swanson)

Implant inserted and bones manipulated into proper alignment

Capsule securely repaired with distal flap drawn down to abduct and pronate toe in good alignment. Extensor tendon then returned to proper position dorsal to joint

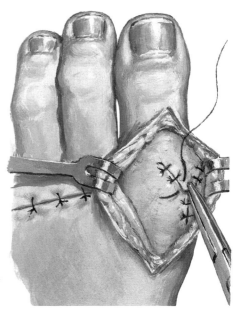

Silicone implant resection arthroplasty is being increasingly used to treat the metatarsophalangeal joint of the great toe in the rheumatoid forefoot. The double-hinged silicone implant of the Swanson design not only imparts stability to the joint but also aligns it and acts as a spacer about which a fibrous joint capsule forms by the process of encapsulation. A good candidate for this procedure is the young patient with moderate-to-marked hallux valgus. Patients undergoing implant arthroplasty of the great toe as opposed to resection arthroplasty must be active enough to benefit from the functional advantages of the implant.

Technique. A Y-shaped (Mercedes-Benz) incision is made in the dorsolateral aspect of the joint capsule; the resulting capsular flap provides additional stability to maintain the alignment of the great toe. The amount of bone removed from the metatarsal head and proximal phalanx is determined by the relative length of the great toe and the requirements for its correct positioning. The metatarsal head is resected distal to the metaphyseal flare, producing a flat, slightly medially beveled surface, which, with the flexible implant in place, imparts a slight varus position to the valgus-oriented great toe. In the markedly splayed forefoot, it is sometimes necessary to remove more bone from the head of the first metatarsal to lessen the possibility of recurrent hallux valgus. In the proximal phalanx, however, bone resection is minimal; just the cartilage and a small amount of bone are removed to produce a flat surface and maintain attachment of the short flexor tendons. If it is necessary to remove more bone, the short flexor tendons are resutured to the base of the proximal phalanx to prevent the development of hammertoes.

After the medullary canals of the metatarsal and phalanx are prepared, the largest implant that fits without excessive bulk at the hinge is inserted "upside down" (in contrast to the orientation of the flexible hinge implant in the metacarpophalangeal joints, Plates 64–66). This reverse positioning allows better dorsiflexion of the great toe. If the metatarsal or the phalanx is too short, the implant stem is shortened to avoid touching the medullary canal, with care not to compromise the implant's stability in the bone. The great toe is secured in the corrected, slightly varus position with a meticulous capsulorrhaphy.

In some patients, the extensor hallucis longus tendon is realigned as part of the procedure. Often, tenotomy of the extensor hallucis longus tendon is carried out at an oblique angle proximal to the level of the metatarsophalangeal joint. This tendon heals and regenerates, with resumption of a relatively normal extensor function in the great toe.

Arthroplasty for the first metatarsophalangeal joint may be combined with procedures to correct other foot deformities, such as metatarsus primus varus and hyperextension and other angular deformities of the great toe (Plate 60).

Modern silicone implants are very durable, and dislocation or fracture of the implant is not a problem if the procedure is performed properly. However, in some cases, abrasion of the implant by rough bone edges can result in an inflammatory reaction called particle-related synovitis, which necessitates removal of the implant. (Particle-related synovitis occurs more often with the nonhinged, or single-stemmed, silicone implant, which we no longer use for reconstruction of the metatarsophalangeal joint of the great toe in the rheumatoid foot.) Removal of the implant leaves a functional resection arthroplasty. □

Postoperative Care After Forefoot Reconstruction

Postoperative Management and Results of Forefoot Reconstruction

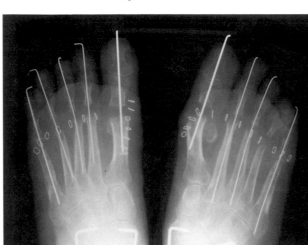

Postoperative radiograph shows toes in good alignment with Kirschner wires in place

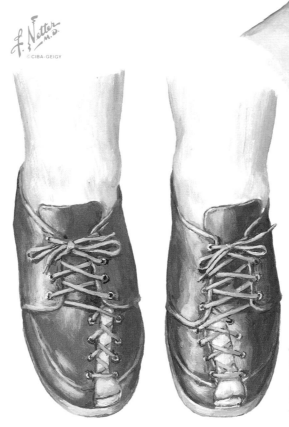

Padded wooden sandal applied over heavy dressing. Curved, raised wooden rim attached to front protects against weight of bedclothes and guards against stubbing of Kirschner wires when patient begins to walk 4 to 5 days later. Cotton padding between toes maintains good alignment. Dressings changed every 2 to 3 days; sutures removed in 2 to 3 weeks and wires in 3 to 4 weeks. Sandals worn until wires removed

Oxford shoes split in front to soles, portion of medial flap cut away, additional eyelets placed, lacing loose. Medial flap opens to avoid pressure on great toe, which might be pushed back into valgus position. After removal of wires, shoes worn until patient asymptomatic

Postoperative Management

Good postoperative care is essential for the success of surgical reconstruction of the forefoot (Plate 55). Before closure, the pneumatic ankle tourniquets are deflated; hemostasis is obtained and small-caliber suction drains are placed in the wound. The circulatory status of each toe is carefully ascertained, and if necessary, the position of the toe or the Kirschner wire is changed to improve circulation. For example, kinking of small vessels may occur when Kirschner wires are used, but often simply pulling the toe gently and thus subjecting the small digital vessels to gentle traction can result in rapid improvement in the circulation. However, if the circulatory status of a toe remains questionable, the wire should be removed. Nonadherent dressings are applied with careful interdigital padding to prevent pressure from adjacent toes and skin maceration; each toe is carefully wrapped to maintain the correct align-

ment. Compression padding is applied around the forefoot.

The heels and pretibial areas, particularly the tibial crest, are routinely padded as well. In rheumatoid arthritis, the skin is exceptionally sensitive to pressure, and potential areas of irritation and ulceration must be protected. Finally, postoperative wooden sandals are applied directly over the surgical bandages and dressings. They will be used after the dressings are changed. The wooden sandal shown on Plate 55 has a raised protective bumper that prevents pressure on both the toes and the protruding Kirschner wires.

Suction drains are removed 24 to 48 hours after surgery. For the first day, the patient remains in

bed with the feet elevated to control postoperative swelling. Standing is permitted on the second to fourth day and walking on the fourth or fifth day; the patient may use a cane or crutches. Initially, walking should be flat-footed, with most of the weight placed on the heels, but with time, more and more weight can be placed directly on the forefoot.

Dressings are changed every 2 to 3 days and sutures or skin clips, now commonly used, are removed 2 to 3 weeks after surgery. If wound healing appears to be slow, the sutures may be taken out a few at a time. As the dressings become lighter, all the toes are taped into the desired position for up to 6 weeks. When Kirschner wire

Results of Forefoot Reconstruction

Postoperative Management and Results of Forefoot Reconstruction

(Continued)

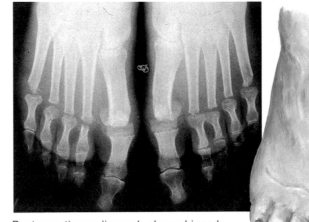

Postoperative radiograph shows hinged silicone implant in great toe, and resection of other metatarsophalangeal joints. Good alignment

6 months after surgery. Toes in good alignment, hallux valgus corrected, incision scars barely noticeable. Painted toenails indicate patient's interest in cosmesis as well as in function

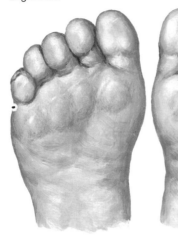

3 months after surgery. Plantar callosities healing well and painless

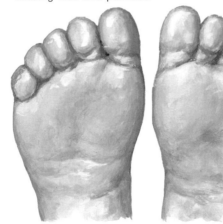

Good functional result after 6 months. Plantar callosities completely healed

After several years, patient can play tennis, dance, wear dress shoes. Must be cautioned against wearing high heels

fixation is used, the taping of toes is eliminated 2 to 3 weeks after surgery, and the wires themselves are removed after 3 to 4 weeks. Maximal recovery after bilateral forefoot reconstruction may be as long as 3 months. After reconstruction, most patients report a dramatic relief of pain.

Proper Shoes. As the swelling subsides and walking becomes more comfortable, the patient can wear a tennis shoe or an oxford shoe, which is split and has additional eyelets to allow more room in the toe box (Plate 55). With time, a regular shoe (often a running shoe) or a sandal can be worn. Women are encouraged to wear sandals; those who must wear dress shoes in the workplace should remove them as often as possible and particularly should seek stylish shoes with adequate room in the forefoot area. Constrictive, pointed shoes must be avoided forever, as wearing incorrect shoes often causes excessive pressure on

the foot or toes and may be directly responsible for recurrent deformities following surgery.

Results

When properly performed using modern refinements, forefoot reconstruction eliminates pain and provides good weight-bearing function (Plate 56). In 85% to 90% of patients, both immediate and long-term results are excellent. Many patients with rheumatoid arthritis who have multiple joint involvement consider surgery of the forefoot the most beneficial of their reconstructive procedures because it permits them to resume important and pleasurable activities, such as walking, tennis, and dancing. Surgery eliminates excessive pressure

points, allowing the painful corns, callosities, and bursae to disappear gradually. In addition to the functional improvement, the cosmetic appearance of the feet is also enhanced, which is particularly important to women. The cosmetic result of an implant resection arthroplasty of the metatarsophalangeal joint of the great toe is superior to that of resection arthroplasty, but the functional results are thought to be about equal.

Postoperative radiographic examinations are still required at regular intervals to detect and monitor midfoot or hindfoot involvement. Radiographs are also essential for assessing the alignment of toes, position of sesamoids, and integrity of the implant. □

Hindfoot Deformities in Rheumatoid Arthritis

Hindfoot Deformities in Rheumatoid Arthritis

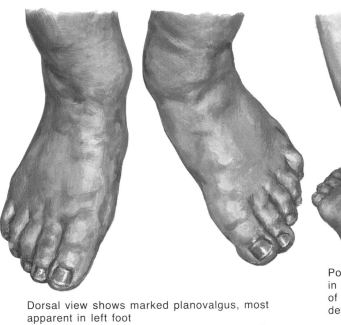

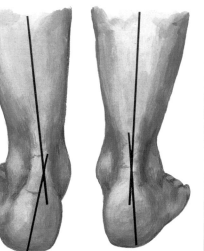

Dorsal view shows marked planovalgus, most apparent in left foot

Posterior view reveals hyperpronation in left foot. In normal foot, midlines of calcaneus and leg are aligned or deviate less than 2°

Medial view of pronated foot reveals flattened longitudinal arch

In some cases, foam-rubber wedge cemented to plastizoate insole may be helpful conservative management

Pronation and flattened arch corrected with orthotic device (ready-made or custom-made), which also provides symptomatic relief in mild cases

Valgus deformity of the hindfoot in rheumatoid arthritis, which resembles paralytic valgus deformity, has an insidious progression. Initially, the inflammatory process affects the talonavicular joint, then spreads to the subtalar joint. Associated spasm of the peroneus tendon increases the valgus position, further contributing to the instability at the talonavicular joint (Plate 57).

Conservative Management

If the deformity remains flexible (ie, amenable to correction with passive exercises), a medial wedge of foam rubber cemented to a soft insole in the shoe provides adequate support; custom-made orthotic devices are also used occasionally. Surgery is indicated when the deformity cannot be corrected with passive exercises or when the pain increases despite appropriate support (Plate 58).

Surgical Procedures

If both the forefoot and hindfoot are involved, forefoot reconstruction should be carried out first because its success rate is better than that of hindfoot surgery; also, the forefoot deformity is usually more painful than the hindfoot problems. Successful results of forefoot surgery often motivate the patient to proceed with surgical correction of the hindfoot deformity at a later date.

Talonavicular Arthrodesis. Pain in the subtalar or talonavicular joint without significant valgus deformity of the hindfoot is the primary indication for talonavicular arthrodesis (Plate 58). A short medial incision is made, and the articular surfaces are denuded. Wire or staple fixation is used to ensure coaptation of bone. Trabecular bone autografts taken from local bones can be used to augment the arthrodesis. The tuberosity of the medial navicular is usually a suitable site for graft material; it is rarely necessary to obtain bone from the iliac crest. The joint is immobilized in a cast for about 8 weeks, but weight-bearing activities can begin earlier.

The progressive nature of rheumatoid arthritis in the hindfoot limits the value of isolated subtalar arthrodesis. Talonavicular fusion performed early has proved more successful.

Surgical Procedures for Hindfoot Deformities

Hindfoot Deformities in Rheumatoid Arthritis

(Continued)

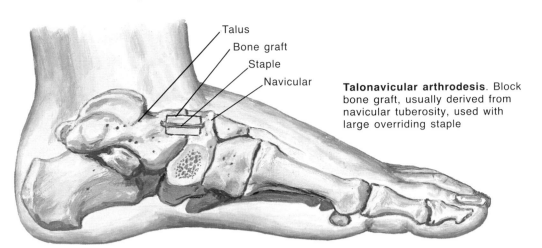

Talus
Bone graft
Staple
Navicular

Talonavicular arthrodesis. Block bone graft, usually derived from navicular tuberosity, used with large overriding staple

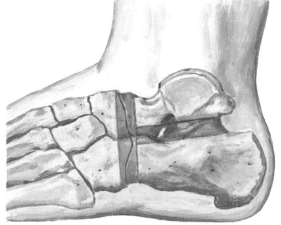

Triple arthrodesis. Bone, including articular surfaces, removed en masse in straight lines (blue-shaded area)

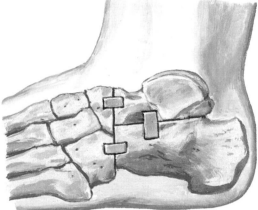

Triple arthrodesis completed. Cut surfaces of trabecular bone apposed and secured with three large staples

Total ankle replacement

Reserved for intractable cases. Often preceded by triple arthrodesis

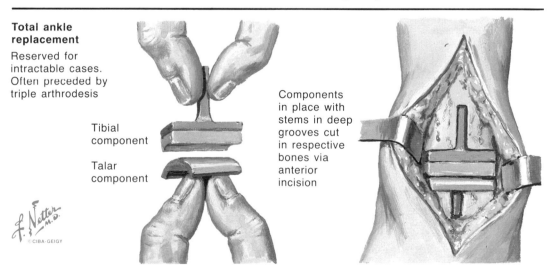

Tibial component

Talar component

Components in place with stems in deep grooves cut in respective bones via anterior incision

Triple Arthrodesis. For painful rheumatoid hindfoot with fixed valgus deformity, triple arthrodesis remains the procedure of choice (Plate 58). The lateral incision over the tarsal sinus often leads to skin problems. A vertical incision from the lateral malleolus to the base of the fifth metatarsal is recommended in combination with a medial incision over the talonavicular joint. As in talonavicular arthrodesis, bone grafts can be used, preferably trabecular bone autografts from the iliac crest or local bones. If used, the bone graft (in the form of dowel grafts or square cubes) should be packed securely into the area to be fused. The joints are then stapled. The hindfoot should be in slightly valgus position, which is the optimal position for weight bearing. In patients with rheumatoid arthritis, it is particularly important to align the hindfoot with the ankle and not the knee, which often has a valgus, external rotation deformity. The joint is at first immobilized in a nonweight-bearing cast, and the patient gradually begins weight-bearing ambulation after 4 to 6 weeks. Union usually occurs in 2 to 4 months.

When multiple hindfoot joints, including the ankle joint, are involved, triple arthrodesis is performed to stabilize the joint, followed later by total ankle replacement or ankle fusion. In severe hindfoot disease with marked osteoporosis in the ankle joint, a pantalar arthrodesis (triple arthrodesis plus ankle fusion) can be successful.

Total Ankle Replacement

Ankle fusion and total ankle replacement are reserved for the ankle with severe rheumatoid involvement. Although arthrodesis of the ankle is a widely used and proven surgical procedure, in the rheumatoid ankle, total joint replacement is preferable because fusion appears to increase pain in the other hindfoot joints. However, total ankle replacement has not been as successful as total hip and knee replacement. Even with the low level of physical activity of many patients with rheumatoid arthritis, a number of prosthetic components have loosened and failed after 5 to 10 years. Furthermore, revision of a failed replacement with fusion is extremely difficult and not always successful. At present, prosthetic components that require fixation with methylmethacrylate cement are rarely used in the ankle. A cementless implant resembling the type shown on Plate 58 is being investigated in clinical trials.

Ankle fusion remains the standard procedure at this time. □

Surgical Procedures for Toe Deformities

Hyperextension Deformity of Great Toe. Arthrodesis of the interphalangeal joint of the great toe is used to correct this type of deformity. An alternative procedure involves fracturing the bone (osteoclasis). After either technique, the toe is maintained in neutral position with internal fixation using a Kirschner wire or a screw.

Flexion Deformity of Lesser Toe. Flexion, or cock-up, deformity (also known as hammertoes) is corrected with excision of the proximal interphalangeal joint, extensor tenotomy, and Kirschner wire fixation. In very mild cases, extensor tenotomy performed through a small incision and passive manipulation of the toe are sufficient.

Keller Operation for Hallux Valgus With Bunion. The Keller operation is used primarily for hallux valgus with severe stiffness and marked osteoarthritis of the first metatarsophalangeal joint. It is not used if the joint can be salvaged with reconstructive surgery, nor is it performed to correct hallux valgus with metatarsus primus varus (Plate 60). Although it relieves pain and corrects the great toe deformity, this procedure produces a weakened, false joint and shortening of the great toe.

The joint is opened and the exostosis removed, the proximal half of the proximal phalanx is resected, and the redundant joint capsule is interposed into the joint and sutured over the metatarsal head. The great toe is bandaged in the corrected position.

Swanson Flexible Implant Resection Arthroplasty for Great Toe. The single-stemmed implant, preferably made of titanium, is used to replace the base of the proximal phalanx when the articular cartilage is destroyed, providing that no bone cysts are present at the metatarsal head and alignment or rotation deformities are not too severe. The procedure is used in cases of hallux rigidus and degenerative hallux valgus. It is not used in rheumatoid arthritis and severe senile hallux valgus. If the intermetatarsal angle is greater than 15°, an associated osteotomy at the base of the first metatarsal is indicated. Complete release of soft-tissue contractures can include release of the lateral capsule and adductor release and lengthening of the extensor hallucis longus tendon.

The double-stemmed flexible hinge implant is used when cartilage loss and degenerative and cystic changes of the metatarsal head necessitate resection of both joint surfaces. This procedure is used to correct a hallux valgus deformity in rheumatoid arthritis, in late stages of degenerative arthritis, in senile hallux rigidus, for revision procedures when both sides of the joint are involved, and for revision of a failed single-stemmed implant arthroplasty. The use of titanium encircling grommets at the proximal and distal surfaces of the silicone hinge has greatly helped to protect the implant from abrasion by sharp bone ends. Correction of all associated soft-tissue contractures and deformities of the first toe ray is essential for a good result. □

Surgical Procedures for Toe Deformities

Hyperextension deformity of great toe

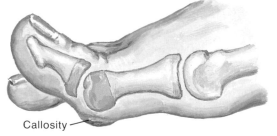

Callosity

Portion of joint resected (blue-shaded areas)

Toe straightened; joint fused and fixed with screw. Callosity heals

Cock-up deformity of lesser toe (metatarsophalangeal joint satisfactory)

Corn

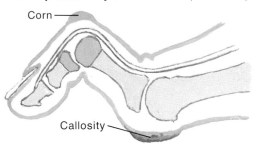

Callosity

Portion of proximal interphalangeal joint resected (blue-shaded areas)

Toe aligned with or without Kirschner wire. Extensor tenotomy over metatarsophalangeal joint. Callosity and corn heal

In very mild cases, transcutaneous extensor tenotomy without bone resection followed by manipulative alignment may suffice

Keller operation for hallux valgus with bunion (other toes satisfactory)

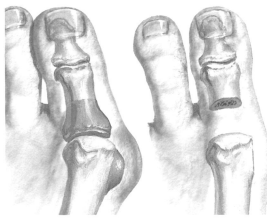

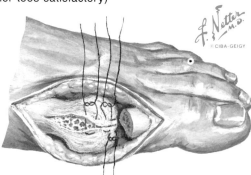

About half of proximal phalanx and exostosis resected (shown in blue) and toe straightened

Capsule reflected from proximal phalanx interposed into joint and sutured over raw area of metatarsal head (pin fixation may be used if necessary)

Swanson flexible implant resection arthroplasty for great toe

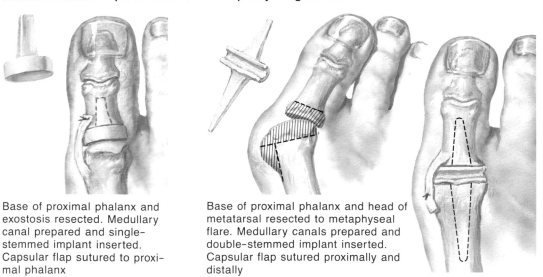

Base of proximal phalanx and exostosis resected. Medullary canal prepared and single-stemmed implant inserted. Capsular flap sutured to proximal phalanx

Base of proximal phalanx and head of metatarsal resected to metaphyseal flare. Medullary canals prepared and double-stemmed implant inserted. Capsular flap sutured proximally and distally

Bunion, Hallux Valgus, and Metatarsus Primus Varus

Hallux Valgus, Bunion, and Metatarsus Primus Varus

A common cause of pain and disability, hallux valgus is an often progressive deformity of uncertain etiology (Plate 60). It is often bilateral and affects women more frequently than men; it is also a familial condition and appears to be related to wearing shoes.

Clinical Manifestations

The deformity has three primary characteristics: (1) outward angulation of the great toe (hallux valgus), (2) medial prominence of the first metatarsal head (bunion), and usually (3) adduction or varus angulation of the first metatarsal (metatarsus primus varus). The marked prominence of the head of the first metatarsal produced by varus deformity is often mistaken for a large exostosis.

Other clinical and radiographic features include medial rotation of the great toe, lateral subluxation of the first metatarsophalangeal joint, exostosis on the medial aspect of the first metatarsal head with or without an overlying thickened and sometimes inflamed bursa, lateral displacement of the flexor hallucis brevis tendons and their sesamoids, and bowstringing of the extensor and flexor hallucis longus tendons.

The joint capsule of the first metatarsophalangeal joint becomes lengthened on the medial side and contracted on the lateral side. Significant degenerative osteoarthritis in this joint, if present, is an important factor in determining appropriate therapy.

Deformities of other toes, particularly the second, are also frequently seen, including corns, claw toe, hammertoe, mallet toe, and dorsal subluxation or dislocation of the metatarsophalangeal joints. The foot often exhibits abnormalities such as painful plantar callosities, pronation, and degenerative changes. These associated symptomatic deformities complicate the treatment of hallux valgus.

Treatment

Conservative management is adequate in many cases of hallux valgus. Therefore, unless the symptoms and deformity are severe, initial therapy should include the use of well-fitting and appropriate shoes, arch supports, protective pads, active and passive exercises, and other measures.

Surgery is indicated if conservative measures do not successfully relieve pain or if the pain and deformity are so severe that nonoperative treatment is judged futile. Surgery is performed primarily for pain relief, not for cosmetic purposes. In an adolescent with minimal symptoms, surgery may be appropriate if severe metatarsus primus varus accompanies early hallux valgus.

Moderate and severe hallux valgus usually comprises both the valgus deviation of the great toe and adduction of the first metatarsal. Yet, the metatarsal deformity is often overlooked or not recognized as a fundamental element of the problem. Thus, it is not logical to attempt surgical correction of the great toe deformity while allowing the metatarsal deviation to persist, and opera-

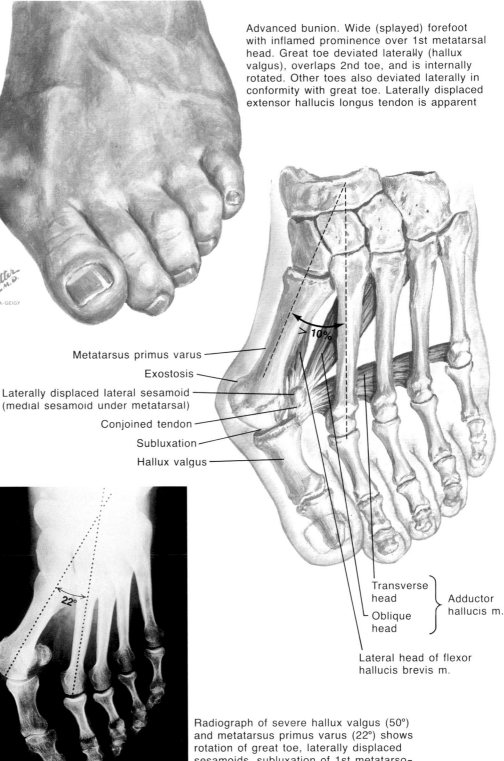

Advanced bunion. Wide (splayed) forefoot with inflamed prominence over 1st metatarsal head. Great toe deviated laterally (hallux valgus), overlaps 2nd toe, and is internally rotated. Other toes also deviated laterally in conformity with great toe. Laterally displaced extensor hallucis longus tendon is apparent

Metatarsus primus varus
Exostosis
Laterally displaced lateral sesamoid (medial sesamoid under metatarsal)
Conjoined tendon
Subluxation
Hallux valgus

Transverse head
Oblique head
Adductor hallucis m.

Lateral head of flexor hallucis brevis m.

Radiograph of severe hallux valgus (50°) and metatarsus primus varus (22°) shows rotation of great toe, laterally displaced sesamoids, subluxation of 1st metatarsophalangeal joint, lateral deviation of toes, and splayed forefoot

tions that do not correct the metatarsal adduction generally produce unsatisfactory results, including recurrence. Adduction of the first metatarsal that results in an intermetatarsal angle of more than 10°, as measured on weight-bearing radiographs, requires surgical correction.

Surgery should include correction of the valgus deformity of the great toe, correction of significant adduction of the first metatarsal, excision of the exostosis and abnormal bursa, and correction of significant associated deformities. The operation should restore the foot to as near normal as possible without interfering with good function. Postoperative care, including use of proper shoes and supports, is essential for optimal results.

McBride Operation for Bunion

The McBride operation is used to correct moderate hallux valgus, but because it revises soft-tissue structures only, it may not be adequate for permanent correction of a significant varus deformity of the first metatarsal (Plate 61). Medial and lateral incisions are made over the first metatarsophalangeal joint. A V-shaped capsular flap is elevated from the exostosis and head of the first metatarsal, leaving its base attached to the proximal phalanx. If necessary, the lateral sesamoid in the flexor hallucis brevis tendon may be enucleated through the lateral incision. The conjoined tendon of the adductor hallucis muscle is

Hallux Valgus, Bunion, and Metatarsus Primus Varus
(Continued)

freed from its insertion into the proximal phalanx and reattached to the lateral surface of the neck of the first metatarsal, thus releasing its rotatory and adducting force on the great toe. A circumferential suture around the necks of the first and second metatarsals may be used to approximate the two metatarsal heads.

The exostosis and thickened bursa are removed through the medial incision, and the capsule of the metatarsophalangeal joint is plicated to maintain the great toe in the correct position. The wounds are closed, and appropriate splints are used for about 3 weeks.

Mitchell Osteotomy-Bunionectomy (Hammond Modification)

The Mitchell osteotomy-bunionectomy corrects the varus deformity in the distal portion of the metatarsal shaft (Plate 61). Because the majority of patients requiring surgical intervention have a significant varus deformity of the first metatarsal, this procedure can be widely used.

The surgical approach for forming the medial capsular flap and for excising the exostosis is the same as in the McBride operation, except that only a medial incision is necessary. An incomplete double osteotomy of the metatarsal neck is performed, and the proximal osteotomy is completed through the lateral cortex. The distal fragment is then displaced laterally until the spur engages against the lateral cortex of the proximal fragment.

In the Hammond modification, instead of a double osteotomy with parallel cuts, the double osteotomy is made with diverging cuts. This produces a slight internal angulation of the fragments, which is important for adequate correction of the metatarsal varus deviation to 10° or less. The hallux valgus is then corrected, and the foot is splinted until the osteotomy is united (6 to 7 weeks).

Arthrodesis of First Metatarsophalangeal Joint (McKeever Operation)

Arthrodesis, a primary technique for hallux valgus, is also used to salvage the foot if other operations for hallux valgus fail (Plate 61). The first metatarsophalangeal joint is completely exposed and dislocated. The head of the first metatarsal is shaped into a blunt point and inserted into a conical hole reamed in the base of the proximal phalanx. With the great toe in the corrected position and the joint held in proper position for ankylosis, a screw is inserted through the proximal phalanx and almost the entire length of the first metatarsal. The foot must be protected until the arthrodesis is solidly healed. Care must be taken to ensure the proper amount of dorsiflexion of the toe, which is determined by the height of the heel usually worn by the patient. Fusion with the toe in the wrong position can be disabling, but properly executed, this procedure corrects the hallux valgus and reduces adduction of the first metatarsal. □

McBride Operation for Bunion
(two-incision technique)

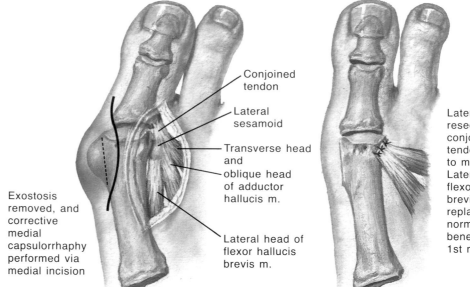

Conjoined tendon

Lateral sesamoid

Transverse head and oblique head of adductor hallucis m.

Lateral head of flexor hallucis brevis m.

Exostosis removed, and corrective medial capsulorrhaphy performed via medial incision

Lateral sesamoid resected, and conjoined adductor tendon transplanted to metatarsal neck. Lateral head of flexor hallucis brevis muscle replaced to its normal position beneath 1st metatarsal

Mitchell Osteotomy-Bunionectomy
(Hammond modification)

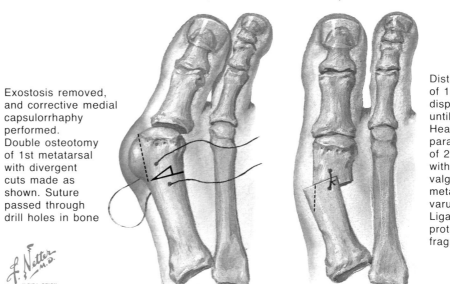

Exostosis removed, and corrective medial capsulorrhaphy performed. Double osteotomy of 1st metatarsal with divergent cuts made as shown. Suture passed through drill holes in bone

Distal fragment of 1st metatarsal displaced laterally until spur engages. Head fragment now parallel to axis of 2nd metatarsal, with fragments in valgus position and metatarsus primus varus corrected. Ligature tied and protrusion of proximal fragment resected

Arthrodesis of 1st Metatarsophalangeal Joint for Hallux Valgus
(McKeever operation)

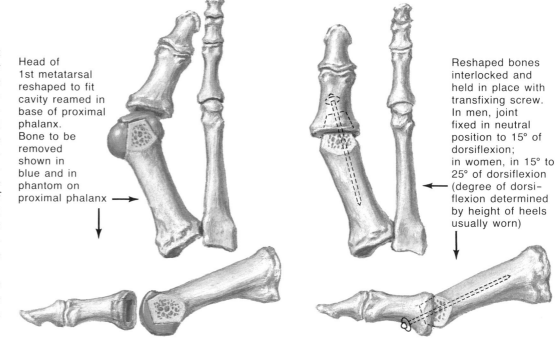

Head of 1st metatarsal reshaped to fit cavity reamed in base of proximal phalanx. Bone to be removed shown in blue and in phantom on proximal phalanx →

Reshaped bones interlocked and held in place with transfixing screw. In men, joint fixed in neutral position to 15° of dorsiflexion; in women, in 15° to 25° of dorsiflexion (degree of dorsiflexion determined by height of heels usually worn)

Deformities of Metacarpophalangeal Joint

Reconstructive Surgery for Deformities of Rheumatoid Hand

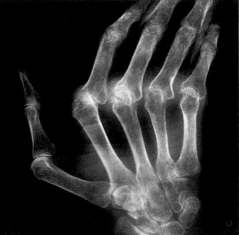

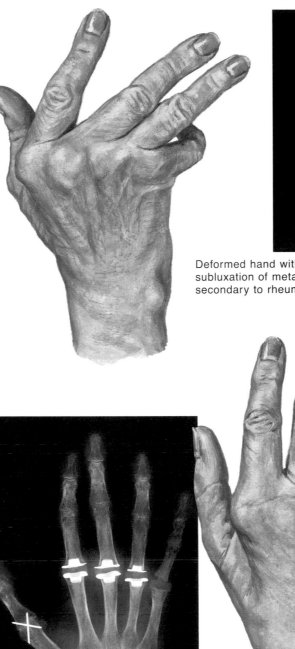

Deformed hand with marked ulnar deviation of fingers and subluxation of metacarpophalangeal joints. Deformities secondary to rheumatoid arthritis

Arthritic diseases may affect any joint, but their effect on the hands can be especially devastating. The disease process attacks the joints, ligaments, and tendons, causing painful and disabling deformities. Fortunately, developments in joint reconstruction and replacement have made it possible to restore hands deformed by crippling arthritis to a nearly normal appearance and useful function.

Ideally, arthroplasty should produce a joint that is pain free, mobile, stable, and durable. Four methods of reconstruction for the joints of the hand have emerged: soft-tissue reconstruction, resection arthroplasty, fixed-axis articulated joint replacement, and flexible implant resection arthroplasty.

Resection arthroplasty can improve motion by shortening skeletal structures, lengthening soft parts, providing new gliding surfaces, and allowing the development of a new supportive fibrous joint capsule. The chief disadvantage of the procedure is the unpredictability of results.

Although *fixed-axis articulated joint replacement* has proved successful in knee and hip joints, results in finger joints have been mixed because of bone resorption and implant loosening.

In *flexible implant resection arthroplasty*, a flexible silicone implant is used as an adjunct to resection arthroplasty. This method was devised in 1962 and has been used successfully in several hundred thousand patients. This discussion emphasizes the techniques of implant resection arthroplasty.

The basic concept of flexible implant resection arthroplasty can be summarized as "bone resection + implant + encapsulation = functional joint." The flexible implant acts as a dynamic spacer, maintaining internal alignment and spacing of the reconstructed joint and supporting the capsuloligamentous system that develops around it. The joint is thus rebuilt through a healing phenomenon called the encapsulation process.

Because the capsuloligamentous system around a new joint is adaptable, a functional balance of mobility and stability can be obtained. When increased mobility is desired, as in finger joint arthroplasty, joint motion must be started soon after surgery. When greater stability is desired, as in reconstruction of the carpal bones and the radiocarpal and first metacarpophalangeal joints, the immobilization period after surgery is longer.

Salvageability of an arthroplasty is most important and requires preservation of enough bone and soft tissue to allow a secondary procedure, if needed. Because minimal bone is removed and the flexible implants are not firmly attached to bone, removal or replacement of the implant or

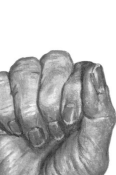

Hand after flexible implant resection arthroplasty with grommets and implants in place. Alignment of digits and flexion and extension capability restored. Good cosmetic and functional result

arthrodesis with a bone graft can be done easily. Secondary correction of the tension of the capsuloligamentous structures can also be done.

Favorable bone remodeling around silicone implants in the metacarpophalangeal and radiocarpal joints is evidenced by maintenance of the shape of the cut end of the bone with metaphyseal cortical thickening and production of new bone around the intramedullary stems. However, irregular, sharp bone edges can occur, especially in severe cases of rheumatoid arthritis, and cause tears in the implant midsection; this can eventually lead to implant failure. Implant fracture may occur when subluxating bone ends impinge on the implant midsection. Bone liner devices

called grommets were devised in 1976 and are being used to shield flexible-hinged implants from sharp bone edges and improve implant durability without losing the favorable bone response. Titanium grommets have proven to be most satisfactory.

General Considerations

The candidate for arthroplasty must be in good general condition. Skin cover and neurovascular status must be adequate. The elements necessary to restore a functioning musculotendinous system and sufficient bone stock to receive and support the implant must be available. In certain patients with progressive rheumatoid arthritis who have

Reconstructive Surgery for Deformities of Rheumatoid Hand

(Continued)

insufficient bone stock to support the implant, a simple resection arthroplasty or arthrodesis with a bone graft is preferable. Surgery is also contraindicated if surgical and postoperative facilities are not adequate.

Proper staging of the reconstructive procedures is important in planning the treatment program. Procedures in the upper limbs should be delayed in patients who also need lower limb reconstruction that will necessitate the use of crutches. After hand reconstruction, patients should avoid excessive manual labor and awkward hand weight bearing when using crutches. The special platform type of crutch is recommended.

In deformities of the metacarpophalangeal joint associated with severe wrist involvement, the wrist should be treated first. In the patient with rheumatoid arthritis, tendon repair and synovectomy of tendon sheaths must precede arthroplasty of the metacarpophalangeal joints by 6 to 8 weeks. If the extensor tendons are ruptured and the metacarpophalangeal joints dislocated, arthroplasty of the metacarpophalangeal joints is done before wrist and tendon reconstruction. If both metacarpophalangeal and proximal interphalangeal joints are involved, the metacarpophalangeal joint is usually treated first. In swan-neck deformity, the metacarpophalangeal and proximal interphalangeal joints are reconstructed at the same stage. In boutonniere deformity, the proximal interphalangeal joint is reconstructed first. Tendon imbalances and joint malalignment must be corrected. Implant arthroplasty for both the metacarpophalangeal and proximal interphalangeal joints of the same digit is usually not recommended.

Several procedures can be performed during one operation, depending on the time available. Surgery for the thumb, proximal interphalangeal and distal interphalangeal joints, wrist, and occasionally, the elbow joint can often be combined. A limb procedure should be limited to no more than 2 hours, and a stellate ganglion block is recommended if the tourniquet time exceeds 1½ hours. Small joints may also be injected with corticosteroids or other agents during surgery.

Deformities of Finger Joints

In the normal hand, a delicate balance exists among the muscles and tendons and the bones and joints through which they interact. The hand has three functional arches, one longitudinal and two transverse. The proximal transverse arch crosses the carpal area, with its center at the capitate. The distal transverse arch is formed by the

Implant Resection Arthroplasty for Metacarpophalangeal Joints

1. Transverse skin incision made over necks of metacarpals to expose extensor tendons. Superficial veins and nerves preserved. Displaced tendon released on ulnar side (see 2) and retracted radially

Long extensor tendon

Metacarpal

Ulnar intrinsic tendon divided

Line of incision through dorsal hood

Central tendon

Lateral tendon

Proximal phalanx

Middle phalanx

2. Long extensor tendon released by incising dorsal hood along tendon's ulnar margin, except in index and little fingers, where incision made between extensor communis and extensor digiti minimi tendons. Ulnar intrinsic tendon divided only if necessary

3. Head of metacarpal resected. Part of flare of metaphysis preserved. Bone ends smoothed. Synovectomy and soft-tissue release completed

4. Medullary canal prepared for implant stem. Air drill with special blunt–tip burr used to prevent cutting through cortex

5. Base of proximal phalanx resected and medullary canal prepared

metacarpal heads and is centered on the head of the third metacarpal. The digits make up the longitudinal arches, each with its apex at the metacarpophalangeal joint.

In rheumatoid arthritis, this balance among the muscles, tendons, and bones is compromised as the inflammatory synovial membrane grows over the surface of the cartilage, into the ligamentous attachments, and into and around the tendons. The result is capsular distention, destruction of cartilage, subchondral erosions, loosening of ligamentous insertions, impaired tendon function, and, finally, joint disorganization. A break in the longitudinal arch system causes collapse deformities of the multiarticular structure of the hand,

disturbing the stability and balance necessary for prehension. Use of the hand in daily activities (functional adaptation) causes further deformity.

Deformities of Metacarpophalangeal Joint

The metacarpophalangeal joint is a key element in finger function. This joint not only flexes and extends but also abducts and adducts; it also has some passive axial rotation. The index finger can pronate up to 45°.

Rheumatoid arthritis commonly involves the metacarpophalangeal joints, resulting in increased ulnar deviation of the fingers, subluxation of extensor tendons, and palmar subluxation of joints (Plate 62). The flexor tendons enter the fibrous

Reconstructive Surgery for Deformities of Rheumatoid Hand

(Continued)

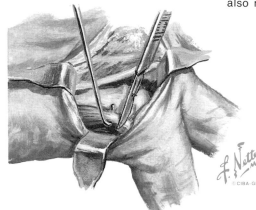

6. After incision of sheath, flexor tendon drawn up and partial synovectomy and release done if indicated

7. In index and middle fingers, radial collateral ligament reconstructed with distal flap made from collateral ligament and radial half of palmar plate. Flap sutured to metacarpal and proximal phalanx through drill holes. Radial capsule also repaired

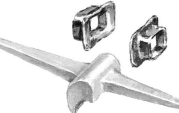

Titanium grommets protect implant from sharp bone ends

8. In little finger, abductor digiti minimi tendon divided. Flexor digiti minimi brevis tendon preserved

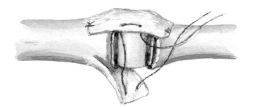

9. In index and middle fingers, drill holes made for capsular and ligamentous closure. Implant and grommets inserted (implant stem shortened if it abuts end of medullary canal)

10. Grommets or bone ends should not impinge on implant midsection. Ulnar edge of capsule sutured to ulnar collateral ligament

11. Capsuloligamentous closure completed for index and middle fingers

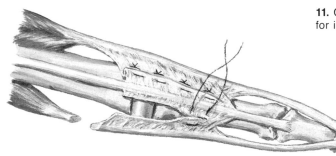

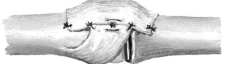

12. Sagittal fibers of dorsal hood reefed in overlapping fashion on radial side to centralize long extensor tendon and maintain correction

sheath at an angle, exerting an ulnar and palmar pull that is resisted in the normal hand. When the rheumatoid process distends and weakens the capsule and ligaments of the metacarpophalangeal joint, the forces generated by the long flexor tendons across the sheath during flexion may elongate these supporting structures. Resistance to the deforming pull of the tendons is gradually lost, and the sheath inlet and tendons are displaced in distal, ulnar, and palmar directions. Eventually, the base of the proximal phalanx moves ulnarly and palmarly. The intrinsic muscles, which normally form a bridge between the extensor and flexor systems and provide direct flexor power across the metacarpophalangeal joint, can also become deforming elements once the disease has lengthened the restraining structures of the metacarpophalangeal joint.

Increased mobility of the fourth and fifth metacarpals, common in rheumatoid arthritis, results from loosening of ligaments at the carpometacarpal joints and dysfunction of the extensor carpi ulnaris tendon (ulnar head syndrome). Flexion of the metacarpophalangeal joints increases the breadth of the transverse arch of the hand, which pulls the extensor tendons in an ulnar direction through the juncture tendons. The extensor tendon expansions (hoods) are loosely fixed and vulnerable to disruption. Ulnar subluxation of the extrinsic extensor tendons compromises the balance of the intrinsic extensor tendons, which in turn increases the tendency for palmar subluxation and ulnar deviation.

Factors that exacerbate ulnar deviation include (1) the normal mechanical advantage of the ulnar intrinsic muscles, (2) the asymmetry and ulnar slope of the metacarpal heads of the index and middle fingers, (3) the asymmetry of the collateral ligaments, (4) the ulnar forces applied on pinch and grasp, and (5) the postural forces of gravity. Wrist deformities and rupture of the extensor tendons play a secondary role in aggravating the joint disturbances.

Pronation deformity of the index finger is common in the rheumatoid hand. In the normal hand, pinch between the thumb and index finger requires a slight supination of the index finger so that the palmar surfaces can meet. In pronation deformity, the less useful lateral surfaces are opposed. During pinch, pronation deformity is seen in all three digital joints, but it is more pronounced in the metacarpophalangeal joint. Arthroplasty of this joint should include reconstruction of the capsuloligamentous and musculotendinous systems (Plates 63–64).

Deformities of Proximal Interphalangeal Joint

The collateral ligament system and the flexor and extensor tendons play an important role in maintaining the normal configuration of the proximal interphalangeal joint. The rheumatoid process compromises the normal anatomy of the joint and may lead to joint stiffness, with or without lateral deviation, or to collapse deformities, most notably boutonniere and swan-neck deformities. Mallet finger is not common in rheumatoid arthritis. Limited joint movement may result from articular factors (adhesions and disorganization of the joint), periarticular factors (adhesions or laxity of ligaments), or tendinous factors (synovial invasion of the flexor tendons and adhesions).

Collapse deformities of the three-joint system of the digit are characterized by hyperextension of one joint and reciprocal flexion of adjacent joints. The deformity occurs when the balance between the tendon and ligament systems is compromised. Axially applied forces further aggravate the deformity, establishing a cycle of deforming forces.

Boutonniere Deformity. This condition is characterized by flexion of the proximal interphalangeal joint and hyperextension of the distal interphalangeal joint (Plate 66). In rheumatoid arthritis, causes of boutonniere deformity include

Implant Resection Arthroplasty for Proximal Interphalangeal Joint

Reconstructive Surgery for Deformities of Rheumatoid Hand

(Continued)

(1) capsular distention of the proximal interphalangeal joint; (2) lengthening of the central long extensor tendon, with lack of extension in the middle phalanx; (3) lengthening of the transverse fibers; (4) palmar subluxation of the lateral bands, which become flexors of the proximal interphalangeal joint; (5) increased extensor pull on the distal phalanx; (6) self-perpetuating collapse deformity; and (7) soft-tissue contracture, joint stiffness, and disorganization.

Swan-Neck Deformity. The term "swan-neck deformity" refers to hyperextension of the proximal interphalangeal joint and flexion of the distal interphalangeal joint (Plate 66). In rheumatoid arthritis, the deformity may result from (1) synovitis of the flexor tendon sheath, which causes difficulty in initiating or completing flexion of the interphalangeal joint; (2) increased flexor pull at the metacarpophalangeal joint; (3) increased pull of the intrinsic muscles to the central tendon; (4) loosened attachments of the palmar ligament (plate) and accessory collateral ligaments of the proximal interphalangeal joint; (5) hyperextension of the proximal interphalangeal joint; (6) stretching of the oblique retinacular ligaments; (7) dorsal subluxation of the lateral bands, which become extensors of the proximal interphalangeal joint; (8) pull of the flexor digitorum profundus tendon, which flexes the distal interphalangeal joint; and (9) joint disorganization and subluxation. Other factors that increase the mechanical advantage of the extensor pull and accentuate the deformity include palmar subluxation of the metacarpophalangeal or wrist joint and contracture of the intrinsic muscles secondary to chronic flexion deformity of the metacarpophalangeal joint.

Deformities of Distal Interphalangeal Joint

In rheumatoid arthritis, deformities of the distal interphalangeal joint are usually secondary to collapse deformities. Specific deformities resulting from synovial invasion are uncommon; however, loosening of the distal attachment of the extensor tendon may cause a mallet or drop finger. Loosening of the collateral ligaments, erosive changes in the subchondral bone, and cartilage destruction in combination with external forces applied during daily activities may lead to joint instability. Complete joint destruction may also occur secondary to the severe resorptive changes seen in arthritis mutilans.

Surgery for Metacarpophalangeal Joint

Flexible implant resection arthroplasty of the metacarpophalangeal joints is carried out for

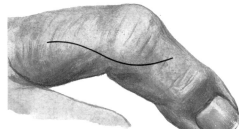

1. Longitudinal, slightly curved incision made over proximal interphalangeal joint

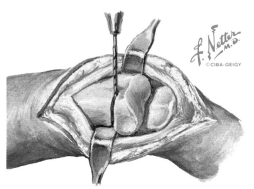

3. Head of proximal phalanx resected using air drill with side-cutting burr

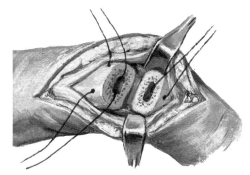

5. Middle phalanx reamed. Sutures passed for reattachment of collateral ligaments and central slip

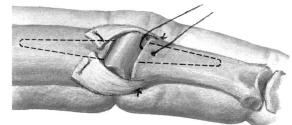

7. With joint extended, bone ends should not impinge on implant midsection. Collateral ligaments reattached

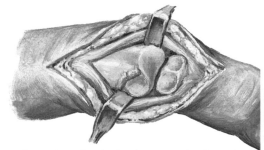

2. Central tendon incised, preserving insertion of middle phalanx, and each half retracted palmarly. Collateral ligament insertions on proximal phalanx preserved

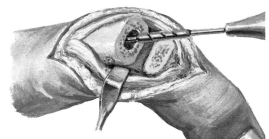

4. Proximal phalanx reamed with blunt-tip burr to avoid perforating cortex. Base of middle phalanx resected

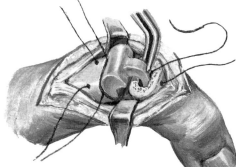

6. Largest implant that can be well seated inserted first into proximal and then into middle phalanx

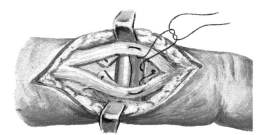

8. Halves of central tendon drawn together and sutured through drill hole in base of middle phalanx

deformities due to rheumatoid arthritis and trauma, with fixed or stiff joints, radiographic evidence of joint destruction or subluxation, ulnar deviation not correctable with soft-tissue surgery alone, contraction of the intrinsic and extrinsic musculature and ligamentous system, and associated stiffness of the interphalangeal joints.

The surgical technique for implant resection arthroplasty for the metacarpophalangeal joint is shown on Plates 63–64. Soft-tissue release must be complete to obtain an appropriate joint space. The ulnar collateral ligament is incised at its phalangeal insertion in all fingers; if severely contracted, it is excised with the palmar ligament. The radial collateral ligaments are preserved

whenever possible and reattached to bone if incised. The ulnar intrinsic tendon, if tight, is sectioned at its myotendinous junction. At the level of the index and middle fingers, it must be preserved if possible, to avoid a postoperative pronation tendency.

Reconstruction of the radial collateral ligament is done for index and middle fingers (Plate 64). The radial collateral ligament and related structures are reattached proximally to the metacarpal neck and distally to the proximal phalanx through small drill holes. The radial half of the palmar plate and the preserved radial capsule are included in this repair. The ulnar edge of the capsule is sutured to the distally released ulnar collateral

Reconstructive Surgery for Deformities of Rheumatoid Hand

(Continued)

ligament. Sutures are placed before the implant is inserted and tied with the finger held in supination and abduction. Although the procedure seems to slightly limit flexion of the metacarpophalangeal joint, this is outweighed by increased lateral and vertical stability and better correction of the pronation deformity.

If grommets are used, the resected surfaces of the metacarpal and proximal phalanx are shaped to obtain a precise press-fit of the grommet sleeve in the medullary canal. Sufficient bone stock must be present to support the grommet. Grommet and implant must be correctly sized (Plates 62 and 64).

After the procedure, a voluminous conforming dressing, including a palmar splint, is applied. During the postoperative period, the limb must be elevated. A meticulous postoperative program of dynamic bracing and therapy is usually started 3 to 5 days after surgery and must be continued for 6 to 8 weeks.

Surgery for Proximal Interphalangeal Joint

Treatment of deformities of this joint includes realignment of the longitudinal arch of the digit (for a complete discussion, see CLINICAL SYMPOSIA, Volume 36, Number 6). Implant resection arthroplasty of the proximal interphalangeal joint is indicated for painful, degenerative, or posttraumatic deformities with destruction or subluxation of the joint and stiffness that cannot be corrected with soft-tissue reconstruction alone. This procedure, however, is seldom indicated for rheumatoid and swan-neck deformities. Implant arthroplasty is preferred for isolated deformities of the proximal interphalangeal joint of the index finger. For deformities of the proximal interphalangeal joints of both the index and middle fingers in an active person, the proximal interphalangeal joint of the index finger is fused in 20° to 40° flexion, and implant arthroplasty is performed for the proximal interphalangeal joint of the middle finger. The more stable index finger can be used in pinch, and the more flexible middle finger can be used in grasp. Flexion of the proximal interphalangeal joints in the ring and little fingers is very important for grasping small objects, and function should be restored if possible.

Implant resection arthroplasty for proximal interphalangeal joints without collapse deformity (with or without lateral deviation) is shown on Plate 65. Good results require adequate release of joint contractures. The collateral ligaments are left intact whenever possible and can be reefed to bone on the weakened side to correct any lateral

Reconstruction of Swan-neck Deformity

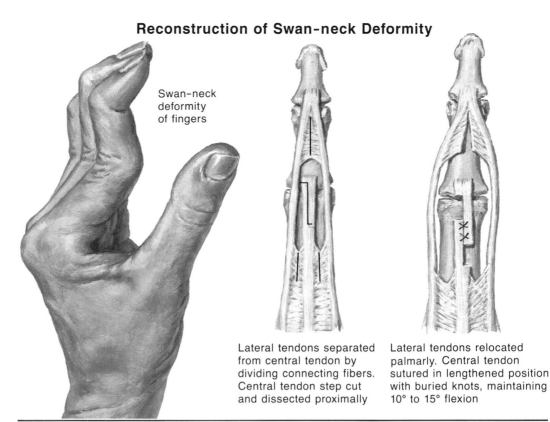

Swan-neck deformity of fingers

Lateral tendons separated from central tendon by dividing connecting fibers. Central tendon step cut and dissected proximally

Lateral tendons relocated palmarly. Central tendon sutured in lengthened position with buried knots, maintaining 10° to 15° flexion

Reconstruction of Boutonniere Deformity

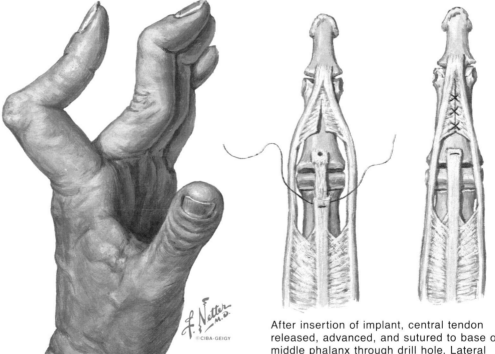

Boutonniere deformity of index finger with swan-neck deformity of other fingers

After insertion of implant, central tendon released, advanced, and sutured to base of middle phalanx through drill hole. Lateral tendons released and relocated dorsally by suturing connecting fibers or overlapping fibers if redundant

deviation or instability. If the joint is severely contracted, more bone is removed. If the contracture persists, the palmar plate and collateral ligaments may be incised proximally or distally, as needed. The collateral ligaments are then reattached to bone.

The hand is dressed as in metacarpophalangeal joint surgery, and 2 or 3 days after surgery, small, padded aluminum splints are applied with the finger in neutral position. Ten days after surgery, a 6- to 8-week program of active exercises is started using a variety of devices, with the metacarpophalangeal joint always supported in extension. The splint can be applied slightly to the radial or ulnar side of the digit to correct any

residual tendency to deviate; it is worn at night and between exercise periods until adequate healing occurs.

In an alternative approach, the central tendon is preserved, and the exposure is made between the lateral band and central tendon on both sides of the joint. The collateral ligaments are released proximally on both sides of the joint, and the palmar plate is released proximally to dislocate the joint laterally for exposure. Bone preparation, implant insertion, and reattachment of the collateral ligaments to bone are carried out as shown on Plate 65. The lateral bands are then sutured back to the central tendon. In this technique, joint motion can be started after 3 to 5 days

Reconstructive Surgery for Deformities of Rheumatoid Hand

(Continued)

Metacarpophalangeal Deformities of Thumb

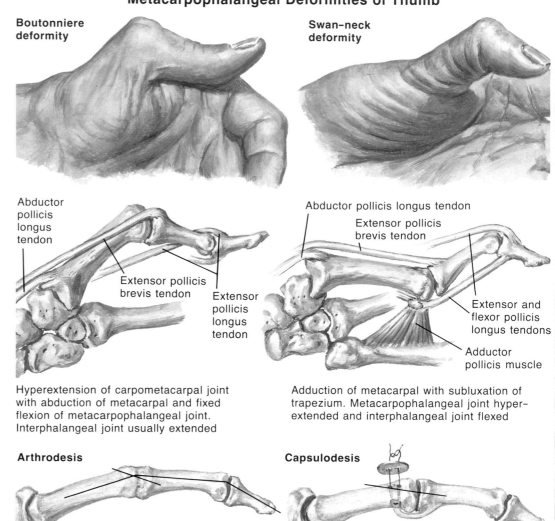

Boutonniere deformity

Hyperextension of carpometacarpal joint with abduction of metacarpal and fixed flexion of metacarpophalangeal joint. Interphalangeal joint usually extended

Swan-neck deformity

Adduction of metacarpal with subluxation of trapezium. Metacarpophalangeal joint hyperextended and interphalangeal joint flexed

because the central tendon has not been disturbed. It is important to protect the repaired collateral ligaments from lateral deviating forces for 6 weeks. Buddy splinting can be useful. A splint is worn at night for 6 to 8 weeks and during the day as needed.

Implant resection arthroplasty for proximal interphalangeal joints with collapse deformity requires adjustment of the tension of the central tendon and lateral bands (Plate 66). Compared with the lateral bands, the central tendon is relatively tight in the swan-neck deformity and must be released, while in the boutonniere deformity, the central tendon is relatively loose and must be tightened.

In swan-neck deformity, flexor synovitis is treated first. If the articular surfaces are preserved, hemitenodesis of the flexor digitorum superficialis tendon to the base of the middle phalanx can be done at the same time to check the hyperextension deformity of the proximal interphalangeal joint. A method for reconstructing the extensor mechanism through a dorsal approach is shown on Plate 66. Usually, it is not necessary to lengthen the central slip in release of the swan-neck deformity. It is important to obtain adequate release of the dorsal capsule, collateral ligaments, and palmar plate. A 10° flexion contracture (or greater) of the proximal interphalangeal joint should be obtained, and associated deformities of the contiguous joints corrected.

In a mild flexible deformity in weak hands, dermadesis is indicated: an elliptic wedge of skin (sufficient to create a 20° flexion contracture) is removed from the flexor aspect of the proximal interphalangeal joint, preserving the underlying vessels and nerves. If the articular surfaces are inadequate, however, fusion of the proximal interphalangeal joint is preferred. Implant arthroplasty is rarely indicated.

Implant resection arthroplasty for boutonniere deformity is accompanied by reconstruction of the extensor tendon mechanism (Plate 66). The collateral ligaments are reefed or reattached to bone as needed (Plate 65). After surgery, extension of the proximal interphalangeal joint and flexion of the distal interphalangeal joint must be maintained. The proximal interphalangeal joint is immobilized in extension with a padded aluminum splint for 3 to 6 weeks; the distal joint is allowed to flex freely. Active flexion and extension exercises are started 10 to 14 days after surgery, and a splint should be worn at night for about 10 weeks.

Arthrodesis

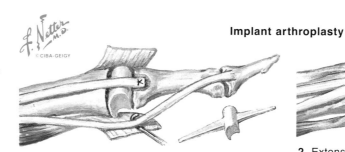

Joint fused in 10° flexion, 5° abduction, and slight pronation. Permanent cross wire and temporary longitudinal Kirschner wire in place

Capsulodesis

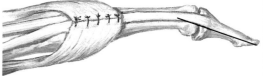

Two drill holes made in metacarpal neck. Concavity made on palmar aspect. Detached proximal end of palmar plate drawn into cavity with pullout wire. Temporary Kirschner wire maintains 10° to 15° flexion

Implant arthroplasty

1. Double-stemmed hinge implant in place. Extensor pollicis brevis tendon sutured to base of proximal phalanx and tension adjusted

2. Extensor pollicis longus tendon advanced distally and centered. Temporary Kirschner wire placed in distal joint. Dorsal hood sutured over both extensor tendons

Surgery for Distal Interphalangeal Joint

If the distal interphalangeal joint is unstable, subluxated, or deviated or if there is articular damage, arthrodesis is the treatment of choice. Contractures of the joint may be treated with soft-tissue release and temporary fixation with Kirschner wire to allow some useful residual movement. Slight flexion movement of the distal interphalangeal joint is very important in finely coordinated activities, but if movement at the proximal interphalangeal joint is good, fixation in a functional position is acceptable. In patients who desire motion and who have adequate bone stock and ligamentous structures, reconstruction of the distal interphalangeal joint with a small flexible-hinged implant can preserve a useful range of motion.

Deformities of Thumb Joints

The thumb is the most important digit of the hand. All three joints of the thumb are important in functional adaptations, and each may be affected primarily or secondarily by imbalances of the other joints (eg, boutonniere and swan-neck deformities). Thus, reconstructive surgery of the thumb must consider the entire thumb (radial) ray; the balance of its musculotendinous system; and the position, mobility, and stability of all its joints. The joints of the thumb may be impaired

Reconstructive Surgery for Deformities of Rheumatoid Hand

(Continued)

ligament. Sutures are placed before the implant is inserted and tied with the finger held in supination and abduction. Although the procedure seems to slightly limit flexion of the metacarpophalangeal joint, this is outweighed by increased lateral and vertical stability and better correction of the pronation deformity.

If grommets are used, the resected surfaces of the metacarpal and proximal phalanx are shaped to obtain a precise press-fit of the grommet sleeve in the medullary canal. Sufficient bone stock must be present to support the grommet. Grommet and implant must be correctly sized (Plates 62 and 64).

After the procedure, a voluminous conforming dressing, including a palmar splint, is applied. During the postoperative period, the limb must be elevated. A meticulous postoperative program of dynamic bracing and therapy is usually started 3 to 5 days after surgery and must be continued for 6 to 8 weeks.

Surgery for Proximal Interphalangeal Joint

Treatment of deformities of this joint includes realignment of the longitudinal arch of the digit (for a complete discussion, see CLINICAL SYMPOSIA, Volume 36, Number 6). Implant resection arthroplasty of the proximal interphalangeal joint is indicated for painful, degenerative, or post-traumatic deformities with destruction or subluxation of the joint and stiffness that cannot be corrected with soft-tissue reconstruction alone. This procedure, however, is seldom indicated for rheumatoid and swan-neck deformities. Implant arthroplasty is preferred for isolated deformities of the proximal interphalangeal joint of the index finger. For deformities of the proximal interphalangeal joints of both the index and middle fingers in an active person, the proximal interphalangeal joint of the index finger is fused in 20° to 40° flexion, and implant arthroplasty is performed for the proximal interphalangeal joint of the middle finger. The more stable index finger can be used in pinch, and the more flexible middle finger can be used in grasp. Flexion of the proximal interphalangeal joints in the ring and little fingers is very important for grasping small objects, and function should be restored if possible.

Implant resection arthroplasty for proximal interphalangeal joints without collapse deformity (with or without lateral deviation) is shown on Plate 65. Good results require adequate release of joint contractures. The collateral ligaments are left intact whenever possible and can be reefed to bone on the weakened side to correct any lateral

Reconstruction of Swan-neck Deformity

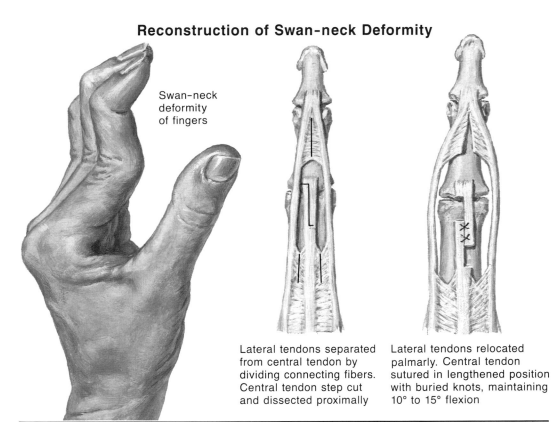

Swan-neck deformity of fingers

Lateral tendons separated from central tendon by dividing connecting fibers. Central tendon step cut and dissected proximally

Lateral tendons relocated palmarly. Central tendon sutured in lengthened position with buried knots, maintaining 10° to 15° flexion

Reconstruction of Boutonniere Deformity

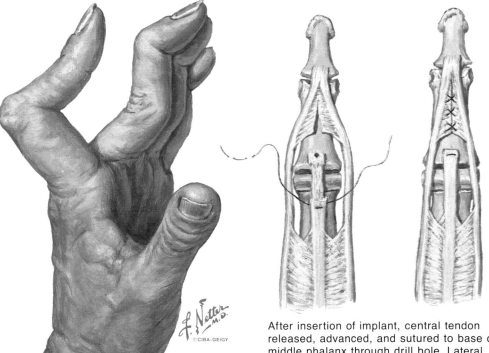

Boutonniere deformity of index finger with swan-neck deformity of other fingers

After insertion of implant, central tendon released, advanced, and sutured to base of middle phalanx through drill hole. Lateral tendons released and relocated dorsally by suturing connecting fibers or overlapping fibers if redundant

deviation or instability. If the joint is severely contracted, more bone is removed. If the contracture persists, the palmar plate and collateral ligaments may be incised proximally or distally, as needed. The collateral ligaments are then reattached to bone.

The hand is dressed as in metacarpophalangeal joint surgery, and 2 or 3 days after surgery, small, padded aluminum splints are applied with the finger in neutral position. Ten days after surgery, a 6- to 8-week program of active exercises is started using a variety of devices, with the metacarpophalangeal joint always supported in extension. The splint can be applied slightly to the radial or ulnar side of the digit to correct any

residual tendency to deviate; it is worn at night and between exercise periods until adequate healing occurs.

In an alternative approach, the central tendon is preserved, and the exposure is made between the lateral band and central tendon on both sides of the joint. The collateral ligaments are released proximally on both sides of the joint, and the palmar plate is released proximally to dislocate the joint laterally for exposure. Bone preparation, implant insertion, and reattachment of the collateral ligaments to bone are carried out as shown on Plate 65. The lateral bands are then sutured back to the central tendon. In this technique, joint motion can be started after 3 to 5 days

Metacarpophalangeal Deformities of Thumb

Reconstructive Surgery for Deformities of Rheumatoid Hand

(Continued)

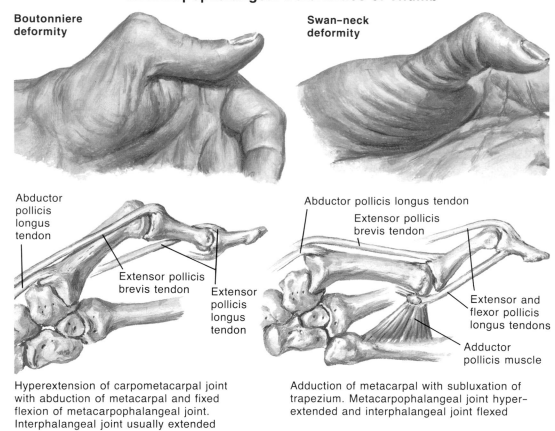

Boutonniere deformity

Swan-neck deformity

Abductor pollicis longus tendon

Extensor pollicis brevis tendon

Extensor pollicis longus tendon

Abductor pollicis longus tendon

Extensor pollicis brevis tendon

Extensor and flexor pollicis longus tendons

Adductor pollicis muscle

Hyperextension of carpometacarpal joint with abduction of metacarpal and fixed flexion of metacarpophalangeal joint. Interphalangeal joint usually extended

Adduction of metacarpal with subluxation of trapezium. Metacarpophalangeal joint hyperextended and interphalangeal joint flexed

because the central tendon has not been disturbed. It is important to protect the repaired collateral ligaments from lateral deviating forces for 6 weeks. Buddy splinting can be useful. A splint is worn at night for 6 to 8 weeks and during the day as needed.

Implant resection arthroplasty for proximal interphalangeal joints with collapse deformity requires adjustment of the tension of the central tendon and lateral bands (Plate 66). Compared with the lateral bands, the central tendon is relatively tight in the swan-neck deformity and must be released, while in the boutonniere deformity, the central tendon is relatively loose and must be tightened.

In swan-neck deformity, flexor synovitis is treated first. If the articular surfaces are preserved, hemitenodesis of the flexor digitorum superficialis tendon to the base of the middle phalanx can be done at the same time to check the hyperextension deformity of the proximal interphalangeal joint. A method for reconstructing the extensor mechanism through a dorsal approach is shown on Plate 66. Usually, it is not necessary to lengthen the central slip in release of the swan-neck deformity. It is important to obtain adequate release of the dorsal capsule, collateral ligaments, and palmar plate. A 10° flexion contracture (or greater) of the proximal interphalangeal joint should be obtained, and associated deformities of the contiguous joints corrected.

In a mild flexible deformity in weak hands, dermadesis is indicated: an elliptic wedge of skin (sufficient to create a 20° flexion contracture) is removed from the flexor aspect of the proximal interphalangeal joint, preserving the underlying vessels and nerves. If the articular surfaces are inadequate, however, fusion of the proximal interphalangeal joint is preferred. Implant arthroplasty is rarely indicated.

Implant resection arthroplasty for boutonniere deformity is accompanied by reconstruction of the extensor tendon mechanism (Plate 66). The collateral ligaments are reefed or reattached to bone as needed (Plate 65). After surgery, extension of the proximal interphalangeal joint and flexion of the distal interphalangeal joint must be maintained. The proximal interphalangeal joint is immobilized in extension with a padded aluminum splint for 3 to 6 weeks; the distal joint is allowed to flex freely. Active flexion and extension exercises are started 10 to 14 days after surgery, and a splint should be worn at night for about 10 weeks.

Arthrodesis

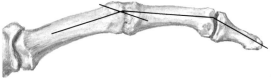

Joint fused in 10° flexion, 5° abduction, and slight pronation. Permanent cross wire and temporary longitudinal Kirschner wire in place

Capsulodesis

Two drill holes made in metacarpal neck. Concavity made on palmar aspect. Detached proximal end of palmar plate drawn into cavity with pullout wire. Temporary Kirschner wire maintains 10° to 15° flexion

Implant arthroplasty

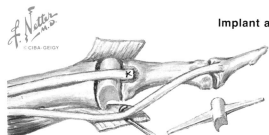

1. Double-stemmed hinge implant in place. Extensor pollicis brevis tendon sutured to base of proximal phalanx and tension adjusted

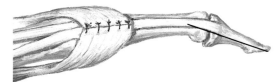

2. Extensor pollicis longus tendon advanced distally and centered. Temporary Kirschner wire placed in distal joint. Dorsal hood sutured over both extensor tendons

Surgery for Distal Interphalangeal Joint

If the distal interphalangeal joint is unstable, subluxated, or deviated or if there is articular damage, arthrodesis is the treatment of choice. Contractures of the joint may be treated with soft-tissue release and temporary fixation with Kirschner wire to allow some useful residual movement. Slight flexion movement of the distal interphalangeal joint is very important in finely coordinated activities, but if movement at the proximal interphalangeal joint is good, fixation in a functional position is acceptable. In patients who desire motion and who have adequate bone stock and ligamentous structures, reconstruction of the

distal interphalangeal joint with a small flexible-hinged implant can preserve a useful range of motion.

Deformities of Thumb Joints

The thumb is the most important digit of the hand. All three joints of the thumb are important in functional adaptations, and each may be affected primarily or secondarily by imbalances of the other joints (eg, boutonniere and swan-neck deformities). Thus, reconstructive surgery of the thumb must consider the entire thumb (radial) ray; the balance of its musculotendinous system; and the position, mobility, and stability of all its joints. The joints of the thumb may be impaired

Reconstructive Surgery for Deformities of Rheumatoid Hand

(Continued)

ligament. Sutures are placed before the implant is inserted and tied with the finger held in supination and abduction. Although the procedure seems to slightly limit flexion of the metacarpophalangeal joint, this is outweighed by increased lateral and vertical stability and better correction of the pronation deformity.

If grommets are used, the resected surfaces of the metacarpal and proximal phalanx are shaped to obtain a precise press-fit of the grommet sleeve in the medullary canal. Sufficient bone stock must be present to support the grommet. Grommet and implant must be correctly sized (Plates 62 and 64).

After the procedure, a voluminous conforming dressing, including a palmar splint, is applied. During the postoperative period, the limb must be elevated. A meticulous postoperative program of dynamic bracing and therapy is usually started 3 to 5 days after surgery and must be continued for 6 to 8 weeks.

Surgery for Proximal Interphalangeal Joint

Treatment of deformities of this joint includes realignment of the longitudinal arch of the digit (for a complete discussion, see CLINICAL SYMPOSIA, Volume 36, Number 6). Implant resection arthroplasty of the proximal interphalangeal joint is indicated for painful, degenerative, or posttraumatic deformities with destruction or subluxation of the joint and stiffness that cannot be corrected with soft-tissue reconstruction alone. This procedure, however, is seldom indicated for rheumatoid and swan-neck deformities. Implant arthroplasty is preferred for isolated deformities of the proximal interphalangeal joint of the index finger. For deformities of the proximal interphalangeal joints of both the index and middle fingers in an active person, the proximal interphalangeal joint of the index finger is fused in 20° to 40° flexion, and implant arthroplasty is performed for the proximal interphalangeal joint of the middle finger. The more stable index finger can be used in pinch, and the more flexible middle finger can be used in grasp. Flexion of the proximal interphalangeal joints in the ring and little fingers is very important for grasping small objects, and function should be restored if possible.

Implant resection arthroplasty for proximal interphalangeal joints without collapse deformity (with or without lateral deviation) is shown on Plate 65. Good results require adequate release of joint contractures. The collateral ligaments are left intact whenever possible and can be reefed to bone on the weakened side to correct any lateral

Reconstruction of Swan-neck Deformity

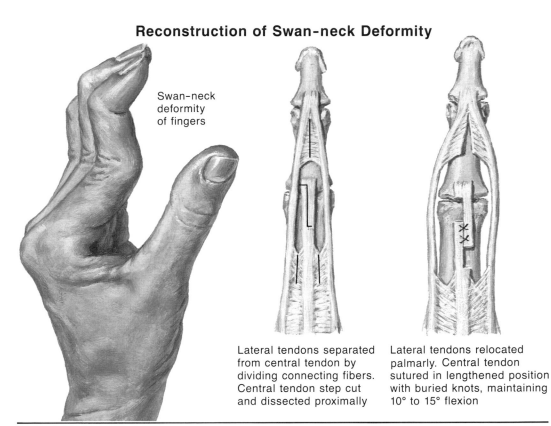

Swan-neck deformity of fingers

Lateral tendons separated from central tendon by dividing connecting fibers. Central tendon step cut and dissected proximally

Lateral tendons relocated palmarly. Central tendon sutured in lengthened position with buried knots, maintaining 10° to 15° flexion

Reconstruction of Boutonniere Deformity

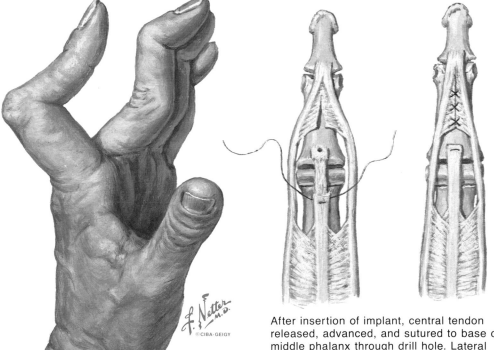

Boutonnniere deformity of index finger with swan-neck deformity of other fingers

After insertion of implant, central tendon released, advanced, and sutured to base of middle phalanx through drill hole. Lateral tendons released and relocated dorsally by suturing connecting fibers or overlapping fibers if redundant

deviation or instability. If the joint is severely contracted, more bone is removed. If the contracture persists, the palmar plate and collateral ligaments may be incised proximally or distally, as needed. The collateral ligaments are then reattached to bone.

The hand is dressed as in metacarpophalangeal joint surgery, and 2 or 3 days after surgery, small, padded aluminum splints are applied with the finger in neutral position. Ten days after surgery, a 6- to 8-week program of active exercises is started using a variety of devices, with the metacarpophalangeal joint always supported in extension. The splint can be applied slightly to the radial or ulnar side of the digit to correct any

residual tendency to deviate; it is worn at night and between exercise periods until adequate healing occurs.

In an alternative approach, the central tendon is preserved, and the exposure is made between the lateral band and central tendon on both sides of the joint. The collateral ligaments are released proximally on both sides of the joint, and the palmar plate is released proximally to dislocate the joint laterally for exposure. Bone preparation, implant insertion, and reattachment of the collateral ligaments to bone are carried out as shown on Plate 65. The lateral bands are then sutured back to the central tendon. In this technique, joint motion can be started after 3 to 5 days

Reconstructive Surgery for Deformities of Rheumatoid Hand

(Continued)

Metacarpophalangeal Deformities of Thumb

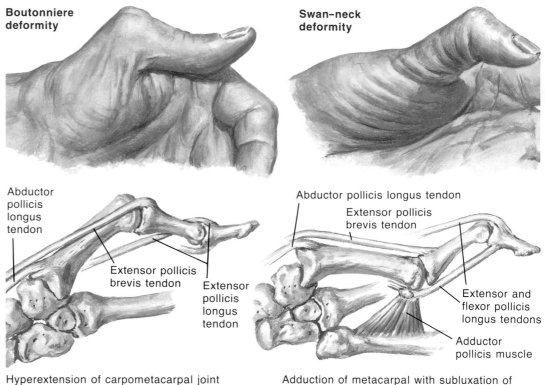

Boutonniere deformity

Abductor pollicis longus tendon

Extensor pollicis brevis tendon

Extensor pollicis longus tendon

Hyperextension of carpometacarpal joint with abduction of metacarpal and fixed flexion of metacarpophalangeal joint. Interphalangeal joint usually extended

Swan-neck deformity

Abductor pollicis longus tendon

Extensor pollicis brevis tendon

Extensor and flexor pollicis longus tendons

Adductor pollicis muscle

Adduction of metacarpal with subluxation of trapezium. Metacarpophalangeal joint hyperextended and interphalangeal joint flexed

Arthrodesis

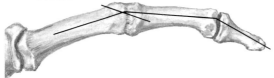

Joint fused in 10° flexion, 5° abduction, and slight pronation. Permanent cross wire and temporary longitudinal Kirschner wire in place

Capsulodesis

Two drill holes made in metacarpal neck. Concavity made on palmar aspect. Detached proximal end of palmar plate drawn into cavity with pullout wire. Temporary Kirschner wire maintains 10° to 15° flexion

Implant arthroplasty

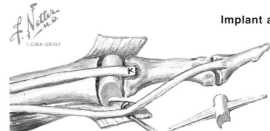

1. Double-stemmed hinge implant in place. Extensor pollicis brevis tendon sutured to base of proximal phalanx and tension adjusted

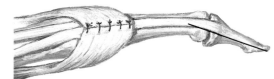

2. Extensor pollicis longus tendon advanced distally and centered. Temporary Kirschner wire placed in distal joint. Dorsal hood sutured over both extensor tendons

because the central tendon has not been disturbed. It is important to protect the repaired collateral ligaments from lateral deviating forces for 6 weeks. Buddy splinting can be useful. A splint is worn at night for 6 to 8 weeks and during the day as needed.

Implant resection arthroplasty for proximal interphalangeal joints with collapse deformity requires adjustment of the tension of the central tendon and lateral bands (Plate 66). Compared with the lateral bands, the central tendon is relatively tight in the swan-neck deformity and must be released, while in the boutonniere deformity, the central tendon is relatively loose and must be tightened.

In swan-neck deformity, flexor synovitis is treated first. If the articular surfaces are preserved, hemitenodesis of the flexor digitorum superficialis tendon to the base of the middle phalanx can be done at the same time to check the hyperextension deformity of the proximal interphalangeal joint. A method for reconstructing the extensor mechanism through a dorsal approach is shown on Plate 66. Usually, it is not necessary to lengthen the central slip in release of the swan-neck deformity. It is important to obtain adequate release of the dorsal capsule, collateral ligaments, and palmar plate. A 10° flexion contracture (or greater) of the proximal interphalangeal joint should be obtained, and associated deformities of the contiguous joints corrected.

In a mild flexible deformity in weak hands, dermadesis is indicated: an elliptic wedge of skin (sufficient to create a 20° flexion contracture) is removed from the flexor aspect of the proximal interphalangeal joint, preserving the underlying vessels and nerves. If the articular surfaces are inadequate, however, fusion of the proximal interphalangeal joint is preferred. Implant arthroplasty is rarely indicated.

Implant resection arthroplasty for boutonniere deformity is accompanied by reconstruction of the extensor tendon mechanism (Plate 66). The collateral ligaments are reefed or reattached to bone as needed (Plate 65). After surgery, extension of the proximal interphalangeal joint and flexion of the distal interphalangeal joint must be maintained. The proximal interphalangeal joint is immobilized in extension with a padded aluminum splint for 3 to 6 weeks; the distal joint is allowed to flex freely. Active flexion and extension exercises are started 10 to 14 days after surgery, and a splint should be worn at night for about 10 weeks.

Surgery for Distal Interphalangeal Joint

If the distal interphalangeal joint is unstable, subluxated, or deviated or if there is articular damage, arthrodesis is the treatment of choice. Contractures of the joint may be treated with soft-tissue release and temporary fixation with Kirschner wire to allow some useful residual movement. Slight flexion movement of the distal interphalangeal joint is very important in finely coordinated activities, but if movement at the proximal interphalangeal joint is good, fixation in a functional position is acceptable. In patients who desire motion and who have adequate bone stock and ligamentous structures, reconstruction of the distal interphalangeal joint with a small flexible-hinged implant can preserve a useful range of motion.

Deformities of Thumb Joints

The thumb is the most important digit of the hand. All three joints of the thumb are important in functional adaptations, and each may be affected primarily or secondarily by imbalances of the other joints (eg, boutonniere and swan-neck deformities). Thus, reconstructive surgery of the thumb must consider the entire thumb (radial) ray; the balance of its musculotendinous system; and the position, mobility, and stability of all its joints. The joints of the thumb may be impaired

Reconstructive Surgery for Deformities of Rheumatoid Hand
(Continued)

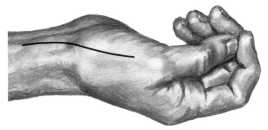

1. Incision centered over trapezium and curved slightly palmarly to parallel flexor carpi radialis tendon (FCR). Branches of superficial radial nerve carefully preserved

Implant Resection Arthroplasty for Trapezium

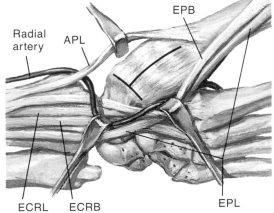

2. Abductor pollicis longus tendon (APL), extensor pollicis brevis tendon (EPB), and radial artery retracted. Capsule over base of 1st metacarpal, trapezium, and scaphoid incised

as a result of osteoarthritis, rheumatoid arthritis, or posttraumatic arthritis. Thumb deformities can be classified as (1) postural, including longitudinal collapse (boutonniere, swan-neck) and fixed positional (adducted retroposed thumb) deformities; (2) unstable, stiff, or painful interphalangeal, metacarpophalangeal, or carpometacarpal joints; and (3) tendon deformities, including contracture, displacement, or rupture of the flexor pollicis longus, extensor pollicis longus or brevis, abductor pollicis longus, or intrinsic tendons.

Postural Deformities. The *boutonniere deformity* is caused primarily by arthritic involvement of the metacarpophalangeal joint. While it is found in 57% of patients with hands affected by rheumatoid arthritis, boutonniere deformity does not usually occur in osteoarthritis. Initially, the capsule and extensor apparatus around the metacarpophalangeal joint are stretched by synovitis. The extensor pollicis longus tendon and adductor expansions are displaced ulnarly, and the lateral thenar expansions are displaced radially. The extensor pollicis brevis tendon attachment to the base of the proximal phalanx is lengthened, and the ability to extend the metacarpophalangeal joint is decreased, causing a flexion deformity of the proximal phalanx. The extensor pollicis longus tendon and extensor insertions of the intrinsic muscles apply all their power to the distal phalanx and produce secondary hyperextension of the interphalangeal joint (Plate 67). Pinch movements further aggravate the deformity. As contractures develop, the deformity becomes fixed. Destructive articular changes compound the deformity, and disorganization and subluxation of the joint may occur.

Swan-neck deformity, in contrast, is far more common in osteoarthritis than in rheumatoid arthritis (Plate 67). It is usually initiated by destructive changes at the carpometacarpal joint, followed by stretching of the joint capsule and radial subluxation of the base of the metacarpal. As motion at the trapeziometacarpal joint during abduction becomes painful, the patient avoids abduction, using the distal joints to compensate for lack of motion at the base of the thumb. An increasing adduction deformity with contracture of the adductor pollicis muscle develops. Effusion in the joint further loosens the capsule, permitting a proximal radial subluxation of the metacarpal. Subluxation may result in hyperextension of the interphalangeal joint, but more frequently, it causes hyperextension of the metacarpophalangeal joint and adduction of the first metacarpal. Further adduction contracture of the metacarpal aggravates the

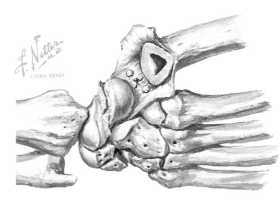

3. Trapezium removed, leaving small flecks of bone to preserve capsuloligamentous support. Holes in capsule sutured. Base of 1st metacarpal resected and medullary canal prepared in triangular shape

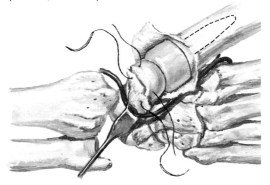

4. Implant inserted with base seated on distal scaphoid. Sutures passed for capsular closure. Partial trapezoidectomy may be required

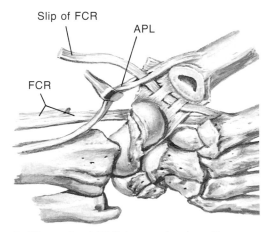

5. Slip made of FCR (preserving insertion on metacarpal) and passed through palmar capsule, abductor pollicis brevis muscle, APL, and lateral capsule. Drill holes in metacarpal for capsular repair

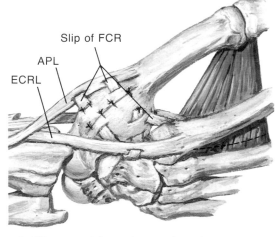

6. Slip passed through capsule, extensor carpi radialis longus tendon (ECRL), then back through capsule and APL. Implant inserted and capsular reinforcement tightened; capsular reflections sutured proximally and distally

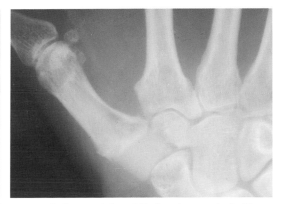

Degenerative arthritis of basal joints of thumb with bony spur between 1st and 2nd metacarpals (left). Four years after trapeziectomy and partial trapezoidectomy, implant in good position over scaphoid (right)

Reconstructive Surgery for Deformities of Rheumatoid Hand

(Continued)

Implant Resection Arthroplasty for Scaphoid

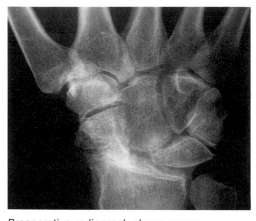

Preoperative radiograph shows severe radioscaphoid involvement with scapholunate separation and degenerative changes between capitate and lunate

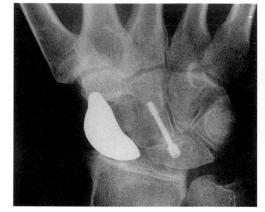

Postoperative radiograph shows titanium scaphoid implant in good position. Lunate relocated and fused to capitate with Herbert screw fixation

hyperextension of the metacarpophalangeal joint and permits collapse of the thumb ray. The interphalangeal joint becomes flexed, as in a swanneck deformity of the finger.

In the *adducted retroposed thumb*, the first metacarpal is retropositioned, adducted, and externally rotated. The deformity is probably initiated by synovitis of the carpometacarpal joint and aggravated by awkward positioning of the thumb, as on a flat surface during acute illness. There seems to be a contracture of the extensor pollicis longus muscle, with adduction and external rotation of the metacarpal and with palmar and radial subluxation of the metacarpal base off the trapezium.

Unstable, Stiff, or Painful Joints. Instability, stiffness, or pain may occur in the interphalangeal, metacarpophalangeal, or carpometacarpal joint, sometimes in association with a collapse deformity of the thumb ray. These deformities are accentuated by forces applied during pinch movements.

Tendon Deformities. In rheumatoid arthritis, tendon deformities are related to muscle contracture, tendon displacement, adhesions, or tendon rupture. Rupture of the extensor pollicis longus tendon is most common, usually occurring within the third extensor compartment in the area of the distal tubercle of the radius. Sudden rupture of the tendon results in a sudden drop of the metacarpophalangeal joint of the thumb and, in some cases, loss of extensor power at the distal phalanx.

Rupture of the flexor pollicis longus tendon usually occurs in the carpal area and must be considered in the diagnosis of hyperextension deformity of the interphalangeal joint of the thumb. Rupture of the abductor pollicis longus and extensor pollicis brevis tendons is rare.

Synovial invasion and stretching of the dorsal hood of the metacarpophalangeal joint may result in displacement and secondary contractures of the tendons of the intrinsic muscles.

Surgery for Interphalangeal Joint

Arthrodesis is usually the preferred treatment for instability of the interphalangeal joint of the thumb; bone grafting is necessary if bone resorption is severe. A flexible hyperextension deformity of the interphalangeal joint, with lateral stability and intact joint surfaces, may require a flexor *hemitenodesis* to prevent hyperextension while allowing some flexion. If bone stock and ligamentous stability are adequate, involvement of the interphalangeal joint may be treated with a single-stemmed condylar replacement or with a flexible-hinged implant as an adjunct to *resection arthroplasty* to preserve some pain-free motion;

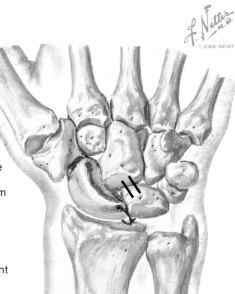

Dorsolateral incision

1. Dissection carried to dorsal capsule between extensor compartments, preserving superficial radial nerve and artery. Capsular flap preserved. Scaphoid removed, leaving thin wafer of bone to maintain continuity of palmar ligaments

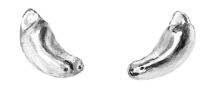

Titanium implants in mirror-image forms for left and right wrists (stemless silicone implants also used)

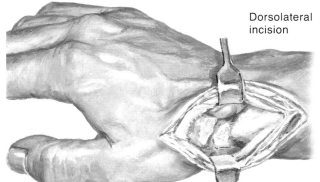

Hamulus of hamate

Pisiform

Palmar ulnocarpal ligament

Lunate

Ulna

Capitate

Trapezium

Tubercle of scaphoid

Palmar radiocarpal ligament

Radius

2. Bone insertions of palmar carpal ligaments. Complete bone removal creates ligamentous defects that must be repaired to provide support for implant

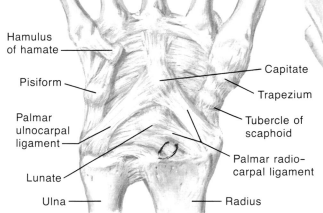

3. Lunocapitate fusion carried out if lunate instability present. Proximal pole of implant sutured to radioscapholunate ligament

this can be important for certain prehensile activities, especially when other joints are disabled.

Surgery for Metacarpophalangeal Joint

Arthrodesis is indicated in joint destruction and collapse deformities to simplify the articular system of the thumb ray, providing the distal and basal joints have adequate mobility (Plate 67). The joint is exposed through a longitudinal dorsal approach, with the extensor hood split longitudinally. The metacarpal head is shaped convexly to fit the concavity formed at the base of the proximal phalanx. A longitudinal wire is placed in a retrograde fashion through the thumb ray and bent in place to the desired position.

Fragments of cancellous bone are used as a graft between the bone ends. A small Kirschner wire is placed obliquely across the joint as the bone ends are firmly pressed together. The small wire is sectioned subcutaneously and removed after 6 to 8 weeks or left in place. The longitudinal wire is removed after 6 to 8 weeks.

Capsulodesis is the treatment of choice in hyperextension deformities of more than 20° with good flexion, lateral stability, and intact articular surfaces (Plate 67). The palmar aspect of the joint is exposed through a lateral incision, and the proximal membranous insertion of the palmar plate is incised. The sesamoids and their tendon attachments are left intact. The periosteum is stripped

Implant Resection Arthroplasty for Trapezium

Reconstructive Surgery for Deformities of Rheumatoid Hand

(Continued)

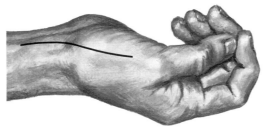

1. Incision centered over trapezium and curved slightly palmarly to parallel flexor carpi radialis tendon (FCR). Branches of superficial radial nerve carefully preserved

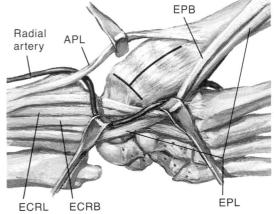

2. Abductor pollicis longus tendon (APL), extensor pollicis brevis tendon (EPB), and radial artery retracted. Capsule over base of 1st metacarpal, trapezium, and scaphoid incised

as a result of osteoarthritis, rheumatoid arthritis, or posttraumatic arthritis. Thumb deformities can be classified as (1) postural, including longitudinal collapse (boutonniere, swan-neck) and fixed positional (adducted retroposed thumb) deformities; (2) unstable, stiff, or painful interphalangeal, metacarpophalangeal, or carpometacarpal joints; and (3) tendon deformities, including contracture, displacement, or rupture of the flexor pollicis longus, extensor pollicis longus or brevis, abductor pollicis longus, or intrinsic tendons.

Postural Deformities. The *boutonniere deformity* is caused primarily by arthritic involvement of the metacarpophalangeal joint. While it is found in 57% of patients with hands affected by rheumatoid arthritis, boutonniere deformity does not usually occur in osteoarthritis. Initially, the capsule and extensor apparatus around the metacarpophalangeal joint are stretched by synovitis. The extensor pollicis longus tendon and adductor expansions are displaced ulnarly, and the lateral thenar expansions are displaced radially. The extensor pollicis brevis tendon attachment to the base of the proximal phalanx is lengthened, and the ability to extend the metacarpophalangeal joint is decreased, causing a flexion deformity of the proximal phalanx. The extensor pollicis longus tendon and extensor insertions of the intrinsic muscles apply all their power to the distal phalanx and produce secondary hyperextension of the interphalangeal joint (Plate 67). Pinch movements further aggravate the deformity. As contractures develop, the deformity becomes fixed. Destructive articular changes compound the deformity, and disorganization and subluxation of the joint may occur.

Swan-neck deformity, in contrast, is far more common in osteoarthritis than in rheumatoid arthritis (Plate 67). It is usually initiated by destructive changes at the carpometacarpal joint, followed by stretching of the joint capsule and radial subluxation of the base of the metacarpal. As motion at the trapeziometacarpal joint during abduction becomes painful, the patient avoids abduction, using the distal joints to compensate for lack of motion at the base of the thumb. An increasing adduction deformity with contracture of the adductor pollicis muscle develops. Effusion in the joint further loosens the capsule, permitting a proximal radial subluxation of the metacarpal. Subluxation may result in hyperextension of the interphalangeal joint, but more frequently, it causes hyperextension of the metacarpophalangeal joint and adduction of the first metacarpal. Further adduction contracture of the metacarpal aggravates the

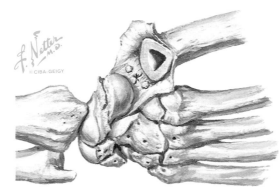

3. Trapezium removed, leaving small flecks of bone to preserve capsuloligamentous support. Holes in capsule sutured. Base of 1st metacarpal resected and medullary canal prepared in triangular shape

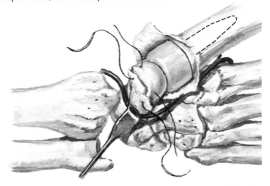

4. Implant inserted with base seated on distal scaphoid. Sutures passed for capsular closure. Partial trapezoidectomy may be required

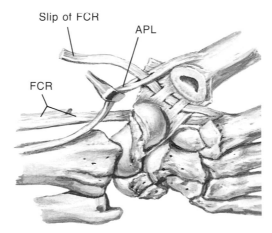

5. Slip made of FCR (preserving insertion on metacarpal) and passed through palmar capsule, abductor pollicis brevis muscle, APL, and lateral capsule. Drill holes in metacarpal for capsular repair

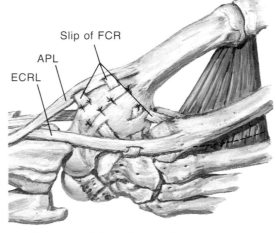

6. Slip passed through capsule, extensor carpi radialis longus tendon (ECRL), then back through capsule and APL. Implant inserted and capsular reinforcement tightened; capsular reflections sutured proximally and distally

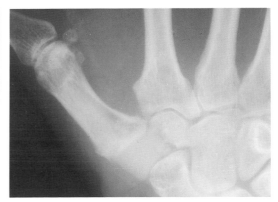

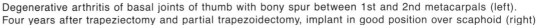

Degenerative arthritis of basal joints of thumb with bony spur between 1st and 2nd metacarpals (left). Four years after trapeziectomy and partial trapezoidectomy, implant in good position over scaphoid (right)

Implant Resection Arthroplasty for Scaphoid

Reconstructive Surgery for Deformities of Rheumatoid Hand

(Continued)

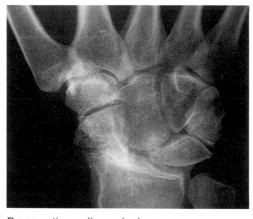

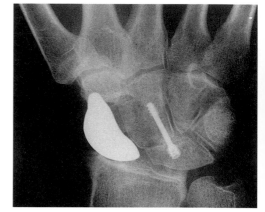

Preoperative radiograph shows severe radioscaphoid involvement with scapholunate separation and degenerative changes between capitate and lunate

Postoperative radiograph shows titanium scaphoid implant in good position. Lunate relocated and fused to capitate with Herbert screw fixation

hyperextension of the metacarpophalangeal joint and permits collapse of the thumb ray. The interphalangeal joint becomes flexed, as in a swan-neck deformity of the finger.

In the *adducted retroposed thumb*, the first metacarpal is retropositioned, adducted, and externally rotated. The deformity is probably initiated by synovitis of the carpometacarpal joint and aggravated by awkward positioning of the thumb, as on a flat surface during acute illness. There seems to be a contracture of the extensor pollicis longus muscle, with adduction and external rotation of the metacarpal and with palmar and radial subluxation of the metacarpal base off the trapezium.

Unstable, Stiff, or Painful Joints. Instability, stiffness, or pain may occur in the interphalangeal, metacarpophalangeal, or carpometacarpal joint, sometimes in association with a collapse deformity of the thumb ray. These deformities are accentuated by forces applied during pinch movements.

Tendon Deformities. In rheumatoid arthritis, tendon deformities are related to muscle contracture, tendon displacement, adhesions, or tendon rupture. Rupture of the extensor pollicis longus tendon is most common, usually occurring within the third extensor compartment in the area of the distal tubercle of the radius. Sudden rupture of the tendon results in a sudden drop of the metacarpophalangeal joint of the thumb and, in some cases, loss of extensor power at the distal phalanx.

Rupture of the flexor pollicis longus tendon usually occurs in the carpal area and must be considered in the diagnosis of hyperextension deformity of the interphalangeal joint of the thumb. Rupture of the abductor pollicis longus and extensor pollicis brevis tendons is rare.

Synovial invasion and stretching of the dorsal hood of the metacarpophalangeal joint may result in displacement and secondary contractures of the tendons of the intrinsic muscles.

Surgery for Interphalangeal Joint

Arthrodesis is usually the preferred treatment for instability of the interphalangeal joint of the thumb; bone grafting is necessary if bone resorption is severe. A flexible hyperextension deformity of the interphalangeal joint, with lateral stability and intact joint surfaces, may require a flexor *hemitenodesis* to prevent hyperextension while allowing some flexion. If bone stock and ligamentous stability are adequate, involvement of the interphalangeal joint may be treated with a single-stemmed condylar replacement or with a flexible-hinged implant as an adjunct to *resection arthroplasty* to preserve some pain-free motion;

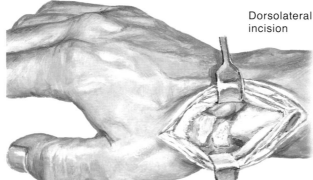

Dorsolateral incision

1. Dissection carried to dorsal capsule between extensor compartments, preserving superficial radial nerve and artery. Capsular flap preserved. Scaphoid removed, leaving thin wafer of bone to maintain continuity of palmar ligaments

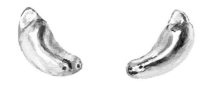

Titanium implants in mirror-image forms for left and right wrists (stemless silicone implants also used)

Hamulus of hamate

Pisiform

Palmar ulnocarpal ligament

Lunate

Ulna

Capitate

Trapezium

Tubercle of scaphoid

Palmar radiocarpal ligament

Radius

2. Bone insertions of palmar carpal ligaments. Complete bone removal creates ligamentous defects that must be repaired to provide support for implant

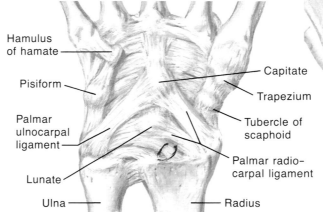

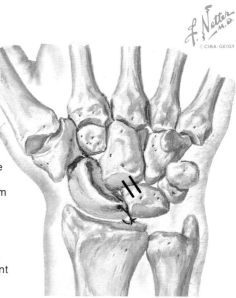

3. Lunocapitate fusion carried out if lunate instability present. Proximal pole of implant sutured to radioscapholunate ligament

this can be important for certain prehensile activities, especially when other joints are disabled.

Surgery for Metacarpophalangeal Joint

Arthrodesis is indicated in joint destruction and collapse deformities to simplify the articular system of the thumb ray, providing the distal and basal joints have adequate mobility (Plate 67). The joint is exposed through a longitudinal dorsal approach, with the extensor hood split longitudinally. The metacarpal head is shaped convexly to fit the concavity formed at the base of the proximal phalanx. A longitudinal wire is placed in a retrograde fashion through the thumb ray and bent in place to the desired position.

Fragments of cancellous bone are used as a graft between the bone ends. A small Kirschner wire is placed obliquely across the joint as the bone ends are firmly pressed together. The small wire is sectioned subcutaneously and removed after 6 to 8 weeks or left in place. The longitudinal wire is removed after 6 to 8 weeks.

Capsulodesis is the treatment of choice in hyperextension deformities of more than 20° with good flexion, lateral stability, and intact articular surfaces (Plate 67). The palmar aspect of the joint is exposed through a lateral incision, and the proximal membranous insertion of the palmar plate is incised. The sesamoids and their tendon attachments are left intact. The periosteum is stripped

Reconstructive Surgery for Deformities of Rheumatoid Hand

(Continued)

from the palmar aspect of the metacarpal neck before the drill holes are made. The pullout suture is removed 3 weeks after surgery and the Kirschner wire after 6 weeks.

Flexible implant resection arthroplasty is used in severely destroyed metacarpophalangeal joints with associated stiffness of the distal or basal joint and in boutonniere deformities in which the metacarpophalangeal joint is destroyed and the distal joint requires fusion. The flexible implant provides adequate stability and increases flexion capability, which is important for finely coordinated movements.

The metacarpophalangeal joint is exposed via a C-shaped incision. Preferably, the extensor hood and the extensor pollicis brevis tendon are split longitudinally. Preparation of bone to receive the implant stems and grommets is similar to that described for the metacarpophalangeal joint of the fingers (Plate 63). If the collateral ligaments are released, they are reattached to bone as described for the proximal interphalangeal joint (Plate 65). The palmar plate is rarely released. If the extensor pollicis brevis tendon is detached, it is reattached to the base of the proximal phalanx (Plate 67). The extensor pollicis longus tendon is advanced distally, and the extensor hood is sutured over both extensor tendons.

Three to 5 days after surgery, a padded aluminum splint is taped over the extended metacarpophalangeal joint. The primary concern after this procedure is stability and retention of some amount of useful flexion. No special exercises are prescribed after the splint is removed 3 to 4 weeks after surgery, but forceful activities are avoided for 6 to 8 weeks.

Treatment of mild-to-moderate boutonniere deformity with less than 10° fixed flexion of the metacarpophalangeal joint involves preserving the joint surfaces and using the same tendon reconstruction technique as in implant arthroplasty. The metacarpophalangeal joint is fixed in full extension with a Kirschner wire for about 4 weeks. If the distal joint is destroyed, implant arthroplasty or arthrodesis is indicated. If the distal joint is adequate but the extensor pollicis longus tendon is contracted, the tendon is lengthened or simply transected distally. The distal joint is then pinned in 10° flexion for 4 to 6 weeks.

Surgery for Basal Joints

The problems presented at the basal joints of the thumb differ in osteoarthritis and rheumatoid arthritis. Accurate diagnosis and evaluation of the location of the arthritic involvement and

Implant Resection Arthroplasty for Lunate

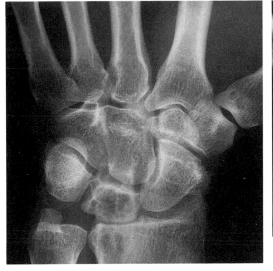

Preoperative radiograph shows stage III Kienböck's disease with associated cyst of radius

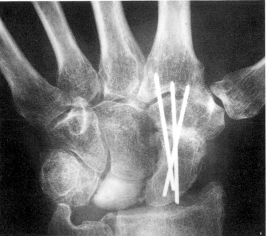

Postoperative radiograph shows silicone lunate implant in position with fusion of scaphoid, trapezium, and trapezoid. Cyst in radius grafted

1. Dorsal incision made between 3rd and 4th compartments of extensor retinaculum, preserving superficial branches of radial and ulnar nerves. Extensor pollicis longus and extensor digitorum tendons retracted. Distal capsular flap preserved. Lunate removed, leaving thin wafer of bone. Palmar capsular defects sutured, and hole made in triquetrum for implant stem

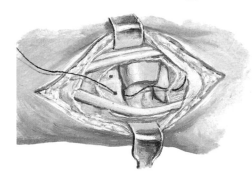

Silicone implants for left and right wrists (stemless titanium implants also used)

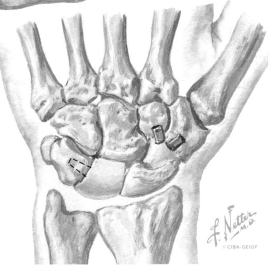

2. Dorsal capsule sutured through two drill holes in distal radius

3. Silicone implant in place with stem in triquetrum (triscaphe fusion may be needed)

alignment of adjacent bones are essential in selecting the appropriate treatment. The pathologic changes may involve the trapeziometacarpal joint alone or also affect the peritrapezial or other carpal bone articulations, with or without resorption or displacement of adjacent carpal bones. Treatment must be selected from several options, including resection arthroplasty of the trapeziometacarpal joint, with or without a convex or concave condylar implant, and resection arthroplasty of the entire trapezium, with or without an implant. In some patients, the distal articulations of the thumb must be stabilized or fused.

Implant resection arthroplasty for the basal joints of the thumb helps maintain a smooth articulating

joint space with improved joint stability, mobility, pain relief, and strength. Meticulous reconstruction of the capsuloligamentous structures around these implants and correction of associated deformities of the thumb ray are essential for a good result.

In osteoarthritis, the destructive changes are usually present in all articulations around the trapezium, and in most patients, total trapeziectomy is necessary to relieve all arthritic pain. When there is adequate bone stock, a trapezium implant can be used as an adjunct to resection arthroplasty. In rheumatoid arthritis, the basal joints of the thumb often exhibit bone resorption or displacement that disturbs the bony elements

Reconstructive Surgery for Deformities of Rheumatoid Hand

(Continued)

Implant Resection Arthroplasty for Radiocarpal Joint

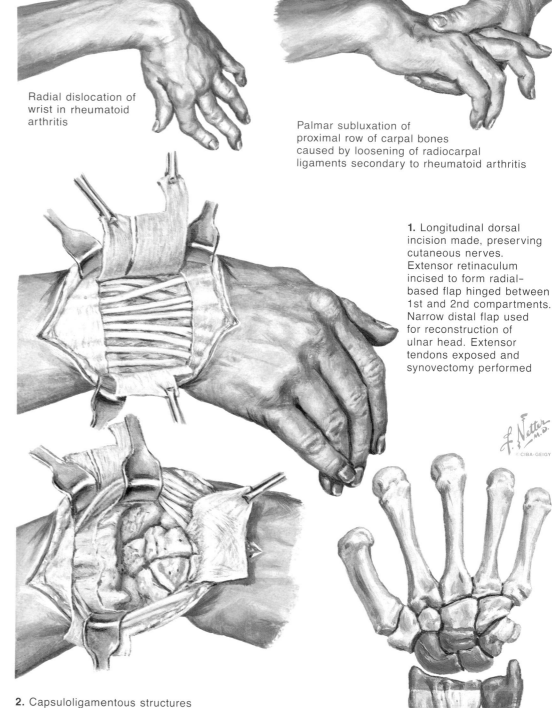

Radial dislocation of wrist in rheumatoid arthritis

Palmar subluxation of proximal row of carpal bones caused by loosening of radiocarpal ligaments secondary to rheumatoid arthritis

1. Longitudinal dorsal incision made, preserving cutaneous nerves. Extensor retinaculum incised to form radial-based flap hinged between 1st and 2nd compartments. Narrow distal flap used for reconstruction of ulnar head. Extensor tendons exposed and synovectomy performed

2. Capsuloligamentous structures elevated as distally hinged flap, exposing carpal bones. Proximal carpal bones usually partially resorbed and dislocated palmarly

3. Bone resection shown in blue. Lunate removed. Part of distal scaphoid, capitate, and triquetrum retained in some cases. End of radius and distal ulna also resected

necessary to receive or support the trapezium implant. Frequently, the trapezium is fused to the scaphoid or the scaphoid is resorbed or shifted ulnarly. Therefore, a simple resection, with or without soft-tissue interposition, or a trapeziometacarpal implant arthroplasty can be used. In certain patients, severe resorptive changes of the metacarpal base and the trapezium produce a result not unlike a resection arthroplasty. If the joint is reasonably stable, mobile, and pain free, surgery is not indicated.

Implant resection arthroplasty for the trapezium is used for conditions due to degenerative or post-traumatic arthritis with localized bony changes (Plate 68). Indications for surgery are (1) localized pain and crepitation during passive circumduction, with axial compression of the thumb (grind test); (2) loss of motion, with decreased pinch and grip strength; (3) radiographic evidence of arthritic changes of the trapeziometacarpal, trapeziotrapezoid, trapezioscaphoid, and trapezium-second metacarpal joints; and (4) unstable, stiff, or painful distal joints of the thumb or swan-neck deformity. As previously noted, the condylar implant is preferred in rheumatoid arthritis.

The trapezium is sectioned with an osteotome and removed piecemeal, with care not to injure the underlying flexor carpi radialis tendon. Osteophytes or irregularities on the distal end of the scaphoid, trapezoid, or bases of the first and second metacarpals are trimmed to ensure proper medialization of the implant. If the trapezoid is shifted radially, a portion of its radial aspect is removed to allow good seating of the implant over the distal scaphoid. The wound is thoroughly irrigated to remove all debris before implant insertion. A secure capsuloligamentous repair around the implant is essential to stabilize the implant over the scaphoid. The radial artery must be carefully protected throughout the procedure. Use of trapezium implants made of the original silicone elastomer without fixation with sutures or Kirschner wires is preferred.

After suture of the capsular flaps, the abductor pollicis longus tendon is advanced distally on the metacarpal, and the extensor pollicis longus tendon is tenodesed over this area. The first dorsal compartment is loosely closed over the abductor pollicis longus and extensor pollicis brevis tendons. The extensor pollicis longus tendon is left subcutaneous. The incision is closed, with care to avoid the branches of the superficial radial nerve. A subcutaneous drain is inserted, and a conforming hand dressing, including an anterior and posterior plaster splint, is applied. The limb is kept

elevated, and a thumb-spica short arm cast is applied after 4 to 6 days and worn for 6 weeks. Guarded motion and pinch and grasp activities using various exercise devices are then started.

Implant resection arthroplasty for the trapeziometacarpal joint is appropriate in severe erosive osteoarthritis and in rheumatoid arthritis with basal joint deformity associated with severe displacement, resorption, or fusion of the contiguous carpal bones. An intramedullary stemmed convex condylar implant is used as an adjunct to resection arthroplasty of the trapeziometacarpal joint; titanium convex condylar implants are preferred in osteoarthritis, and silicone implants made of the original elastomer are used in rheumatoid

arthritis. A concave condylar implant is used when there is inadequate bone stock to allow shaping of the trapezium to receive the convex head of the implant.

The surgical approach and preparation of the first metacarpal are similar to those described for the trapezium implant (Plate 68). A limited resection of the metacarpal base is performed, and a slight concavity is shaped in the distal facet of the trapezium to receive the convex implant. Enough bone should be removed to create a joint space of approximately 4 mm and allow 45° radial abduction of the first metacarpal. The implant stem is inserted into the medullary canal of the first metacarpal. A distally based slip of the

Reconstructive Surgery for Deformities of Rheumatoid Hand

(Continued)

abductor pollicis longus tendon is interwoven through the metacarpal, trapezium, and capsule to provide an excellent stabilizing effect. Because of the narrow joint space, the usual range of motion obtained with the standard trapezium implant cannot be expected. However, the recommended technique results in a stable, pain-free, functioning thumb joint.

Special considerations in reconstruction of the basal joints of the thumb include the following.

Adduction of the first metacarpal, if severe and untreated, unbalances the thumb and seriously affects the result of resection arthroplasty. If the angle of abduction between the first and second metacarpals is not at least 45°, the origin of the adductor pollicis muscle must be released from the third metacarpal through a separate palmar incision.

Hyperextension of the metacarpophalangeal joint of the thumb contributes to the adduction tendency of the metacarpal and prevents proper abduction of the metacarpal and seating of the implant. If hyperextension is less than 10°, a cast is applied postoperatively so that the metacarpal, but not the proximal phalanx, is abducted. If the hyperextension ranges from 10° to 20°, temporary fixation with a Kirschner wire is indicated; if it is greater than 20°, stabilization with either palmar capsulodesis or arthrodesis (Plate 67) is essential. These procedures should be performed at the time the implant is inserted.

In swan-neck deformity associated with loss of flexion at the metacarpophalangeal joint, the metacarpophalangeal joint is fused and the distal joint temporarily pinned in extension.

Deformities of Wrist

Deformities of the wrist are common sequelae in rheumatoid arthritis, osteoarthritis, fractures, and dislocations. Involvement of individual carpal bones or the intercarpal, radiocarpal, or distal radioulnar joint can occur singly or in combination. The goal of reconstructive procedures of the wrist and carpus is to provide pain relief with reasonable stability, strength, and mobility for assistance in hand adaptations. Appropriate evaluation of the specific problem, including severity of disease, patient's age, and functional requirements, is essential in selecting the best treatment from the wide range of available procedures.

Surgery for Scaphoid and Lunate

Treatment of necrosis, fracture or fracture dislocation, and subluxation of the scaphoid or

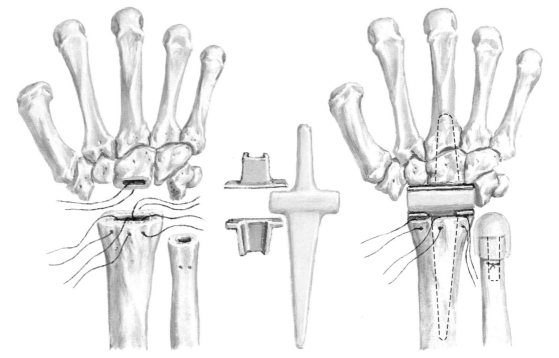

4. Medullary canal of radius prepared for proximal stem of implant. Channel for distal stem reamed through remnant of capitate and 3rd metacarpal. Drill holes made in radius for securing palmar and dorsal capsules. Distal ulna prepared

Silicone implant and titanium grommets

5. Wrist and ulnar head implants in place. Distal grommet placed dorsally and proximal grommet placed palmarly

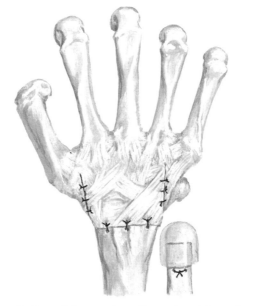

6. Capsuloligamentous flap sutured through drill holes in distal radius

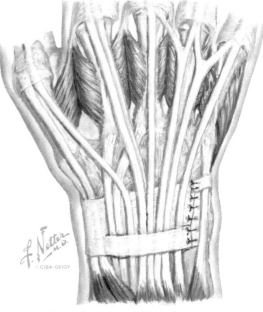

7. Retinacular flap positioned under extensor tendons. Proximal retinacular flap sutured over extensor tendons to prevent bowstringing. Note pulley over extensor carpi ulnaris tendon

lunate includes conservative methods, localized bone grafting, bone resection, implant arthroplasty with or without intercarpal arthrodesis, and wrist implant arthroplasty or fusion. To help select the appropriate treatment, lunate and scaphoid conditions have been classified into six stages based on the severity of disease (see Table 1, page 232). Implant resection arthroplasty for the scaphoid and lunate can achieve good long-term results if the pathologic condition is well identified, the disease is not too advanced, and the proper surgical indications and techniques are followed.

The carpal implants act as articulating spacers to maintain the relationship of the adjacent

carpal bones while preserving wrist mobility. Their use allows stabilization of associated intercarpal instability, which prevents collapse and settling of the carpus. The implants have essentially the same shape as their anatomic counterpart but with more pronounced concavities for greater stability. Implants made of the original silicone elastomer or titanium are preferred to the high-performance silicone elastomer implants. Fixation of silicone implants with sutures or Kirschner wires is no longer used.

Ligamentous instability and carpal collapse are often associated with disorders of the scaphoid or lunate and may be a contraindication to the implant procedure unless firm capsuloligamentous

Implant Resection Arthroplasty for Distal Radioulnar Joint

Reconstructive Surgery for Deformities of Rheumatoid Hand

(Continued)

support can be provided around the implant and a stable relationship of the carpal bones can be obtained.

Because the palmar carpal ligaments are attached to bone, total removal of these bones can create ligamentous defects that cause further implant instability. A subluxated carpal implant is under abnormal shear stress; if it is also submitted to excessive loading forces across the wrist joint, the silicone will wear excessively and the arthroplasty will eventually fail. During excision of a carpal bone, a small wafer of the palmar part of the bone should be retained to preserve the palmar ligaments (Plate 69); if the ligaments are weakened, they should be repaired.

Associated collapse deformities should be treated at the time of implant arthroplasty with intercarpal fusions using trabecular (cancellous) bone grafts (preferably obtained from the ilium) and internal fixation with staples, Kirschner wires, or Herbert screw. If a wrist requiring lunate implant arthroplasty also has scaphoid instability, a scaphotrapeziotrapezoid or scaphocapitate fusion may be considered. Conversely, if lunate instability is present in a wrist requiring scaphoid implant arthroplasty, a lunocapitate or lunotriquetrum fusion may be considered (Plate 70). Cysts in contiguous bones must be treated with curettage and cancellous bone grafting at the time of the procedure. The implant must not be oversized and should not be used if space is inadequate.

If intercarpal fusion was not performed, a plaster cast is used for 6 to 8 weeks; after intercarpal fusion, the cast is used for 8 to 12 weeks. Excessive or abusive motion must be avoided after replacement of a carpal bone. Advanced pathologic changes in carpal bones are not treatable with implants, and implant arthroplasty or fusion of the wrist is the procedure of choice.

Implant resection arthroplasty for the scaphoid (Plate 69 and Table 1, page 232), with or without intercarpal fusion, can be used for comminuted or grossly displaced fractures; avascular necrosis of a fragment; scaphoid subluxation; or pseudarthrosis associated with degenerative and cystic changes of the scaphoid, collapse of the carpal height ($\leq 15\%$), mild-to-moderate lunate dorsiflexion, and mild-to-moderate degenerative changes in contiguous carpal bones. The more severe problems require alternative procedures, including scapholunate replacement, proximal row carpectomy, fusion of proximal carpus to radius, hemiarthroplasty, and total wrist implant resection arthroplasty or arthrodesis.

A longitudinal dorsoradial incision of 7 cm to 10 cm is made across the radiocarpal joint midway between the tip of the styloid process and the radial tubercle. The extensor retinaculum is

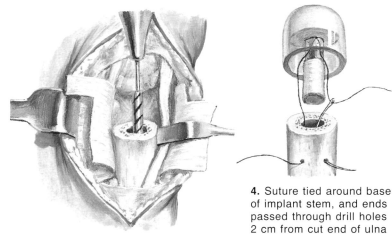

Dorsal cutaneous branch of ulnar nerve preserved

Longitudinal incision centered over head of ulna

1. Extensor retinaculum of 6th compartment incised to form narrow radial-based distal flap and broad ulnar-based proximal flap

ECU

2. Flaps reflected and extensor carpi ulnaris tendon (ECU) retracted. Ulna sectioned at neck. Periosteum not stripped. Joint synovectomy completed

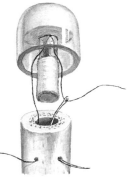

3. Medullary canal of ulna reamed to receive implant stem. Bone end smoothed

4. Suture tied around base of implant stem, and ends passed through drill holes 2 cm from cut end of ulna

5. Implant in place with suture tied securely

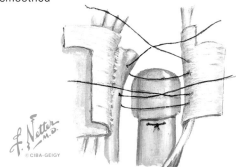

6. Before implant insertion, sutures placed through interosseous ligament and edge of radius to secure distal ulna in reduced position

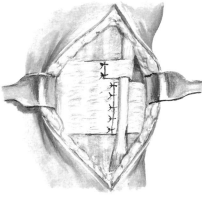

7. Broad proximal flap sutured under ECU and narrow distal flap passed around tendon to act as pulley

incised over the extensor pollicis longus tendon and elevated from the third compartment radially to expose the second compartment. The extensor carpi radialis longus and brevis tendons are mobilized to their insertion for appropriate retraction, and the underlying transverse metacarpal vessels are carefully preserved. The dorsocarpal wrist ligament is incised in a T shape and, with the wrist flexed, elevated from the radius by sharp dissection close to the bone to preserve adequate tissues for reattachment. The scaphoid should be positively identified, with radiographs if necessary, before bone removal begins.

The scaphoid is removed piecemeal with a rongeur, avoiding injury to the underlying palmar

ligaments. A thin wafer of bone is left in the palmar ligaments to ensure their continuity. In the presence of collapse deformities or instability, rotation of the lunate must be corrected and the carpus stabilized with fusion of the lunate to the capitate or the triquetrum, or both, with or without fusion of other involved carpal bones.

Scaphoid implants for left and right wrists are available in seven sizes. Correct sizing is important because if the implant is too large, excessive stress is placed on it. The stem of the silicone scaphoid implant is usually resected, with stability maintained by the integrity of the capsuloligamentous structures. The stemless titanium implant is stabilized with sutures passed through

Reconstructive Surgery for Deformities of Rheumatoid Hand

(Continued)

the carpal ligaments at both the scapholunate and scaphotrapezium areas.

Approximately 1 cm of the posterior sensory branch of the posterior interosseous nerve is resected to provide some sensory denervation of part of the carpal area. The preserved dorsal capsule is firmly sutured, with the knots inverted to prevent adherence to overlying tendons. At least 30° wrist flexion and extension should be obtained. The retinaculum is sutured over the extensor tendons, except for the extensor pollicis longus tendon, which is left free in the subcutaneous tissue.

After the repair is completed, the wound is closed in layers, and small silicone drains are inserted subcutaneously. A dressing, including an anterior and posterior plaster splint, is applied, and the limb is kept elevated for 3 to 5 days. A thumb-spica, scaphoid-type long arm cast is then applied. If the cast is applied immediately, it should be univalved dorsally and must be strong enough to prevent breaking at the wrist area.

The cast is removed in 6 to 8 weeks (8 to 12 weeks if an intercarpal bone fusion was done). Sutures are removed after 2 to 3 weeks through a window made in the cast. Full use of the wrist is resumed at 12 weeks. Radiographs should be obtained postoperatively and during long-term follow-up to check the position of the implant and wrist bones.

The indications for *implant resection arthroplasty for the lunate* (Plate 70 and Table 2, page 232) include avascular sclerosis (Kienböck's disease), localized arthritic changes, and long-standing dislocation. Alternative procedures are indicated in patients with severe decrease in the lunate space, significant intercarpal and radiocarpal arthritic changes, and carpal instability or collapse.

A transverse incision may be used for some uncomplicated deformities, especially in women. A palmar approach is recommended when the lunate is dislocated palmarly. Positive identification of the lunate is essential. If the palmar capsuloligamentous structures are weak, the palmar ulnocarpal and radiocarpal ligaments are sutured together; if necessary, the palmar defect can be repaired with a tendon graft.

A collapse deformity or instability of the carpus requires limited fusion of associated carpal bones to improve the distribution of forces across the wrist joint. Rotatory subluxation of the scaphoid must be corrected and the carpus stabilized with either triscaphe or scaphocapitate fusion using an iliac bone graft. Scaphocapitate fusion is preferred when cystic changes are present in the capitate.

Implants are available in five sizes. The stem of the silicone implant can be removed, if needed. The stemless titanium implant has holes for placement of sutures through the palmar carpal ligaments.

Denervation of the posterior sensory branch of the posterior interosseous nerve; repair of the dorsal capsule, extensor retinaculum, and skin; and postoperative care, casting, and rehabilitation are the same as for implant resection arthroplasty for the scaphoid.

When implant arthroplasty is performed to correct palmar dislocation of the lunate, a palmar exposure is used. The lunate is usually displaced into the carpal canal and easily exposed. The palmar radiocarpal ligament is meticulously repaired to ensure implant stability. A free graft of the palmaris longus tendon can be used to stabilize the carpus on the palmar side and reinforce the radiocarpal ligaments. The graft can be threaded through the ligamentous structures or through drill holes in the radius, scaphoid, and capitate and then back across the lunate implant to the radius. The transverse carpal ligament is left unsutured to decompress the carpal canal.

Surgery for Radiocarpal Joint

The radiocarpal, distal radioulnar, and intercarpal joints can be affected individually or in combination. Synovitis and tendon involvement are common, particularly in rheumatoid arthritis. Therefore, selection of the appropriate treatment depends on the site and extent of involvement, instability, deformity, arthritic destruction, and the patient's requirements. Like lunate and scaphoid deformities, wrist deformities have also been classified into seven stages based on the localization and severity of disease (see Table 2, page 232).

A reconstructive procedure must provide reasonable stability, strength, and mobility to assist in hand adaptations. A flexible-hinged implant for the radiocarpal joint, used as an adjunct to resection arthroplasty, maintains joint space and alignment while supporting the reconstructed capsuloligamentous system (Plates 71–72). The degree of mobility, stability, durability, and biologic tolerance obtained with this technique has been encouraging, and use of titanium grommets has improved durability.

Implant resection arthroplasty for the wrist is indicated in rheumatoid arthritis, osteoarthritis, or posttraumatic arthritis with instability of the wrist caused by subluxation or dislocation of the radiocarpal joint, severe deviation of the wrist that causes musculotendinous imbalance of the digits, stiffness or fusion of the wrist in a nonfunctional position, and stiffness of the wrist. Its use in persons who do heavy manual labor is controversial. If the implant arthroplasty does not meet functional requirements, wrist arthrodesis can be done later.

The technique for *implant resection arthroplasty for the radiocarpal joint* is shown on Plates 71–72. If indicated, reconstruction of the distal ulna is carried out at the same time. Radiocarpal subluxation should be completely reduced. The medullary canal of the third metacarpal is identified by passing a wire or thin broach through the capitate and the base and medullary canal of the third metacarpal. The distal stem of the implant, which should not extend beyond the metaphysis of the third metacarpal, is shortened as needed. If titanium grommets are used, the distal radius and base of the capitate must be prepared further to allow a precise press-fit.

After insertion of the implant and closure, the mobility of the wrist is tested; approximately 30° extension and flexion and 10° ulnar and radial deviation should be possible on passive manipulation. An excessive range of motion, which may increase the potential for implant failure, does not significantly improve wrist function. In patients with significant loss of bone stock or loose ligaments, sutures may need to be added to the palmar, radial, and ulnar cortex of the radius to tighten the capsule in these areas. Adequate ligamentous repair is very important for proper function and durability of the implant.

After the procedure, a voluminous conforming dressing, including a palmar plaster splint, is applied with the wrist in a neutral position. The limb is elevated for 3 to 5 days. A short arm cast that holds the wrist in neutral position is then applied and fitted with outriggers that hold rubber-band slings to support finger extension if the digital tendons have been repaired. The cast is worn for 4 to 6 weeks. A program of flexion-extension exercises is begun to achieve 30% to 40% of normal movements with good stability.

Surgery for Distal Radioulnar Joint

Implant arthroplasty of the ulnar head may be considered for disabilities of the distal radioulnar joint in rheumatoid arthritis, osteoarthritis, or posttraumatic arthritis. Specific indications include pain and weakness in the wrist joint that do not improve with conservative treatment and instability of the ulnar head with radiographic evidence of dorsal subluxation and erosive changes. The procedure can be used to correct sequelae of a failed simple resection.

The goal of *implant resection arthroplasty for the distal radioulnar joint* is to preserve the length of the ulna to help prevent ulnar shift of the carpus and provide greater wrist stability. After resection of the head of the ulna, a stemmed and cuffed intramedullary implant is used to cap the bone end (Plate 73). This helps preserve the anatomic relationships and function of the distal radioulnar joint. The ulnar head implant provides a smooth articular surface for the radioulnar and carpoulnar joints and the overlying extensor tendons. It decreases the occurrence of bone overgrowth and allows reconstruction of the distal radioulnar joint.

The stem of the silicone implant has a polyester retention cord to secure the implant. The last one-third of the stem is covered with polyester velour to provide fixation in the medullary canal by bone ingrowth.

The dorsal cutaneous branch of the ulnar nerve is preserved. Retinacular flaps are created, and synovectomy of the dorsal compartments is carried out. The bone is prepared to receive the implant, the implant is positioned, and the flaps are sutured. The implant stem must fit snugly into the prepared medullary canal, and the cuff should fit loosely over the bone. It is important to release the extensor carpi ulnaris tendon both proximally and distally and repair ruptures of the digital extensor tendons.

The incision is closed and drained. A voluminous, conforming hand dressing, including a plaster palmar splint, is applied with the hand in slight dorsiflexion and worn for 4 to 5 days. The drain is removed 3 days after surgery, and a short arm cast or splint is worn for 3 to 4 weeks. □

Table 1. CLASSIFICATION FOR SCAPHOID PATHOLOGY AND TREATMENTS

Stage	Pathology	Treatment Options
I	Acute scaphoid fractures Acute scaphoid fracture/dislocation	Immobilization Open or closed reduction
II	Nonunion of scaphoid	Bone graft Bone stimulator

III	Avascular necrosis of a fragment with:
	  Carpal height collapse 0%–5%
	  Lunate dorsiflexion minimal
	  (R-L angle 0°–10°)
		Partial scaphoid implant
		replacement
		Scaphoid implant replacement

IV	Comminuted or grossly displaced fracture
	Avascular necrosis with scaphoid degenerative arthritic changes
	Subluxation of scaphoid with degenerative arthritic changes
	Nonunion of scaphoid with cystic changes with:
	  Carpal height collapse 5%–10%
	  Lunate dorsiflexion minimal to moderate (R-L angle 10°–30°)
	  Mild degenerative arthritic changes of contiguous bones (particularly between lunate and capitate)
		Scaphoid implant replacement with/without intercarpal fusions

V	Stage IV pathology of scaphoid with:
	  Carpal height collapse >10%
	  Lunate dorsiflexion moderate to severe (L-R angle >30°)
	  Mild-to-moderate degenerative arthritic changes of contiguous bones
		Scaphoid implant replacement with intercarpal fusions
		Scapholunate implant replacement
		Proximal row carpectomy
		Fusion proximal carpus to radius
		Hemiarthroplasty

VI	Stage IV pathology of scaphoid or previous surgery with:
	  Carpal height collapse >15%
	  Lunate dorsiflexion severe (R-L angle >30°)
	  Severe intercarpal and radiocarpal degenerative arthritic changes
		Total wrist implant arthroplasty
		Wrist arthrodesis
		Ulna impingement treatment PRN

Table 2. CLASSIFICATION FOR AVASCULAR NECROSIS OF LUNATE AND TREATMENTS

Stage	Pathology	Treatment Options

I	Sclerosis of lunate with:
	  Minimal symptoms
	  Normal carpal bone relationships
		Splinting and rest
		Revascularization
		Ulna and radius lengthening/shortening

II	Sclerosis of lunate with cystic changes with:
	  Clinical symptoms
	  Normal carpal bone relationships
		Lunate implant replacement
		Ulna and radius lengthening/shortening

III	Sclerosis, cysts, and fragmentation of lunate with:
	  Scaphoid-radius angle 40°–60°
	  Carpal height collapse 0%–5%
	  Carpal translation minimal
		Lunate implant replacement with/without intercarpal fusions

IV	Sclerosis, cysts, and fragmentation of lunate with:
	  Scaphoid-radius angle <70°
	  Carpal height collapse 5%–10%
	  Carpal translation moderate
		Lunate implant replacement with scaphoid stabilization (distal fusion)
		Intercarpal fusions if early changes in contiguous bones

V	Sclerosis, cysts, and fragmentation of lunate with:
	  Scaphoid-radius angle >70°
	  Carpal height collapse >10%
	  Carpal translation severe
	  Cystic changes in contiguous bones
		Lunate implant replacement and intercarpal fusions
		Scapholunate implant replacement
		Wrist arthrodesis
		Ulna impingement treatment PRN

VI	Sclerosis, cysts, and fragmentation of lunate with:
	  Scaphoid-radius angle >70°
	  Carpal height collapse >15%
	  Carpal translation severe
	  Cystic changes in contiguous bones
	  Significant intercarpal and radio-carpal degenerative arthritic changes
		Total wrist implant arthroplasty
		Wrist arthrodesis
		Ulna impingement treatment PRN

Section IV

Total Joint Replacement

Frank H. Netter, M.D.

in collaboration with

Mack L. Clayton, M.D. and Donald C. Ferlic, M.D.   *Plates 25–26*

Stuart C. Kozinn, M.D., Philip D. Wilson, Jr., M.D., and
Paul M. Pellicci, M.D.   *Plates 1–14*

Alfred B. Swanson, M.D. and Genevieve de Groot Swanson, M.D.   *Plates 27–28*

Russell E. Windsor, M.D. and John N. Insall, M.D.   *Plates 15–24*

Total Hip Replacement

Prostheses

Arthroplasty, or surgical reconstruction of the joints, has revolutionized the treatment of crippling diseases such as osteoarthritis and rheumatoid arthritis, which destroy the joint's smooth cartilage surfaces and lead to painful, decreased motion. Relief of pain and improved hip function are dramatic advantages of reconstruction procedures. Hip arthroplasty not only benefits the older patient, but total hip replacement and other procedures using prostheses now permit young and middle-aged patients with congenital, developmental, arthritic, traumatic, malignant, or metabolic hip disorders to lead active and productive lives.

Treatment with a total hip prosthesis must always be weighed against nonsurgical treatment and other more conservative surgical procedures that do not sacrifice as much bone, such as intertrochanteric (proximal femoral) osteotomy (Plate 14), resurfacing arthroplasty, and arthrodesis. Appropriate selection of patients is essential.

Hip prostheses must function under high mechanical loads for many years, and the strength of materials used is critical. The technique of total hip replacement began as an improvement on the placement of molds or films between degenerated joint surfaces (interpositional arthroplasty). In 1923, Smith-Petersen used a Pyrex cup to cover and reshape an arthritic femoral head in a technique called mold arthroplasty. This brittle cup broke under stress, but the technique led to the development of interpositional molds made of a stronger material, Vitallium, a noncorrosive and relatively inert cobalt-chromium alloy.

In the early 1960s, Sir John Charnley developed the technique of low-friction total hip arthroplasty, still the standard against which all newer variations must be measured. From his work, two important principles have stood the test of time and govern all subsequent modifications. The first is the principle of low friction, that is, a bearing of a highly polished metal alloy against ultrahigh-molecular-weight polyethylene. The second is the principle of rigid fixation of components to bone. For the first, he advocated a small diameter (22.25 mm) bearing, and for the second, the use of methylmethacrylate (acrylic) cement to act as a grouting material by forming an interlocking mechanical bond with the trabecular bone.

The *Charnley prosthesis*, still in use today, has undergone minor modifications. The *Triad prosthesis* comprises a femoral and an acetabular component. The femoral stem is made of a titanium alloy, with a cobalt-chromium head. The acetabular component is made of a high-density polyethylene, and many are covered with a metal shell for improved stress tolerance at the underlying cement-bone junction.

Femoral and acetabular components are made in a variety of sizes, and it is possible to mix and match femoral stems with acetabular cups

Prostheses for Total Hip Replacement

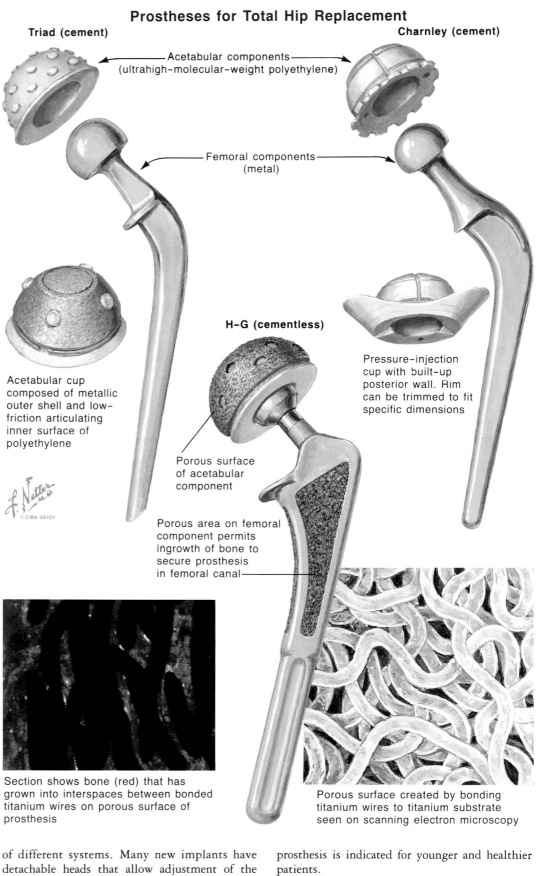

Acetabular components (ultrahigh-molecular-weight polyethylene)

Femoral components (metal)

Triad (cement)

Charnley (cement)

H-G (cementless)

Acetabular cup composed of metallic outer shell and low-friction articulating inner surface of polyethylene

Porous surface of acetabular component

Porous area on femoral component permits ingrowth of bone to secure prosthesis in femoral canal

Pressure-injection cup with built-up posterior wall. Rim can be trimmed to fit specific dimensions

Section shows bone (red) that has grown into interspaces between bonded titanium wires on porous surface of prosthesis

Porous surface created by bonding titanium wires to titanium substrate seen on scanning electron microscopy

of different systems. Many new implants have detachable heads that allow adjustment of the neck length of the prosthesis, making it much easier to correct and equalize leg length.

New designs in total hip prostheses include implants that do not require acrylic cement for fixation to bone. The *Harris-Galante (H-G) prosthesis* is one type of cementless hip replacement. The metal backing of the acetabular cup and the sides of the femoral stem are made of a fine mesh of titanium wires. This porous surface allows the ingrowth of bone trabeculae to produce a "biologic fixation" of prosthesis to bone. However, since good bone quality is needed for implant stability and maximal bone ingrowth, this type of

prosthesis is indicated for younger and healthier patients.

Another type of porous surface is formed by sintering small metal beads onto the solid surface of the prosthetic stem. Bone grows into this surface by a process of intramembranous ossification that is roughly similar to the callus formation seen in a healing fracture. Because bone ingrowth is unpredictable and may not always occur, cementless prostheses are still under clinical investigation.

Femoral stems of other designs are composed of smooth, grooved, or corrugated surfaces that fit tightly into the medullary canal. One advantage of these implants is ease of removal if revision surgery is required. □

Total Hip Replacement

Technique

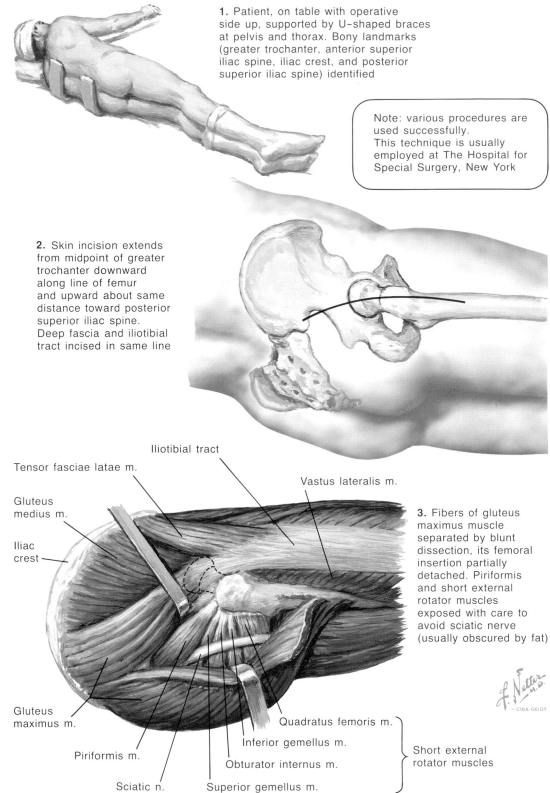

1. Patient, on table with operative side up, supported by U-shaped braces at pelvis and thorax. Bony landmarks (greater trochanter, anterior superior iliac spine, iliac crest, and posterior superior iliac spine) identified

Note: various procedures are used successfully.
This technique is usually employed at The Hospital for Special Surgery, New York

2. Skin incision extends from midpoint of greater trochanter downward along line of femur and upward about same distance toward posterior superior iliac spine. Deep fascia and iliotibial tract incised in same line

Iliotibial tract

Tensor fasciae latae m.

Vastus lateralis m.

Gluteus medius m.

Iliac crest

3. Fibers of gluteus maximus muscle separated by blunt dissection, its femoral insertion partially detached. Piriformis and short external rotator muscles exposed with care to avoid sciatic nerve (usually obscured by fat)

Gluteus maximus m.

Quadratus femoris m. ⎫
Inferior gemellus m. ⎬ Short external rotator muscles
Obturator internus m.
Superior gemellus m. ⎭

Piriformis m.

Sciatic n.

The procedure for total hip replacement begins with preoperative planning, which includes a complete medical work-up of the patient to identify any existing health problems. A rheumatologist or internist often works with the orthopedic surgeon in planning the appropriate medical therapy. The rehabilitation program should also be thoroughly discussed with the patient.

The goal of preoperative planning is to create a graphic representation of a joint that will provide optimal function. The biomechanical principles that govern movement, weight bearing, and impact must be observed. The prosthetic components must be selected carefully to maximize fit and function for each individual.

Lateral and anteroposterior radiographs are taken to determine the bony anatomy and the size of the femoral canal. Then clear plastic templates of each prosthesis are placed on the radiographs to choose the correct size. At this time, any existing deformities must be taken into consideration. Many patients have a limb-length discrepancy, usually a shortening of the painful limb, due to superior displacement of the femoral head resulting from destruction of the joint space. This can be corrected with resection of the femur at the appropriate level and use of an implant with the proper neck length. If a flexion contracture of the hip exists, a more extensive dissection of the soft tissues is necessary.

The acetabulum must be evaluated for dysplasia or deficiency; in such cases, reconstruction with bone grafts, screws, or special devices is carried out (Plate 7). Custom-designed implants are

required if standard-sized implants are inadequate. Patients with congenital dislocation of the hip may need extra-small implants with special angles of the femoral neck. Long-stemmed prostheses are often needed to extend past fracture sites or defect sites in the femur. If a cementless implant is used, it must fit tightly into the femoral canal and pelvis.

Preparation

The patient is placed in the lateral decubitus position (supine if an anterior approach is used) on a fracture table modified for total hip replacement (Plate 2). A number of anatomic exposures can be used for total hip replacement, each of

which has advantages and disadvantages. The posterior, or modified Moore, approach is commonly used for reconstruction of osteoarthritic hips. It allows quick and safe access to the joint without interfering with the abductor mechanism.

The limb is swabbed with iodine solution and draped to allow free movement. The bony landmarks are marked on the skin. The anterior and posterior superior iliac spine, greater trochanter, iliac crest, and shaft of the femur are all palpable.

Incision

A typical incision is centered on the greater trochanter and curves gently posteriorly, in line proximally with the fibers of the gluteus maximus

Technique for Total Hip Replacement (continued)

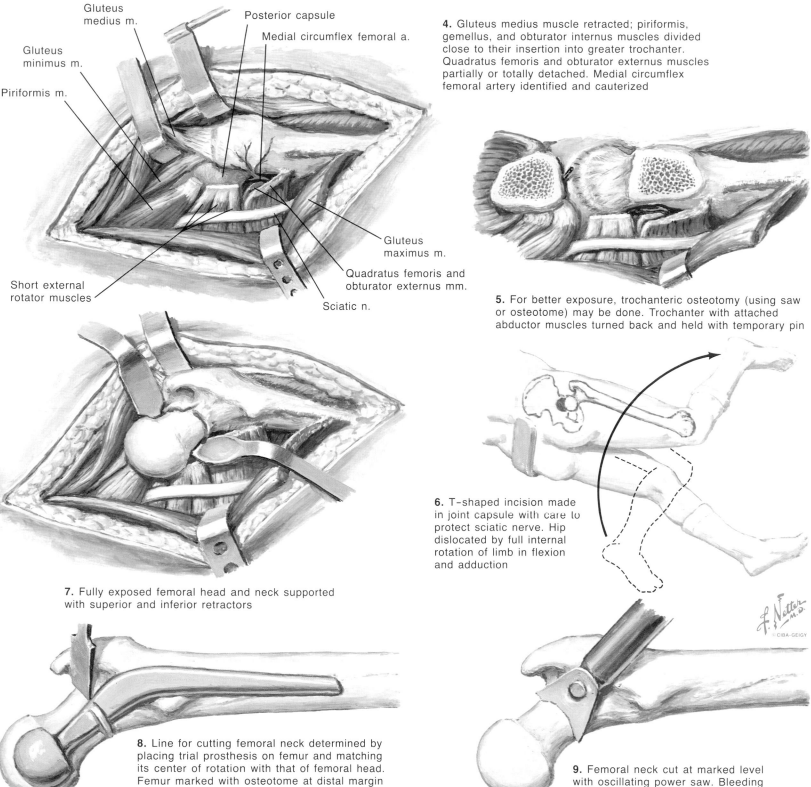

Gluteus medius m.

Gluteus minimus m.

Piriformis m.

Posterior capsule

Medial circumflex femoral a.

Short external rotator muscles

Gluteus maximus m.

Quadratus femoris and obturator externus mm.

Sciatic n.

4. Gluteus medius muscle retracted; piriformis, gemellus, and obturator internus muscles divided close to their insertion into greater trochanter. Quadratus femoris and obturator externus muscles partially or totally detached. Medial circumflex femoral artery identified and cauterized

5. For better exposure, trochanteric osteotomy (using saw or osteotome) may be done. Trochanter with attached abductor muscles turned back and held with temporary pin

6. T-shaped incision made in joint capsule with care to protect sciatic nerve. Hip dislocated by full internal rotation of limb in flexion and adduction

7. Fully exposed femoral head and neck supported with superior and inferior retractors

8. Line for cutting femoral neck determined by placing trial prosthesis on femur and matching its center of rotation with that of femoral head. Femur marked with osteotome at distal margin of prosthetic collar

9. Femoral neck cut at marked level with oscillating power saw. Bleeding controlled with bone wax, if necessary

SECTION IV PLATE 3   Slide 4657

Total Hip Replacement

Technique

(Continued)

muscle (Plate 2). Distally, the incision overlies the femoral shaft. An incision is made in the fascia lata and the fascia over the gluteus maximus muscle. The fibers of the gluteus maximus muscle are separated proximally by blunt incision, without denervating the muscle. The gluteus maximus

tendon is partially released from its insertion into the proximal femur; care must be taken to protect the underlying sciatic nerve. The hip is internally rotated and the piriformis tendon identified.

Dislocation of Hip and Femoral Transection

A retractor is passed above the piriformis and beneath the gluteus medius and minimus muscles to delineate the superior hip capsule; another is placed deeply at the proximal border of the quadratus femoris muscle to outline the inferior joint capsule (Plate 3). The piriformis and short external rotator muscles are removed from their insertions into the trochanter and stripped back to expose the posterior hip capsule, which is incised.

An anterior capsulotomy is optional. It facilitates exposure of the acetabulum and improves mobility of the femur and is desirable when the hip deformity is severe or exposure is cramped for other reasons. In such cases, it may be helpful to expose its femoral insertion in the interval between the tensor fasciae latae and the gluteus medius muscles before making the posterior exposure.

An alternative approach is to remove the greater trochanter and reflect the attached gluteus maximus and minimus muscles superiorly for better exposure of the acetabulum. The trochanter and attached abductor muscles are turned back and held with Steinmann pins placed in the ilium, and the superolateral capsule is reflected (Plate 3).

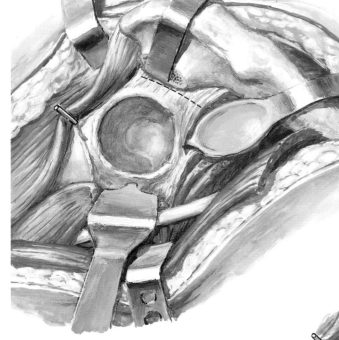

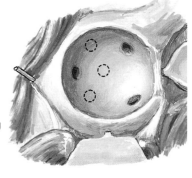

11. Reamer of appropriate size inserted and acetabulum reamed to receive acetabular component

12. Reamers of increasing size used to enlarge acetabulum to fit acetabular cup of preselected size

10. To expose acetabulum, femur with cut neck retracted anteriorly. Gluteus medius and minimis muscles retracted with pin. Posterior capsule and short external rotator muscles retracted with spiked retractor; inferior retractor placed under transverse acetabular ligament. Anterior capsule may also be cut to increase exposure

13. Trial cups tested in acetabulum to ensure appropriate fit

14. Cement fixation holes drilled in iliac, ischial, and pubic areas of acetabulum and additional holes drilled in ilium, followed by irrigation and gauze packing

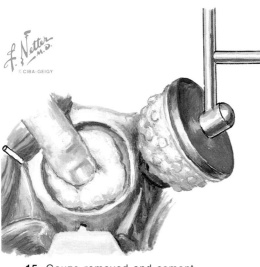

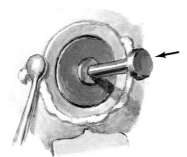

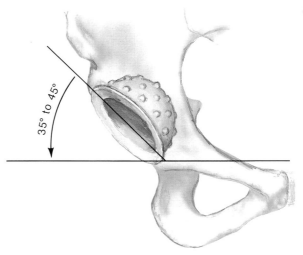

35° to 45°

15. Gauze removed and cement pressurized into acetabulum and applied to cup

16. Cup pressed firmly into place and pressure maintained until cement hardens. Excess cement removed

17. Final position of cup 35° to 45° lateral inclination and 15° anteversion

Total Hip Replacement

Technique

(Continued)

After capsulotomy, the hip is ready for dislocation; it is flexed, internally rotated, and adducted to bring the femoral head and acetabulum into view. The limb is kept in internal rotation and the insertions of the quadratus femoris muscle and the inferior capsule are incised and reflected

so that the lesser trochanter can be visualized. The psoas tendon is identified but not cut. The surgeon is now ready to plan the femoral neck osteotomy.

The trial prosthesis is laid on the femur to check that the implant's center of rotation coincides with that of the femoral head. Existing deformities of the head and neck should be corrected. Measurements upward from the lesser trochanter should be recorded for use in determining the level of the osteotomy, the desired level of the center of motion of the prosthetic femoral head, and the degree of offset. The transection line is marked on the neck of the femur, and a smooth cut is made with an oscillating saw.

Acetabular Component

The femur is retracted anteriorly to expose the acetabulum (Plate 4). Unrestricted exposure of the acetabulum is the key to easy reaming and positioning of the prosthesis. Further exposure is obtained by placing a retractor posteriorly into the ischium (which also protects the sciatic nerve from injury during reaming) and another retractor inferiorly beneath the transverse acetabular ligament. The acetabulum is reamed in a medial direction to remove osteophytes and to define the true medial wall. Larger reamers are then used until the appropriate size is obtained. Trial acetabular cups are inserted, and the one with the

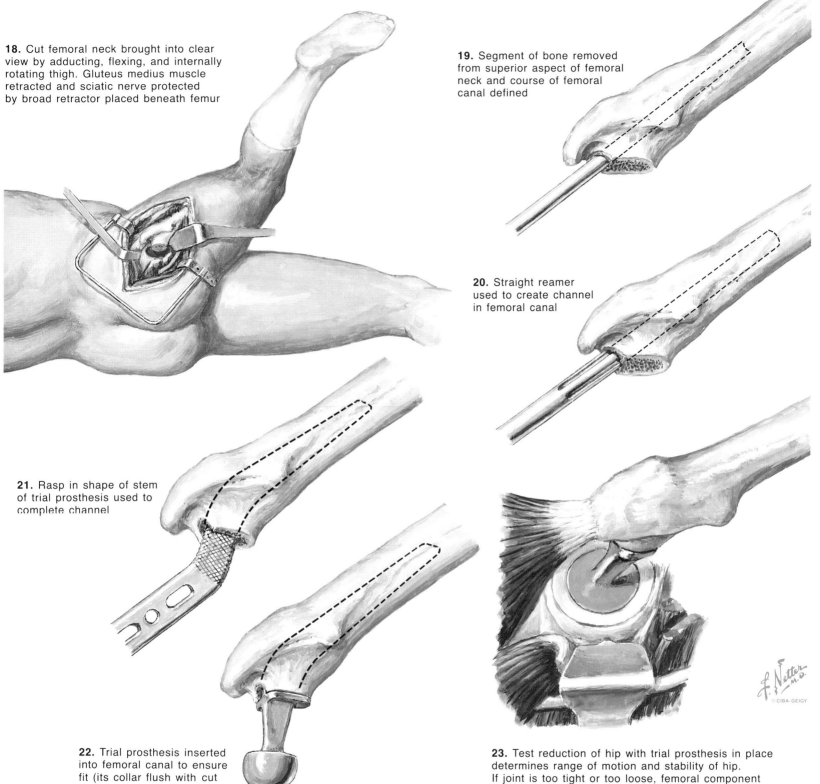

18. Cut femoral neck brought into clear view by adducting, flexing, and internally rotating thigh. Gluteus medius muscle retracted and sciatic nerve protected by broad retractor placed beneath femur

19. Segment of bone removed from superior aspect of femoral neck and course of femoral canal defined

20. Straight reamer used to create channel in femoral canal

21. Rasp in shape of stem of trial prosthesis used to complete channel

22. Trial prosthesis inserted into femoral canal to ensure fit (its collar flush with cut surface of femoral neck)

23. Test reduction of hip with trial prosthesis in place determines range of motion and stability of hip. If joint is too tight or too loose, femoral component with shorter or longer neck required

SECTION IV PLATE 5   Slide 4659

Total Hip Replacement

Technique
(Continued)

best fit is selected. The trial cup must be positioned in the proper degrees of anteversion and of lateral inclination with the horizontal plane. The desired orientation varies with the prosthetic design and should match as closely as possible the recommendation for each type. Generally, the lat-

eral inclination should not exceed 45°, and anteversion should not exceed 30°. It is wise to observe the rule that the greater the lateral inclination, the less should be the anteversion, and vice versa. Three cement fixation holes are prepared in the ilium, ischium, and pubic bone. The acetabulum is then irrigated and dried while the acrylic cement is mixed. When the cement reaches a workable consistency, it is inserted into the acetabulum and pressurized into the trabecular bone. When the cement has reached a doughy consistency, the acetabular cup is correctly positioned with an inserter, pressed into the cement, and held until the cement polymerizes. Extruded cement is then removed.

Femoral Component

A broad retractor is placed beneath the femoral neck to bring it into clear view (Plate 5). During reaming of the femoral canal, the leg is placed so that proper anteversion and valgus positioning of the stem can be achieved. The thigh is flexed, internally rotated, and adducted to achieve the best exposure of the femoral canal; a canal-finding instrument is inserted to determine the correct direction. Straight reamers and then rasps are used to shape the femoral canal. A trial prosthesis is placed in the femur, and the hip is temporarily reduced. Range of motion is tested, noting hip stability at the extremes of motion. If dislocation

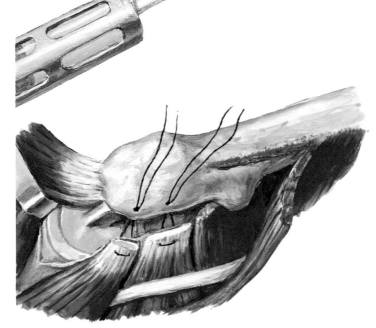

24. Trial prosthesis removed; femoral canal irrigated and dried. Canal closed off distally (about 2 cm beyond stem of prosthesis) with plug from excised femoral head and filled with cement

25. Prosthesis inserted into cement-filled canal must be properly aligned. Extruded cement cleaned away and pressure maintained until cement dries

26. Acetabular cup irrigated and prosthetic head reduced into it. Joint mobility (in all directions) rechecked. Piriformis and short external rotator muscles reattached to trochanter via small holes drilled in its margin

27. Gluteus maximus muscle repaired. Subcutaneous tissue approximated over vacuum drain and skin closed

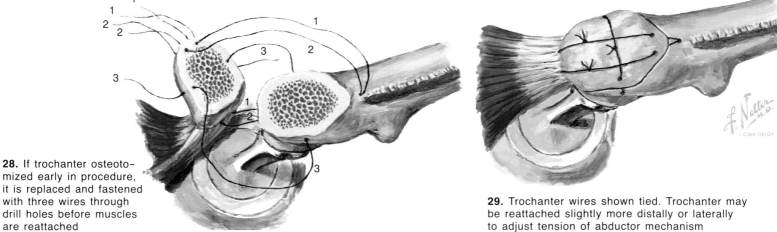

28. If trochanter osteotomized early in procedure, it is replaced and fastened with three wires through drill holes before muscles are reattached

29. Trochanter wires shown tied. Trochanter may be reattached slightly more distally or laterally to adjust tension of abductor mechanism

SECTION IV   PLATE 6   Slide 4660

Total Hip Replacement

Technique

(Continued)

occurs too easily, either component may be incorrectly positioned. If soft-tissue laxity contributes to instability, an implant with a longer neck may be needed.

After stable movement is demonstrated, the trial component is removed. A canal plug is inserted in the femur about 2 cm beyond the implant stem. This allows pressurization of the cement and prevents its flow to the distal femur. The femoral canal is again irrigated to wash out blood and debris and dried while the second batch of cement is mixed.

Cement is injected into the femoral canal, then pressurized; more cement is added and then again pressurized. The implant is then inserted and correctly aligned in a neutral or slightly valgus position in the medial-lateral plane and kept in place until the cement polymerizes. Extruded cement is removed. After the wound is irrigated, the hip is reduced and once again tested for a stable full range of motion.

The posterior capsule, piriformis muscle, and conjoined tendon of the short external rotator muscles are reattached in the trochanter through drill holes (Plate 6). Two suction drains are laid in the wound and brought out through the lateral aspect of the thigh. The gluteus maximus tendon is repaired with interrupted sutures. If a trochanteric osteotomy has been done, the trochanter fragment is replaced and secured with wires. Abductor muscle tension can be increased, if desired, by advancing the bone fragment. The deep fascia lata and gluteus maximus fascia are closed with interrupted sutures, the skin is closed with clips or a continuous nylon suture, and a sterile dressing is applied. □

Total Hip Replacement

Dysplastic Acetabulum and Protrusio Acetabuli

Reconstruction of the dysplastic or deficient acetabulum presents a particularly difficult surgical challenge, because the anatomic landmarks commonly used as reference points may not be in their normal positions. Portions of the bony circumference of the acetabulum may be deficient as a result of old fractures or congenital dysplasia. For example, in a long-standing posterior fracture dislocation of the hip, the posterior wall of the acetabulum is usually severely deficient; in congenital dislocation of the hip, the acetabulum is shallow and poorly developed. If the femoral head has been dislocated for many years, it articulates with the iliac wing in a pseudoacetabulum. The true acetabulum is stunted, small, and shallow, but its anatomic configuration is usually preserved and identifiable once the contracted overlying inferior capsule is reflected.

Dysplastic Acetabulum

Dysplasia of the acetabulum is often seen without actual dislocation of the femoral head. Usually, the acetabulum is shallow and the femur is displaced laterally. The superolateral wall, or roof, of the acetabulum is deficient and must be reconstructed with a bone graft before it can support an acetabular prosthetic component.

Total hip replacement in the patient with congenital hip dislocation is extremely difficult. Because the acetabulum may be deficient in bone mass and the proximal femur malformed, as is common, custom-made prostheses (very small or miniature) are required.

Treatment. A trochanteric osteotomy is usually required for adequate mobilization of the femur and visualization of the acetabulum; this procedure also facilitates reconstruction of the abductor mechanism at a lower point on the femur when the femur has to be shortened. The nerves and vessels are displaced as a result of the proximal displacement of the femur, and to avoid overstretching them, the femur usually has to be shortened. The psoas and rectus femoris tendons may also need to be released for adequate mobilization of the proximal femur.

A bone graft is often used to reinforce the superior acetabulum; it can be fashioned from the resected femoral head. The bone graft is fixed to the ilium with screws and then reamed to receive a small acetabular component, with the pubic bone and ischium used as anterior and posterior landmarks to avoid excessive reaming. When cement fixation is used, the bone graft–prosthesis

Dysplastic Acetabulum

Preoperative view

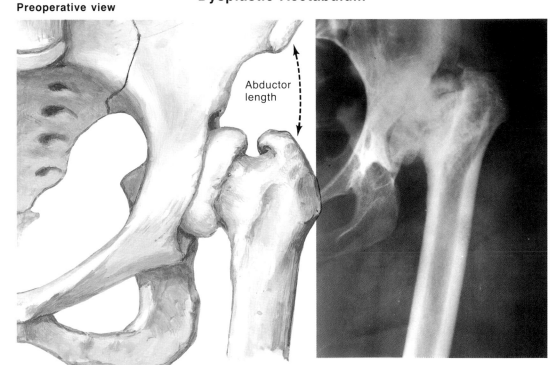

Shallow dysplastic acetabulum with proximal subluxation of femoral head and superolateral deficiency of acetabulum

Postoperative view

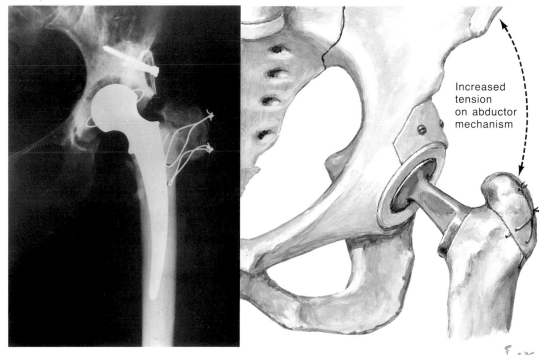

Total hip replacement with reinforcement of superior acetabulum with bone graft from excised femoral head. Bone graft held in place with screws. Limb slightly lengthened and tension in abductor muscle mass increased

interface is "caulked" with chips of trabecular bone to prevent the cement from intruding and inhibiting the incorporation of the bone graft into the acetabulum; then the acetabular prosthesis is cemented into place. Custom-made femoral components with varying angles and neck lengths can be used to achieve a near-normal abductor lever arm.

After a failed total hip replacement, bone autografts or allografts may also be used to reconstruct an acetabulum that is deficient in bone mass. After thorough removal of the loose acetabular component, old cement, and fibrous membrane are thoroughly removed from the bony surface, bone mass deficiencies are repaired. Segmental defects

are preferably reconstructed with autografts fixed to the host bone. Cavitational defects, on the other hand, may be filled with allografts, usually best impacted into the cavity in the form of chips. A smooth surface can be created by reaming in reverse. A bipolar or acetabular prosthesis may be inserted without cement, but it is usually preferable to cover the bone graft bed with a metal protrusio shell and then fix a nonmetal-backed prosthetic socket into the reconstructed complex with cement. Newer cementless fixation techniques can be used as well, but these are still in a phase of clinical trial. When the bone graft heals, pelvic bone mass is increased, making subsequent revision surgery easier.

Total Hip Replacement

Dysplastic Acetabulum and Protrusio Acetabuli

(Continued)

Protrusio Acetabuli

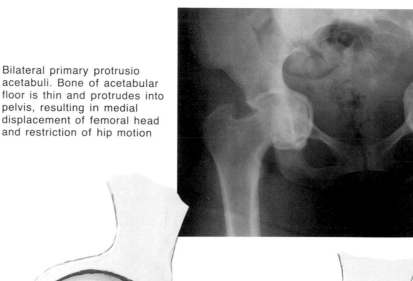

Bilateral primary protrusio acetabuli. Bone of acetabular floor is thin and protrudes into pelvis, resulting in medial displacement of femoral head and restriction of hip motion

Bone graft
Cement
Acetabular prosthesis
Femoral prosthesis

Medial Wall Defect

Another common site of bone mass deficiency is the medial wall, or floor, of the acetabulum. Often discovered during revision surgery, this problem is frequently related to the first procedure, during which the medial wall was perforated and packed with cement.

Treatment. Medial wall deficits have been classified by size into three types: minor (diameter <1 cm); intermediate (diameter <3 cm); and major (diameter >3 cm). All deficits are repaired surgically with one of three types of bone grafts. *Bulk bone* is used to reconstruct major deficits. For example, a large plug is fashioned from a resected femoral head and used to fill a medial wall defect. Screws may be added to further stabilize the graft, and a hemispheric depression can be reamed in the graft. *Chips of trabecular bone* are harvested and used as packing material to fill small deficits, cysts, and cracks. *Pulverized bone* (from reaming or a bone mill) can be made into a soft, pastelike consistency and finger packed into small deficits.

Bulky pieces of bone allograft maintain their structural integrity and may be variously replaced by host living bone through a process called *creeping substitution*; the trabeculae in the bone allograft act as a "trellis" for the ingrowth of live bone. Cementing into a bone graft is possible as long as the host bone–bone graft interface is adequate and intimate.

Protrusio Acetabuli

As a result of any disease that causes bone resorption, the pelvic bones become osteoporotic and soft, and the medial wall of the acetabulum may be gradually displaced medially. Bone remodeling in response to applied load causes varying degrees of superomedial protrusion of the femoral head (Plate 8). Protrusio acetabuli occurs when the femoral head is displaced past the ilioischial line in the pelvis. Other conditions that can cause progressive protrusion of the acetabulum are osteomalacia, rickets, Paget's disease of bone, and infections. Central dislocation of the femur due to trauma can also heal with a protrusion deformity. Arthrokatadysis (Otto's pelvis) is a rare idiopathic form of severe bilateral protrusio acetabuli most often seen in adolescent females. Metastatic carcinoma to the pelvis can lead to pathologic fractures, which result in a protrusion deformity.

Primary manifestations of protrusio acetabuli are thigh pain and decreased range of motion. Lateral and rotatory movements are particularly inhibited by the impingement of the femoral neck

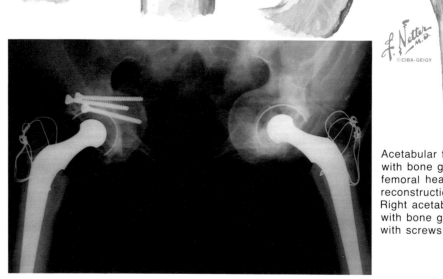

Acetabular floors augmented with bone grafts from excised femoral heads; total hip reconstruction completed. Right acetabulum reinforced with bone graft held in place with screws

against the acetabular labrum, or rim. A classification of protrusion deformities distinguishes cases with an intact medial wall from those with a perforated medial wall. Third-degree protrusio acetabuli is the most severe, occurring when the medial displacement is greater than 5 mm and is coupled with penetration of the medial wall. Protrusio acetabuli prosthetica occurs when a hip prosthesis is gradually displaced through the soft bone of the medial wall. Revision of these deformities is particularly difficult because the cement may be in direct contact with the pelvic vasculature.

Treatment. Like medial wall defects, protrusio acetabuli is treated with various types of bone grafts to reinforce areas deficient in bone mass to ensure that prosthetic components remain in the correct anatomic positions.

A metal ring implant is another method used to support an acetabular cup. Protrusio ring implants rest circumferentially on the intact bony rim of the acetabulum and do not rely on the integrity of the medial wall for support. However, a tailored bone graft is usually placed over a medial wall defect to repair it and add to acetabular bone mass. Large outer-diameter sockets, whether metal backed or not, may be used instead of protrusio rings and serve the same purpose of transferring load from the defective medial wall to the acetabular margins. □

Total Hip Replacement

Complications

Although many complications may follow total hip replacement, their incidence is fortunately low. The most common postoperative complications are deep venous thrombosis, neurologic complications, loosening of prosthetic component, dislocation, fracture, and infection.

The usual risks associated with general anesthesia and stress following any surgical procedure must be discussed with the patient. Since there may be significant blood loss during this procedure, replacement blood must be available. Transient hypotension, an uncommon intraoperative problem specific to hip replacement, occurs in some patients after the compression of cement into the femoral canal. The etiology of this phenomenon is still unclear, but it is theorized that a small amount of unpolymerized monomer in the cement may cause vasodilatation, or perhaps the increased pressure in the femoral canal causes fat embolization. Adequate blood volume must be maintained, and rapid infusion of fluids may be required to restabilize the blood pressure.

Deep Venous Thrombosis. While not unique to total hip replacement, deep venous thrombosis is unusually common in this type of surgery, occurring in 30% to 50% of cases. Most clots are small and asymptomatic and form in the small veins of the lower limb. Thrombosis of the femoral and iliac veins should be treated early with anticoagulants to minimize the risk of pulmonary embolism. At present, venography is the most accurate technique for assessing the patency of lower limb veins. Pulmonary embolism serious enough to cause death occurs in a very small percentage of patients, and postoperative treatment with aspirin or oral warfarin is therefore recommended. Intravenous administration of heparin is not recommended for prophylaxis because of possible bleeding complications. Evaluation of arterial blood gases is required if the patient becomes confused or develops inspiratory chest pain. Although ventilation and perfusion scans can help rule out a significant pulmonary embolism, angiography is the only definitive test. Fat embolism syndrome from disruption of the femoral bone marrow is rare.

Neurologic Complications. Peripheral nerve palsy is seen in about 0.25% of cases. The femoral nerve can be damaged by anteriorly extruded cement, and sciatic nerve palsy may occur secondary to pressure from an expanding hematoma. In hip replacement, the most common cause of sciatic nerve palsy is tension placed on the nerve by overretraction or overlengthening of the limb during surgery. This is usually manifested by extensor-evertor weakness of the foot and ankle or decreased sensation in the distribution of the more labile peroneal portion of the sciatic nerve. While slow improvement usually occurs, complete recovery is uncommon. Rarely, acute dislocation of a total hip replacement causes sciatic nerve injury, necessitating rapid reduction and supportive care.

Loosening of Femoral Component

Loosening of implant revealed by radiolucent zone along stem at cement-bone interface

Thorough removal of old cement and fibrous membrane and irrigation of femoral canal essential before replacement prosthesis can be cemented in. Special instruments, long suction tips, and good headlight or hand-held light source required. Removal and replacement of distal plug in canal necessary to accommodate new longer-stemmed implant

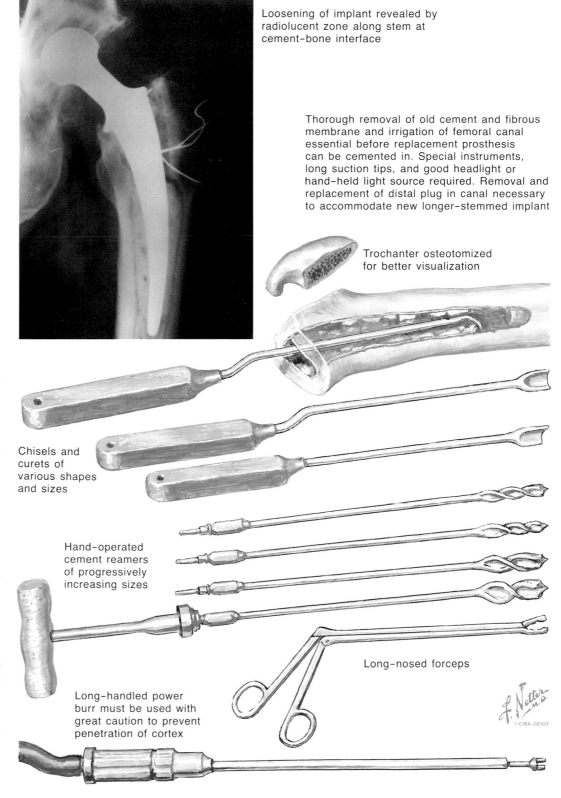

Trochanter osteotomized for better visualization

Chisels and curets of various shapes and sizes

Hand-operated cement reamers of progressively increasing sizes

Long-nosed forceps

Long-handled power burr must be used with great caution to prevent penetration of cortex

Loosening of Femoral Component

Loosening of the femoral component is a late complication that usually occurs 5 to 10 years after total hip replacement (Plate 9). Predisposing factors include age (<50 years); weight (>80 kg); and a high level of physical activity. Varus positioning of the femoral stem, poor cementing technique, and certain femoral stem designs are also associated with increased implant loosening. For example, the curved and diamond-shaped femoral stems are more likely to loosen, possibly because of their tendency to fragment the cement. When gaps remain between the bone and the stem of the prosthesis, because of poor cement infiltration or interposition of blood, a pistonlike movement can occur and lead to progressive loosening.

Early loosening can be diagnosed by characteristic radiographic findings even before clinical symptoms appear. Evidence of loosening is a radiolucent zone at the prosthesis-cement or the cement-bone interface. Histologic studies on tissue samples from this zone show a fibrous-tissue membrane containing acrylic, metallic, or polyethylene debris. Histiocytic cells and areas of granulomatous reaction to foreign bodies are also seen. This membrane may aggravate the implant's loosening by enzymatic osteolysis, or it may merely cushion the enlarging gap between the moving implant and the surrounding bone.

Total Hip Replacement

Complications
(Continued)

Thigh pain, the primary symptom of component loosening, is particularly evident when the patient attempts to walk. The pain, which often radiates to the knee, may begin gradually after an initial pain-free interval. Severe pain or rapidly advancing bone lysis indicates the need for revision surgery. Before a revision procedure is undertaken, however, an aspiration arthrogram and culture should be done to rule out infection, which can also cause loosening (Plate 12).

Correction of a loose implant with revision surgery is far more difficult than the initial total hip replacement. Careful preoperative planning is most essential. If possible, the previous incision should be used to avoid transecting scars that might compromise the vascular supply and result in skin necrosis. If scarring is particularly severe, the sciatic nerve should be exposed to ensure its safety. An intertrochanteric osteotomy facilitates the revision procedure by providing the widest possible exposure of the femoral canal. It also allows the adjustment of abductor muscle tension, which improves the stability of the reconstruction and optimizes postoperative function.

With the abductor muscles retracted superiorly, all scar tissue and pseudocapsule are excised to allow dislocation and mobilization of the proximal femur. Very loose prostheses can easily be removed. Any remaining debris must be removed carefully in a piecemeal fashion with special instruments. The distal cement plug is very difficult to remove and must often be penetrated or reamed with a high-speed power burr or hand-operated cement reamer. Long curets, cement chisels, and pituitary forceps are used for deeper access into the femoral canal. Great care must be taken to avoid perforating the femoral canal, since perforations create stress risers that can induce postoperative fractures. If perforation occurs, a femoral component with a long enough stem to reach at least two femoral cortical diameters below the defect must be used for adequate reinforcement. After the canal is thoroughly cleaned, a new plug is inserted distally. The replacement prosthesis is first placed without cement for a trial reduction. If range of motion is stable and leg length is correct, the implant is then cemented into the femoral canal. Alternatively, a cementless femoral prosthesis can be used, particularly when bone graft repair of an osteolytic, deficient femur is required. After the hip has been reduced, the trochanter is reattached with three or four metal wires that match the alloy of the femoral component.

Fracture of Femoral Component

Occasionally, a femoral component fractures within the femoral canal (Plate 10). This complication, most common in heavy men, is usually due to metal fatigue resulting from imperfect

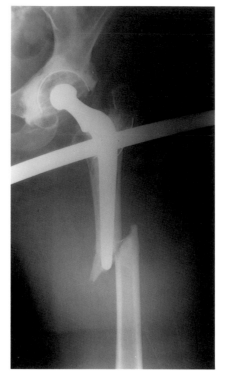

Fracture of femur at stem of femoral component

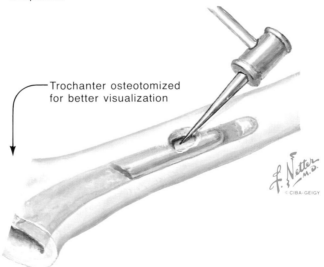

Trochanter osteotomized for better visualization

Proximal fragment of fractured prosthetic stem easy to remove but distal fragment more difficult. Sometimes distal fragment can be withdrawn with special instruments. It may be necessary to cut window in cortex and drive out fragment with punch. Windows in cortex plugged with bone or wire mesh before installing new long-stemmed prosthesis that extends beyond opening. Canal plug replaced more distally

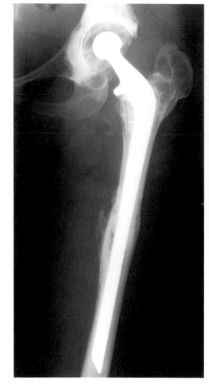

Long-stemmed replacement femoral component in position

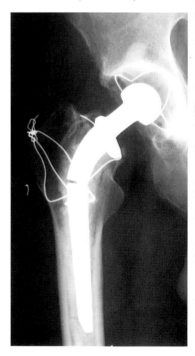

Fracture of femoral component stem

cementing or weight-bearing stress, or both. Often, the proximal half of a stem loosens first, leaving the distal stem rigidly fixed; this can lead to a bending stress, which eventually fractures the stem. Other factors associated with fractures of the femoral component are varus positioning and outmoded designs or methods of manufacture no longer in use. Most fractures occur in the middle third of the stem and start on the lateral side, where tension stresses are highest.

The proximal portion of the stem is relatively easy to remove. If, as is usually the case, the distal portion remains well fixed, it is very difficult to remove. A carbide drill is used to make an extraction hole in the proximal end of the

implant into which is hooked a special T-handled device. Alternatively, a window is created in the cortex of the femur at the level of the distal tip of the implant, and a punch is then used to push the broken tip out of the femoral canal. The window should be anterior and oval, with no sharp corners that could act as stress risers. To prevent later fractures, the stem of the replacement prosthesis should be long enough to extend at least two diameters below the window.

Fracture of Femur

Fracture of the femur can occur around or distal to a cemented femoral prosthesis (Plate 10). Even minor trauma can cause fracture if a significant

Total Hip Replacement

Complications

(Continued)

stress riser is present in the femoral shaft, particularly if the bone is osteoporotic. Any bony defect can act as a concentration point for stress, including screw holes and areas of cortical penetration.

Fractures are treated with open or closed reduction. Oblique fractures distal to the implant stem heal with the limb in traction or in a cast if bone contact is maintained. Since healing can take months, open reduction with internal fixation is often the best treatment. If the implant has loosened, revision with a long-stemmed component is indicated and helps stabilize the fracture site. However, good technique demands that cement, if used, is kept out of the fracture lines, and bone graft should be used to supplement the repair.

Loosening of Acetabular Component and Fracture of Acetabulum

The incidence of acetabular component loosening increases markedly after 12 to 15 years of function (Plate 11). Earlier loosening may be due to poor penetration of cement into the acetabular bone. Improper positioning and bone deficiency above the implant can also accelerate loosening. Obesity and strenuous activities can also lead to mechanical failure of the component. Fracture of the acetabular component is rare. While the average rate of polyethylene wear is very low, relatively high wear does occur, and loosening may result from granulomatous destruction of bone or bearing penetration associated with marginal impingement.

Pain in the inguinal region on weight bearing often heralds a loose acetabular component. Radiographs reveal a radiolucent zone around the implant. Since radiolucent zones may be evident before symptoms appear, radiographic follow-up after surgery is very important.

Revision of the loose component involves removal of the cup and cement. The fibrous membrane is also removed with a curet until a dry surface is obtained. Large defects in the medial wall of the acetabulum must be repaired with bone grafts. The new acetabular component is then cemented into place, or a cementless implant may be used.

A fracture of the acetabulum requires revision if function of the prosthesis is impaired. However, sometimes it is best to let the fracture heal first, because the new component can then be inserted more easily. Fractures of the anterior or posterior bony columns of the acetabulum may be repaired with internal fixation and the use of pelvic plates and screws.

Dislocation of Total Hip Prosthesis

Dislocation of the prosthesis can occur immediately after surgery if the patient moves the limb into a prohibited position (Plate 11). The patient must avoid extremes of internal rotation, flexion, and adduction for about 12 weeks until a thick

Loosening of Acetabular Component

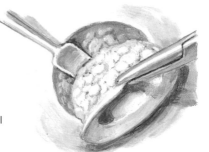

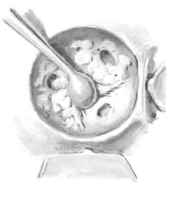

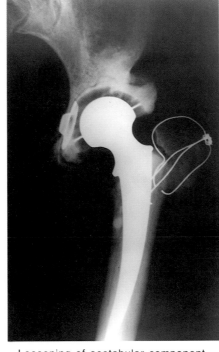

Loosening of acetabular component related to supraacetabular bone deficiency (reconstruction with bone graft necessary)

Loosened (or fractured) cup removed. Thin bony rim of acetabulum must not be damaged. Cup may be removed piecemeal

Old cement and fibrous membrane removed, fixation holes cleaned or rebored, and acetabulum thoroughly irrigated

Dislocation of Total Hip Prosthesis

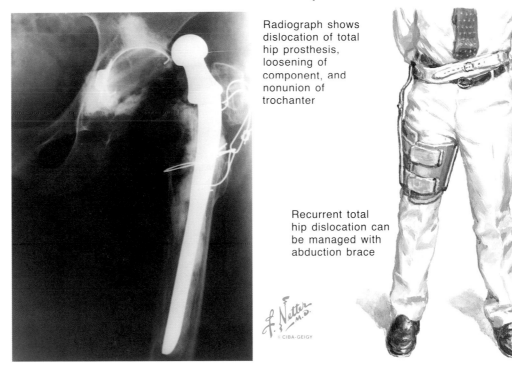

Radiograph shows dislocation of total hip prosthesis, loosening of component, and nonunion of trochanter

Recurrent total hip dislocation can be managed with abduction brace

capsule forms around the prosthetic joint. Treatment of an early dislocation is immediate reduction with the patient under sedation or general anesthesia. If the components are positioned properly, the patient can resume rehabilitation but must avoid the dangerous limb positions. Use of a hip-hinge abduction brace with a flexion stop at 60° is wise because it prevents unguarded movement into the proscribed positions. Recurrent dislocation should be treated according to the cause. If the position of either component is faulty, revision surgery is necessary, or if the myofascial tension is lax, advance osteotomy of the greater trochanter may be indicated when limb length is correct. If the limb is short, the

neck of the femoral component may need to be lengthened.

Nonunion of Greater Trochanter

Most intertrochanteric osteotomies heal uneventfully after repair with internal fixation. However, poor bone contact, osteoporosis, excessive soft-tissue tension, and previous surgery are factors that predispose to nonunion. A positive Trendelenburg sign may indicate a detached and proximally displaced trochanter. If there is no significant disability, no treatment is necessary. Significant weakness of the abductor muscles, thigh pain, or joint instability indicates the need to revise the trochanteric attachment. □

Total Hip Replacement

Infection

Subfascial (deep) infection, whether acute or latent, is a serious complication in joint replacement surgery. It is important to identify the type of infection because prognosis and treatment differ. Also, because any implant can become a focus for infection, patients with a hip prosthesis should be given preventive antibiotics when undergoing dental, urinary, or gastrointestinal procedures.

Any unexplained wound or hip pain in the early postoperative period should arouse suspicion. Acute infections are easiest to diagnose because they manifest classic systemic and local signs of sepsis. Diagnosis of latent infections is more difficult because clinical and radiographic signs are similar to those seen in aseptic loosening of the prosthesis.

Suprafascial Infections. Strong indications of a suprafascial infection are pain at the incision site, inflammation, and drainage in the first 2 weeks after surgery; fever and leukocytosis may also be present. Daily surgical wound care is therefore essential. Suprafascial infections respond well to local drainage and debridement.

Subfascial (Deep) Infections. Symptoms may include swelling of the thigh, increased hip pain, and elevated leukocyte count with an increased proportion of neutrophils. Accurate diagnosis depends on culture of aspirated fluid to isolate the causative organism. Blood cultures are also indicated. If the culture results are positive, surgical debridement and intravenous administration of antibiotics should be instituted immediately.

Acute subfascial infections cause a variety of signs and symptoms, depending on the organism's virulence and the patient's immunologic status. Since long-term postoperative administration of antibiotics can mask the appearance of symptoms, preventive intravenous administration of antibiotics should not be continued for more than 48 hours after surgery. In severe cases, acute fulminant infection and systemic illness, often due to a β-hemolytic streptococcus, can cause septic shock in the first few days after surgery.

Acute deep infections must be treated aggressively with intravenous administration of antibiotics and fluid replacement, as well as immediate open debridement of the implant site. Since most nosocomial gram-positive cocci have become resistant to penicillin, early treatment with a penicillinase-resistant synthetic penicillin or cephalosporin is necessary until the drug sensitivity of the organism is determined. If the infection is controlled early enough, it may be possible to save the prosthesis. When the tissues are inflamed and edematous, "delayed" closure of the suprafascial layers may be desirable, but the deep layers should always be loosely approximated over suction drains. If the infection is intractable or is due to antibiotic-resistant organisms, the prosthesis and cement must be removed. Secondary acute hematogenous infections can occur after months or years, with or without septicemia and sudden onset of hip pain.

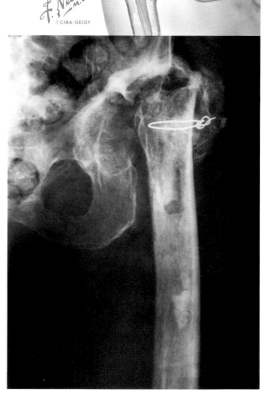

Suprafascial infection
Manifested by incisional pain, inflammation, and/or drainage. Usually responds well to debridement and antibiotics

Subfascial infection
Acute subfascial infection
May be fulminant with severe systemic and febrile manifestations. More commonly mild with few or no systemic symptoms and only mild local signs. Early, deep debridement needed
Latent infection
Pain, weeks or months after surgery. Radiographs may be inconclusive. Prosthesis should be removed

Aspiration for smear and culture
Primary procedure for diagnosis and choice of antibiotics. Staphylococci most common pathogens. Gram-negative infections most difficult to treat

Loosening of component due to infection; note bone lysis around stem

Girdlestone resection arthroplasty may be required after removal of total hip prosthesis

Latent infections do not usually become evident until at least 12 weeks after surgery. They should be suspected if the patient is not recovering normally. Delayed primary infections may be due to bacterial contamination from a remote body source (mouth, urine, bowel), in the perioperative period. There may be no fever or elevated leukocyte count, although the erythrocyte sedimentation rate is usually elevated. In a long-standing infection, radiographs may show osteopenia and a radiolucent zone around the cement. Results of bone scans are positive for both infection and a loosened implant, but the pattern of radioisotope uptake is sometimes specific enough to differentiate between the two conditions.

Treatment. Removal of the prosthesis is the treatment of choice. Intravenous administration of antibiotics to establish adequate bactericidal levels as confirmed by tube dilution sensitivity studies should be instituted for 4 to 6 weeks. Before revision surgery, histologic examination of local tissue is needed to ensure that the infection has been controlled.

Some organisms are so virulent and difficult to eradicate that a new implant can never be placed for fear of recurrent infection. A Girdlestone resection arthroplasty may be the only alternative procedure. Pain, severe limb shortening, and concomitant gross instability of the hip are serious disadvantages. □

Total Hip Replacement

Hemiarthroplasty of Hip

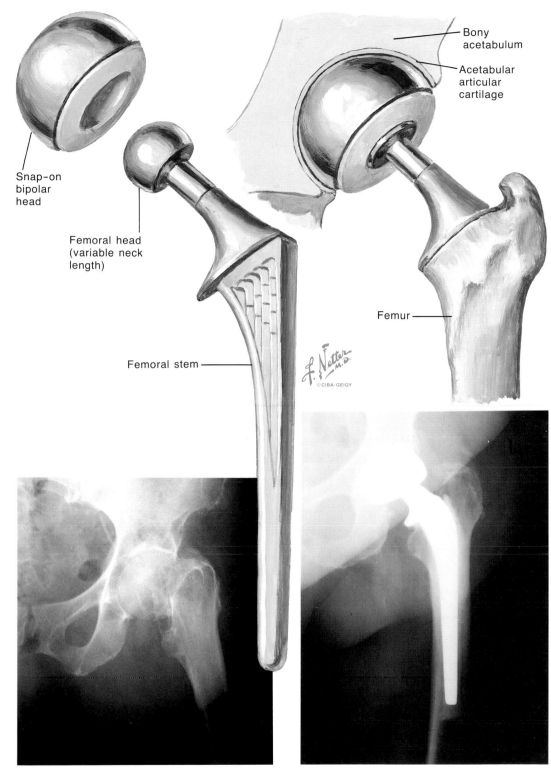

Snap-on bipolar head

Femoral head (variable neck length)

Femoral stem

Bony acetabulum

Acetabular articular cartilage

Femur

Fracture of femoral neck with articular cartilage preserved

Bipolar prosthesis used to restore alignment and function

Hemiarthroplasty, or partial reconstruction, of the hip is a less radical procedure than total hip replacement. It is performed when the acetabular cartilage is intact, and pathology is limited to the femoral side of the joint.

Partial hip replacement is frequently used in patients with metastatic lesions of the proximal femur, especially if there is risk of impending fracture. It is also appropriate for patients with osteonecrosis (avascular necrosis) of the femoral head after collapse of subchondral bone, providing the acetabular cartilage is still intact. The majority of patients with osteonecrosis are young adults. Factors associated with osteonecrosis in the joint include fractures and dislocations, corticosteroid therapy, alcoholism, and (less commonly) Gaucher's disease, sickle cell disease, and Caisson's disease.

Although hemiarthroplasty is appropriate for some fractures of the femoral neck, in children and young adults, every attempt must be made to save the femoral head and neck with internal pin fixation. This treatment may also be desirable in older patients if the fracture is only slightly displaced, impacted, or if it can be stably reduced. Since the main goal of treatment in older patients is early ambulation, hemiarthroplasty may be the treatment of choice even for minimally displaced fractures, especially if the bone is markedly osteoporotic. Displaced fractures of the femoral neck should be treated primarily with hemiarthroplasty or total hip replacement because of the high incidence of complications following treatment with pin fixation.

In 1927, Groves performed the first partial replacement of the hip, using a femoral head prosthesis made of ivory. Since then, other workers, including Bohlman, the Judet brothers, Moore, and Thompson, have used various materials to develop designs of one-piece implants with femoral heads and stems in many sizes and lengths. Unfortunately, an unacceptably high (40%) early rate of failure due to pain, loosening, or acetabular erosion created the frequent need for conversion to a total hip arthroplasty.

Bateman advanced the technique by initiating the clinical application and development of a new generation of bipolar prostheses. The modern bipolar prosthesis has two articulations, both of which contribute to hip motion: (1) the outer bearing is the large bipolar head that rests against the cartilage in the acetabulum; (2) the inner bearing comprises the small femoral head that fits into the polyethylene-lined larger bipolar head. It is hoped that the extra articulation provided by the bipolar prosthesis will result in better long-term preservation of the acetabular cartilage.

The modern bipolar prosthesis can be secured in the femoral canal with or without cement. Cementless designs are fixed with a tight press fit, a decided advantage in young patients since it will facilitate revision surgery when required in the future. Femoral stems with surfaces for bone ingrowth are also available. But to be successful, press-fit and ingrowth techniques of fixation both require a large inventory of variously sized and shaped devices, careful preoperative planning with templates, and precise surgical technique. In older patients with atrophic femurs, however, the stem of the femoral component should be appropriately shaped for rigid fixation with acrylic cement.

Another major advantage of the bipolar prosthesis is the ease with which it can be converted into a total hip replacement. The large bipolar head can be snapped off the smaller head, and an acetabular component can then be cemented into the pelvis. There is no need to replace the femoral component if it remains well fixed and is properly functioning. □

Total Hip Replacement

Intertrochanteric Osteotomy

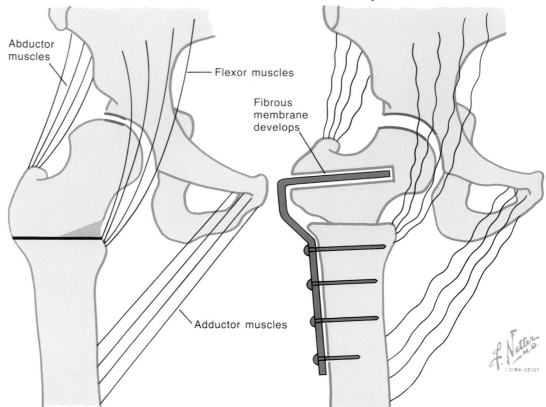

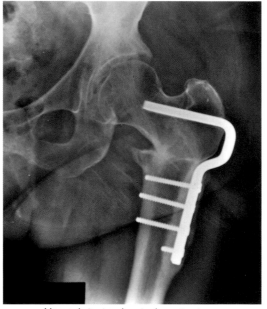

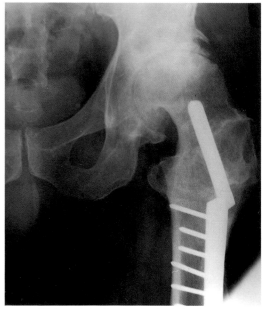

Preoperative view. Heavy black line indicates level of femoral section. Wedge of bone to be resected (blue); weight-bearing area (red) small. Abductor, flexor, and adductor muscles tense

Postoperative view. Wedge of bone excised and femoral neck reset in varus position, resulting in slight shortening of limb. Weight-bearing area increased and muscle tension reduced

Varus intertrochanteric osteotomy

Valgus intertrochanteric osteotomy

Intertrochanteric (proximal femoral) osteotomy is performed to improve the congruity of hip joint surfaces, correct the distribution of weight bearing in the joint, and release the tension exerted on tendons, muscles, and ligaments.

The biomechanical advantages of the procedure are shown in the illustration. In the more common superolateral type of osteoarthritic hip, weight bearing is concentrated on the superolateral aspect of the acetabulum; the adductor, abductor, external rotator, and flexor muscles of the hip are under tension. By removing a wedge of bone from the medial side of the femur at the level of the trochanter and performing a varus derotational osteotomy, all muscle tension is reduced and healthy cartilage is rotated into a weight-bearing position. Since the center of the femoral head is tilted medially, the abductor lever arm is lengthened but the strength of abduction is decreased owing to the shortening of the distance from origin to insertion. Disadvantages of the varus osteotomy are a limp, usually temporary but sometimes permanent, and permanent shortening of the limb. In about 20% of patients, persistence of unacceptable pain may require conversion to a total hip arthroplasty.

Osteotomy is most appropriate for young and middle-aged patients. Its chief advantages are preservation of bone and avoidance of long-term complications related to prostheses. Rigid internal fixation with a blade plate and screws greatly reduces the risk of nonunion. Also, with appropriate administration of antibiotics, the risk of postoperative infection is extremely low.

Osteotomy can also be combined with rotation of the proximal fragment relative to the femoral shaft to correct an excess of femoral anteversion, a problem commonly seen in young patients with valgus deformity of the hips. The addition of an extension component to the osteotomy can compensate for a flexion contracture.

Patients selected for osteotomy must have adequate range of motion in the joint, since this is not improved by the procedure. Preoperative radiographs are taken with the hip widely abducted or adducted to mimic the postoperative position of the joint. If abduction provides for a better fit of the femoral head into the acetabulum, a varus osteotomy is performed. Conversely, if adduction produces better joint congruence, a valgus osteotomy is selected. Radiographic evidence of mechanical overload includes localized bone sclerosis, cysts, and narrowing of joint space. Fluoroscopy, with or without arthrography, can also be carried out to determine maximum congruence in the joint.

Rehabilitation is relatively long and usually includes 8 to 12 weeks of partial weight bearing on crutches. After this, the patient must use a cane and may walk with a limp for an unpredictable length of time. After rehabilitation, young, active patients are able to resume normal activities.

Because total hip replacement is remarkably successful in relieving pain and the rehabilitation period is short, osteotomy is being performed less frequently. It should be considered a temporizing procedure that enables the younger patient to wait 5 to 10 years before undergoing a total hip replacement. This time may be well spent, since research in joint replacement technology continues to produce better prostheses. □

Total Knee Replacement

Prostheses

Arthroplasty for the treatment of severe painful arthritis of the knee originated in the midnineteenth century when Verneuil suggested the interposition of soft tissues to replace the articular surfaces of the knee joint; materials used included pig's bladder, nylon, fascia lata, and prepatellar bursa. Resection arthroplasty was also performed. The joints developed good motion but lacked good mechanical stability. These operations were confined to patients with severe conditions, such as tuberculosis or other infectious processes that destroyed the knee.

Success with femoral mold arthroplasty of the hip prompted the development of a similar metallic device for use in the knee. In 1958, MacIntosh used an acrylic tibial plateau prosthesis, and a metal prosthesis of a similar design was developed by McKeever. Gunston applied Charnley's principle of low-friction arthroplasty of the hip to develop a prosthesis for the knee joint. He used metal femoral runners that articulated with polyethylene tibial components. Each component was fixed in bone with acrylic cement. Freeman developed a single femoral-tibial component to replace the entire surface of each bone. The Freeman-Swanson prosthesis consisted of two components whose stability was determined by a roller-in-trough mechanism. Other designs featured fully constrained hinges that replaced the articular surfaces of the joint and did not require a balanced tension of the collateral ligaments. However, these prostheses loosened early, and the rate of infection increased. Consequently, surface-replacement designs were developed that allowed the knee joint to move in a normal fashion.

Indications and Contraindications

Total knee replacement is performed in patients with severe, incapacitating pain in the knees due to osteoarthritis, osteonecrosis, or rheumatoid arthritis, after conservative management, such as administration of nonsteroidal antiinflammatory drugs (NSAIDs), use of a cane, and weight loss in obese patients, has been exhausted. Arthritis due to trauma, gout, and psoriasis should also first be treated conservatively. Joint destruction secondary to pigmented villonodular synovitis may require total joint replacement after appropriate synovectomies have been performed. More

Total Condylar Knee Prosthesis

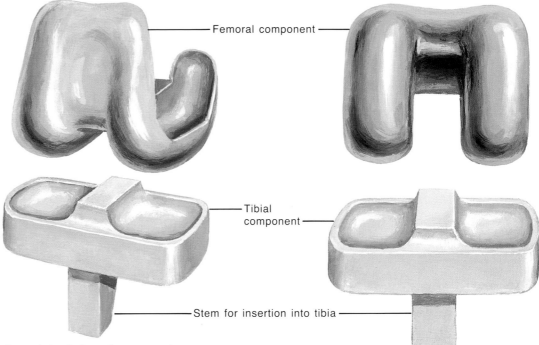

Femoral component

Tibial component

Stem for insertion into tibia

Anterolateral view of components in position of extension

Anterior view of components in position of flexion

Femur

Tibia

Lateral sectional view of knee joint in extension with components in place

Femur

Tibia

Lateral sectional view of knee joint in flexion with components in place

recently, total knee replacement has been successfully used in patients with hemophilic arthritis.

In patients with rheumatoid arthritis, total knee replacement may be done at any age and has been successful in patients with juvenile arthritis. In these patients, growth is limited, and extra-small or custom-made prostheses may be required. In patients with osteoarthritis, total knee replacement should be confined to those over 60 years of age. If one or both collateral ligaments are injured, a constrained design, such as the total condylar III or the constrained posterior stabilized knee prosthesis, should be used rather than the total condylar prosthesis, which requires intact collateral ligaments to provide joint stability.

In older patients with mild narrowing of joint space and patchy articular degeneration in the femorotibial joint, severe patellofemoral arthritis may be successfully treated with total joint replacement. In patients with a previous infection, total knee replacement should be delayed until the infection has been eradicated. If the infection persists, however, and if the infectious organism cannot be adequately treated, then arthrodesis is the treatment of choice.

Knee joint replacement should not be carried out if a sound, painless arthrodesis is in good position. In these patients, arthroplasty is rarely successful, and if it fails, attempts at fusing the knee again may not succeed.

Total Knee Replacement

Prostheses

(Continued)

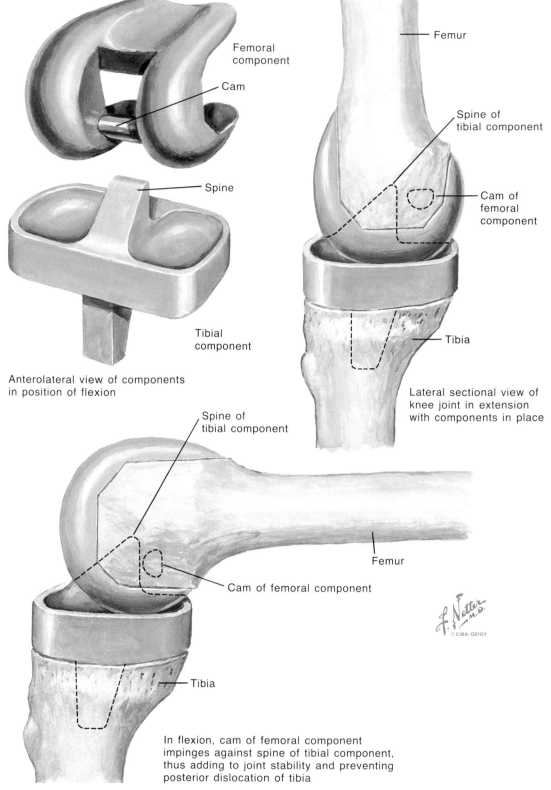

Femoral component

Cam

Spine

Tibial component

Anterolateral view of components in position of flexion

Femur

Spine of tibial component

Cam of femoral component

Tibia

Lateral sectional view of knee joint in extension with components in place

Spine of tibial component

Cam of femoral component

Femur

Tibia

In flexion, cam of femoral component impinges against spine of tibial component, thus adding to joint stability and preventing posterior dislocation of tibia

Total knee replacement should not be performed in patients with severe neuropathic joint disease, recent joint infection, painless paralytic deformities due to antecedent poliomyelitis, or cerebrovascular insufficiency. Nor is it recommended in manual laborers, athletes, or overweight persons, because the excessive mechanical stresses placed on the knee lead to early loosening and subsequent failure of the prosthesis. Patients with posttraumatic osteoarthritis are typically young, and only in rare instances should total knee replacement be considered in this group. In the very young patient, arthrodesis is the procedure of choice.

Total Condylar Prosthesis

The total condylar prosthesis was developed in 1973 at The Hospital for Special Surgery (Plate 15). The term describes a family of prostheses with similar design characteristics that allow unconstrained movement of the knee joint.

The total condylar prosthesis requires balancing the tension of the collateral ligaments to stabilize the knee joint in flexion and extension. With appropriate design of the prosthesis and stable symmetric balancing of the collateral ligaments, the cruciate ligaments are not necessary for function of the knee joint. The total condylar prosthesis allows only 90° of knee flexion, which can be increased by flexing the position of the femoral component. A total condylar design in which the posterior cruciate ligament is retained has been developed at the Brigham and Women's Hospital. This design allows greater flexion of the knee joint and improves the ability to climb stairs.

Posterior Stabilized Condylar Prosthesis

The posterior stabilized condylar prosthesis, a modification of the total condylar design, retains more of the function of the posterior cruciate ligament (Plate 16). The central spine of the prosthesis is smaller and has a slightly different shape. It is positioned in such a way that the spine engages the cam of the femoral component at 75° of flexion. Thereafter, with further flexion, the cam of the femoral component imposes a progressive roll-back at the femoral condyle to prevent posterior impingement, a mechanism similar

to that found in the knee with an intact posterior cruciate ligament. The standard version is designed to reach 120° of flexion. (A special type that allows 140° of flexion is available in Asia; it is compatible with the life-style in that region.) This prosthesis functions the same way as the total condylar prosthesis, except that the amount of flexion is significantly improved.

Results

A 10-year follow-up study of 100 patients with the total condylar knee prosthesis indicated that 93% of the prostheses functioned well, did not require revision, and lasted the remainder of the patient's life. Mechanical complications were rare

(2%), usually occurring in the first 2 to 3 years after surgery. Follow-up studies 2 to 8 years after replacement surgery with a posterior stabilized prosthesis reported good-to-excellent results in 96% of patients.

Both types of prostheses were originally developed to replace the surfaces of the patella, tibia, and femur. The patella should be replaced in all patients with rheumatoid arthritis, but replacement of the patella in the osteoarthritic knee remains controversial. However, studies show that clinical results are more predictably good if the patella is resurfaced. At The Hospital for Special Surgery, resurfacing of the patella is routinely done in total knee arthroplasty. □

Technique for Total Knee Replacement

Total Knee Replacement

Technique

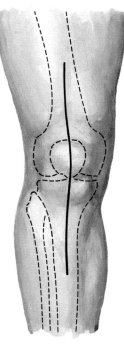

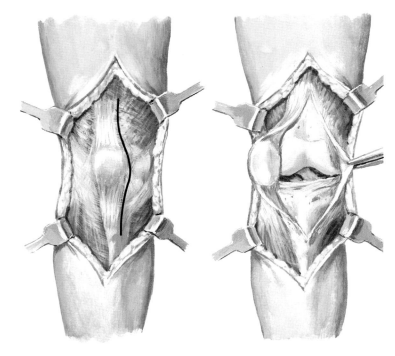

1. Longitudinal 10 to 12 in. skin incision centered on patella

2. Capsular incision skirts medial margin of patella and courses distally through periosteum medial to tibial tuberosity

3. Patella reflected laterally by raising patellar ligament in continuity with periosteum

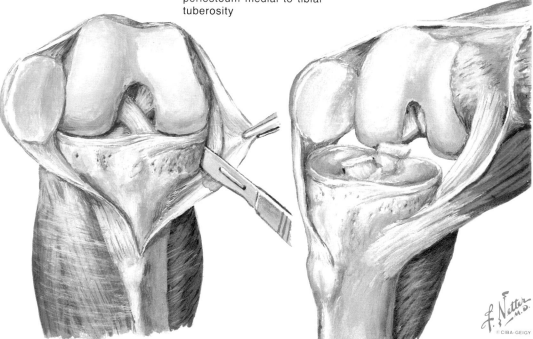

4. Medial flap raised by detaching tibial collateral ligament and pes anserinus subperiosteally, aided by external rotation of tibia

5. Cruciate ligaments divided, and tibia subluxated anteriorly

A 10- to 12-in. longitudinal incision is centered on the anterior surface of the patella. This incision affords the best medial and lateral exposure of the knee without placing undue tension on the skin (Plate 17). The capsule is incised directly over the medial margin of the patella so that the incision is as straight as possible. The medial placement is done to prevent wound dehiscence during knee flexion in the postoperative period. The periosteum 1 cm medial to the tibial tuberosity is left intact to help prevent avulsion of the patellar ligament from the tibial tuberosity. Every effort should be made to prevent avulsion, because reattachment of the patellar ligament is difficult and may result in limitation of knee extension.

The patella is reflected laterally by raising the patellar ligament about 5 mm in continuity with the periosteum. Any scar tissue should be removed from the lateral femoral gutter to facilitate eversion of the patella. The capsular incision should extend far enough proximally to allow eversion of the patella, but care must be taken to avoid dissecting across the quadriceps femoris tendon.

A medial flap is raised by detaching the tibial (medial) collateral ligament and pes anserinus tendon subperiosteally, which allows the superficial and deep portions of the tibial collateral ligament to remain intact. External rotation of the tibia may facilitate dissection of the posteromedial aspect of the bone, and the anterior portions of the remaining menisci may be incised to obtain a better exposure. External rotation of the tibia enables the patella to remain everted with minimal tension on the patellar ligament. The insertion of the pes anserinus tendon is reflected subperiosteally to obtain a wide, clear exposure of the medial tibial plateau.

The anterior cruciate ligament is then divided and the tibia subluxated anteriorly. Any large osteophytes on the lateral and medial femoral condyles or the intercondylar notch are removed with an osteotome. This facilitates excision of the anterior and posterior cruciate ligaments from their respective attachments on the femur.

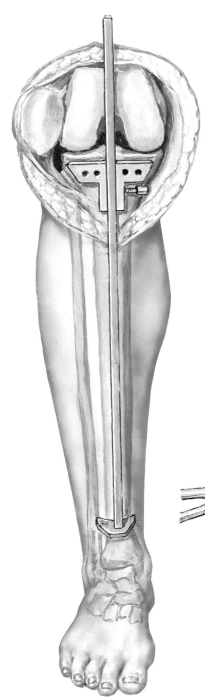

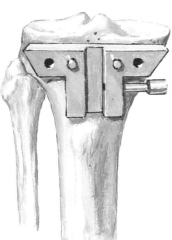

7. Cutting block adjusted to just below articular surface of tibia, fixed on alignment bar with thumbscrew, and nailed to tibia. Alignment bar removed

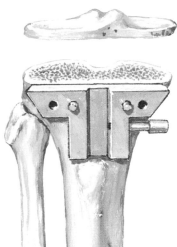

8. With cutting block as guide, articular surface of tibia resected with oscillating saw

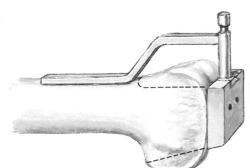

9. For resection of anterior and posterior femoral condyles, template of appropriate size selected after testing with detachable arm that rests on femur. Correct size allows resection of equal amounts of each condyle anteriorly and posteriorly

11. Posterior and anterior femoral condyles resected. Note square cut anteriorly and inclined cut posteriorly

10. With joint distracted, template placed parallel to cut surface of tibia and nailed to femur. Because of unequal tension of collateral ligaments, more of one condyle may need to be removed

12. Largest spacer that fits flexion gap selected. Spacers range from 7.5 to 30 mm in thickness and serve as guide in setting tensor for resection of correct amount of distal femoral condyles

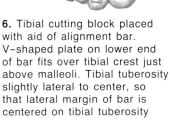

6. Tibial cutting block placed with aid of alignment bar. V-shaped plate on lower end of bar fits over tibial crest just above malleoli. Tibial tuberosity slightly lateral to center, so that lateral margin of bar is centered on tibial tuberosity

Total Knee Replacement

Technique

(Continued)

A tibial cutting block is placed on the anterior aspect of the tibia with the aid of an alignment bar (Plate 18). A V-shaped plate, located at the lower end of the bar, fits snugly on the skin overlying the tibial crest just above the malleolar line. The lateral margin of the bar is centered over the midpoint of the tibial tuberosity. The tibial crest is another point of reference for the correct positioning of the tibial cutting block horizontal to the long axis of the tibia. The cutting block should be placed so that no more than 5 mm of bone can be resected from the tibia. The bone mass in this subchondral region is very strong, and removal of more bone exposes the mechanically weaker trabecular bone. The alignment bar is removed, while the cutting block remains fastened to the tibia with pins. The articular surface of the proximal tibia is resected with an oscillating saw, and the remainder of the surgical procedure follows from this tibial cut. It is most important to make the tibial cut at 90° to the long axis of the tibia.

Flexion Gap. The anterior and posterior portions of the femoral condyles are resected using a femoral cutting guide. The guide is placed with the help of a detachable arm that rests on the anterior aspect of the femur and helps to protect the anterior femoral cortex from being cut with the oscillating saw. (It is important to avoid making notches on the femoral cortex, because they create an area of stress concentration that may be

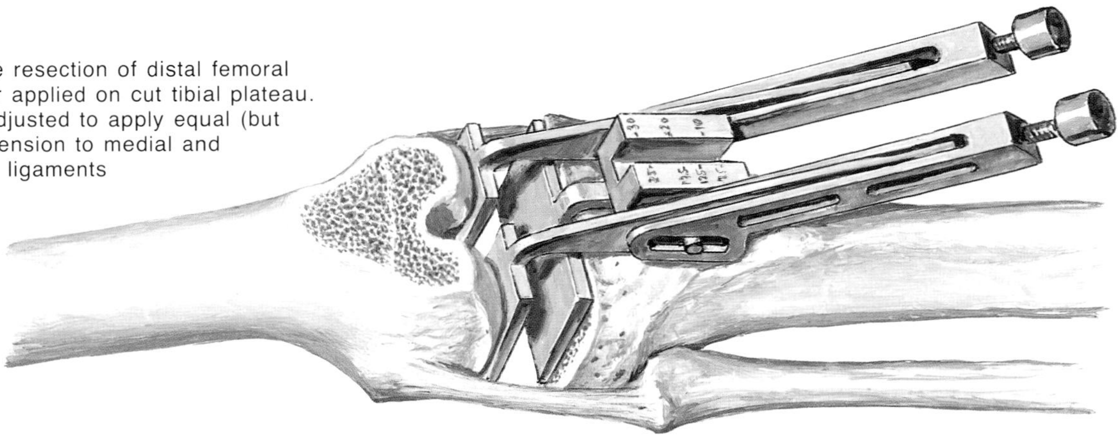

13. For accurate resection of distal femoral condyles, tensor applied on cut tibial plateau. Thumbscrews adjusted to apply equal (but not excessive) tension to medial and lateral collateral ligaments

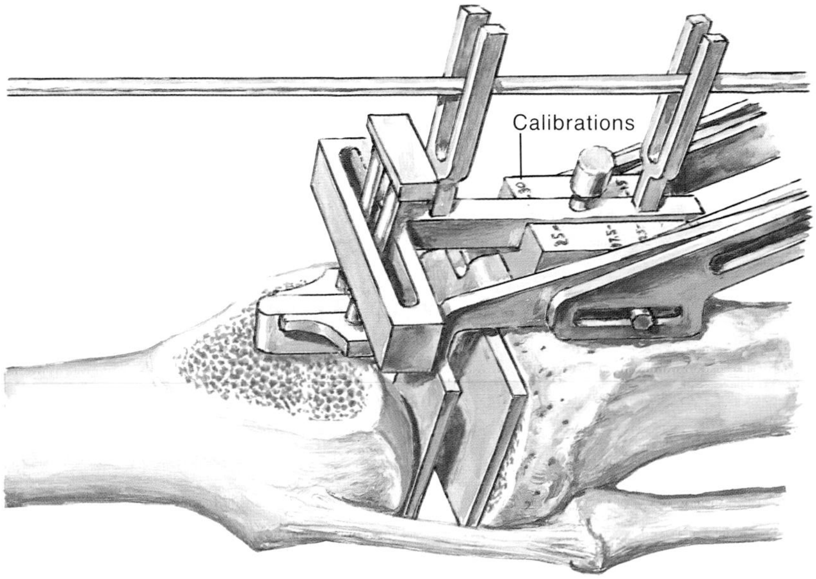

Calibrations

14. Additional tensor component to hold cutting block added and set at level matching thickness of spacer that best fits flexion gap. Calibrations on original tensor unit correspond to thicknesses of various spacers

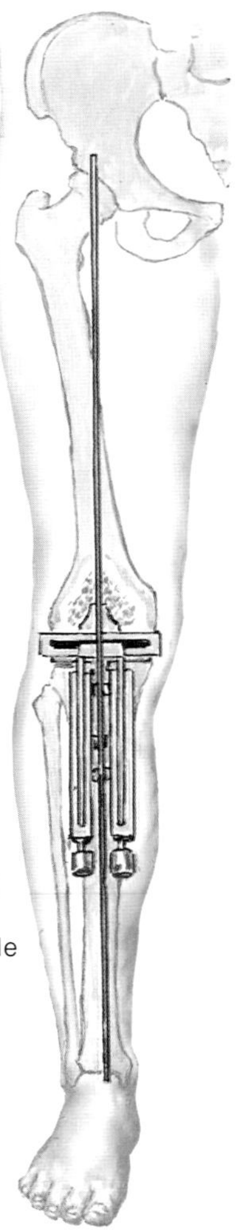

15. Alignment measured with rod passing over head of femur and middle of ankle joint

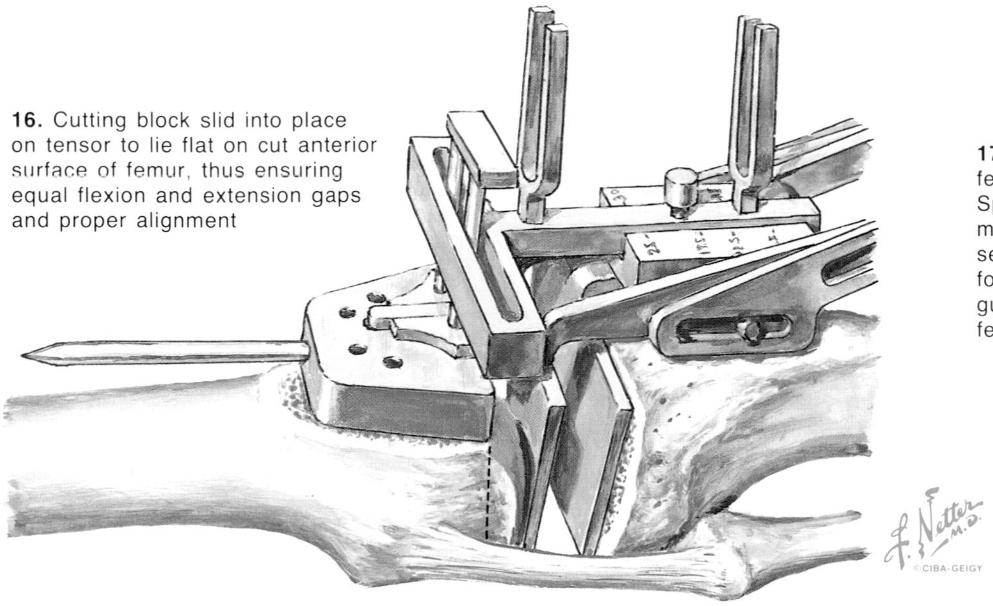

16. Cutting block slid into place on tensor to lie flat on cut anterior surface of femur, thus ensuring equal flexion and extension gaps and proper alignment

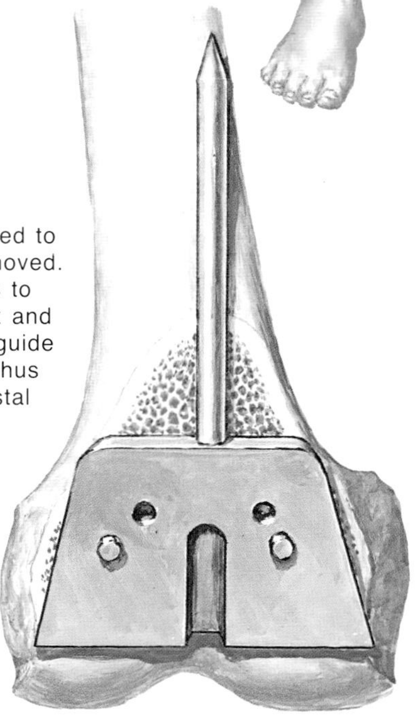

17. Cutting block nailed to femur and tensor removed. Spike on block points to medial femoral cortex and serves as additional guide for alignment. Block thus guides excision of distal femoral condyles

Total Knee Replacement

Technique

(Continued)

susceptible to pathologic fractures of the femur if the patient suffers a fall.) The femoral cutting block should be positioned to allow an equal amount of bone to be removed from the anterior and posterior parts of the condyles. The template may be placed parallel to the cut surface of the tibia, ensuring that equal tension on the collateral ligaments is obtained. Occasionally, more bone may have to be removed from one condyle than from the other. However, after an extensive release of the collateral ligaments is done to balance tension on them, the cutting block is placed on the femur so that equal amounts of bone are removed from the posterior portion of both femoral condyles. After the block is fixed to the femur with pins, the detachable arm is removed, and the resections are carried out. An appropriately sized spacer is then placed in the gap created by the femoral and tibial resections, and an alignment rod is placed through it to check the tibial resection (Plate 18). The overall alignment and size of the components are evaluated when there is equal tension on the collateral ligaments. This flexion gap determines the amount of bone that must be subsequently removed from the distal femur to create an extension gap that matches it in size.

Extension Gap. With the knee in extension, a tensor device is placed between the femur and tibia, and the collateral ligaments are tensed (Plate 19). At the same time, the alignment is

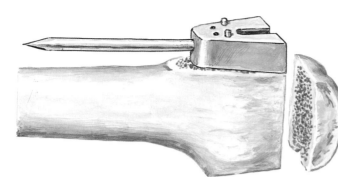

18. Distal femoral condyles resected, using cutting block nailed to femur as guide

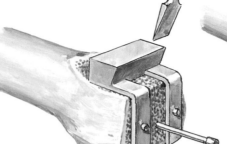

19. Femoral notch guide pinned to femur. Guide also used to ensure accuracy of anterior and distal cuts in femur

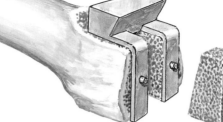

20. Medial and lateral cuts of femoral notch made with saw, and proximal cut with osteotome (angle conforms to notch guide). Bone fragment and notch guide removed. Template reapplied to check accuracy of anterior and posterior cuts

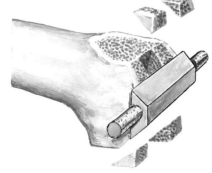

21. Chamfer guide pinned into holes used for notch guide, and end of femur beveled to conform to shape of inside of prosthesis

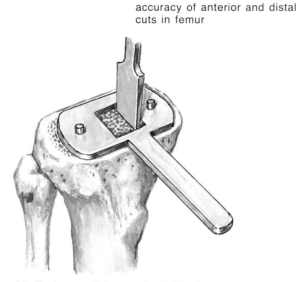

22. To form well in proximal tibia for stem of tibial component, template pinned to cut tibial plateau, and initial cuts made with osteotome

23. Well in tibia completed by tamping down trabecular bone with punch of same size and shape as stem of tibial component. (Well thus rectangular with anteriorly inclined posterior wall)

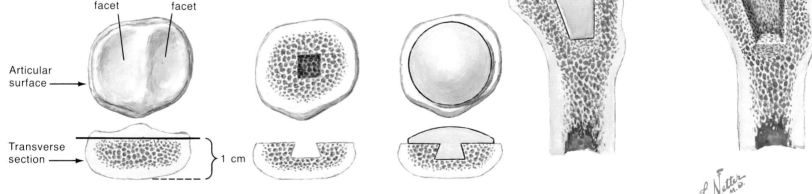

Medial facet   Lateral facet

Articular surface

Transverse section

1 cm

24. Articular surface of patella resected to leave flat surface. Equal amounts to be removed from medial and lateral facets, but at least 1 cm of bone must be left to ensure adequate strength. Small, shallow cavity cut or drilled into surface, its edges slightly undercut, to receive stem of patellar component, which is cemented in place

Total Knee Replacement

Technique

(Continued)

checked to ensure that the normal valgus angle of 7° to 10° has been obtained. Thus, the tensor performs three functions: (1) it tenses the collateral ligaments, (2) it assesses the correct mechanical alignment of the joint, and (3) it determines the level of the distal femoral resection. The cutting block, which guides the excision of the distal femur, is mounted on the proximal aspect of the tensor device, and the resection is completed.

Insertion of Components. The goal of the surgical procedure is to restore the normal mechanical axis of the knee. Once this critical phase is accomplished, the individual components are fitted (Plate 20). A femoral notch guide is used to remove a portion of bone from the center of the femur for placement of the femoral component.

With the aid of a chamfer guide, the end of the femur is beveled to match the internal surface of the prosthesis. A well is fashioned in the proximal tibia to receive the fixation peg. The trabecular bone is tamped down into the well with an impactor, which prevents excess cement from extruding distally into the shaft of the tibia. The articular surface of the patella is then resected to create a flat surface on which the patellar component is cemented (Plate 20). The patellar component glides on the femoral component.

Trial prostheses are placed to verify the fit of each component and the accuracy of the mechanical alignment of the knee. The joint is taken through a range of motion from 0° to 120° to

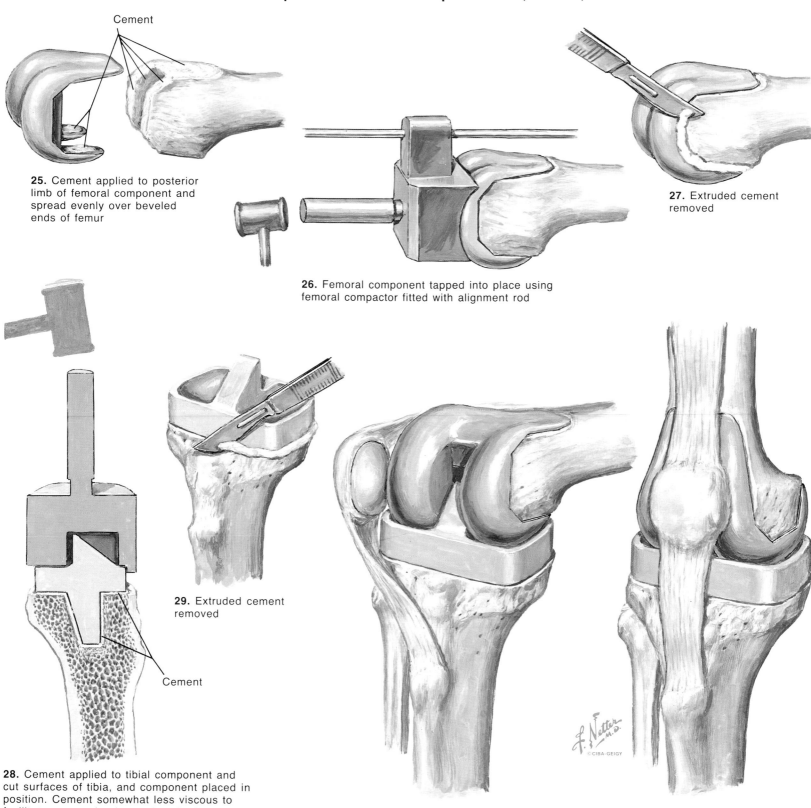

25. Cement applied to posterior limb of femoral component and spread evenly over beveled ends of femur

26. Femoral component tapped into place using femoral compactor fitted with alignment rod

27. Extruded cement removed

28. Cement applied to tibial component and cut surfaces of tibia, and component placed in position. Cement somewhat less viscous to facilitate penetration into trabecular bone (sagittal section)

29. Extruded cement removed

30. With all components in place, joint reduced in flexion and thoroughly irrigated

31. Knee extended and wound closed over suction drain

SECTION IV PLATE 21   Slide 4675

Total Knee Replacement

Technique

(Continued)

assess the balance of the collateral ligaments. The tourniquet is then released in order to obtain hemostasis and is reinflated after the limb is exsanguinated with an Esmarch bandage. The trabecular bone surfaces are irrigated with saline solution mixed with polymyxin and neomycin and are dried, and the prosthetic components are fixed into the bone with methylmethacrylate (acrylic) cement (Plate 21). The femoral and patellar components are inserted first, then the tibial component; separate batches of cement are prepared for each component. After the cement has cured, the wound is irrigated with a saline and antibiotic solution, suction drains are placed, and the wound is closed in layers. A bulky dressing is applied to the knee. In some patients, the limb is placed in a continuous passive motion machine to initiate early flexion of the knee.

Postoperative Care. Typically, the patient is hospitalized for 10 to 14 days. Physical therapy is started on the second day after surgery, and active assisted motion is encouraged. Patients can begin to ambulate with a walker and then with a cane; they can be discharged as soon as they can flex the knee 90°, ascend steps, and use a cane. For as long as the prosthesis remains in place, patients must be given antibiotics 48 hours before any dental procedure and urinary or gastrointestinal surgery to protect against the hematogenous seeding of bacteria, which can localize at the site of the prosthesis. □

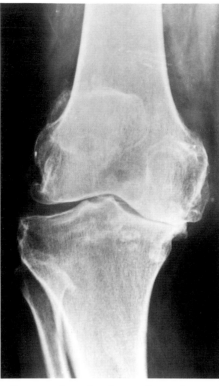

Bilateral
tibia vara
with severe
osteoarthritis

Preoperative standing radiograph
shows varus deformity of knee with
sloping defect of medial tibial plateau

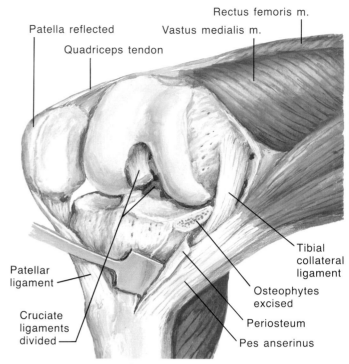

Patella reflected
Quadriceps tendon
Rectus femoris m.
Vastus medialis m.

Patellar
ligament

Cruciate
ligaments
divided

Tibial
collateral
ligament

Osteophytes
excised

Periosteum

Pes anserinus

Medial release. Superficial tibial collateral
ligament and pes anserinus (insertion of gracilis,
sartorius, and semitendinosus muscles) stripped
from upper medial tibia together with periosteal
flap; osteophytes excised

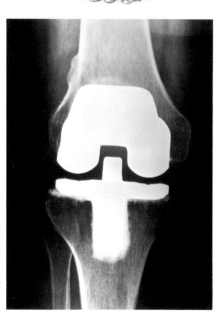

Postoperative radiograph shows good
alignment after medial release
and total knee replacement

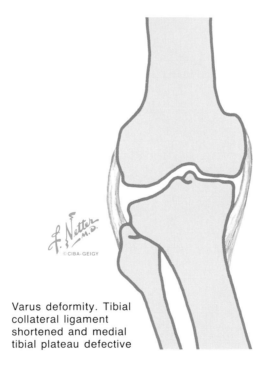

Varus deformity. Tibial
collateral ligament
shortened and medial
tibial plateau defective

Release of tibial
collateral ligament
from tibia permits
balanced alignment

Surgical Treatment of Varus and Valgus Deformities of Knee

Medial Release for Varus Deformity of Knee

Severe varus deformity in a knee that is to
undergo total knee arthroplasty sometimes requires
a full release of the tibial (medial) collateral ligament (Plate 22). Long-term follow-up studies
show that if the knee remains in a varus position,
the mechanical stresses placed on the tibial component are uneven. This leads to early loosening
and subsequent failure of the prosthesis. It is
impossible to fully balance the tibial collateral
ligament without releasing it distally. The release
is achieved by first elevating the pes anserinus and
semimembranosus muscle insertions subperiosteally. After the posterior aspect of the tibial plateau is resected, an osteotome is used to lift the
distal insertion of the superficial and deep tibial
collateral ligaments. During healing, the tibial collateral ligament reattaches itself at a more proximal level, resulting in good joint stability and
obviating the need for a constrained prosthesis.

Lateral Release for Valgus Deformity of Knee

In severe valgus deformity, the lateral structures of the knee are released to return the knee
joint to its normal valgus alignment of 7° to 10°
(Plate 23). The proximal attachment of the fibular (lateral) collateral ligament and popliteus tendon are released first. The periosteum of the
lateral side of the femur is then stripped proximally. If a flexion contracture is present, the
insertion of the lateral head of the gastrocnemius
muscle is released. In very severe valgus deformities of more than 40°, the iliotibial tract must
also be released.

Surgical Treatment of Varus and Valgus Deformities of Knee

(Continued)

Lateral Release for Valgus Deformity of Knee

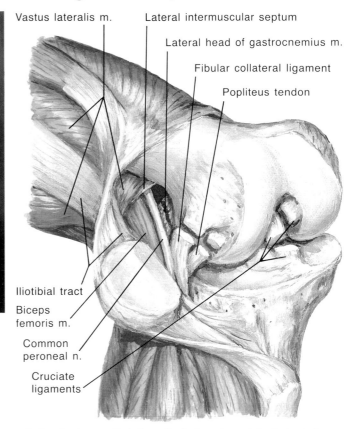

Vastus lateralis m.
Lateral intermuscular septum
Lateral head of gastrocnemius m.
Fibular collateral ligament
Popliteus tendon
Iliotibial tract
Biceps femoris m.
Common peroneal n.
Cruciate ligaments

Lateral release. Patella reflected and cruciate ligaments cut. Fibular collateral ligament, lateral capsule, popliteus tendon, and part of lateral head of gastrocnemius muscle divided. If further release required, lower fibers of vastus lateralis muscle and iliotibial tract may also be severed. Common peroneal nerve carefully preserved

Preoperative standing radiograph shows severe valgus deformity

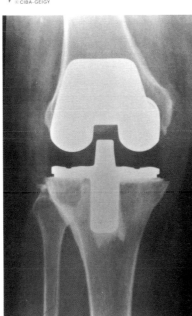

Postoperative radiograph after lateral release and total knee replacement reveals good alignment with functional stability

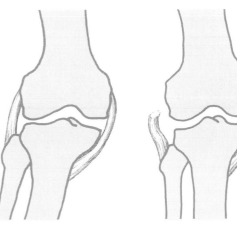

Preoperative view   Postoperative view

Lateral release done at femoral level (in contrast to medial release, which is at tibial level). Release of lateral tension corrects valgus deformity

When the valgus deformity is combined with a flexion contracture, there is an increased risk of postoperative peroneal nerve palsy. After many years of being in a valgus and flexed position, the peroneal nerve is contracted, and correction of a severe valgus deformity stretches it to the point that the blood supply to the nerve is compromised. It is best treated by removing the bulky dressing and flexing the knee, which can be done in the recovery room. The early postoperative use of continuous passive motion machines has almost totally prevented this problem. If care is taken to look for this complication, peroneal nerve function is usually restored quite rapidly. Exploration of the nerve may cause damage and is not recommended in most cases. Peroneal nerve palsy occurs in less than 1% of patients with valgus knee deformities who undergo total knee replacement.

High Tibial Osteotomy for Varus Deformity of Knee

High tibial osteotomy is a time-proven operation performed in patients with varus deformity and unicompartmental osteoarthritis (Plate 24). Coventry obtained excellent results by removing a wedge of bone based laterally at the level of the tibia proximal to the tibial tuberosity. In 1875, Volkmann contributed the first report of tibial osteotomy. Osteotomy has also been successfully used in revision surgery to correct a faulty primary procedure.

Osteotomy is performed in a patient with medial compartment osteoarthritis and a varus

deformity of the knee. The varus deformity should not be greater than 15°, since the ligamentous laxity seen in a greater deformity would compromise the postoperative result. Osteotomy is indicated for patients under 60 years of age, although in other countries, it is performed in older patients as well. (In the United States, total knee replacement is the preferred treatment in patients over age 60.) High tibial osteotomy may also be performed in patients with Blount's disease (tibia vara), poliomyelitis, or other dysplasias of the proximal tibia.

Osteotomy is not recommended in patients with varus deformity of the knee greater than 15°, valgus deformity greater than 10°, instability of

Surgical Treatment of Varus and Valgus Deformities of Knee

(Continued)

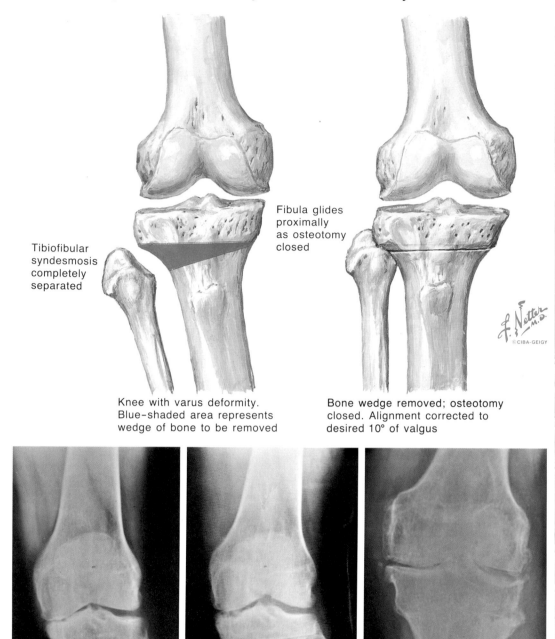

High Tibial Osteotomy for Varus Deformity of Knee

Tibiofibular syndesmosis completely separated

Fibula glides proximally as osteotomy closed

Knee with varus deformity. Blue-shaded area represents wedge of bone to be removed

Bone wedge removed; osteotomy closed. Alignment corrected to desired 10° of valgus

Preoperative standing radiograph reveals varus deformity

Postoperative standing radiograph shows good result; 10° of valgus

Severe joint deterioration 3 years after surgery. Total knee replacement indicated

the collateral ligaments, associated patellofemoral arthritis, fixed flexion contracture greater than 20°, and range of motion less than 70°.

A preoperative standing anteroposterior radiograph is taken, and the mechanical axis is measured. Tibial osteotomy should result in an ideal alignment of 5° to 10° valgus. The amount of bone to be removed must be measured carefully. In a woman, 1° of correction is obtained by resecting a 1-mm wedge of bone; in a man, 8° of correction is obtained by removing a 10-mm wedge of bone.

A lateral incision is made at the level of the tibial tuberosity and proximal fibula. The anterior muscle compartment is lifted subperiosteally over the proximal aspect of the tibia, and the tibiofibular syndesmosis is separated so that the fibula can be moved proximally after the osteotomy is closed. When the base of the proposed wedge is identified, sharp osteotomes are used to remove an appropriately sized wedge of bone. The gap is then closed and the alignment checked with an alignment rod to ensure that the mechanical axis of 10° valgus has been obtained. The wound is irrigated and then closed in layers. A cylinder cast is applied with three-point fixation to maintain the valgus alignment.

Postoperative care begins with gradual weight bearing with crutches. A follow-up anteroposterior radiograph is taken after 2 weeks to make sure that the correct alignment is preserved.

Results

Long-term follow-up studies have shown that high tibial osteotomy results in a significant relief of pain for 2 to 12 years. Full range of motion is preserved, and there is no risk of complications associated with a prosthetic device. However, the same long-term studies revealed deterioration with time at the rate of 1% per year. This procedure should be regarded as one that affords temporary relief of pain until total knee replacement is required. Studies indicate that total knee replacement after osteotomy is not significantly superior to knee arthroplasty without prior osteotomy. Total knee replacement, if necessary, is usually performed about 6 years after the osteotomy. Therefore, although high tibial osteotomy is the procedure of choice in young patients, in older patients, the advantages and disadvantages of osteotomy versus total knee replacement should be carefully evaluated. □

Total Shoulder Replacement

Prosthetic replacement of the shoulder was first carried out by Pean in 1893 to treat a patient with glenohumeral destruction due to tuberculosis. Currently, the two principal types of devices used in shoulder joint replacement are constrained and nonconstrained implants. The constrained implant consists of glenoid and humeral components that are connected to each other and also fixed to the bone; it is used to treat the dislocated shoulder or one with inadequate musculature or bone mass. However, owing to mechanical forces acting on the glenoid cavity, the failure rate for this type of implant is high. The mainstay of shoulder replacement surgery is the nonconstrained implant, which consists of articulating glenoid and humeral components. It is used in the shoulder destroyed by arthritis or by trauma, where bone integrity cannot be reestablished and the humeral head has to be removed. In the patient with an arthritic shoulder, total shoulder arthroplasty affords excellent pain relief.

Preoperative Planning

Evaluation of the patient begins with a thorough medical work-up. Levels of function and pain are measured and recorded. Range of motion and active forward elevation (a more useful motion than abduction) are tested with the patient in the upright position.

Radiographs are taken in the anteroposterior, axillary lateral, and true anteroposterior glenohumeral views. The standard anteroposterior view is used to evaluate the acromioclavicular joint, which may need to be excised. The axillary lateral view determines the presence of subluxation or insufficiency of the anterior or posterior portion of the glenoid cavity. The true anteroposterior view accurately shows the extent of destruction of the articular surfaces because it eliminates the usual overlap of the humeral head on the glenoid cavity.

If the glenoid cavity is intact—as, for example, in the patient with acute fracture or aseptic necrosis—hemiarthroplasty with only the humeral component may suffice. The entire shoulder joint is replaced in all patients with rheumatoid arthritis, because bone mass is usually inadequate and the metal humeral head may eventually erode the glenoid cavity.

Technique

A deltopectoral incision is made from the clavicle to the insertion of the deltoid muscle on the humerus (Plate 25). The deltoid muscle is not released from its insertion because this will delay rehabilitation. The cephalic vein is ligated. The coracoid process is drilled for later reattachment and divided with an osteotome; it remains attached medially so that it will not retract distally and compromise its neurovascular trunk. If additional

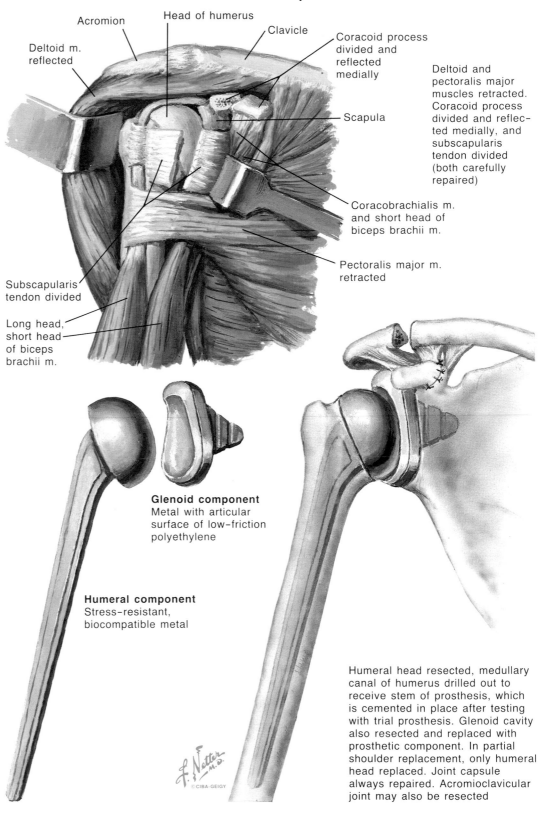

Total Shoulder Replacement

Acromion — Head of humerus — Clavicle — Coracoid process divided and reflected medially

Deltoid m. reflected

Scapula

Deltoid and pectoralis major muscles retracted. Coracoid process divided and reflected medially, and subscapularis tendon divided (both carefully repaired)

Coracobrachialis m. and short head of biceps brachii m.

Pectoralis major m. retracted

Subscapularis tendon divided

Long head, short head of biceps brachii m.

Glenoid component
Metal with articular surface of low-friction polyethylene

Humeral component
Stress-resistant, biocompatible metal

Humeral head resected, medullary canal of humerus drilled out to receive stem of prosthesis, which is cemented in place after testing with trial prosthesis. Glenoid cavity also resected and replaced with prosthetic component. In partial shoulder replacement, only humeral head replaced. Joint capsule always repaired. Acromioclavicular joint may also be resected

exposure is required, the superior half of the pectoralis major tendon may be divided near its insertion; it may also be useful to strip away the anterior part of the insertion of the deltoid muscle. The rotator cuff is examined. The tendinous portion of the subscapularis muscle is divided, leaving enough of the tendon attached distally for later repair. If an internal rotation contracture of the shoulder is present, the subscapularis muscle is divided by beveling the tendon so that it can be lengthened at closure.

The joint is opened. The articular surface of the humeral head is resected, with the cut placed at 35° of retroversion. Care should be taken to remove only the amount of bone needed to ensure

a good fit of the prosthesis, leaving enough for reattachment of the rotator cuff or the subscapularis muscle. The biceps brachii tendon, if intact, is left as an anterior stabilizer. The joint is debrided to allow visualization of the true glenoid cavity. For better exposure, a retractor is placed over the humeral head and behind the glenoid cavity.

If the glenoid cavity is eroded posteriorly or if it is excessively retroverted, it may need reconstruction with a bone graft taken from the humeral head. The glenoid cavity and the medullary canal of the humerus are prepared for the prostheses. Usually, the humeral head is set in 35° of retroversion, although this angle may be modified depending on the condition of the joint.

Exercises Following Total Shoulder Replacement

Total Shoulder Replacement
(*Continued*)

A trial reduction is carried out. A canal plug is placed a little beyond the end of the implant stem, the cement is injected under pressure, and the implant is inserted; alignment and range of motion are checked. If necessary, the rotator cuff is repaired by inserting the torn edges into bone, by mobilizing the superior half of the subscapularis muscle, or by using a graft. The subscapularis muscle is repaired and the coracoid process reattached. Any osteophytes found under the acromioclavicular joint are removed with a rongeur. If the distal end of the clavicle is arthritic, it may be excised. If impingement is found at this stage, the coracoacromial ligament may be excised and an anterior acromioplasty performed.

Suction drains are placed and the wound closed. The patient's arm is placed against the chest in a sling that immobilizes the shoulder, unless the type of repair to the rotator cuff requires the shoulder to be in abduction. In this case, a foam rubber humeral splint is used.

Rehabilitation

Successful management of the reconstruction procedure depends on the patient's willingness to follow the rehabilitation program. The program is designed for the type of surgical repair, condition of the muscles, and the patient's needs and rate of progress. A physical therapist monitors the patient closely for at least 3 weeks after surgery, and for a period up to 2 years after discharge.

Immediately after surgery, the patient is encouraged to move the hand, wrist, forearm, and elbow. Thereafter, the physical therapy program is divided into three stages (Plate 26).

Stage I (day 4–week 2). In the 2 weeks after surgery, only passive and assisted forward flexion exercises are performed. Excessive external rotation exercises should be avoided to protect the surgical repair. To protect the repair of the subscapularis muscle, all forward flexion exercises must be carried out with the arm in internal rotation and adduction. On the fourth day, pendulum exercises and passive range-of-motion exercises are begun.

After 1 week, active assisted exercises with a pulley and stick are introduced. The sling may be discarded during the day (for controlled activities).

Stage II (week 3–week 5). At the beginning of the fourth week, gentle active exercises are started. If the deltoid muscle was not detached during surgery, active motion is regained quite rapidly. In the fifth week, external rotation exercises are added.

Stage III (week 6 and beyond). Isometric rotational exercises with resistance to external and internal rotation provided by the opposite hand are initiated 6 weeks after surgery.

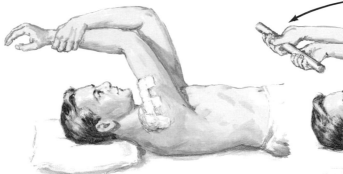

Passive flexion exercises started 4 to 5 days after surgery. Lying supine, grasp wrist of operated limb with other hand and progressively draw it overhead

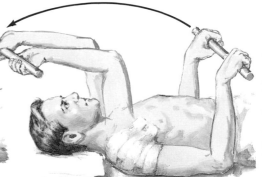

Assisted flexion exercises using rod or cane started about 1 week after surgery

Pendulum exercises also started about 1 week after surgery. Bend forward, supported by good hand on table, and gently swing operated limb in small circles in both directions

Internal rotation exercises begun 8 to 10 days after surgery. Grasp wrist of operated limb behind back with good hand and pull it upward

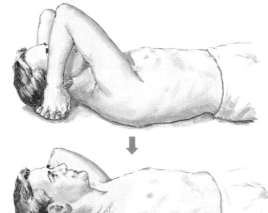

External rotation exercises started about 1 month after surgery. Elbow passively flexed, as in first exercise. Clasp hands and draw behind neck, and spread elbows flat on table or bed

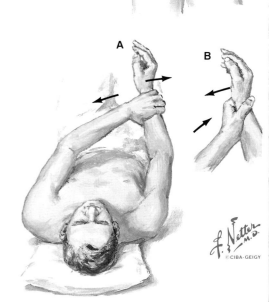

Isometric rotational exercises with resistance from opposite hand started after 20 to 25 days. Hand positions for A: resistance to external rotation; B: resistance to internal rotation

Complications

Complications following shoulder arthroplasty include dislocation or subluxation, loosening of the glenoid component, fracture of the humerus during reaming of the medullary canal or manipulation, infection, and damage to the axillary or musculocutaneous nerves. The incidence of clinical loosening of the implant stem is not significant. Follow-up studies indicate that patients with total shoulder replacement achieve greater forward elevation than those with replacement of the humeral component only. In the latter group, some medial migration and joint pain are occasionally seen, leading to revision surgery with total shoulder arthroplasty. ☐

Elbow Reconstruction

Many methods have been advocated for surgical reconstruction of diseased or destroyed elbow joints. They include surgical synovectomy, arthrodesis, osteotomy, resection arthroplasty with or without interpositional materials, and implant replacement.

Surgical synovectomy of the elbow in patients with rheumatoid arthritis helps relieve pain and retard or prevent further destruction of cartilage and bone. Because the radiocapitular joint is usually involved in long-standing disease, the radial head is usually excised; this facilitates the exposure for synovectomy through the same incision. A radial head silicone implant may or may not be used (Plate 27). A second medial incision is made if there is evidence of synovial thickening medially. A posterior transolecranon approach may also be used. The medial collateral ligament must be preserved. If entrapment of the posterior interosseous nerve is present, the nerve must be decompressed. Ulnar nerve entrapment may require decompression by dividing the cubital tunnel or transposing the nerve anteriorly.

Elbow fusion, or *arthrodesis*, is rarely indicated in rheumatoid arthritis because some elbow motion is needed to help compensate for restricted motion in the shoulder, wrist, and digits. However, arthrodesis may be indicated when destruction of the elbow by trauma or disease is an isolated joint problem. Because bilateral ankylosis of the elbows is a severely disabling condition and other, more functional reconstruction methods are available, bilateral elbow arthrodesis should never be considered.

Currently, *osteotomy* about the elbow to improve joint function is not indicated in patients with arthritis, except to correct deformities such as cubitus valgus or varus.

Resection arthroplasty of the elbow remains popular in some centers. Its main disadvantage is instability, especially in patients with rheumatoid arthritis who may lack muscle strength to stabilize the pseudarthrosis. In addition, severe bone resorption may develop, leading to a flail elbow. Bony ankylosis can also occur.

Interpositional arthroplasty incorporates the use of materials such as the J-K membrane (chromicized autogenous fascia lata), the OMS membrane (chromicized small-intestinal serosa of the horse), autogenous fascia lata, dermal graft, or silicone membrane.

Implant replacement may be required at the capitular-radioulnar and ulnohumeral joints. Disabilities of the capitular-radioulnar joint can be treated with radial head resection arthroplasty with or without a radial head implant (Plate 27). Treatment of disabilities of the ulnohumeral joint has included implant hemiarthroplasty (now no longer used) to replace the distal humerus or proximal ulna, and replacement of both sides of the joint with a linked or unlinked prosthesis, with or without the use of a radial head component.

Simple *resection of the radial head* provides relief in many cases. However, muscle pull and extrinsic forces stretch the interosseous membrane and

Radial Head Implant Arthroplasty

Dorsolateral incision. Extensor aponeurosis incised, radiohumeral joint opened, and hypertrophied synovium excised. Diseased radial head resected with side-cutting burr of air drill

Radiograph shows implant in place with good functional result

Implant inserted over resected radius. Implant stem placed securely in reamed medullary canal

Total Elbow Replacement

Swanson constrained (linked) prosthesis

Disassembled implant shows polyethylene bushing used to decrease particle formation from metal-to-metal contact. Stems inserted and cemented into reamed medullary canals of humerus and ulna

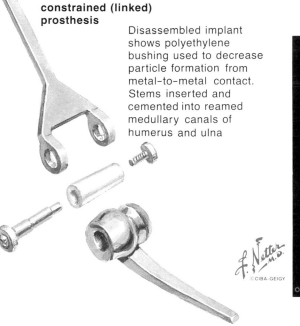

Radiograph shows functioning implant in place

the annular and quadrate ligaments, allowing proximal displacement of the radial shaft. This results in stretching and widening of the distal radioulnar joint, causing pain and instability followed by limitation of wrist motion, radial deviation of the hand, and prominence of the distal end of the ulna. Stretching of the interosseous membrane also limits motion, especially supination.

Radial head resection also increases the valgus deviation of the elbow. Destruction of the annular and quadrate ligaments, as in rheumatoid arthritis, or removal of an excessively large segment of the proximal end of the radius also increases this deformity. These complications can be prevented by leaving the annular and quadrate ligaments

intact when the radial head is resected and inserting a space-occupying implant.

Radial Head Implant Arthroplasty

Indications for radial head implant arthroplasty (Plate 27) are (1) pain and decreased motion secondary to the incongruity of joint surfaces; (2) radiographic evidence of joint destruction or subluxation; and (3) replacement after radial head resection for rheumatoid arthritis, osteoarthritis, posttraumatic arthritis, or fracture. The procedure is not indicated in children, persons with dislocation of the radius on the ulna that does not allow radiohumeral articulation, and persons with inadequate bone stock.

Elbow Reconstruction
(Continued)

The implant preserves the joint space and the relationships of the radiohumeral and proximal radioulnar joints after excision of the radial head. Implants are made in various sizes, with radial heads of various lengths. A titanium radial head is preferred for more active patients with post-traumatic conditions and healthy bone stock.

The radiohumeral joint is exposed between the anconeus and extensor carpi ulnaris muscles, with care to preserve the motor branch of the radial nerve. The radial head is resected at the epiphyseal-metaphyseal junction, preserving the annular and quadrate ligaments. Synovectomy of the antero-lateral and posterior aspects of the elbow joint is performed, and excrescences and marginal osteophytes are trimmed. The medullary canal of the radius is shaped to fit the implant stem. Bone resection and preparation must be sparing. The implant must be properly sized for snug articulation with the capitulum on flexion, extension, and rotation. If ulnar nerve entrapment or significant medial synovitis is present, an additional medial exposure is made to complete the synovectomy and release or transpose the ulnar nerve anteriorly. If the medial collateral ligament has been incised, it should be repaired.

Following wound closure, a bulky conforming dressing, including a posterior plaster splint, is applied with the elbow at 90° of flexion and the forearm in 0° rotation.

Total Elbow Replacement

Fixation with methylmethacrylate cement has made total elbow replacement with hinged prostheses possible. Early designs featured metal-to-metal hinges cemented into the medullary canals. This type of fixation involved complete resection of the epicondyles, with sacrifice of the proximal attachments of the collateral ligaments. Many of these attempts failed because of component loosening and endosteal bone resorption.

Since the late 1960s, many implant designs have emerged, based on different articular mechanisms and methods of fixation into the humerus. These implants are divided into linked and unlinked types. The original metal-to-metal hinge designs have been supplanted by metal-to-high–density polyethylene hinge types.

Linked prostheses are indicated in patients with excessive bone destruction and ligamentous destruction or instability. Motion and stability are derived from the mechanical characteristics of the implant. Most failures are related to loosening of the humeral or ulnar component. The hinge mechanism is classified as constrained or semiconstrained on the basis of the absence or presence of side-to-side laxity.

The Swanson linked prosthesis has a constrained hinge, high-density polyethylene bushing, condylar-sparing design, and intercondylar fixation to decrease rotation of the humeral component (Plate 27).

Total Elbow Replacement (continued)

Wadsworth unconstrained (unlinked) prosthesis

— Humeral component

Ulnar component —

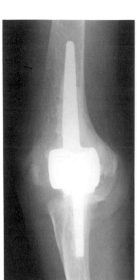

Preoperative radiograph of elbow shows destructive changes due to rheumatoid arthritis

Postoperative radiograph shows prosthesis in place

Coonrad semiconstrained (linked) prosthesis

— Humeral component

Anterior flange —

Ulnar component —

Preoperative radiograph shows loss of bone stock in distal humerus and proximal ulna

Postoperative radiograph shows prosthesis with long-stemmed humeral component in place

The Coonrad titanium-to-polyethylene hinge prosthesis has a semiconstrained, or lax, articulation that allows some side-to-side laxity and intercondylar fixation (Plate 28). In the Morrey modification of the Coonrad implant, a band of porous coating was added to the stems for fixation by bony ingrowth, and an anterior flange was added to the lower humeral stem for insertion of a bone graft anteriorly at the site of maximum stress. Humeral stems are available in longer lengths to add further resistance to rotation.

Unlinked prostheses essentially have an unconstrained hinge and require the presence of adequate bone stock and intact or reconstructed collateral ligaments. Implant failure is usually due to instability. The first unconstrained implant designs were shell-fit surface replacements with unstemmed humeral components. Modifications included stemmed ulnar and radial components. Because loosening of the unstemmed component was frequently due to poor bone stock, it appeared that shell-fit surface replacements should include intramedullary stems. Because the bone stock at the trochlea is often inadequate, unlinked stemmed prostheses with a solid trochlea and stemmed humeral and ulnar components were developed. The Wadsworth-2 prosthesis is included in this category (Plate 28). Other designs have solid trochlea implants with both intramedullary and condylar fixation. □

Selected References

Section I

Plates

AITKEN GT: *Proximal femoral focal deficiency—definition, classification, and management.* In AITKEN GT (ed): *Proximal Femoral Focal Deficiency. A Congenital Anomaly.* Washington, NAS Publication, 1969, pp 1–22   99–111

AITKEN GT (ed): *Proximal Femoral Focal Deficiency. A Congenital Anomaly.* Washington, NAS Publication, 1968   46–49

AITKEN GT, FRANTZ CH: *Management of the child amputee.* Instr Course Lect 1960, 17:246–295   46–49

ALBERS-SCHÖNBERG H: *Eine seltene, bisher nicht bekannte Strukturanomalie des Skelettes.* Fortschr a d Geb Röntgenstrahlen d Nuklearmed Erganzungsband 1915–1916, 23:174   23

ALBERS-SCHÖNBERG H: *Röntgenbilder einer seltenen Knochenkrankung.* München Med Wehnschr 1904, 51:365   22

ALBERTSSON MA, GILLQUIST J: *Discoid lateral menisci: a report of 29 cases.* J Arthros Rel Surg 1988, 4:211–214   71

AMERICAN ACADEMY OF ORTHOPAEDIC SURGEONS: *Atlas of Limb Prosthetics: Surgical and Prosthetic Principles.* St Louis, CV Mosby, 1981   46–49

ANDERSON M, GREEN WT, MESSNER MB: *Growth and predictions of growth in the lower extremities.* J Bone Joint Surg 1963, 45A:1–14   84

ANDERSON M, MESSNER MB, GREEN WT: *Distribution of leg lengths of normal femur and tibia in children from one to eighteen years of age.* J Bone Joint Surg 1964, 46A:1197–1202   84

ANDREN L, VON ROSEN S: *The diagnosis of dislocation of the hip in newborns and the primary results of immediate treatment.* Acta Radiol 1958, 49:89   50–56

ANTON JI, REITZ GB, SPIEGEL MB: *Madelung's deformity.* Ann Surg 1938, 108:411–439   43

APPLE JS, MARTINEZ S, HARDAKER WT, et al: *Synovial plicae of the knee.* Skeletal Radiol 1982, 7:251–254   72

AUSTIN GE, GOLD RH, MIRRA JM, et al: *Long-limbed campomelic dwarfism. A radiologic and pathologic study.* Am J Dis Child 1980, 134:1035–1042   1–16

AXELSSON R: *Behandling av Lunatomalacia.* Göteborg, Elanders Boktvyckar Akticbolag, 1971   41

AYMÉ S, PREUS M: *Spondylocostal/spondylothoracic dysostosis: the clinical basis for prognosticating and genetic counseling.* Am J Med Genet 1986, 24:599–606   1–16

BARLOW TG: *Early diagnosis and treatment of congenital dislocation of the hip.* J Bone Joint Surg 1962, 44B:292   50–56

Section I (continued)

Plates

BEALS RK: *Hypochondroplasia. A report of five kindreds.* J Bone Joint Surg 1969, 51A:728   1–16

BLECK EE, BERZINS UJ: *Conservative management of pes valgus with plantar flexed talus, flexible.* Clin Orthop 1977, 122:85–94   92

BLOUNT WP: *Unequal leg length.* Instr Course Lect 1960, 17:218–245   84–86

BOUGH BW, REGAN BF: *Medial and lateral synovial plicae of the knee: pathological significance, diagnosis and treatment by arthroscopic surgery.* Ir Med J 1985, 78:279–282   72

BOWKER JH, THOMPSON EB: *Surgical treatment of recurrent dislocation of the patella.* J Bone Joint Surg 1964, 46A:1451–1461   68

BOXALL D, BRADFORD DS, WINTER RB, et al: *Management of severe spondylolisthesis in children and adolescents.* J Bone Joint Surg 1979, 61A:479–495   37

BOYER DW, MICKELSON MR, PONSETI IV: *Slipped capital femoral epiphysis. Long-term follow-up study of one hundred and twenty-one patients.* J Bone Joint Surg 1981, 63A:85–95   66–67

BRADDOCK GT: *Experimental epiphysial injury and Freiberg's disease.* J Bone Joint Surg 1959, 41B:154–159   97

BRADFORD DS, MOE JH, MONTALVO FJ, et al: *Scheuermann's kyphosis and roundback deformity. Results of Milwaukee brace treatment.* J Bone Joint Surg 1974, 56A:740–758   35

BURKE SW, FRENCH HG, ROBERTS JM, et al: *Chronic atlantoaxial instability in Down syndrome.* J Bone Joint Surg 1985, 67A:1356–1360   24–25

BURWELL RG, DANGERFIELD PH, HALL DJ, et al: *Perthes' disease. An anthropometric study revealing impaired and proportionate growth.* J Bone Joint Surg 1978, 60B:461–477   57–65

CAHILL BR: *Treatment of juvenile osteochondritis dissecans and osteochondritis dissecans of the knee.* Clin Sports Med 1985, 4:367–384   73–74

CAHILL BR, BERG BC: *99m-technetium phosphate compound joint scintigraphy in the management of juvenile osteochondritis dissecans of the femoral condyles.* Am J Sports Med 1983, 11:329–335   73–74

CALDWELL GD: *Surgical correction of relaxed flatfoot by the Durham flatfoot plasty.* Clin Orthop 1953, 2:227–233   92

CAMPBELL CJ, PAPADEMETRIOU T, BONFIGLIO M: *Melorheostosis: a report of the clinical, roentgenographic and pathological findings in fourteen cases.* J Bone Joint Surg 1968, 50A:1281–1304   23

CANALE ST, GRIFFIN DW, HUBBARD CN: *Congenital muscular torticollis. A long-term follow-up.* J Bone Joint Surg 1982, 64A:810–816   27–28

CARLETON A, ELKINGTON J St C, GREENFIELD JG, et al: *Maffucci's syndrome (dyschondroplasia with haemangiomata).* Quart J Med 1942, 11:203–228   82

CARROLL NC, GRANT CG, HUDSON R, et al: *Experimental observations on the effects of leg lengthening by the Wagner method.* Clin Orthop 1981, 160:250–257   84–86

CARSON WG, LOVELL WW, WHITESIDES TE JR: *Congenital elevation of the scapula. Surgical correction by the Woodward procedure.* J Bone Joint Surg 1981, 63A:1199–1207   40

CATTELL HS, FILTZER DL: *Pseudosubluxation and other normal variations in the cervical spine in children. A study of one hundred and sixty children.* J Bone Joint Surg 1965, 47A:1295–1309   24–25

Section I (continued)

Plates

CATTERALL A, PRINGLE J, BYERS PD, et al: *A review of the morphology of Perthes' disease.* J Bone Joint Surg 1982, 64B:269–275   57–65

CHUNG SMK: *The arterial supply of the developing proximal end of the human femur.* J Bone Joint Surg 1976, 58A:961–970   57–65

CHUNG SMK, BATTERMAN SC, BRIGHTON CT: *Shear strength of the human femoral capital epiphyseal plate.* J Bone Joint Surg 1976, 58A:94–103   66–67

CLARK MW, D'AMBROSIA RD, FERGUSON AB: *Congenital vertical talus: treatment by open reduction and navicular excision.* J Bone Joint Surg 1977, 59A:816–824   90

COCCHI V: *Hereditary diseases with bone changes.* In SHINZ HR, BAENSCH WE, FRIEDL E, et al: *Roentgen Diagnostics,* Vol I. New York, Grune & Stratton, 1951   22

COLEMAN SS: *Treatment of congenital dislocation of the hip in the infant.* J Bone Joint Surg 1965, 47A:590   50–56

COLEMAN SS, CHESNUT WJ: *A simple test for hindfoot flexibility in the cavovarus foot.* Clin Orthop 1977, 123:60–62   91

COLEMAN SS, STELLING FH 3RD, JARRETT J: *Pathomechanics and treatment of congenital vertical talus.* Clin Orthop 1970, 70:62–72   90

COLEMAN SS, STEVENS PM: *Tibial lengthening.* Clin Orthop 1978, 136:92–104   84–86

CONWAY JJ, COWELL HR: *Tarsal coalition: clinical significance and roentgenographic demonstration.* Radiology 1969, 92:799–811   93–94

COOPER RR, PONSETI IV: *Metaphyseal dysostosis: description of an ultrastructural defect in the epiphyseal plate chondrocytes.* J Bone Joint Surg 1973, 55A:485–495   1–16

COVENTRY MB, HARRIS LE: *Congenital muscular torticollis in infancy; some observations regarding treatment.* J Bone Joint Surg 1959, 41A:815–822   27–28

COWELL HR: *Diagnosis and management of peroneal spastic flatfoot.* Instr Course Lect 1975, 24:94–103   93–94

COWELL HR: *The significance of early diagnosis and treatment of slipping of the capital femoral epiphysis.* Clin Orthop 1966, 48:89–94   66–67

CRAWFORD AH: *Neurofibromatosis in children.* Acta Orthop Scand (Suppl) 1986, 218:1–60   17–19

CRAWFORD AH: *Pediatric Orthopaedic Surgery.* Burbank CA, Science Image Comm, 1981   84–86

CRAWFORD AH: *Neurofibromatosis in the pediatric patient.* Orthop Clin North Am 1978, 9:11–23   17–19

CRAWFORD AH, GABRIEL KR: *Foot and ankle problems.* Orthop Clin North Am 1987, 18:649–666   96

CROSSAN JF, WYNNE-DAVIES R, FULFORD GE: *Bilateral failure of the capital femoral epiphysis: bilateral Perthes disease, multiple epiphyseal dysplasia, pseudoachondroplasia, and spondyloepiphyseal dysplasia congenita and tarda.* J Pediatr Orthop 1983, 3:297–301   1–16

CROWE FW, SCHULL WJ, NEEL JN: *Pathological and Genetic Study of Multiple Neurofibromatosis.* Springfield IL, Charles C Thomas, 1956   17–19

CURTIS D: *Heterozygote expression in Grebe chondrodysplasia* (letter). Clin Genet 1986, 29:455–456   1–16

DE BASTIANI G, ALDEGHERI R, RENZI-BRIVIO L, et al: *Limb lengthening by callus distraction (callotasis).* J Pediatr Orthop 1987, 7:129–134   87

THOMPSON GH, CARTER JR, SMITH CW: *Late onset tibia vara: a comparative analysis.* J Pediatr Orthop 1984, 4:185–194 — 78–79

THOMPSON GH, SALTER RB: *Legg-Calvé-Perthes disease. Current concepts and controversies.* Orthop Clin North Am 1987, 18:617–635 — 57–65

THOMPSON GH, SALTER RB: *Legg-Calvé-Perthes disease.* Clin Symp 1986, 38(1):1–31 — 57–65

THOMPSON GH, WESTIN GW: *Legg-Calvé-Perthes disease. Results of discontinuing treatment in the early reossification phase.* Clin Orthop 1979, 139:70–80 — 57–65

TODOROV AB, SCOTT CI JR, WARREN AE, et al: *Developmental screening tests in achondroplastic children.* Am J Med Genet 1981, 9:19–23 — 1–16

TROJAK JE, POLMAR SH, WINKELSTEIN JA, et al: *Immunologic studies of cartilage-hair hypoplasia in the Amish.* Johns Hopkins Med J 1981, 148:157–164 — 1–16

TURCO VJ: *Resistant congenital club foot—one-stage posteromedial release with internal fixation. A follow-up report of a fifteen-year experience.* J Bone Joint Surg 1979, 61A:805–814 — 88–89

UMBER JS, MOSS SW, COLEMAN SS: *Surgical treatment of congenital pseudarthrosis of the tibia.* Clin Orthop 1982, 166:28 — 77

VERRES JL, HERZENBERG JE: *Management of kyphoscoliosis associated with neurologic deficit.* In TARLOV E (ed): *Surgical Treatment of Diseases of the Thoracic Spine.* Park Ridge IL, American Association of Neurological Surgeons. In press — 36

VON ROSEN S: *Diagnosis and treatment of congenital dislocation of the hip joint in the newborn.* J Bone Joint Surg 1962, 44B:284 — 50–56

WALKER BA, SCOTT CI JR, HALL JG, et al: *Diastrophic dwarfism.* Medicine 1972, 51:41–59 — 1–16

WARKANY J: *Congenital Malformations: Notes and Comments.* Chicago, Year Book Med Publishers, 1975 — 82

WAUGH W: *The ossifications and vascularization of the tarsal navicular and their relation to Köhler's disease.* J Bone Joint Surg 1958, 40B:765–777 — 98

WEAVER JK: *Bipartite patellae as a cause of disability in the athlete.* Am J Sports Med 1977, 5:137–143 — 68

WEINSTEIN SC: *Legg-Calvé-Perthes disease.* Instr Course Lect 1983, 32:272–291 — 57–65

WESTH RN, MENELAUS MB: *A simple calculation for the timing of epiphyseal arrest: a further report.* J Bone Joint Surg 1981, 63B:117–119 — 84–86

WHITEHOUSE D: *Diagnostic value of the café-au-lait spot in children.* Arch Dis Child 1966, 41:316–319 — 17–19

WILES P, ANDREWS PS, BREMNER RA: *Chondromalacia of the patella: a study of the later results of excision of the articular cartilage.* J Bone Joint Surg 1960, 42B:65–70 — 69

WILES P, ANDREWS PS, DEVAS MB: *Chondromalacia of the patella.* J Bone Joint Surg 1956, 38B:95–113 — 69

WILKIE DPD: *Congenital radial ulnar synostosis.* Br J Surg 1913–1914, 1:366 — 44

WILKINSON JA: *Prime factors in the etiology of congenital dislocation of the hip.* J Bone Joint Surg 1963, 45B:268 — 50–56

WILLERT HG, HENKEL HL: *Klinik und Pathologie der Dysmelie: die Fehlbildungen an den oberen Extremitaten bei der Thalidomid-Embryopathie.* New York, Springer-Verlag, 1969 — 99–111

WILLIAMS PF: *The management of arthrogryposis.* Orthop Clin North Am 1978, 9:67–88 — 20

WILSON PD, JACOBS B, SCHECTER L: *Slipped capital femoral epiphysis: an end-result study.* J Bone Joint Surg 1965, 47A:1128–1145 — 66–67

WILTSE LL, WIDELL EH JR, JACKSON DW: *Fatigue fracture: the basic lesion in isthmic spondylolisthesis.* J Bone Joint Surg 1975, 57A:17–22 — 37

WINTER RB, MOE JH, WANG JF: *Congenital kyphosis. Its natural history and treatment as observed in a study of 130 patients.* J Bone Joint Surg 1973, 55A:223–256 — 36

WOODWARD JW: *Congenital elevation of the scapula. Correction by release and transplantation of muscle origins; a preliminary report.* J Bone Joint Surg 1961, 43A:219–228 — 40

WYNNE-DAVIES R: *Genetics and malformations of the hand.* Hand 1971, 3:184–192 — 99–111

WYNNE-DAVIES R, HALL CM, APLEY AG (eds): *Atlas of Skeletal Dysplasias.* Edinburgh, Churchill Livingstone, 1985, pp 131–144 — 1–16

YONENOBU K, TADA K, SWANSON AB: *Arthrogryposis of the hand.* J Pediatr Orthop 1984, 4:599–603 — 99–111

YOUNG ID, MOORE JR: *Severe pseudoachondroplasia with parental consanguinity.* J Med Genet 1985, 22:150–153 — 1–16

ZADEK I, GOLD AM: *The accessory tarsal scaphoid.* J Bone Joint Surg 1948, 30A:957–968 — 95

Section II

DAHLIN DC: *Bone Tumors. General Aspects and Data on 6,221 Cases,* ed 3. Springfield IL, Charles C Thomas, 1978 — 1–34

ENNEKING WF: *Musculoskeletal Tumor Surgery.* New York, Churchill Livingstone, 1983 — 1–34

HUVOS AG: *Bone Tumors. Diagnosis, Treatment and Prognosis.* Philadelphia, WB Saunders, 1979 — 1–34

Section III

General References

CRENSHAW AH: *Campbell's Operative Orthopaedics,* Vol 4, ed 7. St Louis, CV Mosby, 1987, pp 2525–2620

FREYBERG RH: *Rheumatoid arthritis: the natural history, diagnosis, prognosis and management.* Med Times 1967, 95:724–753

KATZ WA (ed): *Rheumatic Diseases.* Philadelphia, JB Lippincott, 1977

KELLEY WN, HARRIS ED JR, RUDDY S, et al (eds): *Textbook of Rheumatology,* ed 2. Philadelphia, WB Saunders, 1985

KRUSEN FH, KOTTKE FJ, ELLWOOD PM JR: *Physical Medicine and Rehabilitation,* ed 2. Philadelphia, WB Saunders, 1971

MCCARTY DJ JR (ed): *Arthritis and Allied Conditions,* ed 10. Philadelphia, Lea & Febiger, 1985

POLLEY HF, HUNDER GG: *Rheumatological Interviewing and Physical Examination of the Joints,* ed 2. Philadelphia, WB Saunders, 1978

SCHUMACHER HR JR, KLIPPEL JH, ROBINSON DR (eds): *Primer on Rheumatic Diseases.* Atlanta, Arthritis Foundation, 1988

WYNGAARDEN JB, SMITH LH JR: *Textbook of Medicine,* ed 16. Philadelphia, WB Saunders, 1982

ANSELL B: *Juvenile arthritis.* Practitioner 1986, 230:343–350 — 17–20

BERG E, et al: *Non-Operative Care of the Painful Rheumatoid Foot* (exhibit). Chicago, American Academy of Orthopaedic Surgeons, 1978 — 50–59

BOLLET AJ: *Nonsteroidal antiinflammatory drugs.* In KELLEY WN, HARRIS ED JR, RUDDY S, et al (eds): *Textbook of Rheumatology,* Vol I, ed 2. Philadelphia, WB Saunders, 1985 — 1–13

BOYD HB, ANDERSON LD: *A method for reinsertion of the distal biceps brachii tendon.* J Bone Joint Surg 1961, 43A:1041–1043 — 45

BREWER EJ JR, BASS J, BAUM J, et al: *Current proposed revision of JRA criteria.* Arthritis Rheum 1977, 20(Suppl):195–199 — 17–20

BREWER EJ JR, GIANNINI EH, PERSON DA: *Juvenile Rheumatoid Arthritis,* ed 2. Philadelphia, WB Saunders, 1982 — 17–20

BUNNELL S: *Surgery of the Hand,* ed 4. Philadelphia, JB Lippincott, 1964 — 47–48

CAMPBELL WC: *Operative Orthopaedics,* ed 4. St Louis, CV Mosby, 1963 — 45, 47, 49

CASSIDY JT, LEVINSON JE, BASS JC, et al: *A study of classification criteria for a diagnosis of juvenile rheumatoid arthritis.* Arthritis Rheum 1986, 29:274–281 — 17–20

CLAYTON ML: *Results of Surgery in Rheumatoid Feet.* Excerpta Medica Intl Congress Series No. 165, Oct 1967 — 50–59

CLAYTON ML: *Surgery of the lower extremity in rheumatoid arthritis.* J Bone Joint Surg 1963, 45A:1517–1536 — 50–59

CLAYTON ML: *Surgery of the forefoot in rheumatoid arthritis.* Clin Orthop 1960, 16:136–140 — 50–59

CLAYTON ML: *Surgery of the forefoot in rheumatoid arthritis.* Arthritis Rheum 1959, 2:84–86 — 50–59

CLAYTON ML, LEIDHOLT JD, SMYTH CJ: *Surgery of the Forefoot in Rheumatoid Arthritis* (motion picture). Chicago, American Academy of Orthopaedic Surgeons — 50–59

COOPERATIVE CLINICS COMMITTEE OF THE AMERICAN RHEUMATISM ASSOCIATION: *A controlled trial of cyclophosphamide in rheumatoid arthritis.* N Engl J Med 1970, 283:883–889 — 1–13

DECKER JL, MALONE DG, HARAOUI B, et al: *NIH conference. Rheumatoid arthritis: evolving concepts of pathogenesis and treatment.* Ann Intern Med 1984, 101:810–824 — 1–13

DU TOIT GT: *Internal derangement of the knee.* Instr Course Lect 1955, 12:9–34 — 49

EHRLICH GE: *Total Management of the Arthritic Patient.* Philadelphia, JB Lippincott, 1973 — 1–13, 21–37

ELBAR JE, THOMAS WH, WEINFELD MS, et al: *Talonavicular arthrodesis for rheumatoid arthritis of the hindfoot.* Orthop Clin North Am 1976, 7:821–826 — 50–59

FAHEY JJ, BOLLINGER JA: *Trigger-finger in adults and children.* J Bone Joint Surg 1954, 36A:1200–1218 — 47

FINK CW: *Clinical, genetic and therapeutic aspects of juvenile arthritis.* Clin Rheumatol 1983, 1:100–115   17–20

FINK CW, KUSTER RM: *Treatment of rheumatic diseases.* In EICHENWALD HF, STRODER J (eds): *Practical Pediatric Therapy.* Deerfield Beach FL, Verlag Chimie International, 1985   17–20

FINKELSTEIN H: *Stenosing tendovaginitis at the radial styloid process.* J Bone Joint Surg 1951, 33B:96   46

FLEMING A, BENN RT, CORBETT M, et al: *Early rheumatoid disease. II. Patterns of joint involvement.* Ann Rheum Dis 1976, 35:361–364   1–13

FLEMING A, CROWN JM, CORBETT M: *Early rheumatoid disease. I. Onset.* Ann Rheum Dis 1976, 35:357–360   1–13

FREIBERGER RH, KILLORAN PJ, CARDONA G: *Arthrography of the knee by double contrast method.* Am J Roentgenol 1966, 97:736–747   1–13

FREYBERG RH: *Nonarticular rheumatism.* Bull NY Acad Med 1951, 27:245–258   36

FREYBERG RH, ZIFF M, BAUM J: *Gold therapy for rheumatoid arthritis.* In HOLLANDER JL, MCCARTY DJ JR (eds): *Arthritis and Allied Conditions,* ed 8. Philadelphia, Lea & Febiger, 1972, pp 455–482   1–13

FUNK FJ JR: *Surgery of the foot in rheumatoid arthritis.* Semin Arthritis Rheum 1971, 1:25   50–59

FUNK FJ JR: *Surgery of the foot in rheumatoid arthritis.* J Med Assoc Ga 1959, 58:8   50–59

FURLONG R: *Injuries of the Hand,* ed 1. Boston, Little Brown, 1957   47

GATTER RA: *A Practical Handbook of Joint Fluid Analysis.* Philadelphia, Lea & Febiger, 1984   15–16

GILCREEST EL, ALBI P: *Unusual lesions of muscles and tendons of the shoulder girdle and upper arm.* Surg Gynec & Obst 1939, 68:903–917   45

GSCHWEND N: *Surgical Treatment of Rheumatoid Arthritis.* Stuttgart, Georg Thieme Verlag, 1980   50–59

HAMMOND A: *Mitchell osteotomy-bunionectomy for hallux valgus and metatarsus primus varus.* Instr Course Lect 1972, 21   60–61

HAMMOND A: *Complete acromionectomy in the treatment of chronic tendonitis of the shoulder.* J Bone Joint Surg 1971, 53A:173   38–41

HAMMOND A: *Operative treatment of hallux valgus and metatarsus primus varus.* Surg Clin North Am 1952, 32:733   60–61

HAMMOND A, TORGERSON WR JR, DOTTER WE, et al: *The painful shoulder: a preliminary report.* Instr Course Lect 1971, 20:83   42–43

HEALEY LA: *Polymyalgia rheumatica.* In HOLLANDER JL, MCCARTY DJ JR (eds): *Arthritis and Allied Conditions,* ed 8. Philadelphia, Lea & Febiger, 1972, pp 885–889   1–13

HENCH PS, KENDALL EC, SLOCUMB CH, et al: *Effect of a hormone of the adrenal cortex (17-hydroxy-11-dehydrocorticosterone, compound E) and of pituitary adrenocorticotropic hormone on rheumatoid arthritis. Preliminary report.* Mayo Clin Proc 1949, 24:181–197   1–13

HOFFMAN P: *An operation for severe grades of contracted or clawed toes.* Am J Orthop Surg 1912, 9:441   50–59

HOLLANDER JL: *Arthrocentesis technique and intrasynovial therapy.* In MCCARTY DJ JR (ed): *Arthritis and Allied Conditions,* ed 10. Philadelphia, Lea & Febiger, 1985, pp 541–553   14

HOOD LE, WEISSMAN IL, WOOD WB (eds): *Immunology.* Menlo Park CA, Benjamin/Cummings, 1978, p 11   1–13

HOWARD LD JR: *Dupuytren's contracture: a guide for management.* Clin Orthop 1959, 15:118–126   48

HOWELL DS: *Etiopathogenesis of osteoarthritis.* In MCCARTY DJ JR (ed): *Arthritis and Allied Conditions,* ed 10. Philadelphia, Lea & Febiger, 1985, pp 1400–1407   1–13

HOWELL DS, MUNIZ O, PITA JC, et al: *Extrusion of pyrophosphate into extracellular media by osteoarthritic cartilage incubates.* J Clin Invest 1975, 56:1473–1478   1–13

JACOBS JC, BERDON WE, JOHNSTON AD: *HLA-B27-associated spondyloarthritis and enthesopathy in childhood. Clinical, pathologic, and radiographic observations in 58 patients.* J Pediatr 1982, 100:521–528   17–20

JAFFEE HL: *Tumors and Tumorous Conditions of the Bones and Joints,* ed 1. Philadelphia, Lea & Febiger, 1958   49

KELLER WL: *Surgical treatment of bunions and hallux valgus.* NY Med J 1904, 80:741   60–61

LARMON WA: *Pigmented villonodular synovitis.* Med Clin North Am 1965, 49:141–150   49

LEÃO L: *De Quervain's disease; a clinical and anatomical study.* J Bone Joint Surg 1958, 40A:1063–1070   46

LIPSCOMB PR: *Tumors of the tendons and tendon sheaths including ganglia and xanthomas.* Instr Course Lect 1954, 11:50–56   47

LIPSCOMB PR: *Nonsuppurative tenosynovitis and paratendinitis.* Instr Course Lect 1950, 7   46

LUCK JV: *Dupuytren's contracture. Pathogenesis and surgical management: a new concept.* Instr Course Lect 1959, 16   48

MARMOR L: *Rheumatoid deformity of the foot.* Arthritis Rheum 1963, 6:749–755   50–59

MARTEL W, SEEGER JF, WICKS JD, et al: *Traumatic lesions of the discovertebral junction in the lumbar spine.* Am J Roentgenol 1976, 127:457–464   1–13

MCBRIDE ED: *The McBride bunion hallux valgus operation.* J Bone Joint Surg 1967, 49A:1675–1683   60–61

MCEWEN C, LINGG C, KIRSNER JB: *Arthritis accompanying ulcerative colitis.* Am J Med 1962, 33:923–941   1–13

MCEWEN C, ZIFF M, CARMEL P, et al: *The relationship to rheumatoid arthritis of its so-called variants.* Arthritis Rheum 1958, 1:481–496   1–13

MCKEEVER DC: *Arthrodesis of the first metatarsophalangeal joint for hallux valgus, hallux rigidus and metatarsus primus varus.* J Bone Joint Surg 1952, 34A:129–134   60–61

MCLAUGHLIN HL: *Repair of major cuff ruptures.* Surg Clin North Am 1963, 43:1535–1540   44

MCLAUGHLIN HL: *The selection of calcium deposits for operation; the technique and results of operation.* Surg Clin North Am 1963, 43:1501–1504   38–41

MCLAUGHLIN HL: *Trauma,* ed 1. Philadelphia, WB Saunders, 1959   45

MCLAUGHLIN HL: *On the "frozen" shoulder.* Bull Hosp Jt Dis 1951, 12:383–393   42–43

MCLAUGHLIN HL: *Lesions of the musculotendinous cuff of the shoulder; observations on the pathology, course and treatment of calcific deposits.* Ann Surg 1946, 124:354–362   38–41

MCMASTER PE: *Pigmented villonodular synovitis*

with invasion of bone. Report of six cases. J Bone Joint Surg 1960, 42A:1170–1183   49

MITCHELL CL, FLEMING JL, ALLEN R, et al: *Osteotomy-bunionectomy for hallux valgus.* J Bone Joint Surg 1958, 40A:41–60   60–61

MOSELEY HF: *Shoulder Lesions,* ed 3. Edinburgh, ES Livingstone, 1969   42–44

MOSKOWITZ RW: *Clinical and laboratory findings in osteoarthritis.* In MCCARTY DJ JR (ed): *Arthritis and Allied Conditions,* ed 10. Philadelphia, Lea & Febiger, 1985, pp 1408–1432   1–13

MOSKOWITZ RW, GOLDBERG VM, BERMAN L: *Synovitis as a manifestation of degenerative joint disease. An experimental study.* Arthritis Rheum 1976, 19:813   1–13

NEER CS 2nd: *Anterior acromioplasty for the chronic impingement syndrome in the shoulder. A preliminary report.* J Bone Joint Surg 1972, 54A:41   38–41

NEVIASER JS: *Musculoskeletal disorders of the shoulder region causing cervicobracheal pain. Differential diagnosis and treatment.* Surg Clin North Am 1963, 43:1703–1714   42–43

PEDIATRIC RHEUMATOLOGY COLLABORATIVE STUDY GROUP (PRCSG): *Methodology and studies of children with juvenile rheumatoid arthritis.* J Rheumatol 1982, 9:107–155   17–20

PETTY RE: *Current knowledge of the etiology and pathogenesis of chronic uveitis accompanying juvenile rheumatoid arthritis.* Rheum Dis Clin North Am 1987, 13:19–36   17–20

PHELPS P, MCCARTY DJ JR: *Crystal-induced arthritis.* Postgrad Med 1969, 45:87–93   1–13

POTTER TA: *Rheumatoid Arthritis of the Foot* (exhibit). Denver, AMA Meeting, 1961   50–59

PUTNAM FW: *Immunoglobulins. I. Structure.* In PUTNAM FW (ed): *The Plasma Proteins: Structures, Function and Genetic Control.* New York, Academic Press, 1977   1–13

RAUNIO P, LAINE H: *Synovectomy of the metatarsophalangeal joints in rheumatoid arthritis.* Acta Rheumatol Scand 1970, 16:12–17   50–59

ROBINSON DR, MCGUIRE MB, LEVINE L: *Prostaglandins in the rheumatic diseases.* Ann NY Acad Sci 1975, 256:318–329   1–13

ROPES MW, BAUER W: *Synovial Fluid Changes in Joint Disease.* Cambridge MA, Harvard University Press, 1953   15–16

ROPES MW, BENNETT GA, COBB S, et al: *1958 revision of diagnostic criteria for rheumatoid arthritis.* Bull Rheum Dis 1958, 9:175–176   1–13

ROSENBERG AM, OEN KG: *The relationship between ocular and articular disease activity in children with juvenile rheumatoid arthritis and associated uveitis.* Arthritis Rheum 1986, 29:797–800   17–20

ROWE CR: *Ruptures of the rotator cuff: selection of cases for conservative treatment.* Surg Clin North Am 1963, 43:1531–1534   44

RYAN LM, MCCARTY DJ JR: *Calcium pyrophosphate crystal deposition disease; pseudogout; articular chondrocalcinosis.* In MCCARTY DJ JR (ed): *Arthritis and Allied Conditions,* ed 10. Philadelphia, Lea & Febiger, 1985, p 1515   35

SCHMID FR: *Principles of diagnosis and treatment of infectious arthritis.* In HOLLANDER JL, MCCARTY DJ JR (eds): *Arthritis and Allied Conditions,* ed 8. Philadelphia, Lea & Febiger, 1972, pp 1203–1217   29

SCHUMACHER HR JR: *Synovial fluid analysis.* In KELLEY WN, HARRIS ED, RUDDY S, et al:

Section III (continued) — Plates

Textbook of Rheumatology. Philadelphia, WB Saunders, 1989 — 15–16

SCHUMACHER HR JR, SIECK MS, ROTHFUSS S, et al: *Reproducibility of synovial fluid analyses. A study among four laboratories.* Arthritis Rheum 1986, 29:770–774 — 15–16

SCULL E: *Chloroquine and hydroxychloroquine therapy in rheumatoid arthritis.* Arthritis Rheum 1962, 5:30–36 — 1–13

SHORT CL, BAUER W, REYNOLDS WE: *Rheumatoid Arthritis.* Cambridge MA, Harvard University Press, 1957 — 1–13

SIGLER JW: *Psoriatic arthritis.* In HOLLANDER JL, MCCARTY DJ JR (eds): *Arthritis and Allied Conditions,* ed 8. Philadelphia, Lea & Febiger, 1972, pp 724–735 — 27

SMITH-PETERSEN MN, AUFRANC OE, LARSON CB: *Useful surgical procedures for rheumatoid arthritis involving joints of the upper extremity.* Arch Surg 1943, 46:764–770 — 50–59

SMYTH CJ: *Diagnosis and treatment of gout.* In HOLLANDER JL, MCCARTY DJ JR (eds): *Arthritis and Allied Conditions,* ed 8. Philadelphia, Lea & Febiger, 1972, pp 1112–1139 — 1–13

STEINBROCKER O, NEUSTADT DH: *Aspiration and Injection Therapy in Arthritis and Musculoskeletal Disorders.* Hagerstown MD, Harper & Row, 1972 — 14

SUSMAN MH, CLAYTON ML: *Surgery of the rheumatoid foot.* Ann Acad Med Singapore 1983, 12:225–232 — 50–59

SWANSON AB: *Flexible implant arthroplasty in the hand.* Clin Plast Surg 1976, 3:141–157 — 62–73

SWANSON AB: *Flexible Implant Resection Arthroplasty in the Hand and Extremities.* St Louis, CV Mosby, 1973 — 62–73

SWANSON AB: *Disabling arthritis at the base of the thumb: treatment by resection of the trapezium and flexible (silicone) implant arthroplasty.* J Bone Joint Surg 1972, 54A:456–471 — 62–73

SWANSON AB: *Flexible implant arthroplasty for arthritic finger joints. Rationale, technique and results of treatment.* J Bone Joint Surg 1972, 54A:435–455 — 62–73

SWANSON AB: *Implant arthroplasty in disabilities of the great toe.* Instr Course Lect 1972, 21 — 60–61

SWANSON AB: *A flexible implant for replacement of arthritic or destroyed joints in the hand.* NY Univ Inter-Clin Inform Bull 1966, 6:16–19 — 62–73

SWANSON AB, DE GROOT SWANSON G: *Congenital limb malformations, classification and treatment.* In FLYNN JE (ed): *Hand Surgery,* ed 4. Baltimore, Williams & Wilkins, 1989 — 62–73

SWANSON AB, DE GROOT SWANSON G: *Flexible implant resection arthroplasty: a method for reconstruction of small joints in the extremities.* Instr Course Lect 1978, 27:27–60 — 62–73

SWANSON AB, DE GROOT SWANSON G, LEONARD J: *Postoperative rehabilitation program in flexible implant arthroplasty of the digits.* In HUNTER J, SCHNEIDER L (eds): *Rehabilitation of the Hand.* St Louis, CV Mosby, 1978, pp 477–495 — 62–73

TAYLOR H: *Cysts of the fibrocartilages of the knee joint.* J Bone Joint Surg 1935, 17:588–596 — 49

VAHVANEN VA: *Rheumatoid arthritis in the plantar joints. A follow-up study of triple arthrodesis on 292 adult feet.* Acta Orthop Scand 1967, 107(Suppl):3 — 50–59

Section III (continued) — Plates

VAINIO K: *The rheumatoid foot; a clinical study with pathological and roentgenological comments.* Ann Chir Gyn Fenn 1956, 45(Suppl):1–107 — 50–59

VANE JR: *Mode of action of aspirin and similar compounds.* In ROBINSON HJ, VANE JR (eds): *Prostaglandin Synthetase Inhibitors.* New York, Raven Press, 1974 — 1–13

WARD JR, WILLIAMS HJ, EGGER M, et al: *Comparison of auranofin, gold sodium thiomalate, and placebo in the treatment of rheumatoid arthritis. A controlled clinical trial.* Arthritis Rheum 1983, 26:1303–1315 — 1–13

WATSON-JONES R: *Fractures and Joint Injuries,* ed 4. Baltimore, Williams & Wilkins, 1955 — 44

WEISSMANN G: *Activation of neutrophils and the lesions of rheumatoid arthritis.* J Lab Clin Med 1982, 100:322–333 — 1–13

WEISSMANN G: *The role of lysosomes in inflammation and disease.* Ann Rev Med 1967, 18:97–112 — 1–13

WEISSMANN G, SERHAN C, KORCHAK HM, et al: *Neutrophils: release of mediators of inflammation with special reference to rheumatoid arthritis.* Ann NY Acad Sci 1982, 389:11–24 — 1–13

WILLIAMS RC JR: *A second look at rheumatoid factor and other "autoantibodies."* Am J Med 1979, 67:179–181 — 1–13

WINCHESTER RJ: *Genetic aspects of rheumatoid arthritis.* Springer Semin Immunopathol 1981, 4:89–102 — 1–13

ZVAIFLER NJ: *The immunology of joint inflammation in rheumatoid arthritis.* Adv Immunol 1973, 13:265–268 — 1–13

Section IV

AMSTUTZ HC, HOY AL, CLARK I: *UCLA anatomic total shoulder arthroplasties.* Clin Orthop 1981, 155:7–20 — 25–26

BARRETT WP, FRANKLIN JL, JACKINS SE, et al: *Total shoulder arthroplasty.* J Bone Joint Surg 1987, 69A:865–872 — 25–26

CLAYTON ML, FERLIC DC, JEFFERS PD: *Prosthetic arthroplasties of the shoulder.* Clin Orthop 1982, 164:184–191 — 25–26

COFIELD RH: *Total shoulder arthroplasty with the Neer prosthesis.* J Bone Joint Surg 1986, 66A:899–906 — 25–26

COONRAD RW: *History of total elbow arthroplasty.* In INGLIS AE (ed): *Symposium on Total Joint Replacement of the Upper Extremity.* St Louis, CV Mosby, 1982, pp 75–90 — 27–28

COONRAD RW: *Seven-year follow-up of Coonrad total elbow replacement.* In INGLIS AE (ed): *Symposium on Total Joint Replacement of the Upper Extremity.* St Louis, CV Mosby, 1982, pp 91–99 — 27–28

HEDLEY A, KOZINN SC: *Experimental work on porous coating.* In HUNGERFORD DS, KRACKOW KA, KENNA RV (eds): *Total Knee Arthroplasty.* Baltimore, Williams & Wilkins, 1984 — 1–14

INSALL JN (ed): *Surgery of the Knee.* New York, Churchill Livingstone, 1984 — 15–24

INSALL JN, HOOD RW, FLAWN LB, et al: *The total condylar knee prosthesis in gonarthrosis. A five- to nine-year follow-up of the first one hundred consecutive replacements.* J Bone Joint Surg 1983, 65A:619–628 — 15–24

Section IV (continued) — Plates

INSALL JN, LACHIEWICZ PF, BURSTEIN AH: *The posterior stabilized condylar prosthesis: a modification of the total condylar design. Two- to four-year clinical experience.* J Bone Joint Surg 1982, 64A:1317–1323 — 15–24

JACKSON JP, WAUGH W (eds): *Surgery of the Knee Joint.* Philadelphia, JB Lippincott, 1984 — 15–24

NEER CS II, WATSON KC, STANTON FJ: *Recent experience in total shoulder replacement.* J Bone Joint Surg 1982, 64A:319–377 — 25–26

PEAN JE: *Prosthetic repair of bone fragments.* Clin Orthop 1973, 94:4–7 — 25–26

PELLICCI P, SALVATI EA: *Complications of hip surgery. Part II—adult patients.* Contemp Orthop 1985, 10:27–39 — 1–14

POST M, HASKELL SS, JOBLON M: *Total shoulder replacement with a constrained prosthesis.* J Bone Joint Surg 1980, 62A:327–335 — 25–26

RANAWAT CS: *Preoperative planning for total hip arthroplasty.* In DORR L (ed): *Revision of Total Hip and Knee Replacements.* Baltimore, University Park Press, 1984 — 1–14

RANAWAT CS: *Triad Total Hip Surgical Technique.* New Brunswick NJ, Johnson & Johnson, 1982 — 16–25

SALVATI EA: *Infection complicating total hip replacement.* In PROCEEDINGS OF THE HIP SOCIETY: *The Hip.* St Louis, CV Mosby, 1976 — 1–14

SALVATI EA, WILSON PD JR, JOLLEY M, et al: *A ten year follow-up study of our first one hundred consecutive total hip replacements.* J Bone Joint Surg 1981, 63A:753–766 — 1–14

SCOTT RD: *Use of a bipolar prosthesis with bone grafting in acetabular reconstruction.* Contemp Orthop 1984, 9:35–41 — 1–14

SCOTT RD, TURNER RH, LEITZES SM, et al: *Femoral fractures in conjunction with total hip replacement.* J Bone Joint Surg 1975, 57A:494–501 — 1–14

SOUTER WA: *The evolution of total replacement arthroplasty of the elbow.* In KASHIWAGI D (ed): *Elbow Joint.* Amsterdam, Elsevier, 1985, pp 255–268 — 27–28

SWANSON AB: *Elbow joint implant resection arthroplasty.* In SWANSON AB: *Flexible Implant Resection Arthroplasty of the Hand and Extremities.* St Louis, CV Mosby, 1973, pp 276–286 — 27–28

SWANSON AB: *Synovectomy of the elbow and implant replacement of the radial head.* In SWANSON AB: *Flexible Implant Resection Arthroplasty of the Hand and Extremities.* St Louis, CV Mosby, 1973, pp 265–275 — 27–28

SWANSON AB, HERNDON JH: *Surgery of arthritis.* In WADSWORTH TG (ed): *The Elbow.* London, Churchill Livingstone, 1982, pp 303–345 — 27–28

SWANSON AB, JAEGER SH, LA ROCHELLE D: *Comminuted fractures of the radial head. The role of silicone-implant replacement arthroplasty.* J Bone Joint Surg 1981, 63A:1039–1049 — 27–28

WADSWORTH TG: *Non-constrained elbow arthroplasty.* In KASHIWAGI D (ed): *Elbow Joint.* Amsterdam, Elsevier, 1985, pp 313–32 — 27–28

WILSON PD JR, COVENTRY MB, CROFT JD JR: *Total hip replacement in the United States. A consensus conference.* JAMA 1982, 248:1817–1821 — 1–14

WOOLSON ST, HARRIS WH: *Complex total hip replacement for dysplastic or hypoplastic hips using miniature or microminiature components.* J Bone Joint Surg 1983, 65A:1099–1108 — 1–14

Subject Index

Boldface numbers refer to terms that appear on plates

INFORMATION ON CIBA COLLECTION VOLUMES

THE CIBA COLLECTION OF MEDICAL ILLUSTRATIONS has enjoyed an enthusiastic reception from members of the medical community since the publication of its first volume. The remarkable illustrations by Frank H. Netter, M.D., and text by leading specialists make these books unprecedented in their educational, clinical, and scientific value.

Volume 1: I **NERVOUS SYSTEM: Anatomy and Physiology**
"...this volume must remain a part of the library of all practitioners, scientists and educators dealing with the nervous system."
Journal of Neurosurgery

Volume 1: II **NERVOUS SYSTEM: Neurologic and Neuromuscular Disorders**
"...Part I is a 'work of art.' Part II is even more grand and more clinical!
...This is a unique and wonderful text...rush to order this fine book."
Journal of Neurological & Orthopaedic Medicine & Surgery

Volume 2 **REPRODUCTIVE SYSTEM**
"...a desirable addition to any nursing or medical library."
American Journal of Nursing

Volume 3: I **DIGESTIVE SYSTEM: Upper Digestive Tract**
"...a fine example of the high quality of this series."
Pediatrics

Volume 3: II **DIGESTIVE SYSTEM: Lower Digestive Tract**
"...a unique and beautiful work, worth much more than its cost."
Journal of the South Carolina Medical Association

Volume 3: III **DIGESTIVE SYSTEM: Liver, Biliary Tract and Pancreas**
"...a versatile, multipurpose aid to clinicians, teachers, researchers, and students..."
Florida Medical Journal

Volume 4 **ENDOCRINE SYSTEM and Selected Metabolic Diseases**
"...another in the series of superb contributions made by CIBA..."
International Journal of Fertility

Volume 5 **HEART**
"The excellence of the volume...is clearly deserving of highest praise."
Circulation

Volume 6 **KIDNEYS, URETERS, AND URINARY BLADDER**
"...a model of clarity of language and visual presentation..."
Circulation

Volume 7 **RESPIRATORY SYSTEM**
"...far more than an atlas on anatomy and physiology. Frank Netter uses his skills to present clear and often beautiful illustrations of all aspects of the system..."
British Medical Journal

Volume 8: I **MUSCULOSKELETAL SYSTEM: Anatomy, Physiology, and Metabolic Disorders**
"...the overall value of this monumental work is nearly beyond human comprehension."
Journal of Neurological & Orthopaedic Medicine & Surgery

Volume 8: II **MUSCULOSKELETAL SYSTEM: Developmental Disorders, Tumors, Rheumatic Diseases, and Joint Replacement**
"...destined to become a primary reference source for medical and allied health disciplines everywhere."

Copies of all CIBA COLLECTION books may be purchased directly from the Medical Education Division, CIBA-GEIGY Corporation, 14 Henderson Drive, West Caldwell, New Jersey 07006. In countries other than the United States, please direct inquiries to the nearest CIBA-GEIGY office.